Medical Management of Vulnerable and Underserved Patients:

Principles, Practice, and Populations

Section Editors

PRINCIPLES

Andrew B. Bindman, MD

Chief, Division of General Internal Medicine, San Francisco General Hospital

Professor, Department of Medicine, University of California, San Francisco

Kevin Grumbach, MD

Chief, Family and Community Medicine, San Francisco General Hospital

Professor and Chair, Department of Family and Community Medicine, University of California, San Francisco

PRACTICE

Alicia Fernandez, MD

Associate Professor of Clinical Medicine, Department of Medicine, University of California, San Francisco, San Francisco General Hospital

Dean Schillinger, MD

Associate Professor of Clinical Medicine, Department of Medicine, University of California, San Francisco, San Francisco General Hospital

POPULATIONS

Teresa J. Villela, MD

Director, San Francisco General Hospital Family and Community Medicine Residency Program; Associate Clinical Professor and Vice Chair, Department of Family and Community Medicine, University of California, San Francisco

Margaret B. Wheeler, MS, MD

Director, San Francisco General Hospital Primary Care Internal Medicine Residency, University of California, San Francisco Internal Medicine Residency Program

Associate Clinical Professor of Medicine, Department of Medicine, University of California, San Francisco

Medical Management of Vulnerable and Underserved Patients:
Principles, Practice, and Populations

Talmadge E. King, Jr., MD

Chief, Medical Services, San Francisco General Hospital

Constance B. Wofsy Distinguished Professor and Vice Chairman, Department of Medicine, University of California, San Francisco

Margaret B. Wheeler, MS, MD

Director, San Francisco General Hospital Primary Care Internal Medicine Residency, University of California, San Francisco Internal Medicine Residency Program

Associate Clinical Professor of Medicine, Department of Medicine, University of California, San Francisco

McGraw-Hill

Medical Publishing Division

*New York   Chicago   San Francisco   Lisbon   London   Madrid   Mexico City
Milan   New Delhi   San Juan   Seoul   Singapore   Sydney   Toronto*

Notice

Medicine is an ever-changing science. As new research and clinical experience broaden our knowledge, changes in treatment and drug therapy are required. The editors and the publisher of this work have checked with sources believed to be reliable in their efforts to provide information that is complete and generally in accord with the standards accepted at the time of publication. However, in view of the possibility of human error or changes in medical sciences, neither the editors, authors, nor the publisher nor any other party who has been involved in the preparation or publication of this work warrants that the information contained herein is in every respect accurate or complete, and they disclaim all responsibility for any errors or omissions or for the results obtained from use of the information contained in this work. Readers are encouraged to confirm the information contained herein with other sources. For example and in particular, readers are advised to check the product information sheet included in the package of each drug they plan to administer to be certain that the information contained in this book is accurate and that changes have not been made in the recommended dose or in the contraindications for administration. This recommendation is of particular importance in connection with new or infrequently used drugs.

Talmadge E. King, Jr.: *I thank Mozelle for her love, support, and encouragement and to Talmadge and Almetta King for teaching me the value of hard work and education. In addition, I thank my daughters, Consuelo and Malaika, for their loving support and understanding during my work on this book.*

Margaret B. Wheeler: *To David for his unstinting support; Alma for her joyful presence; Chuck, Jan, Kate, and Krissy Wheeler for their encouragement always; and Alicia, Teresa, and Emilia for extending the family.*

Andrew B. Bindman: *I thank my parents, Arthur and Bernice, who have encouraged me to contribute toward making a constructive difference in people's lives. I also thank my wife, Rebecca, and our three wonderful children, Sarah, Julia, and Jacob, who have made an enormous positive impact on my own life.*

Alicia Fernandez: *To my parents, Hector and Paulina B. Fernandez, with gratitude. For Emilia, Alma, and Jesse, who will, in their own ways, carry on. And for my patients, with appreciation for lessons learned.*

Kevin Grumbach: *With appreciation to my family, colleagues, students, and patients, for all they have taught me.*

Dean Schillinger: *I thank George Schillinger for demonstrating the potential for resilience in the face of vulnerability and for imbuing me with a belief that doctoring requires the head, hands and heart; Zahava Schillinger for instilling in me the confidence and diligence to accomplish my goals; Nahum Joel for conveying his passion regarding science and the pursuit of social justice; and Ariella Hyman for partnering with me in this struggle.*

Teresa J. Villela: *To Amado, Carolina, Elvira, Marcelo, Florentina, Gilberto, and Rosario, with great respect and gratitude, and to my brothers and sisters for all they have taught me.*

CONTENTS

CONTRIBUTORS

Nancy Adler, PhD

Professor, Vice-Chair, Department of Psychiatry, Director, Center for Health and Community, University of California, San Francisco
Chapter 1: Vulnerable Populations and Health Disparities: An Overview

John R. Balmes, MD

Professor, Division of Occupational & Environmental Medicine, Department of Medicine, University of California, San Francisco; Chief, Division of Occupational & Environmental Medicine, Department of Medicine, San Francisco General Hospital
Chapter 21: Work, Living Environment, and Health

Ann Smith Barnes, MD

Assistant Professor, Department of Medicine, Baylor College of Medicine; Ben Taub General Hospital, Houston, Texas
Chapter 31: Obesity as a Clinical and Social Problem

Patricia Barreto, MD, MPH

Assistant Clinical Professor of Pediatrics, Division of Child Health Policy & Community Pediatrics, Department of Pediatrics, David Geffen School of Medicine, University of California, Los Angeles
Chapter 17: Underserved Children: Preventing Chronic Illness and Promoting Health

Ellen Beck, MD

Clinical Professor, Department of Family & Preventive Medicine, Director, Community Education, Division of Family Medicine, Department of Family & Preventive Medicine, University of California, San Diego
Chapter 16: Health and the Community

Neal Benowitz, MD

Professor, Medicine, Psychiatry & Biopharmaceutical Sciences, Chief, Division of Clinical Pharmacology, University of California San Francisco; Program Leader, Tobacco Control Program, UCSF Comprehensive Cancer Center, San Francisco, California
Chapter 34: Tobacco Use

Kirsten Bibbins-Domingo, PhD, MD

Assistant Professor of Medicine, Epidemiology, & Biostatistics, University of California, San Francisco; Attending Physician, Division of General Internal Medicine; San Francisco General Hospital
Chapter 8: Assessing and Promoting Medical Adherence

JudyAnn Bigby, MD

Associate Professor of Medicine, Division of General Medicine & Primary Care, Department of Medicine, Harvard Medical School; Director, Community Health Programs, Brigham and Women's Hospital, Boston, Massachusetts
Chapter 9: Navigating Cross-Cultural Communication

Andrew B. Bindman, MD

Chief, Division of General Internal Medicine, San Francisco General Hospital; Professor, Department of Medicine, University of California, San Francisco
Chapter 1: Vulnerable Populations and Health Disparities: An Overview
Chapter 2: Health Care Disparities: An Overview

Thomas S. Bodenheimer, MD

Professor, Department of Family & Community Medicine, University of California, San Francisco
Chapter 36: Chronic Disease

Paula A. Braveman, MD, MPH

Professor of Family & Community Medicine, Director, Center on Social Disparities in Health, Department of Family & Community Medicine, University of California, San Francisco
Chapter 1: Vulnerable Populations and Health Disparities: An Overview

Paul G. Brunetta, MD

Co-Founder, Tobacco Education Center, University of California, San Francisco Mt. Zion Medical Center; Medical Director, Genentech, Inc., San Francisco, California
Chapter 34: Tobacco Use

Alice Hm Chen, MD, MPH

Assistant Clinical Professor of Medicine, Division of General Internal Medicine, Department of Medicine, University of California, San Francisco; Medical Director, General Medicine Clinic, San Francisco General Hospital
Chapter 26: Providing Care to Patients Who Speak Limited English

Helen Chen, MD

Associate Clinical Professor of Medicine, Division of Geriatrics, Department of Medicine, University of California, San Francisco; Director, Geriatrics & Extended Care Service Line, San Francisco VA Medical Center
Chapter 20: The Hidden Poor: Care of the Elderly

LaVera M. Crawley, MD, MPH

Acting Assistant Professor (Research), Center for Biomedical Ethics, Department of Pediatrics, Stanford University School of Medicine, Palo Alto, California
Chapter 22: Care of the Dying Patient

Jeffrey M. Critchfield, MD

Vice-Chief of Medical Services, Clinical Affairs, San Francisco General Hospital; Assistant Clinical Professor, Division of Rheumatology, Department of Internal Medicine, University of California, San Francisco
Chapter 39: Care of Ill Socially Complicated Patients in the Hospital

Allison Diamant, MD, MSHS

Assistant Professor, Deparment of Medicine, David Geffen School of Medicine, University of California, Los Angeles
Chapter 27: Sexuality as Vulnerability: The Care of Lesbian and Gay Patients

Janet Victoria Diaz, MD

Pulmonary and Critical Care Fellow, Division of Pulmonary and Critical Care Medicine, Department of Internal Medicine, University of California, San Francisco, San Francisco General Hospital
Chapter 21: Work, Living Environment, and Health

M. Robin DiMatteo, PhD

Professor of Psychology, Department of Psychology, University of California, Riverside
Chapter 8: Assessing and Promoting Medical Adherence

Joanne Donsky, MSW

Associate Clinical Professor, Department of Family and Community Medicine, University of California, San Francisco, San Francisco General Hospital
Chapter 16: Health and the Community

Christopher Dunn, PhD

Associate Professor, Psychiatry & Behavioral Sciences, University of Washington School of Medicine, Seattle, Washington
Chapter 7: Promoting Behavior Change

Alicia Fernandez, MD

Associate Professor of Clinical Medicine, Department of Medicine, University of California, San Francisco, San Francisco General Hospital
Chapter 15: Case Management/Multidisciplinary Care Models

Christopher B. Forrest, MD, PhD

Associate Professor of Health Policy and Management, Johns Hopkins Bloomberg School of Public Health, Baltimore, Maryland
Chapter 3: Financing and Organization of Healthcare for Vulnerable Populations

Kevin Grumbach, MD

Chief, Family and Community Medicine, San Francisco General Hospital; Professor and Chair, Department of Family and Community Medicine, University of California, San Francisco
Chapter 1: Vulnerable Populations and Health Disparities: An Overview
Chapter 2: Health Care Disparities: An Overview

Neal Halfon, MD, MPH

Professor of Pediatrics, Public Health, & Public Policy, Director of University of California, Los Angeles Center for Healthier Children Families & Communities
Chapter 17: Underserved Children: Preventing Chronic Illness and Promoting Health

Hali Hammer, MD

Associate Clinical Professor, Department of Family & Community Medicine, University of California, San Francisco; Medical Director, Family Health Center, San Francisco General Hospital
Chapter 12: Group Medical Visits for Underserved Populations

Elizabeth Harleman, MD

Assistant Clinical Professor, Departments of Internal Medicine & Obstetrics, Gynecology & Reproductive Sciences, University of California, San Francisco; Associate Program Director, University of California San Francisco Internal Medicine Residency Program
Chapter 29: Women's Health: Reproduction and Beyond in Poor Women

Suzanne Harris, RN

Co-Founder & Nurse Administrator, Tobacco Education Center, University of California, San Francisco Medical Center at Mt. Zion, San Francisco, California; Coordinator, San Francisco General Hospital Smoking Cessation & Relapse Prevention Program
Chapter 34: Tobacco Use

Clemens Hong, MD, MPH

Resident, San Francisco General Primary Care Residency, University of California Internal Medicine Residency Program
Chapter 34: Tobacco Use

Virginia W. Huang, MPH

PhD Candidate, Division of Health Services Research, Department of Health Policy & Management, Johns Hopkins Bloomberg School of Public Health, Baltimore, Maryland
Chapter 3: Financing and Organization of Healthcare for Vulnerable Populations

Lisa I. Iezzoni, MD, MSc

Professor of Medicine, Division of General Medicine & Primary Care, Beth Israel Deaconess Medical Center, Harvard Medical School, Boston, Massachusetts
Chapter 37: Disability and Patients with Disabilities

Elizabeth A. Jacobs, MD, MPP

Assistant Professor of Medicine, Collaborative Research Unit, Division of Primary Care & General Internal Medicine, Department of Medicine, John H. Stroger, Jr. Hospital of Cook County Hospital & Rush University Medical Center, Chicago, Illinois
Chapter 26: Providing Care to Patients Who Speak Limited English

Sharad Jain, MD

Associate Professor, Division of General Internal Medicine, Department of Medicine, University of California, San Francisco; Assistant Chief, Medical Services, VA Medical Center, San Francisco, California
Chapter 24: Care of the Homeless Patient

Yeva Johnson, MD

Assistant Clinical Professor, Department of Family & Community Medicine, University of California, San Francisco; Infection Control Physician, Bioterrorism & Infectious Disease Emergencies Unit, Communicable Disease Control & Prevention Section, San Francisco Department of Public Health
Chapter 32: Chronic Pain Management in Vulnerable Populations

Seijeoung Kim, RN, PhD

Postdoctoral Fellow, School of Public Health Division of Epidemiology & Biostatistics, University of Illinois at Chicago
Chapter 14: Applying Principles and Practice of Quality Improvement to Better Care for the Underserved

Leigh Kimberg, MD

Assistant Clinical Professor of Medicine, Division of General Internal Medicine, Department of Medicine, San Francisco General Hospital, University of California, San Francisco; Attending Physician, Maxine Hall Health Center, San Francisco, California
Chapter 30: Intimate Partner Violence

Talmadge E. King Jr., MD

Chief, Medical Services, San Francisco General Hospital; Constance B. Wofsy Distinguished Professor and Vice Chairman, Department of Medicine, University of California, San Francisco
Chapter 2: Health Care Disparities: An Overview

Margot Kushel, MD

Assistant Professor of Medicine in Residence, Division of General Internal Medicine, Department of Internal Medicine, University of California, San Francisco, San Francisco General Hospital; Attending Physician, San Francisco General Hospital
Chapter 37: Disability and Patients with Disabilities
Chapter 24: Care of the Homeless Patient

C. Seth Landefeld, MD

Professor of Medicine, Chief, Geriatrics Division, Director, Center on Aging, University of California, San Francisco; Associate Chief of Staff/Geriatrics & Extended Care, San Francisco VA Medical Center
Chapter 20: The Hidden Poor: Care of the Elderly

Daniel S. Lessler, MD, MHA

Associate Professor of Medicine, Division of General Internal Medicine, Department of Medicine, University of Washington School of Medicine; Associate Medical Director, Harborview Medical Center, Seattle, Washington
Chapter 7: Promoting Behavior Change

Lee Lipsenthal, MD

Founder, Finding Balance in a Medical Life, San Anselmo, California
Chapter 40: Caring for Oneself While Caring for Others

Bernard Lo, MD

Professor of Medicine, Director, Program in Medical Ethics, Department of Medicine, University of California, San Francisco
Chapter 5: Principles in the Ethical Care of Underserved Patients

Susana Morales, MD

Associate Professor of Clinical Medicine, Weill Medical College of Cornell University, New York, New York
Chapter 25: Immigrant Health Issues

Matthew Nealon, DDS

Associate Dentist, Dental Department, Native American Health Services, San Francisco, California
Chapter 35: Dental Care: The Forgotten Need

Meg D. Newman, MD

Associate Professor of Clinical Medicine, University of California, San Francisco; Director, HIV Clinical Scholars Fellowship, Centers for Disease Control and Prevention-University of California, San Francisco National Clinicians' Consultation Center
Chapter 38: HIV/AIDS: Impact on Vulnerable Populations

Thomas P. O'Toole, MD

Associate Dean for Curriculum, Professor of Medicine, Department of Medicine, Georgetown University School of Medicine, Washington, D.C.
Chapter 41: Advocacy

Michael K. Paasche-Orlow, MD, MA, MPH

Assistant Professor of Medicine, Division of General Internal Medicine, Department of Medicine, Boston University School of Medicine, Boston, Massachusetts
Chapter 10: Improving the Effectiveness of Patient Education: A Focus on Limited Health Literacy

Ruth M. Parker MD

Professor of Medicine, Division of General Medicine, Department of Medicine, Emory University School of Medicine, Atlanta, Georgia
Chapter 10: Improving the Effectiveness of Patient Education: A Focus on Limited Health Literacy

Victor H. Perez, MD, MPH

Assistant Clinical Professor of Pediatrics, Division of Child Health Policy & Community Pediatrics, Department of Pediatrics, David Geffen School of Medicine, University of California, Los Angeles
Chapter 17: Underserved Children: Preventing Chronic Illness and Promoting Health

John D. Piette, PhD

Career Scientist, VA Ann Arbor Healthcare System; Associate Professor of Internal Medicine, University of Michigan, Ann Arbor
Chapter 13: Applying Interactive Health Technologies for Vulnerable Populations

Michael B. Potter, MD

Associate Professor of Clinical Family & Community Medicine, Department of Family & Community Medicine, University of California, San Francisco
Chapter 32: Chronic Pain Management in Vulnerable Populations

Douglas R. Price-Hanson, MD

Assistant Clinical Professor of Medicine, Psychiatrist, Division of General Internal Medicine, Department of Internal Medicine, University of California, San Francisco, San Francisco General Hospital; Staff Physician, Tom Waddell Health Center, San Francisco, California
Chapter 28: The Medical Treatment of Patients with Psychiatric Illness

Francisco Ramos-Gomez, DDS, MS, MPH

Associate Professor, Department of Orofacial Sciences, Division of Pediatric Dentistry, University of California, San Francisco Center to Address Disparities in Children's Oral Health
Chapter 35: Dental Care: The Forgotten Need

Marisa Rogers, MD, MPH

Assistant Professor of Clinical Medicine, Division of General Medicine, Department of Internal Medicine, University of Pennsylvania School of Medicine, Penn Presbyterian Medical Center, Philadelphia
Chapter 31: Obesity as a Clinical and Social Problem

F. Joseph Roll, MD

Associate Professor of Clinical Medicine, Department of Medicine, University of California, San Francisco, San Francisco General Hospital
Chapter 33: Principles of Caring for Alcohol and Drug Users

Sara Rosenbaum, JD

Hirsh Professor & Chair, Department of Health Policy, School of Public Health and Health Services, George Washington University, Washington, D.C.
Chapter 4: Legal Issues in the Care of Underserved Populations

Anne Rosenthal, MD

Clinical Instructor, Division of General Internal Medicine, Department of Medicine, University of California, San Francisco; Associate Physician, National HIV/AIDS Clinician's Consultation Center, Department of Family & Community Medicine, University of California, San Francisco; Attending Physician, Maxine Hall Health Center, Department of Public Health, San Francisco, California
Chapter 27: Sexuality as Vulnerability: The Care of Lesbian and Gay Patients

George William Saba, PhD

Professor of Clinical Family & Community Medicine, University of California, San Francisco; Associate Director, Director of Behavioral Science, Division of Family Practice Residency, Department of Family & Community Medicine, San Francisco General Hospital
Chapter 6: Creating a Context for Effective Intervention in the Clinical Care of Vulnerable Patients
Chapter 19: The Family as the Context for Care

Ellen M. Scarr, RNC, MS, FNP, WHNP

Clinical Professor, Department of Family Health Care Nursing, University of California, San Francisco; Nurse Practitioner, Department of Pediatrics, Young Women's Clinic Nurse Practitioner, San Francisco County Department of Jail Health Services, County Jail
Chapter 18: Adolescence and its Vulnerabilities

Gordon D. Schiff, MD

Director, Clinical Quality Research & Improvement, Division of General Medicine, Department of Medicine, Cook County Hospital; Associate Professor of Medicine, Rush Medical College, Chicago, Illinois
Chapter 14: Applying Principles and Practice of Quality Improvement to Better Care for the Underserved

Dean Schillinger, MD

Associate Professor of Clinical Medicine, Department of Medicine, University of California, San Francisco, San Francisco General Hospital
Chapter 6: Creating a Context for Effective Intervention in the Clinical Care of Vulnerable Patients
Chapter 13: Applying Interactive Health Technologies for Vulnerable Populations

Michelle Schneidermann, MD

Assistant Clinical Professor of Medicine, Division of General Internal Medicine, Department of Internal Medicine, University of California, San Francisco; Medical Director, High User Case Management Program, Department of Medicine, San Francisco General Hospital
Chapter 15: Case Management/Multidisciplinary Care Models

Margaret A. Scott, RN, MSN, FNP

Assistant Clinical Professor, School of Nursing, Department of Family Health Care Nursing, University of California, San Francisco
Chapter 18: Adolescence and its Vulnerabilities

William B. Shore, MD, FAAFP

Clinical Professor, Director of Predoctoral Education, Permanente Medical Group Teaching Chair in Primary Care, Department of Family & Community Medicine, University of California, San Francisco
Chapter 18: Adolescence and its Vulnerabilities

Jody Steinauer, MD, MAS

Assistant Clinical Professor, Department of Obstetrics, Gynecology, & Reproductive Services, University of California, San Francisco, San Francisco General Hosptial
Chapter 29: Women's Health: Reproduction and Beyond in Poor Women

Cam-Tu Tran, MD, MS

Associate Clinical Professor, Department of Pediatrics, University of California, San Francisco; Director, Pediatric Healthy Lifestyle Clinic at San Francisco General Hospital
Chapter 31: Obesity as a Clinical and Social Problem

Jacqueline P. Tulsky, MD

Professor of Clinical Medicine, Positive Health Program, Department of Medicine, University of California, San Francisco, San Francisco General Hospital,
Chapter 23: Clinical Care for Persons with a History of Incarceration

Teresa J. Villela, MD

Director, San Francisco General Hospital Family and Community Medicine Residency Program; Associate Clinical Professor and Vice Chair, Department of Family and Community Medicine, University of California, San Francisco
Chapter 6: Creating a Context for Effective Intervention in the Clinical Care of Vulnerable Patients
Chapter 19: The Family as the Context for Care
Chapter 36: Chronic Disease

Alexander Y. Walley, MD

Fellow, Division of General Internal Medicine, Department of Medicine, Boston University School of Medicine; Medical Director, Acute Treatment Services, Staff Physician, Adult Medicine, Dimock Community Health Center, Boston, Massachusetts
Chapter 33: Principles of Caring for Alcohol and Drug Users

Emily A. Wang, MD

Resident Physician, Department of Medicine, University of California, San Francisco
Chapter 23: Clinical Care for Persons with a History of Incarceration

Margaret B. Wheeler, MS, MD

Director, San Francisco General Hospital Primary Care Internal Medicine Residency, University of California, San Francisco Internal Medicine Residency Program; Associate Clinical Professor of Medicine, Department of Medicine, University of California, San Francisco
Chapter 11: The Home Visit/Mobile Outreach
Chapter 36: Chronic Disease
Chapter 38: HIV/AIDS: Impact on Vulnerable Populations

Mary C. White, RN, MPH, PhD

Professor, Department of Community Health Systems, School of Nursing, University of California, San Francisco
Chapter 23: Clinical Care for Persons with a History of Incarceration

Sara E. Wilensky, JD, MPP

Assistant Research Professor, Department of Health Policy, School of Public Health and Health Services, George Washington University, Washington, D.C.
Chapter 4: Legal Issues in the Care of Underserved Populations

Mark V. Williams, MD, FACP

Professor of Medicine, Director of the Hospital Medicine Unit, Department of Medicine, Emory University School of Medicine, Atlanta, Georgia
Chapter 39: Care of Ill Socially Complicated Patients in the Hospital

Dan Wlodarczyk, MD

Professor of Clinical Medicine, Division of General Internal Medicine, Department of Medicine, University of California, San Francisco; Attending Physician, Division of Primary Care, Department of Public Health, San Francisco Department of Public Health
Chapter 11: The Home Visit/Mobile Outreach

Naomi Wortis, MD

Director of Community Programs, Assistant Clinical Professor, Department of Family & Community Medicine, University of California, San Francisco; Attending Physician, Silver Avenue Family Health Center, Division of Community Primary Care, San Francisco Department of Public Health
Chapter 16: Health and the Community

Barry D. Zevin, MD

Assistant Clinical Professor, Division of General Internal Medicine, Department of Medicine, University of California, San Francisco; Medical Director, Tom Waddell Health Center, San Francisco Department of Public Health
Chapter 32: Chronic Pain Management in Vulnerable Populations

PREFACE

It has been widely documented that populations of lower socioeconomic status and from minority racial and ethnic backgrounds have worse health and often receive a lower standard of health care. When worse health outcomes can be attributed to inequity in the targets or distribution of resources, they are termed disparities in health or health care. Increased mortality, morbidity and burden of disease and other adverse health experiences are observed when illness, social conditions, and social policy conspire to undermine health and create barriers to care.

As healthcare providers, there is perhaps no more distressing medical research than that which suggests that healthcare workers and the healthcare system contribute to disparities in in health for vulnerable populations. Studies reveal that healthcare workers feel ill-prepared when caring for vulnerable patients, especially those who are chronically ill, the elderly, addicted, mentally ill, victims of violence, or from minority or disadvantaged backgrounds—patients whose numbers are on the rise and patients for whom we are not currently providing adequate care. Consequently, healthcare workers may be the 3rd factor in the a "triple jeopardy" vulnerable patients face when it comes to health care: not only are these patients more likely to be ill and to have difficulty accessing care, but when they do, the care they receive is more likely to be sub-optimal.

Fortunately, training healthcare workers to care for vulnerable patients makes a difference. With training, they are more willing to work with these populations and provide better care. Nevertheless, while the need to teach healthcare workers of all health professions how to care for vulnerable patients may seem obvious, it is often overlooked. Medical faculty members are often uncomfortable teaching patient-centered, efficient, effective and equitable care to these frequently complex patients. They feel incompetent to teach students and residents a set of skills that range from cross-cultural communication to caring for patients with addictions. Thus, developing curricula in competencies critical to caring for vulnerable patients is one of the most pressing tasks in clinical education today, one that is increasingly being embraced by national and local educational, accreditation and regulatory bodies.

The purpose of this book is to offer the theoretical background and practical knowledge required to teach health care providers to care for vulnerable, underserved patients both at the individual and system levels.[1] In this book, we give the readers an understanding of the complex nature of the problem of caring for vulnerable, underserved patients, an appreciation of the need to address disparities at multiple levels, and suggestions for practical approaches to improve the care of vulnerable populations. We aim to "enable" healthcare workers, students, and other interested parties to contribute to the solution. We focus on issues of patient care that are common amongst underserved patients and suggest ways to use our materials as teaching tools for health professions trainees in both didactic and clinical settings.

Our book is intended as a basis for teaching the core principles and skills required to care for our most complex patients—the vulnerable and underserved—where our

---

[1](Although these terms are often used interchangeably, traditionally, "underserved" refers to patients whose barriers to healthcare are due to lack accessible services, e.g., for geographic or financial reasons. "Vulnerable" patients are those whose impediments to care are social or medical, that is, related to culture, education, transportation, language, homelessness, legal status or difficult health problems such as chronic disease, mental illness, substance use or HIV)

clinical skills must be the most astute. Our text is appropriate both for students (medical students, nurses, pharmacists, physician's assistants, public health, and other health care practitioners) in classes introducing them to clinical, community, or social medicine, and in their initial practical experiences, including, but not limited to, primary care rotations and clerkships in family medicine, pediatrics, internal medicine, women's medicine and psychiatry. As teaching hospitals are the major providers of care to uninsured, poor and minority patients in the United States, the book is also intended as a resource for teachers and trainees who practice in these settings as well as public health care settings internationally. Post-graduate trainees (e.g. residents and fellows) from all disciplines could use this text for didactics in behavioral and clinical medicine, and quality improvement. Finally, it can also serve as a rapid, yet comprehensive reference for all practitioners.

The book is organized into three sections: *Principles, Practice* and *Populations*. Chapters in each section discuss ways in which both the individual practitioner and the health care system may be more responsive to patients in order to assure or "enable" patients with these characteristics to receive accessible, high quality care, thereby reducing the health care disparities associated with vulnerability. Each chapter features both *Critical Concepts* and *Common Pitfalls,* and ends with a *Core Competency* highlighting important concepts and skills for quick and easy referencing.

Putting together a book of this scope and magnitude was no easy task and involved making certain decisions that not all readers may agree with. For example, while trying to keep the length of the book as manageable as possible, we were forced to exclude some relevant topics and decided to allow some overlap of content in those areas that are most critical. In addition, we welcomed differences of opinion among authors, provided the issues were clearly stated and the reasons for the author's opinion documented.

The first section, entitled *Principles,* lays out the theoretical groundwork of the book. Topics discussed include: overview of the concepts of medical vulnerability and disparities in health and health care; financing and organization of health care for vulnerable populations; laws and regulations governing the care of medically underserved populations and ethical dilemmas that arise in the clinical care of medically underserved populations. The second section, *Practice,* considers overarching themes and skills necessary to care for patients and how population medicine and systems approaches to caring for vulnerable patients can improve care. Topics discussed include: the importance of building a therapeutic alliance and assessing for vulnerability; supporting health behavior change and adherence; principles of effective communication when cultural or literacy barriers may exist; models of care delivery to improve the effectiveness of medical care, such as mobile outreach, group medical visits, community-oriented care, and use of interactive health technologies; and quality improvement and case management programs. The third section, *Populations,* examines particular conditions or social circumstances that can lead to worse care. Chapters consider approaches to patients with histories of chronic disease, mental illness, intimate partner violence and addiction, for example. Care of patients with limited English proficiency, history of incarceration, gay and lesbian patients, children, adolescents and the elderly are subjects of others. In addition, this section addresses common situations that uniquely complicate the care of vulnerable populations such as environmental and occupational illnesses; the care of socially complicated hospitalized patients; end-of-life health care; chronic pain management; dental health; the care of adults with HIV/AIDS and patients with disabilities. We end with chapters that address preventing practitioner burnout and promoting physician advocacy.

We are deeply appreciative to the authors for their outstanding contributions to this book. We would also like to acknowledge the support and patience of the staff at Lange. We especially wish to recognize the efforts of Isabel Noguiera for believing in the project and to Janet Foltin, Christie Naglieri and James Shanahan for bringing it to fruition. Special acknowledgment goes to Amy Markowitz and Amy Wollman for their editorial assistance. We appreciate the expert staff support from Cliff Wilson, Nikki Bengal and Salwa Mrabe. A grant from the Health Resources and Services Administration (HRSA) helped us bring this project to fruition. Finally, we are forever grateful to our patients for allowing us to participate in their care, our students for inspiring us to do better and our families for their generous support.

Talmadge E. King, Jr., MD
Margaret B. Wheeler, MS, MD
Andrew B. Bindman, MD
Alicia Fernandez, MD
Kevin Grumbach, MD
Dean Schillinger, MD
Teresa J. Villela, MD

PART 1

Principles

Andrew B. Bindman, MD, and Kevin Grumbach, MD, editors

CHAPTERS

1 VULNERABLE POPULATIONS AND HEALTH DISPARITIES: AN OVERVIEW

2 HEALTH CARE DISPARITIES: AN OVERVIEW

3 FINANCING AND ORGANIZATION OF HEALTHCARE FOR VULNERABLE POPULATIONS

4 LEGAL ISSUES IN THE CARE OF UNDERSERVED POPULATIONS

5 PRINCIPLES IN THE ETHICAL CARE OF UNDERSERVED PATIENTS

Chapter 1

Vulnerable Populations and Health Disparities: An Overview

Kevin Grumbach, MD, Paula Braveman, MD, MPH, Nancy Adler, PhD, and Andrew B. Bindman, MD

Objectives

- Define the terms vulnerable populations and health disparities.
- Distinguish among differences in health, health disparities, and health care disparities.
- Understand the relationship between social vulnerability and health disparities, and the pathways mediating this association.
- Recognize the ethical and human rights principles underlying efforts to reduce health disparities.
- Identify actions health professionals may take to change the social conditions that create vulnerability and produce health disparities.

"Vulnerable" derives from the Latin word for wounded. In a sense, medically vulnerable populations are those that are wounded by social forces placing them at a disadvantage for their health. Vulnerability is visible in the variation in the incidence, prevalence, and outcomes of health conditions across social groups.

This chapter provides an overview of the concept of medical vulnerability. It begins by introducing the notion of health disparities and distinguishing it from simple differences in health. It describes evidence of health disparities, particularly by race/ethnicity and socioeconomic status (SES). It then discusses conceptual models for understanding the pathways between social vulnerability and poor health status. It concludes by suggesting that health professionals have a responsibility not only to develop their skills to respond effectively to the health care needs of vulnerable patients, but also to take action to change the fundamental social conditions that produce vulnerability.

WHAT ARE HEALTH AND HEALTH CARE DISPARITIES?

Webster's dictionary defines a disparity as a difference. "Difference" sounds like a neutral concept. Why should there be concern about differences in health among different people? After all, it is only logical that different people have different states of health, requiring different kinds and quantities of care. For example, elderly people are expected to be less healthy than young adults. People who ski are more likely to suffer leg fractures than people who do not.

Concern for health disparities, then, is not a wholesale concern for all differences in health. It is a particular concern for a subset of differences that seem particularly unfair because of social injustice. Although few readers of this book probably were moved to righteous indignation by the health differences cited in the preceding paragraph, the following observations are likely to prompt qualitatively different reactions: A child born to an African-American mother in the United States is

3

2.5 times as likely to die before reaching her or his first birthday as a child born to a white mother.[1] A study of 22 countries in Europe and North America found that 11-year-old children in the most economically disadvantaged households and communities were eight times more likely to have poor self-rated health compared with their counterparts in the most economically advantaged households and communities.[2]

HEALTH DISPARITIES

"Health disparities" is a shorthand term denoting a specific kind of health difference between more and less privileged social groups. It refers to differences that are systematic,[3] not random or occasional, and that are at least theoretically amenable to social intervention. The social groups being compared are differentiated by their underlying social position; that is, their relative position in social hierarchies defined by wealth, power, and/or prestige; this includes socioeconomic, racial/ethnic, gender, and age groups and those defined by disability, sexual orientation, or other characteristics reflecting social privilege or stigma.[4,5]

HEALTH CARE DISPARITIES

Disparities in health care, as opposed to health, refer to the systematic differences in health care received by people based on these same social characteristics. Although disparities in health care account for only a relatively small proportion of disparities in health, they are of particular importance to health care providers and are discussed in greater detail in the next chapter.

ROLE OF RACE/ETHNICITY AND SOCIOECONOMIC CLASS IN HEALTH DISPARITIES

Although there is some disagreement about which factors are the most significant predictors of health disparities, the majority of the research evidence suggests that race/ethnicity and socioeconomic class are among the most important.[6-9]

RACE/ETHNICITY

Race and ethnicity often are combined and referred to as one concept. Nevertheless, the concept of race as commonly used tends to emphasize geographic origin, whereas ethnicity incorporates the concept of culture.[10]

The classification of both racial and ethnic groups is relatively arbitrary and, apart from a small number of genes that encode skin color, has little biologic basis. Advances in genomics have exposed the concept of race as predominantly a social construct, rooted in historical biases and social stratification based on ancestry and superficial phenotype rather than emanating from fundamental genetic differences among populations perceived to be of different "races." There is no gene or set of genes that is exclusive to one race and that can be used to define those belonging to a race. Stated another way, one cannot look at a person's DNA and tell definitively that she or he is Chinese, African American, Latino, or white. The genetic variation among people within a racial and ethnic group is much greater than the variation across groups.[11]

Despite the lack of definitive genetic determinants, race and ethnicity have important influences on health. Based on historical conventions, the 2000 US Census identified five major racial groups: African American or black, American Indian or Alaska native, Asian, native Hawaiian or other Pacific Islander, and white.

The National Institutes of Health have found important differences based on these categories of race and ethnicity in such diverse health indicators as infant mortality, cancer mortality, coronary heart disease mortality, prevalence of diabetes, end-stage renal disease, and stroke (Table 1-1).[6] Two clear observations can be made about these health outcomes categorized by race and ethnicity. First, African Americans experience the greatest morbidity and mortality on every reported indicator, and the gap often is substantial. For example, African Americans experience 13.9 deaths for every 1000 live births, compared with Asian or Pacific Islanders, who experience 5.1 deaths.

Second, there is no other group that shows consistently poor health outcomes across all indicators. Whites show poorer outcomes than groups other than African Americans on many of the reported health indicators (e.g., overall cancer mortality). American Indians and Alaska natives have the second highest rates of infant mortality, and Hispanics or Latinos have the second highest prevalence of diabetes. Asian Americans and Pacific Islanders show the most favorable profile.

One limitation of these conclusions is that they are based on large groupings by race and ethnicity. These broad categories may obscure substantial variation in health within some of the groups. Members of the same major ethnic group from different countries and areas of origin have different degrees of disadvantage and health risk. For example, Asian-Pacific Islanders as a group have the lowest rate of infant deaths (5.1 per 1000 births) compared with other groups. However, infant mortality for Hawaiians (8.7 per 1000 births) is more than twice that of Chinese (3.2). Among Latinos and Hispanics, infant mortality rates range from a low of 4.2 deaths among Cubans to a high of 8.7 deaths among Puerto Ricans. The importance of looking at subgroups also may differ by disease. For example, Asian-Indians have the lowest rates of all-cause mortality, yet

Table 1-1. Health Disparities of Certain Conditions in Selected Populations

| Health Condition and Specific Example | White | African American | NIH Categories of Race/Ethnicity | | American Indian and Alaska Native |
			Hispanic/ Latino	Asian and Pacific Islander	
Infant mortality: rate per 1000 live births	5.9	13.9	5.8	5.1	9.1
Cancer mortality: rate per 100,000	199.3	255.1	123.7	124.2	129.3
Lung cancer: age-adjusted death rate	38.3	46.0	13.6	17.2	25.1
Female breast cancer: age-adjusted death rate	18.7	26.1	12.1	9.8	10.3
Coronary heart disease: mortality rate per 100,000	206	252	145	123	126
Stroke: mortality rate per 100,000	58	80	39	51	38
Diabetes: diagnosed rate per 100,000	36	74	61	DSU	DSU
End-stage renal disease: rate per million	218	873	DNA	344	589

DNA, Data have not been analyzed; DSU, data are statistically unreliable.
Source: NIH Health Disparities Strategic Plan, Fiscal Years 2004–2008, vol 1. Bethesda, MD: NIH, U.S. Dept. of Health & Human Services.

they have relatively high rates of coronary heart disease compared with other Asian groups.[12]

SOCIOECONOMIC STATUS

Social class shows a strong association with health independent of race and ethnicity.[7] In general, social class is inversely associated with longevity. There is no standardized method for defining or measuring social class, and this information is not routinely collected as a part of health care encounters. Some of the typical dimensions of social class used in research studies include occupation, income, and education level, which are all components of what is generally referred to as socioeconomic status (SES).

Some of the most compelling evidence about the association between SES and health comes from the Whitehall study in the United Kingdom. This research on British civil servants demonstrated a linear association of higher occupational grade with lower 10-year mortality.[13] This was a striking finding because significant differences in mortality occurred in a population in which all participants were employed and had health care coverage. Despite the relative homogeneity of the group, those in higher occupational grades had significantly lower rates of a number of diseases as well as lower mortality.

In the United States, it has been more difficult to investigate whether a similar SES and health gradient exists. Public health monitoring and epidemiologic surveys frequently collect information on race and ethnicity but less often include information on income or education. Data from the few large studies in the United States that have examined socioeconomic factors in health show that the difference in mortality between those at the top versus the bottom of the SES hierarchy are large, and even greater than those between racial and ethnic groups. For example, the National Longitudinal Mortality Survey showed a difference between those with an income of less than $10,000

(in 1980 dollars) and those earning $25,000 or more of 7.9 years and 8.6 years, respectively, among whites and African Americans. This is almost double the difference in life expectancy between whites and African Americans, which is 4.4 years.[14] Analyses of the SES gradient generally reveal a sharp drop in mortality as income increases from the most extreme categories of poverty toward more moderate poverty, and a continued but more gradual drop in mortality as incomes rises above this moderate poverty level (Fig. 1-1).[15] It should

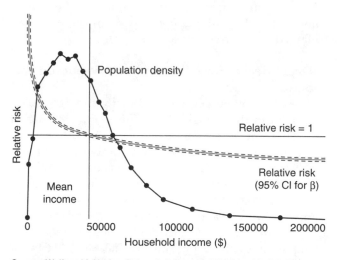

Source: Wolfson M, Kaplan G, Lynch J, Ross N, & Backlund E. (1999). Permission pending from BMJ.

Figure 1-1. Relative risk of dying and population distribution for US individuals by household income ($). The downward sloping curves (close together) show the estimated relation between household income and the relative risk of mortality, plus a 95% confidence interval, after controlling for age and gender. The relation is highly significant both statistically and substantively and is clearly consistent with a diminishing returns individual level relation between income and risk of mortality. The other "humped" curve shows the resulting distribution of individuals by household income for the whole of the United States.

be noted that a relatively small proportion of the US population is at the very bottom of the income distribution, where the steepest drop occurs. Individuals in this population are of most concern because they are at highest risk and greatest disadvantage; however, on a population basis, more individuals are affected by health disparities at somewhat higher levels of income. Thus, these factors continue to play a role in the risk of mortality and morbidity well into the middle class, where a majority of the US population resides.

Impact of Education

In contrast to the relationship between income and health, which demonstrates a continued drop in mortality as income increases (albeit with a sharper drop in the lower portion of the distribution), the association between mortality and education is more discontinuous. For all-cause mortality and each of the specific causes, the death rates are lower for those with more education. To the extent that education provides information, knowledge, and skills that improve health, each additional year of education should contribute somewhat equally to improved health. However, educational attainment also serves a credentialing function. As a result, there is a greater benefit of achieving years of schooling that result in a degree or credential than of additional years that do not. Thus, the benefit of completing the 12th year of schooling, which results in a high school degree, is greater than the benefit of completing any other single year of high school (referred to as the "sheepskin" effect).

Dual Effect of Race/Ethnicity and Socioeconomic Status

The overlap between race/ethnicity and SES makes it difficult to disentangle the relative contributions of each of these factors toward health.[16] Both African Americans and Hispanics are overrepresented in lower SES categories. Data from the 2000 census reveal that 49% to 50% of Hispanics and 26% to 30% of African Americans have less than a high school education, compared with 13% to 14% of whites. Similarly, there are large differences in income by race/ethnicity. For example, in 2000 the median income was $29,645 for African Americans, whereas it was $47,777 for whites. If one uses a measure of net worth (wealth) instead of income, the economic differences by race/ethnicity are even more dramatic.

For some health outcomes, differences between African Americans and whites become nonsignificant once analyses control for income. For other health outcomes, although the difference among groups is substantially reduced, there is still a residual effect associated with race/ethnicity.[9] Some part of this difference may have to do with other socioeconomic differences between African Americans and whites beyond household income, such as differences in wealth rather than simply annual income.

As social scientists continue to investigate the complex interplay among race/ethnicity, statuses, and health status, the prevailing wisdom is that *both* race/ethnicity *and* SES matter.[7] Race/ethnicity can confer a vulnerability rooted in experiences of racism and social oppression that is not completely reducible to socioeconomic disadvantage. At the same time, focusing exclusively on disparities by racial and ethnic groups overlooks the contribution of socioeconomic inequalities to these disparities. The following section examines in greater detail the pathways through which social vulnerabilities such as minority race/ethnicity or low SES translate into poor health status.

HEALTH DISPARITIES AND PATHWAYS OF VULNERABILITY

Phyllis Gripman has been driving a bus for 22 years. The stress of keeping on schedule despite traffic congestion and impatient commuters contributes to her poorly controlled blood pressure. She often skips taking her diuretic medication when working. Not infrequently, passenger complaints about the bus service are coupled with derogatory comments about the fact that she is a woman and African American.

Tho Van fled his native Cambodia to escape the Pol Pot regime. He has nightmares reliving watching his brother being tortured to death. He often must rely on his daughter to translate during his medical visits. He avoids discussing his nightmares in front of his daughter. He worries about his teenage son, who has joined a gang and is truant from school.

Walter Jones has been homeless since his discharge from the army following the Gulf War. He has been in and out of rehabilitation programs for his heroin addiction. He is managing to stay clean while in a methadone maintenance program. He initiated evaluation for other medical problems at the Veteran's Administration medical center, but did not follow up for treatment after he overheard a physician refer to him as "that noncompliant homeless drug addict who's wasting our time and money."

These three examples identify individuals with social characteristics that make them vulnerable to experiencing health disparities. Viewed within the framework of health disparities, defined in the preceding as health differences between more and less privileged groups, "vulnerability" consists of those social characteristics, such as minority race/ethnicity and low SES, that are associated with health disparities. How do these characteristics ultimately result in inferior health status?

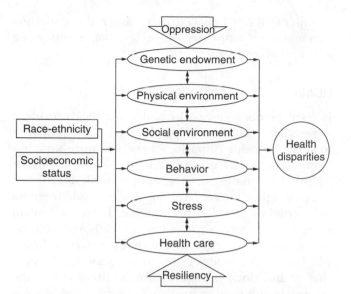

Figure 1-2. A conceptual model that synthesizes ideas from a variety of models proposed to explain the pathways between demographic characteristics and health status. This model proposes that poor health culminates from several major forces.

The conceptual model displayed in Figure 1-2 synthesizes ideas from a variety of models that have been proposed to explain the pathways between demographic characteristics and health status.[17–23]

This model proposes that poor health culminates from several major forces:

1. *Genetic endowment.* Everyone is born with a genetic endowment that offers relative protection against, or vulnerability to, certain conditions. Ms. Gripman, the bus driver, may have inherited a disposition to develop essential hypertension. Mr. Jones, the homeless veteran, may have a genetic susceptibility to opiates that abetted his addiction to heroin.

2. *Physical environment.* The air, water, food, toxins, and physical dangers to which one is exposed may have a profound impact on health. Minorities and the poor are more likely to reside in neighborhoods and work settings with unhealthful physical environments; therefore, this is a socially mediated influence on their health (see Chap. 21). For example, housing is often crowded, noise is pervasive, pollutants and toxins are prevalent, and facilities for exercise are sparse. Mr. Jones' lack of housing is a particularly glaring example of vulnerability in his physical environment.

3. *Social environment.* Vulnerable populations also often face an oppressive social environment, including factors such as institutional and other forms of racism, housing segregation, and low levels of social capital (generally defined as the resources that come from strong community and interpersonal relationships).

Communities with greater social capital and collective efficacy (i.e., more able to organize and garner resources) have lower morbidity and mortality.[24,25] Mr. Van's experience of political violence and social disruption as a refugee from Cambodia poignantly represents a social environment that has adverse effects on health and the receipt of health care (see Chap. 25).

4. *Behavior and lifestyle.* Unhealthful behaviors such as smoking and substance use are more prevalent among people with less education, and sedentary lifestyles and high-fat diets are more common among African Americans and those with low SES.[8,26] The reasons for these high rates of prevalence are complex but also are heavily influenced by differences in physical and social environments, chronic stress, and delivery of health care (see Chaps. 31 and 33).

5. *Chronic stress.* Researchers also have begun to identify the toxic effects of chronic stress related to lack of economic and social resources or experiences of discrimination. The concept of "allostatic load" was developed by McEwen and colleagues[27] to describe the biological processes involved in responses to chronic stress. Allostatic load scores have been found to be higher among African Americans than whites and greater among those with less than more education.[28] Allostatic load scores, in turn, have been shown in a sample of older adults to predict physical and cognitive decline, the onset of new cardiovascular disease, and mortality over a 7-year period.[29,30] The types of occupational stresses experienced by Ms. Gripman also have been associated with unfavorable health outcomes.[31]

6. *Health care.* Inadequate access to and quality of health care is a final pathway to health disparities. Inferior health care may result from several types of deficiencies in the health care system. There may be structural inequalities in the distribution of health care resources, such as physicians and hospitals, across communities. The interpersonal process of delivering care may be deficient because of factors such as discrimination or lack of cultural or non-English language competence among health care workers. For example, a clinic with greater availability of interpreters and culturally appropriate mental health services might afford Mr. Van greater opportunity for effective treatment of his posttraumatic stress disorder, resulting in better health status and well-being (see Chaps. 9 and 10).

Although Figure 1-2 presents this model in a relatively linear form, it is important to recognize that the forces producing health disparities function in a more dynamic, multidirectional manner involving interactions and feedback loops among all the elements displayed. For example, chronic stress from war trauma may have contributed to Mr. Jones' adoption of unhealthful behaviors such as alcohol and drug use as a mechanism to cope with stress. Poor health or a chronic medical condition, such as Ms. Gripman's hypertension, may increase stress levels. Moreover, these factors all operate at multiple levels, ranging from the individual to the broader community and social institutions. The cumulative negative force of these pathways may be viewed as representing the social vulnerability that produces health disparities.

In contrast, individual and collective resiliency—the capacity to develop positively despite harmful environments and experiences—represents the positive vector of these pathways that may act as a countervailing force and produce better health outcomes. One example of the positive effects that can result from individual and collective resiliency is reflected in the finding that first-generation immigrants appear to have a health advantage across virtually every group.[32] This may partially result from the "healthy immigrant" effect, in which there is differential selection for those who have the characteristics (including better health) that allow them to emigrate to the United States.[33] It also may reflect protective effects of traditional diets, supportive social networks, or other health practices of first-generation immigrants. The finding of lower mortality among older Mexican Americans living in neighborhoods with a higher density of Mexican Americans supports this view.[34] The researchers attributed this difference to the protective effects of the concentration, which may buffer Mexican Americans from the "unhealthful aspects of US culture."

ETHICAL AND HUMAN RIGHTS PRINCIPLES

Ethical and human rights principles underlie the notion of health disparities. "Distributive justice," that is, normative ethical principles designed to allocate resources in limited supply relative to demand, is especially relevant to health disparities.[35]

DISTRIBUTIVE JUSTICE

The ethicist John Rawls has provided a framework for considering the principle of distributive justice and its application to health disparities. In defining how one would know what was a just allocation of resources to different groups in a society, Rawls[36] introduced the notion of "the veil of ignorance." In his view, policies allocating resources should be made as if one were operating behind a "veil of ignorance" about the social group into which one had been born. If I did not know whether I would be born rich or poor, black or white, male or female, into a family living in a rural area or one in an urban area, how would I recommend allocating

resources? Rawls believed that, under those circumstances, most people would prefer that resources be allocated according to need.

HUMAN RIGHTS AND RIGHT TO HEALTH

Human rights frameworks and principles provide a universally recognized frame of reference for initiatives to reduce health disparities between more and less advantaged social groups. When the term "human rights" is encountered, most people think of civil and political rights, such as freedom of speech and freedom from cruel or arbitrary punishment. However, human rights also encompass economic, social, and cultural rights, such as the right to a decent standard of living, which in turn includes rights to adequate food, water, shelter, and clothing requisite for health as well as the right to health itself.

In addition, almost every country in the world has signed one or more agreements that include health-related rights. The right to health is a cornerstone underlying efforts to reduce health disparities. The World Health Organization's constitution[37] defined the right to health as the right of everyone to enjoy the highest possible level of health. The right to health can be operationalized as the right of all social groups (defined by social position) to attain the level of health enjoyed by the most privileged group in society. The right to health thus provides the basis for comparing the health experienced by different social groups, always using as the reference group the most privileged group in a given category.

RACISM AND HEALTH

One final conceptual framework useful for understanding vulnerability derives from a model developed by Jones for understanding racism and its impact on health.[38] Jones proposes that racism operates at three levels: institutionalized, personally mediated, and internalized. *Institutionalized racism* refers to the structural elements of racism that are "codified in our institutions of customs, practice and law so there need not be an identifiable perpetrator." Examples are housing segregation, school inequality, and the history of Jim Crow laws in the United States. *Personally mediated racism* is the prejudice and discrimination experienced in daily encounters, ranging from overt racial slurs to the less explicit racism of the prejudicial judgments made by teachers, clinicians, shopkeepers, and other social contacts. *Internalized racism* is defined as "acceptance by members of the stigmatized races of negative messages about their own abilities and intrinsic worth." Internalized racism manifests itself as lack of self-esteem and devaluing of the sense of self-worth.

Although developed for understanding racism, Jones model is applicable to all the "-isms" that create social vulnerability. For example, the levels proposed by Jones apply to sexism. Sexism operates at an institutional level (e.g., objectification of women by mass media and entertainment, inadequate laws and lax enforcement to protect women against violence and sexual abuse), interpersonal level (e.g., prejudice in hiring and promotion decisions), and internalized level (e.g., victimization, lowered expectations for achievement). The same principles apply to vulnerabilities based on social class, sexual orientation, immigrant status, and other characteristics.[7]

TREATING VULNERABILITY: ADDRESSING THE ROOT CAUSES

For health professionals to successfully attend to the health needs of vulnerable populations, they must recognize how vulnerability manifests itself at each of these levels for each patient's particular constellation of vulnerabilities. Social consciousness is required to identify the factors that perpetuate vulnerability at the institutional level, whether in health care organizations or other community institutions; to change these conditions requires translating awareness into social advocacy. Insight and reflection are necessary to enhance awareness of the biases and misassumptions—both obvious and subtle—that reinforce vulnerability at the personally mediated level. Finally, for clinicians to effectively care for vulnerable populations also requires healing of patients' internalized wounds—the despair and devaluation of self-worth that thwart healthful living and healthy relationships.

What health care providers can do to reduce health care disparities—in other words, to increase and improve health care for socially vulnerable and underserved patients—is addressed throughout this book. Subsequent chapters comprehensively discuss approaches to delivering more accessible, effective, and responsive health care and social services to vulnerable patients. However, the most effective treatment for the problems of vulnerable patients would be to change the fundamental social conditions that are the sources of vulnerability and primary determinants of health disparities.

Is it appropriate to expect health care professionals to engage in arenas (e.g., health care policy making) for which they are not trained? Without becoming policy makers themselves, health professionals have made major contributions to health care policy debates by speaking out in diverse forums, contributing their time to support other activities of groups advocating for policies to reduce health care disparities, and/or providing financial support for such groups (see Chap. 41).

At some time nearly every health care provider has experienced the frustration of providing an effective treatment for a patient's health problem, only to send the patient back to the same circumstances in the physical or social environment that caused or triggered the illness. An example is treating an asthma attack and then discharging the patient to the same substandard housing permeated with allergens. Virtually every clinician knows the frustration of prescribing regimens of medications, diet, and/or exercise to patients whose life circumstances make the successful implementation of those care plans very unlikely. For example, people who live in neighborhoods without stores that sell affordable fresh produce or in which outdoor exercise is unsafe or infeasible do not have the same opportunities to follow recommended regimens as those who live in more health-promoting neighborhoods.

However, most health care professionals probably feel that fulfilling their own personal professional expectations as providers of high-quality health care, informed by the latest evidence, is difficult enough without adding expectations that they change their patients' life circumstances as well. In addition, most probably feel ill-equipped to change circumstances outside of the realm of health care, in which they are trained and experienced. However, there are many realistic ways in which physicians and other health care providers can contribute to reducing disparities in health, beyond their influence on reducing disparities in health care. Providers can become involved in local community initiatives to improve living conditions for vulnerable groups; for example, efforts to bring farmers' markets, community gardens, and other sources of affordable fresh produce into poor neighborhoods; initiatives to improve the quality of public education, create recreational opportunities for children in public schools, or increase public pressure toward ridding neighborhoods of crime. With a modest investment of time, providers can lend support at crucial moments, such as by speaking at a hearing before the local city commission to highlight the likely health benefits of such initiatives. A health care professional's endorsement can play an important role, inspiring community members to persevere in a difficult effort and lending credibility to the effort.

CONCLUSION

Patients like Ms. Gripman, Mr. Van, and Mr. Jones need excellent health professionals who understand the needs and circumstances of vulnerable populations and can deliver high-quality care to vulnerable patients. A public health perspective compels health professionals to not only heal the wounds of vulnerability, but also eradicate the primary causes of those wounds. Health professionals do not need to become policy makers, or abandon health care delivery, to make significant contributions to efforts to alter the fundamental conditions breeding vulnerability and producing health disparities.

KEY CONCEPTS

- Vulnerable populations are those with a disadvantaged position in social hierarchies defined by wealth, power, and/or prestige, placing them at risk for poor health.
- Health disparities are systematic differences in health status that are associated with social vulnerability and are at least theoretically amenable to social intervention.
- Several different pathways mediate the association between social vulnerability and health disparities, including genetic endowment, physical environment, social environment, behavior and lifestyle, chronic stress, and health care.
- The ethical principle of distributive justice and international human rights principles provide a universally recognized frame of reference for initiatives to reduce health disparities.
- In addition to acting to reduce health disparities through their role in delivering high-quality health care to vulnerable populations, health professionals also can make meaningful contributions to improving the fundamental social conditions that create vulnerability and produce health disparities.

ACKNOWLEDGMENT

The authors acknowledge the contributions of Sofia Gruskin, JD, MIA, of the Francois Xavier Bagnoud Center for Human Rights, Harvard University School of Public Health to the development of many of the concepts presented in this chapter.

DISCUSSION QUESTIONS

1. Review the data on health disparities shown in Table 1-1.
   a. What are some of the reasons that African Americans as a group have such poor health status relative to whites? Consider the different pathways mediating vulnerability and health status (e.g., social environment, physical environment) in suggesting the various mechanisms possibly mediating the association between African American race/ethnicity and poor health.
   b. The infant mortality rates for Latinos and non-Latino whites are nearly identical, despite Latinos as a group having much lower incomes and educational status than whites. What might be the factors that confer a "protective effect" for Latino birth outcomes and infant health in the face of socioeconomic disadvantage?
2. Many public health advocates call for the complete elimination of health disparities in the United States. Is this goal reasonable and feasible, or will societies always have inequities in health because of differences in income, education, occupation, and related aspects of SES among different members of a society?
3. Try to locate some data on public health measures in your own county, city, or community. (Your local or state health department may be a source of information comparing neighborhoods or social groups on health indicators such as infant mortality rates, age-adjusted mortality rates, cancer deaths, and preventable hospitalizations.) Use these data to identify a vulnerable social group (e.g., homeless persons, minorities) or a vulnerable neighborhood that appears to experience a health disparity. What are the most important factors in your local community contributing to this health disparity? Develop an action plan for how you and your colleagues could address these factors and improve the health of the identified vulnerable population. Make sure to consider interventions outside of the formal health care system in developing your action plan.

RESOURCES

http://www.cdc.gov/omh/AboutUs/disparities.htm
  Centers for Disease Control. Healthy People 2010: Goal of Eliminating Racial and Ethnic Health Disparities.

http://www.kaiseredu.org/topics_reflib.asp?id=329&parentid=67&rID=1
  Kaiser Family Foundation. Race, Ethnicity and Health Care: The Basics.

http://www.macses.ucsf.edu/
  MacArthur Foundation Research Network on Socioeconomic Status and Health.

http://www.sph.umich.edu/miih/index2.html
  The Michigan Initiative on Inequalities in Health.

http://www.ucsf.edu/csdh/
  The UCSF Center on Social Disparities in Health.

REFERENCES

1. U.S. Department of Health and Human Services, Health Resources and Services Administration, Maternal and Child Health Bureau. *Child Health USA 2003*. Rockville, MD: U.S. Department of Health and Human Services, 2003. Accessed August 21, 2005. Available at: http://www.mchb.hrsa.gov/chusa03/

2. Torsheim T, et al. Material deprivation and self-rated health: A multilevel study of adolescents from 22 European and North American countries. *Soc Sci Med* 2004:1.

3. Starfield B. Improving equity in health: a research agenda. *Int J Health Serv* 2001;31:545.

4. Braveman P, Gruskin S. Defining equity in health. *J Epidemiol Commun Health* 2003;57:254.

5. Braveman P, Egerter S, Cubbin C, et al. An approach to studying social disparities in maternal and infant health and health care. *Am J Public Health* 2004;94:2139.

6. National Institutes of Health. *NIH Health Disparities Strategic Plan, fiscal years 2004–2008*, vol 1. Bethesda, MD: National Institutes of Health, 2006.

7. Fiscella K, Williams D. Health disparities based on socioeconomic disparities: Implications for urban health care. *Am J Acad Med* 2004:1139.

8. Pamuk E, et al. *Socioeconomic status and health chartbook: Health United States.* Hyattsville, MD: National Center for Health Statistics.1998. Accessed August 21, 2005. Available at: http://www.cdc.gov/nchs/data/hus/hus98ncb.pdf

9. Williams DR, Jackson PB. Social sources of racial disparities in health. *Health Affairs* 2005;24:325.

10. Burchard E, et al. The importance of race and ethnic background in biomedical research and clinical practice. *N Engl J Med* 2003;348:1170.

11. Freeman H. Commentary on the meaning of race in science and society. *Cancer Epidemiol Biomarkers Prev* 2003; 12:232s.

12. Palaniappan L, Wang Y, Fortmann S. Coronary heart disease mortality for six ethnic groups in California, 1990–2000. *Ann Epidemiol* 2004;14:499.

13. Marmot M, Rose G, Shipley M, et al. Employment grade and coronary heart disease in British civil servants. *J Epidemiol Commun Health* 1978;32:244.

14. Lin CC, Rogot E, Johnson NJ, et al. A further study of life expectancy by socioeconomic factors in the National Longitudinal Mortality Study. *Ethn Dis* 2003;13:240.

15. Wolfson M, et al. Relation between income inequality and mortality: Empirical demonstration. *BMJ* 1999;319:953.

16. Isaacs S, Schroeder S: Class: The ignored determinant of the nation's health. *N Engl J Med* 2004;351:1137.

17. McGinnis J, Foege W. Actual causes of death in the United States. *JAMA* 1993;270:2207.

18. Kaplan G. What is the role of the social environment in understanding inequalities in health? *Ann NY Acad Sci* 1999;896:116.

19. Hertzman C. Population health and human development. In: Keating DP, Hertzman C, eds. *Developmental health and the wealth of nations: Social, biological, and educational dynamics.* New York: Guildford Press, 1999:21.

20. Brunner E, Marmot M. Social organization, stress and health. In: Marmot M, Wilkinson RG, eds. *Social determinants of health.* Oxford, UK: Oxford University Press, 1999:17.

21. House JS, Williams DR. Understanding and reducing socioeconomic and racial/ethnic disparities in health. In:

Smedley BD, Syme L, eds. *Promoting health: Intervention strategies from social and behavioral research.* Washington, DC: National Academics Press, 2001:81.

22. Krieger N. Embodying inequality: A review of concepts, measures, and methods for studying health consequences of discrimination. *Int J Health Serv* 1999;29:295.

23. Williams DR. Race and health: Basic questions, emerging directions. *Ann Epidemiol* 1997;7:322.

24. Kawachi I, Berkman L. Social cohesion, social capital, and health. In: Berkman LF, Kawachi I, eds. *Social epidemiology.* New York: Oxford University Press, 2000:174.

25. Cohen D A, et al. Neighborhood physical conditions and health. *Am J Public Health* 2003;93:467.

26. Krebs-Smith S, et al. U.S. adults' fruit and vegetable intakes, 1989 to 1991: A revised baseline for the Healthy People 2000 objective. *Am J Public Health* 1995;85:1623.

27. McEwen B. Protective and damaging effects of stress mediators. *N Engl J Med* 1998;338:171.

28. Seeman T, et al. Racial/ethnic and socioeconomic disparities in health: How socioeconomic status gets "under the skin." National Press Club, Washington, DC, 2004. Accessed February 10, 2004. Available at: http://www.macses.ucsf.edu/News/Teresa%20Seeman-transcript.pdf

29. Seeman T, McEwen B, Rowe J, et al. Allostatic load as a marker of cumulative biological risk: McArthur studies of successful aging. *PNAS* 2001;98:4770.

30. Karlamangla A, et al. Allostatic load as a predictor of functional decline: MacArthur Studies of Successful Aging. *J Clin Epidemiol* 2002;55(7):696.

31. Greiner BA, Krause N, Ragland D, et al. Occupational stressors and hypertension: A multi-method study using observer-based job analysis and self-reports in urban transit operators. *Soc Sci Med* 2004;59:1081.

32. Singh G, Miller B. Health, life expectancy, and mortality patterns among immigrant populations in the United States. *Can J Pub Health* 2004;95:114.

33. Thomas D, Karagas M. Migrant studies. In: Schottenfeld D, Fraumeni JF, eds. *Cancer epidemiology and prevention,* 2nd ed. New York: Oxford University Press, 1996:236.

34. Eschbach K, et al. Neighborhood context and mortality among older Mexican Americans: Is there a barrio advantage? *Am J Pub Health* 2004;94:1807.

35. Peter F, Evans T: Ethical dimensions of health equity. In: Evans T, Whitehead M, Diderichsen F, et al, eds. *Challenging inequalities in health: From ethics to action.* New York: Oxford University Press, 2001:24.

36. Rawls J. Justice as fairness. *Philos Pub Affairs* 1985;14:223.

37. World Health Organization Constitution of the World Health Organization; as adopted by the International Health Conference. June 19–22, 1946. Accessed August 21, 2005. Available at: http://www.ldb.org/iphw/whoconst.htm

38. Jones C. Levels of racism: A theoretic framework and a gardener's tale. *Am J Public Health* 2000;90(8):1212.

Chapter 2

Health Care Disparities: An Overview

Andrew B. Bindman, MD, Kevin Grumbach, MD, and Talmadge E. King Jr., MD

Objectives

- Define the term health care disparities.
- Describe the patient and provider factors that influence access to and the use of health care services.
- Review the characteristics of patients who are at increased risk for health care disparities.
- Identify actions health professionals can take to eliminate health care disparities.

The previous chapter defined *health disparities* as systematic, yet potentially modifiable, differences in health between more and less privileged social groups. This chapter focuses more narrowly on health *care* disparities. After defining this term, the factors that contribute to health care disparities, the patients affected by these inequities in access to and quality of care, and strategies to eliminate health care disparities are discussed.

QUALITY OF CARE AND HEALTH CARE DISPARITIES

The Institute of Medicine has defined quality as "... the degree to which health services for individuals and populations increase the likelihood of desired health outcomes and are consistent with current professional knowledge."[1] Quality can be impaired in different ways, such as overuse, underuse, and misuse. There are major deficiencies on all of these accounts in the quality of care provided by the US health care system. For example, there are major deficiencies in the quality of care provided to patients with common chronic diseases: two-thirds of patients with high blood pressure are inadequately treated; the majority of diabetics have glycohemoglobin (A1C) levels >7% and half have total serum cholesterol levels ≥200 mg/dL; half of patients hospitalized with congestive heart failure are readmitted within 90 days of discharge.

Furthermore, many studies have shown that, compared to whites, racial and ethnic minority patients experience even greater deficits in the quality, intensity, and comprehensiveness of diagnostic procedures and treatment choices afforded to them. These disparities in health care among populations persist in most instances even after controlling for health insurance, sex, age, income, education, severity of disease, and comorbidity. These health care disparities reflect systematic differences in access to or quality of care between more and less privileged groups that cannot be explained by the differences in the need for care or preference for care among the individuals in these groups (Fig. 2-1).

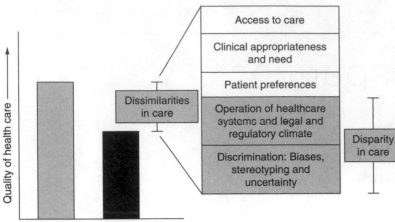

Figure 2-1. Model of health care disparities. The Gomes and McGuire model views health care disparities as resulting from characteristics of the health care system, the society's legal and regulatory climate, discrimination, bias, stereotyping, and uncertainty. Not all dissimilarities in care are considered a disparity in care. (Adapted from: Gomes C, McGuire T. Identifying the sources of racial and ethnic disparities in health care use. Boston: Department of Health Care Policy, Harvard Medical School, 2001. Cited in: Smedley BA, Stith A, Nelson A, eds. *Unequal treatment: Confronting racial and ethnic disparities in health care.* Washington, DC: National Academy Press; LaVeist TA, Isaac L. Examples of racial disparities in health care. Baltimore, 2005. Available online at: http://www.rwjf.org/files/newsroom/interactives/ExofRacialDisparitiesRWJF.ppt#261,2,Overview)

MEASURES OF QUALITY: PROCESSES OR OUTCOMES OF CARE

William Mason and Peter Dixon are admitted to the same hospital on the same day with the same diagnosis: non-ST wave elevation myocardial infarction. Mr. Mason, a white business executive, is promptly rushed to the cardiac catheterization suite where he receives coronary angioplasty and stenting. He is discharged home on aspirin, clopidogrel, a statin, a beta-blocker, and an angiotensin converting enzyme inhibitor. Three months later, he is able to garden without experiencing angina. Mr. Dixon, an African American who is an intermittently employed construction worker, is admitted to the coronary care unit but does not receive a coronary arteriogram during his hospital stay. He is discharged home on a statin and calcium channel blocker. Two weeks later, he is readmitted with unstable angina.

Applying a quality of care framework developed by Donnabedian, health care disparities can be observed to occur in the *processes* or *outcomes* of care.[2] Processes of care are the actions health care providers take to diagnose, treat, and manage patients' health care needs. Health outcomes, such as morbidity and mortality, are, in part, consequences of these health care actions. Mr. Mason had a process of care that was more consistent with evidence-based guidelines than the care received by Mr. Dixon. The inferior process of care received by Mr. Dixon contributed to him having a worse clinical outcome (recurrence of symptomatic coronary heart disease) than Mr. Mason. Of particular concern are the types of health care disparities illustrated in this case that contribute to differences in health outcomes (health disparities).

Most investigators agree that health care processes have a relatively modest role in explaining health disparities—perhaps explaining only 10% to 15% of the variation in health outcomes among different groups.[3] On the other hand, health disparities resulting from health care disparities clearly are in the purview of the people working in the health care system and are amenable to change. Health professionals have a particular obligation to eliminate disparities in access to and quality of care that contribute to inferior health outcomes for vulnerable populations.

BEHAVIORAL MODEL APPLIED TO HEALTH CARE DISPARITIES

Why is a patient like Mr. Dixon less likely than a patient like Mr. Mason to receive high-quality care? One of the most frequently used models for conceptualizing access to care is the behavioral model developed to explain differences in care received by different people or groups of people.[4] The behavioral model proposes analyzing the care people receive by looking at three fundamental categories of factors: *need, predisposing characteristics,* and *enabling resources.* Gelberg and colleagues have revised the model based on their work with homeless populations, proposing a behavioral model for vulnerable populations that includes both traditional categories and vulnerable domains (Table 2-1).[5]

Need for Care

It is axiomatic that people with a greater need for health care, all other things being equal, make greater use of health care services. For example, a patient with diabetes has a greater than average need for health

Table 2-1. The Behavioral Model Applied to Vulnerable Populations

Need	
Traditional Domains	**Vulnerable Domains**
Perceived health	Perceived health
General population health conditions	Vulnerable population health conditions
Evaluated health	Evaluated health
General population health conditions	Vulnerable population health conditions

Predisposing Characteristics	
Traditional Domains	**Vulnerable Domains**
Demographics	Social structure
Age	Country of birth
Gender	Acculturation/immigration/literacy
Marital status	Sexual orientation
Veteran status	Childhood characteristics
Health beliefs	Residential history/homelessness
Values concerning health and illness	Living conditions
Attitudes toward health services	Mobility
Knowledge about disease	Length of time in the community
Social structure	Criminal behavior/prison history
Ethnicity	Victimization
Education	Mental illness
Employment	Psychological resources
Social networks	Substance abuse
Occupation	
Family size	
Religion	

Enabling Resources	
Traditional Domains	**Vulnerable Domains**
Personal/family resources	Personal/family resources
Regular source of care	Competing needs
Insurance	Hunger
Income	Public benefits
Social support	Self-help skills
Perceived barriers to care	Ability to negotiate system
Community resources	Case manager/conservator
Residence	Transportation
Region	Telephone
Health services resources	Information sources
	Community resources
	Crime rates
	Social services resources

Source: Gelberg L, Andersen RM, Leake BD. The Behavioral Model for Vulnerable Populations: Application to medical care use and outcomes for homeless people. Health Serv Res 2000;34(6):1273–1302.

care. How much need depends on the severity of the diabetes, and whether there are complications or other chronic conditions. Having diabetes per se does not necessarily constitute a disparities-related vulnerability (although it is certainly a risk factor for adverse health outcomes such as heart disease and kidney failure). On the other hand, some clinical conditions may in and of themselves confer a social vulnerability. Prime examples are the socially stigmatizing conditions of mental illness and substance use.

In the preceding case, might there have been some difference between Mr. Dixon's and Mr. Mason's clinical presentation that made it appear that Mr. Dixon had less clinical need for urgent coronary stenting?

Predisposing Characteristics

Predisposing characteristics refer to health beliefs and culture, care-seeking behaviors, trust in health care and other social institutions, and related characteristics that may influence whether, when, and from whom an individual decides to obtain health care when needed. Health education may assist individuals to make well-informed decisions about using health care services.

Patients from vulnerable groups such as ethnic minorities may understandably be less trusting of the health care system. In addition, medical institutions often lack trustworthiness, in part, because they make no attempt to gain the trust of vulnerable groups. Consequently, it is understandable that individuals from these groups may be less willing to seek medical care or adhere to recommended treatment. One glaring example of the lack of trustworthiness of the health care system is the Tuskegee Syphilis Experiment.[6] Between 1932 and 1972, the US Public Health Service conducted an unethical study at the Tuskegee Institute in Alabama in which African-American patients with syphilis were left untreated in order to observe the "natural" progression of syphilis—despite the discovery in the 1940s of penicillin as a highly effective treatment for this infection. African Americans cite the Tuskegee experiment as one reason for concern that medical research may exploit rather than aid them.[7] Personal experience of racism contributes even more significantly to mistrust of medical care.[8]

The human resources deployed in the health care system also may contribute to minority patients' mistrust of the health care system and predisposition against using health care services. African Americans, Latinos, and Native Americans are underrepresented within the physician workforce. African Americans, Latinos, and American Indians comprised 23% of the nation's adult population in 2000, but only 9% of the physicians, 12% of the registered nurses, and 4% of the dentists in the United States.[9] African-American patients cared for by African-American physicians report that their physicians include them more in medical decision making and that they are more satisfied with their care than those who are cared for by non–African-American physicians.[10] Similarly, Spanish-speaking patients are more satisfied with the care they receive from Spanish-speaking physicians.[11]

Is it possible that both Mr. Mason and Mr. Dixon were offered urgent cardiac catheterization by their physicians, but Mr. Dixon might have declined to have the procedure performed because of less trust in his physicians and nurses?

Enabling Resources

Enabling resources are factors that promote access to effective health care. These resources may be at the community or personal level. *Community-level* enabling resources are the assets of the local health care system and other social services. The presence of a community clinic that provides financial assistance for low-income patients or has interpreters on site are enabling resources that contribute to improving access to care, particularly in low-income and minority communities where private physicians are less likely to practice.[12] The

access to care barriers associated with the scarcity of physicians in certain communities can be compounded by the lack of another community "enabler," reliable transportation.

Among the most obvious and fundamental resources that make care easier for a person to access are *financial resources*: health insurance and the financial means to pay for those health care costs not covered by insurance. Individuals from racial and ethnic minority groups are more likely than whites to be uninsured, a situation that contributes to racial and ethnic disparities in health care. In 2004, 37% of Latinos, 20% of African Americans, 17% of Asians, and 11% of non-Latino whites were uninsured.[13] Differences in average income between racial and ethnic groups explain much, but not all, of the differences in rates of health insurance by race and ethnicity.

Lack of health insurance is the single greatest impediment to access to care in the United States and results in unnecessary morbidity for affected individuals and inefficient use of health care resources.[14] Numerous studies have demonstrated that the uninsured are less likely than those with health insurance to have a regular source of health care, have fewer physician visits, are less likely to receive appropriate preventive services, and are more likely to delay receiving needed medical care. The uninsured are 30% to 50% more likely than privately insured persons to have some deterioration in their health resulting from a chronic condition such as diabetes or asthma that ultimately necessitates a hospitalization that could have been prevented with timely ambulatory care.[15]

Other research has demonstrated that the uninsured present for care with more advanced stages of cancer, including breast, colorectal, prostate, and skin cancers. Delay in diagnosis is one of the reasons that the uninsured have shorter life expectancies than insured persons. The Institute of Medicine estimates that the age-specific mortality rate is 25% higher in the uninsured than the privately insured population.[16]

Not surprisingly, socioeconomic class is a strong predictor of health insurance status. Although 80% of the uninsured live in families with a working adult, the majority of uninsured persons have family incomes falling at the lower end of the income scale. As a result, these individuals have few personal financial resources to allow them to overcome barriers to care associated with the lack of health insurance. In many cases, health insurance coverage is only available to low-income persons on an emergency basis through Medicaid when these individuals become so ill that they require hospitalization. Patients with a chronic disease who only have episodic health insurance coverage for hospitalizations are less likely than those with continuous coverage to receive appropriate treatment in the ambulatory setting that could prevent the pain and suffering associated with complications of their illness.[17]

Might it have been the case that Mr. Dixon was uninsured, and that is why his physicians did not provide the same resource-intensive care received by Mr. Mason?

HEALTH CARE DISPARITIES: THE EVIDENCE

As discussed in Chapter 1, race/ethnicity and socioeconomic status are powerful predictors of a person's health status. These same factors are also strongly associated with access to health care and quality of care. There is ample evidence indicating that the differences in care received by Mr. Mason, a high-income white man, and Mr. Dixon, a working-class African-American man, are indicative of pervasive differences in processes of care in the United States based on race/ethnicity and class.

RACE/ETHNICITY

Individuals from minority groups are less likely than whites to have a regular source of care or to have had a doctor visit in the past year. Minorities are also more likely to report delays in receiving needed care. Summarizing a series of national access to care indicators, the Agency for Health Research and Quality determined that access to care is generally better for non-Latino whites than for members of all other racial and ethnic groups in the United States. The Agency found that, compared with whites, Latinos had worse access to care on 90%, Native Americans on 50%, African Americans on 40%, and Asians on 30% of the measures.[18]

The National Healthcare Disparities Report applied quality indicators for preventive, prenatal, neonatal, cancer, and cardiac care, as well as care for chronic conditions such as diabetes, asthma, and HIV/AIDS—measures that extend beyond more general indicators of access to care (e.g., ability to obtain medical care when needed) to assess whether patients received specific services appropriate to their medical needs (Fig. 2-2). Results indicate that African Americans received poorer quality of care than whites for about two-thirds of the measures. Latinos, Native Americans, and Asians also were less likely than non-Latino whites to receive a high quality of care. The reasons for these differences remain ill-defined but it has recently been shown that the US health care system's organization contributes to discriminatory care. For example, minority patients commonly receive care concentrated within a relatively small group of physicians who report that they do not have access to the full range of clinical resources needed to provide quality care.[19]

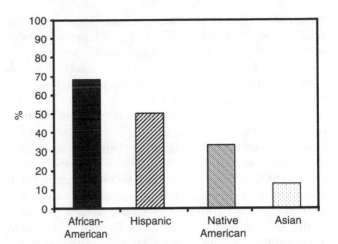

Figure 2-2. Racial and ethnic groups experienced poorer quality of care compared with whites. To quantify disparities systematically, a subset of 38 measures of effectiveness of health care were assessed and the percent of measures for which members of selected racial groups experience poorer quality of care were compared with whites (Hispanic and non-Hispanic) in 2001. Poorer quality of care indicated that for a particular measure, the group did not receive as high a quality care as whites and that the relative difference was at least 10% and statistically significant ($p < 0.05$). Compared with whites, African Americans received poorer quality of care for about 66% of quality measures; American Indians and Alaska Natives about 33%; Asians about 10%; and Hispanics (comparison group is non-Hispanic white) about 50%. (Modified from: Agency for Healthcare Research and Quality. 2004 National Healthcare Disparities Report. Accessed September 3, 2005. Available online at: http://www.qualitytools.ahrq.gov/disparitiesreport)

HEALTH INSURANCE

Do these differences in health care according to race/ethnicity simply reflect the fact that minorities are less likely than whites to have private health insurance? Indeed, differences in access to care are attributable to differences in their health insurance status; however, these differences persist even among individuals with the same type of insurance coverage. For example, within Medicare, a public health insurance program for the elderly that is designed to provide a uniform benefit to its beneficiaries, minorities (most particularly individuals who are African American) are less likely to have a regular source of care and make visits to the physician.[20] Thus, the evidence suggests that patients like Mr. Mason and Mr. Dixon often receive unequal care even when they have the same type of health insurance.

SOCIOECONOMIC STATUS

Although less research has examined health care disparities associated with an individual's socioeconomic status, the limited findings are consistent with the notion that those with less social privilege experience worse quality of care. Findings from the National Healthcare Disparities Report indicate that individuals who are poor (<100% of the federal poverty level, i.e., yearly income <$18,850 for a family of four) receive lower quality of care on approximately 60% of the indicators than those with higher incomes (≥400% of the federal poverty level). This report did not assess the degree to which differences in health insurance coverage might have explained these socioeconomic differences in the receipt of high-quality health care. However, a small number of separate studies, primarily in the area of cardiac care, have explored this issue in greater detail. In one study of Medicare patients hospitalized for an acute myocardial infarction, higher income was associated with a higher rate of evidence-based treatment and lower 1-month and 1-year mortality rates.[21] In this study, African-American race, as well as insurance status, did not fully account for the association between income and the processes or outcomes of care. A similar result was found in a Canadian study of patients hospitalized for acute myocardial infarction. Higher income was associated with greater use of specialized cardiac services and lower 1-year mortality rates despite the fact that all of the patients were covered under the same universal health insurance program.[22]

NEED AND PREDISPOSING FACTORS

If differences in health care according to race/ethnicity and socioeconomic status are not entirely attributable to differences in a dominant "enabling" factor such as health insurance, could non–health care system factors explain these differences? For example, perhaps there are differences in health care needs, such as disease severity, or predisposing factors, such as patient beliefs and preferences, that might account for the differences found in the National Healthcare Disparities Report. Rather than representing health care disparities, might these observed differences in the use of health care simply represent a health care system responding reasonably to patients with differing needs and interests?

Many of the findings on health care differences that appear in The National Healthcare Disparities Report and similar analyses are based on data obtained from patient surveys and administrative records (e.g., billing records) that lack clinical detail about patients' clinical needs and preferences for care. Some studies have found that the magnitude of the differences in patterns of care is diminished sometimes after more thoroughly accounting for differences in the need and preferences for care across patient groups. However, in most cases, the differences in care patterns persist. For example,

studies in emergency departments have demonstrated that African Americans and Latinos are less likely than whites to receive opiates for pain management of broken limbs.[23–26] Although these studies did not specifically investigate patient preferences, the findings suggest that physicians' assessments of patients' need for care are influenced by more than physiologic information and may be influenced, consciously or subconsciously, by race or ethnicity. Some studies of patients with acute coronary syndromes, similar to the coronary events experienced by Mr. Mason and Mr. Dixon, have examined detailed information on coronary anatomy and failed to find clinical differences in underlying disease status that would explain the difference in rates of revascularization for African-American and white patients.[27–29]

Other studies have compared rates of refusal of recommended major procedures between white and minority patients and found relatively small differences in refusal rates that do not explain the observed differences in the use of these health care services across racial and ethnic groups.[28,30] Thus, research suggests that differences in rates of patient refusal of invasive procedures rarely explain why patients like Mr. Dixon tend to be less likely than patients like Mr. Mason to undergo coronary revascularization.

A final consideration is whether some disparities represent inappropriately *excessive* care for privileged patients rather than inappropriately *low* use among vulnerable populations. Several studies have investigated this question for patients with coronary heart disease. Investigators demonstrated that white patients were more likely than African-American patients with the same severity of illness to receive coronary artery bypass surgery.[31] Comparing the results of white and African-American Medicare patients who received coronary artery bypass surgery against well-established clinical criteria has revealed that some white patients were more likely than African-American patients to be inappropriately "overtreated" using surgery.[32] However, the degree of undertreatment among African-American patients was substantially greater than the amount of overtreatment among white patients. Furthermore, one study has shown that African-American patients with cardiovascular disease had a higher mortality than white patients because the African-American patients received lower use of appropriate surgical treatments.[29] Even for low-cost cardiovascular treatments such as prescribing of aspirin, African Americans are less likely to receive appropriate therapy than white patients for all levels of coronary heart disease risk.[33]

After conducting an extensive literature review of studies comparing the use of health care services across racial and ethnic groups, and across a wide spectrum of clinical conditions, the authors of the Institute of Medicine report *Unequal Treatment,* concluded that they were "struck by the consistency of the research findings: even among better controlled studies, the vast majority indicated that minorities are less likely than whites to receive needed services, including clinically necessary procedures."[34,35] The report also concluded that most of the differences in care could not be explained by differences in patient preferences or the need for care. They concluded that discrimination and health system characteristics (e.g., lack of interpreters or fragmentation in care) are the main basis for the differences in care that minorities receive.

BIAS, STEREOTYPING, AND RACISM

It is difficult for research to directly and objectively measure the attitudes and motivations underlying the behavior of clinicians. Thus, determining whether health care disparities can be attributed to bias, stereotyping, or racism tends to be a "diagnosis of exclusion." However, the Institute of Medicine's *Unequal Treatment* report raises serious concern that health care disparities may result from bias, stereotyping, or even racism among people working in the health care system, especially given that the lower-quality health care received by racial and ethnic disparities cannot be explained by differences in the need for care, or patient preferences. This sort of bias and stereotyping are presumed to be subconscious.

ADDRESSING HEALTH CARE DISPARITIES

The Institute of Medicine has proposed a broad set of recommendations at the policy, health system, provider, and patient levels that can contribute to eliminating health care disparities (see Core Competency).[35] These recommendations include strategies such as increasing the diversity of the health care workforce, structuring payment systems so that they support equitable distribution of health care resources, and increasing patient education programs that can empower patients, particularly those from vulnerable groups, to take a greater role in their own medical decision making. This book explores many of the actions that can be taken by health policy decision makers, health professionals, educators, and researchers to eliminate disparities in health care. It is clear that improvement has and can be accomplished. This section summarizes some of the key approaches that health professionals can adopt to reduce health care disparities.

RECOGNIZE HEALTH CARE DISPARITIES AS A PROBLEM

Although many health care professional organizations have endorsed a position that all patients, regardless of race, ethnic origin, nationality, primary language, or religion, deserve high-quality health care,[36] considerable evidence documents that many inequities exist in actual practice. One recent study found that physicians, medical students, and members of the public have very different views about health care disparities, with physicians being the least likely to agree that there is unfairness in the health care system based on a patient's race or class.[37] Thus, one of the first steps in eliminating health care disparities is to inform health professionals of the problem so that effective interventions can be established to reduce the inequities.

UNIVERSAL HEALTH INSURANCE

Despite dozens of attempts in the United States in the past century to pass legislation establishing a universal, national health insurance program, the United States remains the only developed nation without universal coverage.[38] Extensive research documents the critical role of health insurance for gaining access to high-quality care. The Institute of Medicine estimates that a lack of health insurance accounts for 18,000 deaths annually in the United States.[16] Minorities and low-income individuals are particularly likely to be uninsured, compounding the health care vulnerability of these groups. Consequently, participating in advocacy efforts for health care financing reform is one way to address disparities. A more short-term strategy is for health professionals to educate themselves about the current array of public and private insurance programs in the United States, in order to more effectively assist individual patients to navigate the health care financing bureaucracy and successfully obtain the coverage they may be entitled to receive (see Chap. 4).

ACCESS AND DELIVERY OF HEALTH SERVICES

Although obtaining health insurance is a necessary step toward the elimination of health care disparities, it is not sufficient. Even when insured, vulnerable populations still face deficiencies in the enabling resources that would permit them to receive equitable delivery of health services. Some of these deficiencies may be related to inequalities in the distribution and availability of facilities and technology, such as the preferential location of specialty hospital units in higher-income urban neighborhoods rather than in inner-city and rural communities.

The quality of health care providers available to different groups of patients may vary as well. One analysis of racial differences in Medicare patients' outcomes after coronary artery bypass graft surgery found that the increased mortality among African-American patients compared with whites disappeared after controlling for the quality of the hospital care where patients were obtaining their procedures.[39] Health care organizations should reach out to surrounding community members and involve community representatives in planning and quality improvement initiatives.[36]

PROVIDERS IN UNDERSERVED AREAS

One of the most important of the non–insurance-related enabling resources are the human resources of the health care system: the physicians, nurses, pharmacists, dentists, physician assistants, and many other essential health care workers. Health care disparities related to human resource enabling factors may result from geographic maldistribution, at least in part. Research has shown that communities in California with a relatively high proportion of minority residents have a much lower supply of physicians, dentists, nurse practitioners, and physician assistants than neighborhoods that have fewer minority residents.[12,40,41] This research also has shown that African-American and Latino health professionals are much more likely than their white counterparts to work in underserved communities with fewer health care resources. Similarly, health professionals who grew up in rural communities are more likely to ultimately practice in rural communities than those who grew up in urban areas. Thus, one strategy for addressing health care disparities related to maldistribution of human resources is to recruit more underrepresented minorities and students from rural backgrounds into the health professions.

CLEAR COMMUNICATION AND CULTURALLY COMPETENT CARE

Providers' assessments of patients' need for care have a subjective component and patients' preferences for care are somewhat dependent on the information patients receive from providers. Thus, one strategy is to improve health professionals' cultural competence so that they can more effectively evaluate and communicate with diverse patient populations. This might be accomplished by increasing the racial, ethnic, and socioeconomic diversity of health professionals and incorporating within health professions training programs curricula on the interpersonal and communications skills necessary for effectively caring for vulnerable populations.

GUIDELINES OR STANDARDS IN THE PROCESS OF CARE

Implementation of evidence-based clinical guidelines that establish an explicit standard of care that is applied to all patients with the same clinical status or

health care need appears to be a way to reduce disparities. A study of end-stage renal disease patients found that disparities by race in the adequacy of dialysis treatment diminished after the adoption of an evidence-based treatment guideline.[42] This study suggests that guidelines, along with monitoring and feedback of clinical performance benchmarked to an evidence-based guideline, may reduce the degree of subjective judgment and potential bias in clinicians' clinical decision making, thereby helping to mitigate health care disparities. A related and promising approach is for health care delivery organizations and payers of care to define explicit guidelines or standards in the process of care for certain conditions, and to monitor processes of care for different patient populations with these conditions based on race/ethnicity, socioeconomic status, or other characteristics to ensure that all groups are achieving an equivalently high standard of quality.

CONCLUSION

The evidence for the existence of health care disparities is overwhelming. Disparities exist in access to care and in the quality of care that is delivered once patients access the health care system. Recognizing health care disparities as a problem is an important first step, but recognition alone will not bring about positive change. Recent studies on the trends in health care disparities over time indicate inadequate progress nationwide in reducing disparities in the management of acute myocardial infarctions or in the use of major procedures within the Medicare program.[43,44] Still there have been some reports of improvement in Medicare and Medicaid managed care,[45,46] and the emergence of some successful strategies.

KEY CONCEPTS

- Health care disparities reflect systematic differences in access to or quality of care between more and less privileged groups that cannot be explained by the differences in the need for care or preference for care among the individuals in these groups.
- Minorities and low-income individuals suffer health care disparities in part because they have less access to high-quality care.
- Even among those patients who have accessed care and whose needs have become visible to the health care system, there are systematic differences in the receipt of services by groups of patients who vary by characteristics of social privilege.

- Provider bias, stereotyping, and perhaps even racism may contribute to health care disparities.
- Recognizing health care disparities as a problem is an important first step, but providers need to participate in a broad range of changes at the policy, system, and provider level in order to eliminate them.

CORE COMPETENCY

Institute of Medicine Recommendations for Addressing Health Care Disparities General Recommendations

- Increase awareness of racial and ethnic disparities in health care among the general public and key stakeholders.
- Increase health care providers' awareness of disparities.

Legal, Regulatory, and Policy Interventions

- Avoid fragmentation of health plans along socioeconomic lines.
- Strengthen the stability of patient–provider relationships in publicly funded health plans.
- Increase the proportion of underrepresented US racial and ethnic minorities among health professionals.
- Apply the same managed care protections to publicly funded HMO enrollees that apply to private HMO enrollees.
- Provide greater resources to the US Department of Health and Human Services Office for Civil Rights to enforce civil rights laws.

Health Systems Interventions

- Promote the consistency and equity of care through the use of evidence-based guidelines.
- Structure payment systems to ensure an adequate supply of services to minority patients, and limit provider incentives that may promote disparities.
- Enhance patient-provider communication and trust by providing financial incentives for practices that reduce barriers and encourage evidence-based practice.
- Support the use of interpretation services where community needs exist.
- Support the use of community health workers.
- Use multidisciplinary treatment and preventive care teams.

Patient Education and Empowerment

- Implement patient education programs to increase patients' knowledge of how to best access care and participate in treatment decisions.

Cross-Cultural Education in the Health Professions

- Integrate cross-cultural education into the training of all current and future health professionals.

Data Collection and Monitoring

- Collect and report data on health care access and use by patients' race, ethnicity, socioeconomic status, and (where possible) primary language.
- Include measures of racial and ethnic disparities in performance measurement.
- Monitor progress toward the elimination of health care disparities.
- Report racial and ethnic data by Office of Management and Budget categories, but use subpopulation groups where possible.

Research Needs

- Conduct further research to identify sources of racial and ethnic disparities and assess intervention strategies.
- Conduct research on ethical issues and other barriers to eliminating disparities.

Source: Institute of Medicine. Insuring America's Health. Washington, DC: National Academies Press, 2004.

DISCUSSION QUESTIONS

1. African-American women are less likely to get breast cancer than white women, yet African-American women are more likely to die from this disease. Does this represent a health care disparity? How would you determine if the problem results from access barriers or the quality of care women receive once they have been diagnosed with cancer?
2. Should you include information on a patient's race in the history and physical examination? Should you include other information on the patient's social class such as education, occupation, or income? In what ways do you think it is helpful or harmful for patient care to include this information?
3. Are there health care disparities where you practice medicine? How well does your practice setting meet the healthcare needs of everyone in your community? Which groups of patients are excluded? Within the practice do you think some patients receive suboptimal care? How might you assess your practice to determine if there are health care disparities? What policy, system, and provider level changes do you think would be most useful for eliminating health care disparities in your practice setting?

RESOURCES

http://www.ahrq.gov
Agency for Health Research and Quality.

http://www.amsa.org/hp/uhcres.cfm
American Medical Students Association.

http://nursingworld.org/readroom/rwjpaper.htm
American Nurses Association.

http://www.kff.org
Kaiser Family Foundation Commission on Medicaid and the Uninsured.

http://www.pnhp.org
Physicians for a National Health Program.

http://www.census.gov/hhes/www/hlthins/hlthins.html
U.S. Census Bureau.

REFERENCES

1. Lohr K, ed. *Medicare: A strategy for quality assurance.* Washington, DC: Institute of Medicine, National Academies Press, 1990.
2. Donabedian A. Evaluating the quality of medical care. *Milbank Mem Fund Q* 1966;44(Suppl):166–206.
3. Adler NE, Boyce WT, Chesney MA, et al. Socioeconomic inequalities in health. No easy solution. *JAMA* 1993;269: 3140–3145.
4. Andersen R, Aday LA. Access to medical care in the U.S.: Realized and potential. *Med Care* 1978;16:533–546.
5. Gelberg L, Andersen RM, Leake BD. The Behavioral Model for Vulnerable Populations: Application to medical care use and outcomes for homeless people. *Health Serv Res* 2000;34:1273–1302.
6. White RM. Unraveling the Tuskegee study of untreated syphilis. *Arch Intern Med* 2000;160(5):585–598.
7. Corbie-Smith G, Thomas S, Williams M, et al. Attitudes and beliefs of African Americans toward participation in medical research. *J Gen Intern Med* 1999;14:537–546.
8. Brandon D, Isaac L, LaVeist T. The legacy of Tuskegee and trust in medical care: Is Tuskegee responsible for race differences in mistrust of medical care? *J Natl Med Assoc* 2005;97:951–956.
9. Grumbach K, Coffman J, Rosenoff E, et al. *Strategies for improving the diversity of the health professions.* Woodland Hills, CA: The California Endowment, 2003.
10. Cooper-Patrick L, Gallo JJ, Gonzales JJ, et al. Race, gender, and partnership in the patient-physician relationship. *JAMA* 1999;282:583–589.
11. Saha S, Komaromy M, Koepsell TD, et al. Patient-physician racial concordance and the perceived quality and use of health care. *Arch Intern Med* 1999;159: 997–1004.
12. Komaromy M, Grumbach K, Drake M, et al. The role of black and Hispanic physicians in providing health care for underserved populations. *N Engl J Med* 1996;334: 1305–1310.
13. U.S. Census Bureau. Health Insurance Coverage: 2004. Accessed September 13, 2005. Available online at: http://www.census.gov/hhes/www/hlthins/hlthin04/hlth04asc.html
14. Hargraves JL, Hadley J. The contribution of insurance coverage and community resources to reducing racial/ethnic disparities in access to care. *Health Serv Res* 2003; 38:809–829.
15. Hadley J. Sicker and poorer: The consequences of being uninsured: a review of the research on the relationship between health insurance, medical care use, health, work, and income. *Med Care Res Rev* 2003;60(2 Suppl): 3S–75S; discussion 76S–112S.
16. Institute of Medicine. *Insuring America's health.* Washington, DC: National Academies Press, 2004.
17. Harman JS, Manning WG, Lurie N, et al. Association between interruptions in Medicaid coverage and use of inpatient psychiatric services. *Psychiatr Serv* 2003;54: 999–1005.
18. Agency for Healthcare Research and Quality. 2004 National Healthcare Disparities Report. 2004. Accessed September 3, 2005. Available online at: http://www.qualitytools.ahrq.gov/disparitiesreport
19. Bach PB, Pham HH, Schrag D, et al. Primary care physicians who treat blacks and whites. *N Engl J Med* 2004; 351:575–584.
20. Gornick ME, Eggers PW, Reilly TW, et al. Effects of race and income on mortality and use of services among Medicare beneficiaries. *N Engl J Med* 1996;335:791–799.
21. Rao SV, Schulman KA, Curtis LH, et al. Socioeconomic status and outcome following acute myocardial infarction in elderly patients. *Arch Intern Med* 2004;164:1128–1133.
22. Alter DA, Naylor CD, Austin P, et al. Effects of socioeconomic status on access to invasive cardiac procedures and on mortality after acute myocardial infarction. *N Engl J Med* 1999;341:1359–1367.
23. Todd KH, Deaton C, D'Adamo AP, et al. Ethnicity and analgesic practice. *Ann Emerg Med* 2000;35:11–16.
24. Todd KH, Samaroo N, Hoffman JR. Ethnicity as a risk factor for inadequate emergency department analgesia. *JAMA* 1993;269:1537–1539.
25. Kasiske BL, London W, Ellison MD. Race and socioeconomic factors influencing early placement on the kidney transplant waiting list. *J Am Soc Nephrol* 1998;9:2142–2147.
26. Young CJ, Gaston RS. Renal transplantation in black Americans. *N Engl J Med* 2000;343:1545–1552.
27. Conigliaro J, Whittle J, Good CB, et al. Understanding racial variation in the use of coronary revascularization procedures: The role of clinical factors. *Arch Intern Med* 2000;160:1329–1335.
28. Hannan EL, van Ryn M, Burke J, et al. Access to coronary artery bypass surgery by race/ethnicity and gender among patients who are appropriate for surgery. *Med Care* 1999;37:68–77.
29. Peterson ED, Shaw LK, DeLong ER, et al. Racial variation in the use of coronary-revascularization procedures. Are the differences real? Do they matter? *N Engl J Med* 1997;336:480–486.
30. Ayanian JZ, Cleary PD, Weissman JS, et al. The effect of patients' preferences on racial differences in access to renal transplantation. *N Engl J Med* 1999;341:1661–1669.
31. Ayanian JZ, Udvarhelyi IS, Gatsonis CA, et al. Racial differences in the use of revascularization procedures after coronary angiography. *JAMA* 1993;269:2642–2646.
32. Schneider EC, Leape LL, Weissman JS, et al. Racial differences in cardiac revascularization rates: Does "overuse" explain higher rates among white patients? *Ann Intern Med* 2001;135:328–337.
33. Sahar E, Folsom A, Romm F, et al. Patterns of aspirin use in middle-aged adults: The Atherosclerosis Risk in Communities (ARIC) Study. *Am Heart J* 1996;131:915–922.

34. Institute of Medicine. Unequal Treatment: What Health Care Providers Need to Know About Racial and Ethnic Disparities in Health Care. 2002. Accessed October 10, 2005. Available online at: http://www.iom.edu/Object.File/Master/4/175/0.pdf

35. Institute of Medicine. *Unequal treatment.* Washington, DC: National Academies Press, 2003.

36. American College of Physicians. *Racial and ethnic disparities in health care.* Philadelphia: American College of Physicians, 2003.

37. Wilson E, Grumbach K, Huebner J, et al. Medical student, physician and public perceptions of health care disparities. *Fam Med* 2004;36:715–721.

38. Bodenheimer T, Grumbach K. *Understanding health policy: A clinical approach.* Norwalk, CT: McGraw Hill-Lange, 2004.

39. Barnato AE, Lucas FL, Staiger D, et al. Hospital-level racial disparities in acute myocardial infarction treatment and outcomes. *Med Care* 2005;43:308–319.

40. Mertz E, Grumbach K. Identifying communities with low dentist supply in California. *J Pub Health Dent* 2001;61:172–177.

41. UCSF Center for California Health Workforce Studies and the Office of Statewide Health Planning and Development. *Nurse practitioners, physician assistants and certified nurse midwives in California.* Sacramento, CA: Office of Statewide Health Planning and Development, 2000.

42. Sehgal AR. Impact of quality improvement efforts on race and sex disparities in hemodialysis. *JAMA* 2003;289:996–1000.

43. Vaccarino V, Rathore SS, Wenger NK, et al. Sex and racial differences in the management of acute myocardial infarction, 1994 through 2002. *N Engl J Med* 2005;353:671–682.

44. Jha AK, Fisher ES, Li Z, et al. Racial trends in the use of major procedures among the elderly. *N Engl J Med* 2005;353:683–691.

45. Trivedi AN, Zaslavsky AM, Schneider EC, et al. Trends in the quality of care and racial disparities in Medicare managed care. *N Engl J Med* 2005;353:692–700.

46. Bindman AB, Chattopadhyay A, Osmond DH, et al. The impact of Medicaid managed care on hospitalizations for ambulatory care sensitive conditions. *Health Serv Res* 2005;40:19–38.

Chapter 3

Financing and Organization of Health Care for Vulnerable Populations

Virginia W. Huang, MPH, and Christopher B. Forrest, MD, PhD

Objectives

- Review the financing and organization of health care for vulnerable populations.
- Describe how the structure of health care insurance coverage leaves so many individuals uninsured.
- Demonstrate that most uninsured persons are employed but have no employer-sponsored insurance benefits.
- Describe how the organization and financing of the health care safety net does not adequately meet all the needs of vulnerable populations.
- Summarize the arguments for increasing the numbers of primary care safety net providers to improve the access for vulnerable populations.

John Walsh is a 56-year-old African-American man with essential hypertension and type II diabetes. Since being laid off from full-time work 2 years ago, Mr. Walsh and his dependents, a wife and two children, are uninsured after losing their employer-sponsored health care insurance. Neither of his part-time jobs as a security guard and a delivery man offers any health insurance.

Mr. Walsh and his family members have slipped through the cracks of the fragmented US system of health care insurance coverage. There are approximately 45 million uninsured people in the United States. Of this total, 70% are families with at least one full-time working adult.[1,2] Absence of insurance creates major barriers to health care access. Members of one or more vulnerable populations—such as low-income, minority status, non-native English speaking, and those in poor health—are more likely to be uninsured, and disproportionately receive their health care from an imperfect patchwork of safety net providers.

Despite the substantial barriers to health care associated with this lack of insurance, the high cost of care and the dearth of providers serving vulnerable populations and communities, the United States has made no systematic effort to finance and organize health care to overcome them. The voluntary system of employer-sponsored health insurance creates substantial gaps for many Americans. Despite the absence of a coherent and logical system of care, a "safety net" system exists to care for those who do not have the means to pay. The providers who make up this safety net system rely on a range of public and private funds to finance the care.

This chapter describes the financing and organization of health care in the United States, identifies the contours and gaps in the safety net, and describes the challenges that are placing significant strain on this already fragile and underfunded system. The chapter concludes with an analysis of safety net providers and the importance of bolstering primary care to improve access to needed services for vulnerable populations.

HEALTH CARE FINANCING

EMPLOYER-SPONSORED HEALTH CARE INSURANCE

Most industrialized and many developing nations provide health care coverage to their populations as a form of social security. The United States is an outlier in this regard. The majority of Americans (60%) obtain coverage through a voluntary system of employer-sponsored health care insurance benefits. About half of those covered by employer-sponsored health insurance (49%) are dependents of workers.[3] Another 9% of Americans purchase private insurance directly from insurance companies, rather than through an employer. Although the majority of Americans obtain health coverage through private insurance, private insurance accounts for only approximately one-third of US health care expenditures. Medicaid and Medicare together account for another one-third; and a variety of other smaller public programs, out-of-pocket costs, and charity care contributes to the remaining one-third (Fig. 3-1).

GOVERNMENT PROGRAMES FOR HEALTH CARE COVERAGE

Health care policy in the United States has largely been created via an "incrementalist" approach by which government confers health benefits to defined categories of the population.[4] Medicare, the Indian Health Service, and the Veterans Administration's (VA) medical system are programs sponsored by the federal government, and are entitlements where, respectively, all US citizens aged 65 years and older, Native American/Alaskan natives, and veterans, are guaranteed insurance coverage. These three programs contrast with Medicaid, which is a means-tested insurance benefit that has demographic and income requirements that limit its eligibility to a subset of poor individuals (Fig. 3-2).

Medicare

Medicare is a federal program insuring the elderly, disabled, and those with end-stage renal disease (ESRD) (see Chap. 37). The program was created in 1965 through Title XVIII of the Social Security Act. All elderly US citizens aged 65 years and older who have paid into Social Security for at least 10 years are guaranteed coverage under Part A ("hospital insurance"). Inpatient services, skilled nursing facilities, hospice care, and some home health care are paid through this program, funded through a payroll tax.

Medicare Part B ("medical insurance") provides limited coverage of outpatient services and requires beneficiaries to pay a monthly premium as well as additional out-of-pocket costs when they use services. Many elderly individuals unable to pay for Part B premiums are eligible to have state Medicaid programs pay their Part B premiums, as well as some of their other out-of-pocket costs. Individuals who receive both Medicare and Medicaid coverage are termed "dual-eligible."

Medicare Part C, The 1997 Balanced Budget Act instituted Medicare Part C, called Medicare+Choice, allows beneficiaries to opt into managed care plans in lieu of enrolling in Medicare Part A and Part B.

Medicare Part D, The Medicare Prescription Drug, Improvement and Modernization Act (MMA) of 2003, added Medicare Part D, a voluntary prescription drug

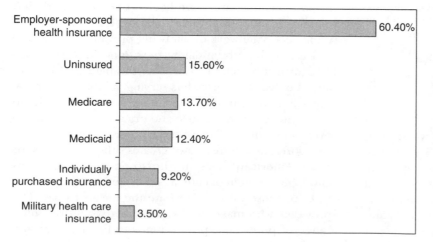

Figure 3-1. Health Care Insurance Coverage in the United States, 2002. Categories are not mutually exclusive; persons can be in more than one insurance category. Military health care insurance includes the following abbreviations: CHAMPUS, Comprehensive Health and Medical Plan for Uniformed Services)/Tricare; CHAMPVA, Civilian Health and Medical programs of the Department of Veteran Affairs. (*Source:* US Census Bureau, Current Population Survey, 2003–2004 Annual Social and Economic Supplements.)

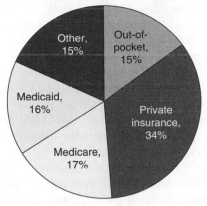

Total in billions, $1,299.5

Figure 3-2. National Health Care Source of Funds, 2000. (*Source:* Centers for Medicare and Medicaid Services. 2002 Data Compendium [Online]. Available at: http://www.cms.hhs.gov/researchers/pubs/datacompendium/2002/02pg15.pdf)

benefit.[5] Before the MMA, Medicare did not provide any coverage for medications prescribed in outpatient settings.

Medicaid

Medicaid was created in 1965 under Title XIX of the Social Security Act. Unlike Medicare—which is funded by federal and beneficiary funds—Medicaid is funded by federal and state revenues, but not beneficiary premiums. The amount of federal matching funds a state receives takes into consideration the profile of a state's vulnerable populations. Federal guidelines govern the administration of the programs but allow for substantial flexibility in coverage and implementation, rendering each state's Medicaid program unique.

Medicaid beneficiaries must meet the residency standards of the state and federal immigration standards, be a member of a population eligible for coverage (e.g., pregnant women, children, disabled persons, etc.), and satisfy income and asset requirements. As a result of these "categorical" eligibility criteria, the main classes of Medicaid beneficiaries are low-income children, pregnant women, low-income disabled individuals (who must first meet state requirements for Supplemental Security Income [SSI]), low-income parents, and low-income elderly with Medicare. Thus, although there is a common misperception that Medicaid provides coverage for all low-income persons, in fact it does not. For example, in many states the income limits are set well below the federal poverty level or a single homeless man would not be eligible on the basis of homelessness alone but would need to meet other qualifying eligibility criteria, such as having a disability. In addition, the program does not cover childless

adults and all illegal and certain legal immigrants. States often choose to cover specific vulnerable groups such as people with tuberculosis or people who "spend down" their assets; that is, they meet categorical requirements and have health care expenses that offset their income to the point of becoming eligible. The spend-down designation is commonly employed for nursing home residents.

Medicaid coverage is more comprehensive than the vast majority of private insurance. Covered benefits include inpatient and outpatient hospital services; office visits; Early and Periodic Screening Diagnosis and Treatment (EPSDT) for children and adolescents (under 21 years), which pays for a variety of preventive care services; nursing facilities for adults (21 years and over); family planning; labs; x-ray; and prescription drugs.[6]

State Children's Health Insurance Program

The State Children's Health Insurance Program (SCHIP) was created in 1997 under the Balanced Budget Act. Under this legislation, states were offered new funds to expand Medicaid to cover children above Medicaid income thresholds but below 200% of poverty level. Some states have chosen to extend this program beyond children to include the uninsured parents of eligible children.[7] SCHIP benefits are generally similar to those of Medicaid. Over the past decade, expansions in Medicaid eligibility and enactment of SCHIP have reduced rates of uninsured children.

INDIVIDUALLY PURCHASED PRIVATE INSURANCE

> With his two part-time jobs Mr. Walsh makes an income too high for his family to qualify for Medicaid or SCHIP. He chooses not to purchase health care insurance on the individual market, because it is completely unaffordable given his current income.

One important benefit of employer-sponsored health care insurance for the consumer is that the employer generally subsidizes the premium charges. Just like auto insurance, individuals can purchase health insurance directly from an agent or insurance company. However, as Mr. Walsh learned, premiums for this type of insurance are extraordinarily high. Because of the smaller pooling of risk that occurs when people are insured on an individual basis, the premium charges for individual policies are substantially higher than those for employees who obtain their health insurance from an employer as part of a large group insurance policy.

Also, preexisting health conditions, such as diabetes and hypertension, can drive premium costs even higher, which may have been the case with Mr. Walsh, who has both hypertension and diabetes. The probability of anyone in fair or poor health buying individual insurance is 50% lower than people in excellent health.[8] Even if Mr. Walsh purchased insurance, his preexisting conditions could limit his benefits. Insurance companies also may choose not to cover any costs related to treatment of preexisting conditions putting him, and patients like him, at risk of being underinsured;[9] that is, having insurance coverage with large gaps in what it will pay for, including coverage for conditions that may be affecting their health profoundly.

FINANCIAL PRESSURES ON THE SAFETY NET

RISING PREMIUM COSTS

Between 2000 and 2004, the average cost of private health insurance premiums increased by 10.9% to 13.9% annually, far outpacing the increases in general inflation and wages in the United States during this period.[10] Higher medical costs result in employers dropping private insurance coverage for their workers and retirees.[11]

Employer-sponsored insurance coverage is eroding for all classes of working Americans, but certain subgroups have been hit particularly hard. From 1979 to 1998, the percentage of workers covered by employer-sponsored health insurance decreased from 72% to 60%.[12] Low-wage workers experienced the greatest declines: 42% had job-based insurance in 1979, but just 20% were covered in 1998. Among high-income employees, the change in coverage decreased from 90% to 80%. Over the past several years, employees have begun shouldering larger shares of premium costs as employer contributions have failed to keep pace with the rate of increase in premium costs.

For retirees eligible for Medicare, supplemental private insurance coverage typically contributes toward covering services that Medicare does not: medications, ambulatory care, and long-term care. Losing this supplemental coverage can undermine the financial accessibility of these services for those with chronic illness.

UNINSURANCE AND UNDERINSURANCE

One of Mr. Walsh's daughters has severe persistent asthma. She is not being managed consistently by a primary care doctor, and is taken frequently the emergency department (ED) for urgent treatment. The costs of medical care have become a large financial strain on the family. Because of these cost concerns, Mr. Walsh has not seen a primary care physician for his own health problems.

Currently, there are 45 million uninsured people in the United States. In addition, 20% of all insured persons have benefits that do not adequately cover their health needs (i.e., they are underinsured).[1,13] This lack of insurance is bad for health. Uninsured persons receive fewer services of all types, and are more likely to delay needed care. For example, the uninsured are less likely than the insured to be screened for cancer, and thus present with more advanced stages of cancer and experience higher mortality rates than people with insurance. Access barriers to primary care, also increases the use of emergency departments for non-urgent care or because of delayed treatment.[9,12]

The ill effects of being uninsured extend beyond delaying care: Poor health that results from lack of insurance reduces income by an estimated 15% to 30%, and people with lower incomes are less likely to have health insurance.[14,15] Uninsured families are at risk of economic catastrophe from a medical episode. Half of all bankruptcies filed are related to medical expenses.[16,17]

Those most likely to be uninsured are those who can least afford to be so. Eight out of ten uninsured persons are from working families. Sixty-six percent are in low-income families, earning less than 200% of the federal poverty level ($37,700 for Mr. Walsh's family of four in 2004). Minorities are more likely to be uninsured; over 33% of Hispanics, 25% of Native Americans, 22% of African Americans, and 20% of Asian Americans are uninsured compared with 14% of white Americans.[3]

Common Pitfalls in Access to Health Care

- Health care coverage is largely based on employment.
- Health care coverage is not based on need or considered a public good.
- Participation in employer-sponsored health care insurance is voluntary.
- Incremental changes rather than systematic and comprehensive reforms characterize health policy making in this country.

ORGANIZATION OF THE HEALTH CARE SAFETY NET

Mr. Walsh lacerates his ankle and presents to the ED. His wound is sutured and he is prescribed antibiotics. The medication costs $80 and he decides not to fill the prescription. The next week he returns to the ED with a septic joint, and now requires a hospital admission. This hospital does not admit uninsured patients and the public hospital to which the ED doctor tries to transfer him, only accepts patients with a higher level-of-care need. Ultimately, Mr. Walsh is admitted to a local, private community hospital.

The admitting doctor starts antibiotics, but an orthopedic surgeon refuses to operate on Mr. Walsh, because of concern about the high risk of being sued for a poor outcome. Mr. Walsh fears he is not improving and leaves against medical advice. His family drives him to the public hospital ED where he is admitted and operated upon the next day.

SAFETY NET PROVIDERS: WHO ARE THEY?

Financing programs, such as Medicaid and SCHIP, as well as the providers of health care to vulnerable patients comprise the safety net. The composition of providers in a safety net varies greatly among communities and depends on factors such as a state's Medicaid policies, the socioeconomic composition of a community, the competitiveness of the local health care market, and the existence of other programs for the poor and uninsured or special needs populations.[18-20] Thus, a diverse group of practitioners, physician organizations, hospitals, and programs provide services to vulnerable populations and can range from pharmaceutical programs for indigent patients, to private physicians serving Medicaid patients, community health centers, free clinics, and hospitals providing uncompensated care. Hence, in most communities the health care safety net is not a formalized network of coordinated services. As a result, navigating the system is difficult for both patients and providers, and experiences like Mr. Walsh's are all too typical.

CORE SAFETY NET PROVIDERS AND THEIR FUNDING

An Institute of Medicine report coined the phrase "core safety net providers" to refer to practitioners and health care organizations that include a substantial share of the uninsured, Medicaid beneficiaries, and other vulnerable populations among the patients they serve.[19] Also called "providers of last resort," core safety net providers share two characteristics. First, their organizational missions mandate serving vulnerable populations within the community or they are legally required to serve patients regardless of ability to pay. Second, these providers tend to bear a disproportionate share of the burden for uncompensated and publicly financed care.[19]

The uncompensated care given by the safety net providers can be indirectly funded by shifting costs to other payers or using uncompensated health care workers (e.g., volunteer physicians and nurses) to provide some of the care. In cost-shifting, financial resources such as profits from insured patients are shifted to subsidize the cost of uncompensated care. Additionally, various

government programs provide some financial support for care to the uninsured who are unable to fully pay. In 2001, an estimated $35 billion in care was provided by the health care system to the uninsured. Ultimately, funding from government programs financed approximately $30.6 billion of this cost (Fig. 3-3).[21]

Medicaid and Medicare have special funding streams for safety net providers. Both programs provide payments called Disproportionate Share Hospital (DSH) payments to hospitals with a high volume of uninsured and low-income patients. These payments supplement regular Medicare and Medicaid payments. Hospitals receive these funds when they exceed a designated threshold of hospital bed days for patients covered by these programs. This funding might be adequate to fund the cost of providing care to the uninsured if they were appropriately distributed. However, National Association of Public Hospitals member institutions report that 60% lose money on Medicaid patients and 84% lose money on Medicare patients even with the supplemental payments.[22]

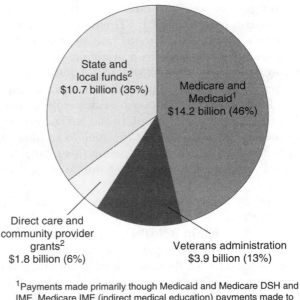

[1]Payments made primarily though Medicaid and Medicare DSH and IME. Medicare IME (indirect medical education) payments made to teaching hospitals and their residency programs in recognition for the role of teaching hospitals as core safety net providers. Medicare and Medicaid DSH (disproportionate hospital share payments) are payments made to hospitals serving a disproportionately large share of the low-income and uninsured patients.

[2]Federal monies at the Indian Health Service, Maternal Child Health Bureau, Bureau of Primary Health Care, National Health Service Corps, HIV/AIDS Bureau applied to uncompensated care.

Figure 3-3. Distribution of government expenditure on $30.6 billion in financing care for the uninsured, 2001. (*Source:* Hadley J, Holahan J. Who pays and how much? The cost of caring for the uninsured. *Health Affairs*, 2003. Web exclusive supplement: w3-66-81.)

Medicare also pays teaching hospitals two types of payments for medical education: Direct Graduate Medical Education (DGME) and Indirect Medical Education (IME) payments. Medicare DGME and IME are paid to these hospitals to subsidize medical education and safety net care, partly in recognition that teaching hospitals disproportionately serve vulnerable populations and rely on physicians in training to provide much of this care.[21-24]

Public, Nonprofit, and Teaching Hospitals

Public, nonprofit, and teaching hospitals are the main providers of hospital safety net care. In 2002, there were a total of 5794 registered hospitals in the United States. Of these, 52% were nonprofit community hospitals (defined as nonprofit and nonfederal general and specialty hospitals), and 20% were public hospitals (federal hospitals, state and local government community hospitals).[25] About 44% of community hospitals are located in rural areas,[25] although these rural hospitals typically have far fewer patient care beds than urban hospitals. In rural areas, where there are shortages of providers,[26] hospitals often serve as the source for both ambulatory and acute care. There are an estimated 1230 teaching hospitals, excluding some specialty care hospitals (e.g., psychiatric, cancer, rehabilitation).[23] Teaching hospitals usually have a nonprofit tax status, are located in urban areas, and are associated with academic medical centers; some are government owned (including a small number of teaching Veterans Administration hospitals). Teaching hospitals play a critical role as major safety net providers and are often the only providers of expensive and unprofitable care, such as trauma care and burn units.[19,27] In many teaching hospitals, up to 51% of total revenues come from Medicaid and Medicare.

There are approximately 1300 public hospitals in the United States.[25] A survey by the National Public Hospital Association (NAPH) found that care for patients who cannot pay, uncompensated care, accounts for 21% of their members' total costs, compared with 6% of total costs at private hospitals.[24] The majority of NAPH members' revenue is from Medicare, Medicaid, and state and local sources (71% of total revenue in 2002); 33% of their uncompensated care costs are covered by Medicaid DSH and Medicare DSH and IME payments.[24] Nevertheless, 90% of NAPH members lost money on care given to Medicaid and Medicare beneficiaries. The ratio of the payments from the programs to the hospital costs for providing care, or the payment-to-cost ratios were 0.77 and 0.81, respectively. Without DGME and IME payments, the Medicare payment-to-cost ratio would have

been 0.65.[24] In 2000, almost half of the National Association of Public Hospitals members experienced negative margins.

Emergency Departments

ED visits account for approximately 10% of all ambulatory care in the United States. The Emergency Medical Treatment and Active Labor Act of 1985 (EMTALA) was enacted to prevent "patient dumping" of uninsured patients from EDs. This legislation guarantees screening and stabilizing treatment in the ED regardless of the patient's ability to pay (see Chap. 4). Because the legislation is an unfunded mandate, hospitals must absorb the cost of uncompensated care. As a result, in the early 1990s many hospitals began closing their EDs to limit their exposure to these costs.[26,28,29] The number of EDs has reduced by 12% between 1993 and 2003.[30] Although there has been a slight increase in patient visits, the rate of visits has remained relatively the same. However, a larger proportion of ED visits are for illness-related conditions and from elderly minorities and ED physicians report seeing more nonurgent cases that could have been treated in primary care settings.[31] Currently, EDs are experiencing overcrowding problems that can have an impact their effectiveness as safety net providers of urgent care. Fewer EDs and a reduced number of inpatient hospital beds (resulting from a hospital nursing shortage in part) hindering the flow patients out of EDs into hospital admissions are the determinants of the current ED overcrowding problem.[26,29]

Health Clinics

Community clinics that serve vulnerable populations may be funded by charitable contributions, local or state government, the federal government, or hospital systems. The Federally Qualified Health Center (FQHC) program deserves special attention, because it is the main federal policy directly aimed at improving access to primary care for vulnerable populations. A clinic receives the FQHC designation through the federal Section 330 grant of the Health Center Consolidation Act of 1996. FQHCs are required to be nonprofit, freestanding clinics, located in medically underserved areas, and must provide primary care regardless of ability to pay. About half are located in rural areas. In addition, FQHCs must provide enabling services such as onsite availability of medications, transportation, translation services, or in-house lab testing in order to lower access barriers to care. Community Health Centers (CHCs), migrant health centers, Health Care for the Homeless Programs, and the Public Housing Primary Care Programs all fall under the FQHC designation.[32]

There were a total of 890 FQHCs in 2003,[33] and the number is growing because of federal initiatives to increase the capacity of the health center safety net. About 4% of primary care visits in the United States occur at FQHCs. Sixty-six percent of FQHC patients are uninsured or Medicaid beneficiaries, which contrasts with 19% of patients at private physicians' offices.[34] Patients in ethnic minority groups comprise a large share of primary care at CHCs: 66% of primary care visits versus 15% in physicians' offices and 37% in hospital outpatient departments.

Although CHCs exist to provide primary care services for vulnerable persons in the United States, there are too few to fulfill all primary care needs of vulnerable subgroups. In general, neither expanding the number of safety net providers nor expanding coverage of the uninsured alone will resolve the access problems of the uninsured. A $2 billion investment in either the community health center program or an expansion of health insurance coverage would result in similar but only marginal gains in access.[35] For example, even if the number of safety net providers were increased and distributed so as to improve access for the uninsured by increasing proximity to care, the percentage of uninsured with unmet medical needs would still range between 10% to 30%.[36]

The National Health Service Corps

A program of the Bureau of Health Professions in the Health Resource and Service Administration, the National Health Services Corps (NHSC) began in 1970 under the Emergency Health Personnel Act in order to improve access to medical care for populations in Health Professional Shortage Areas (HPSAs).[37] A HPSA may be a geographic area, population group, or facility with a shortage of primary medical, dental, or mental health providers.[38] The NHSC is one of the main federal programs recruiting providers to work in medically underserved communities by providing direct financial incentives.

The NHSC aims to attract these providers through two programs: a loan repayment program, and a scholarship program, both of which provide financial aid to students or practitioners of primary care disciplines in exchange for terms of service in a HPSA. Currently, there are approximately 2700 clinicians consisting of allopathic or osteopathic physicians, dentists, mental health professionals, nurse practitioners, nurse midwives, and physician assistants who are participating in the program.[39] However, in 2000 the program only covered 0.5% of the physician workforce and each year there are more requests from HPSA areas than providers available to fill the positions.[37]

Physicians

Private physicians contribute to safety net care by providing charity care or volunteering at safety net clinics. Private physicians' offices receive no direct subsidies for uninsured care and yet provide an estimated $5.1 billion in reduced-price or free care.[21] In a 2001 national survey, most physicians (71%) said they provided charity care, but this proportion was lower than in 1998.[40]

Charity care in private physicians' offices is not necessarily available for all patients. A survey of general internists found that most of their uninsured patients were established patients who recently lost coverage.[41] Although most primary care physicians are willing to accept uninsured patients, their payment policies for uninsured patients vary widely and may make care inaccessible.[42] Between 1998 and 2001 the number of providers willing to serve Medicaid patients declined from 87% to 85%, and fewer were willing to accept new Medicaid patients.[40] Reasons given by physicians for not participating in Medicaid include low reimbursement, too much paperwork, Medicaid cases being more medically and socially complex, time intensity, and negative perceptions about Medicaid patients (i.e., noncompliant, ungrateful, have more psychosocial problems).[43,44] Approximately half of generalists and specialists in one survey cited additional risk of being sued as a factor in the decision to not serve uninsured and Medicaid patients,[44] although low income patients are not in fact more likely to file malpractice claims.

Additionally, health insurance status can affect the content of care. The disparity in access and use of services between the uninsured and insured are well established. Overall, the uninsured are less likely than the insured to receive preventive services, are more likely to be diagnosed with late stage disease, and receive less treatment after diagnosis of disease.[15] Studies suggest that physicians are more likely to recommend services for insured than uninsured patients with similar clinical presentations; this may be at least partly explained because physicians know that few services are available to the uninsured.[36,40,46]

Not surprisingly, physicians find it difficult to refer uninsured and Medicaid-eligible patients to other physicians. Both general internists with private offices and providers at CHCs say it is very difficult to obtain needed medical services beyond what can be provided at the office visit for their uninsured patients. Physicians believe they must rely on personal relationships as opposed to formal processes to connect the uninsured to needed specialty care.[41,47] Also, 25% of the physician faculty at US academic health centers report that they were rarely able to provide nonurgent admissions for their uninsured patients, and for 13% of respondents, there were formal policies limiting care to uninsured patients at their institutions.[48]

CONCLUSION

The patchwork health care financing system in the United States leaves many individuals, such as Mr. Walsh and his family, vulnerable to the negative effects of being uninsured. Mr. Walsh's difficulty finding adequate primary care and paying for prescription drugs resulted in use of expensive and uncoordinated hospital-based care. The existing acute care safety net too often addresses only complications of underlying disorders, rather than preventing those problems in the first place.

The solutions to the problem of ensuring the availability of quality health care for all Americans—providing insurance coverage for all and strengthening the primary care infrastructure in this country—are complex. Nonetheless, the many people in this country whose health suffers because of an inadequately financed and uncoordinated safety net create an imperative for action now. Because of their hands-on experience in health care, health professionals are in a unique position to advocate for strategies that will bolster the safety net and address the needs of the most vulnerable in US society.

KEY CONCEPTS

The Health Care Safety Net

- Safety net characteristics
—Public financing or charity care serves low-income persons unable to obtain private insurance.
—Providers are those who deliver services to large numbers of patients with significant access problems.
—Medical resources are available despite the ability to pay.
—Uncompensated care is paid for by cost-shifting from other payers.
—The composition of the safety net varies across communities.
- Most safety net funding comes from a mix of federal, state, and local government programs.
- Core safety net providers:
—Disproportionately bear the burden of safety net care.
—Usually are legally obligated or have mission to serve regardless of ability to pay.
- Despite access to a safety net provider, referral care is challenging to arrange.

CORE COMPETENCY
Understanding Medicaid Eligibility

Why?

- Receipt of Medicaid improves access to care for low-income patients.
- Medicaid covers many services that are not covered by Medicare; that is, pays the Medicare premium and deductible (and in some cases, the coinsurance), and prescriptions.
- Medicaid covers long-term care.
- Receipt of Medicaid improves revenues for institutions providing lots of uncompensated care.
- Improved revenues for these institutions allow provision of care and better care to larger numbers of patients.

Who is eligible?
Low-income:

- Children under 18
- Pregnant women
- Working parents (particularly single mothers)
- Patients with very severe physical and mental disabilities
- Elderly low-income Medicare beneficiaries
- All beneficiaries who receive SSI cash benefits
- Migrant workers, even if they travel are still eligible.
- Home address is not required, hence homeless are eligible.
- Limited eligibility only for emergency care:
—Those otherwise eligible for benefits (e.g., low-income children and pregnant women) but who are either undocumented persons or short-term (<5 years) legal residents.

DISCUSSION QUESTIONS

1. As a primary care practitioner, if Mr. Walsh were your patient who became newly uninsured, what would you do? What ethical dilemmas might you encounter?
2. Who are the safety net providers in your community? What local funds or programs exist to support your safety net providers?
3. As providers, one of the ways to help your vulnerable patients is to get involved in advocacy. In what safety net related issues can a provider be involved at the organizational, city/county, state, or federal levels?

RESOURCES

Center for Studying Health System Change: www.hschange.org
The Kaiser Family Foundation, Commission on Medicaid and the Uninsured: www.kff.org

Lewin ME, Altman S, eds. *America's health care safety net.* Washington, DC: National Academies Press, 2000.

Reports from the Institute of Medicine, Committee on the Consequences of Uninsurance:

- *Coverage matters: Insurance and health care.* Washington, DC: National Academy Press, 2001
- *Care without coverage: Too little, too late,* 2002
- *Health insurance is a family matter,* 2002
- *A shared destiny: Community effects of uninsurance,* 2003
- *Hidden costs, value lost,* 2003

ACKNOWLEDGMENT

This work was supported in part by Grant No. 6 U30 CS 00189-05 S1 R1 of the Bureau of Primary Health Care, Health Resources and Services Administration, Department of Health and Human Services, to the Primary Care Policy Center for the Underserved at Johns Hopkins University.

REFERENCES

1. DeNavas-Walt C, Proctor BD, Mills RJ, et al. *Income, poverty, and health insurance coverage in the United States, 2003.* (Current population reports, P60-226). Washington, DC: US Government Printing Office, 2004.
2. Hoffman C, Wang M. *Health insurance coverage in America: 2002 data update.* Kaiser Commission on Medicaid and the Uninsured, Publication No. 4154, 2003. [Online]. Available at: http://www.kff.org/uninsured/4154.cfm
3. *The uninsured: A primer, key facts about Americans without health insurance.* Kaiser Family Foundation, 2003.
4. Starr P. *The social transformation of American medicine.* New York: Basic Books, 1989.
5. Centers for Medicare and Medicaid Services. *Medicare Information Resource, 2004a.* [Online]. Available at: http://www.cms.hhs.gov/medicare
6. Centers for Medicare and Medicaid Services. *Medicare Information Resource, 2004b.* [Online]. Available at: http://www.cms.hhs.gov/medicaid
7. Centers for Medicare and Medicaid Services. *Medicare Information Resource, 2004c.* [Online]. Available at: http://www.cms.hhs.gov/schip/researchers_default.asp
8. Hadley J, Reschovsky JD. Health and the cost of nongroup insurance. *Inquiry* 2003b;40(3): 235–253.
9. Institute of Medicine. *Coverage matters: Insurance and health care.* Washington, DC: National Academies Press, 2001.
10. Kaiser Family Foundation, Health Research and Educational Trust. *Employer Health Benefits Annual National Survey 2004. 2004a.* [Online]. Available at: http://www.kff.org/insurance/7148/index.cfm
11. Fronstin P, Reno V. Recent trends in retiree benefits and the role of COBRA coverage. National Academy of Social Insurance, Health and Income Security Brief No. 4, 2001. [Online]. Available at: http://www.nasi.org/usr_doc/risks_brief_4.pdf
12. Medoff JL, Shapiro HB, Calabrese M, et al. *How the new labor market is squeezing workforce health benefits.* Center for National Policy, The Commonwealth Fund, June 2001 [Online]. Available at: http://www.cmwf.org
13. Kaiser Family Foundation. *Underinsured in America: Is health coverage adequate?* 2002. [Online]. Available at: http://www.kff.org/uninsured/loader.cfm?url=/commonspot/security/getfile.cfm&PageID=14136
14. Institute of Medicine. *Care without coverage: Too little, too late.* Washington, DC: National Academy Press, 2002a.
15. Hadley J. Sicker and poorer: The consequences of being uninsured. *Med Care Res Rev* 2003a;60(Suppl 2):35–75s.
16. Institute of Medicine. *Health insurance is a family matter.* Washington, DC: National Academy Press, 2002b.
17. Himmelstein DU, Warren E, Thorne D, et al. MarketWatch: Illness and injury as contributors of bankruptcy. *Health Affairs,* web exclusive 2005;W5(63–73).
18. Baxter R, Mechanic RE. The status of local health care safety nets. *Health Affairs* 1997;16(4), 7–23.
19. Lewin ME, Altman S, eds. *America's health care safety net.* Washington, DC: National Academies Press, 2000.
20. Norton SA, Lipson DJ. *Public policy, market forces, and the viability of safety net providers.* Washington, DC: The Urban Institute, 1998.
21. Hadley J, Holahan J. How much medical care do the uninsured use and who pays for it? *Health Affairs,* web exclusive 2003c;1:W66–W81.
22. Tolbert J, ed. *Safety net financing: A policy source book for healthcare executives.* Washington, DC: National Association of Public Hospitals and Health Systems, June 2003.
23. American Association of Medical Centers. All you ever wanted to know about teaching hospitals (presentation). [Online]. Available at: http://www.aamc.org/members/shared/priselachospitals.ppt
24. Singer I, Davison L, Tolbert J, et al. *America's SafetyNet Hospitals and Health Systems, 2002.* Washington, DC: National Association of Public Hospitals and Health Systems, 2004.
25. American Hospital Association. *Fast Facts on U.S. Hospitals from Hospital Statistics, 2004.* Available at: http://www.aha.org/aha/resource_center/fastfacts/fast_facts_US_hospitals.html
26. Institute of Medicine. *A shared destiny: Community effects of uninsurance.* Washington, DC: National Academy Press, 2003.
27. Moy E, Valente E, Levin RJ. Academic medical centers and the care of underserved populations. *Acad Med* 1996; 71(12):1370–1377.
28. Gordon JA, Billings J, Asplin BR, et al. Safety net research in emergency medicine. *Acad Emerg Med* 2001;8(11): 1021–1029.
29. Burt CW, McCaig LF. Trends in hospital emergency department utilization: United States 1992–99. National Center for Health Statistics, 2001. *Vital Health Stat* 13(150).
30 McCaig LF, Burt CW. *National hospital ambulatory medical care survey: 2003 emergency department summary.* Hyattsville, MD: National Center for Health Statistics, 2005.
31. Siegel B. The emergency department: Rethinking the safety net for the safety net. *Health Aff (Millwood)* 2004:Jan-Jun;Suppl Web Exclusives: W4-146-8.

32. Bureau of Primary Health Care. FY 2003 UDS National Roll-Up. 2004b. [Online]. Accessed at: http://bphc.hrsa.gov/uds/data.htm

33. Bureau of Primary Health Care. Community Health Center Program Information. 2004a. [Online]. Available at: http://bphc.hrsa.gov/programs/CHCPrograminfo.asp

34. Forrest CB, Whelan E. Primary care safety net delivery sites in the United States. *JAMA* 2000;284(16):2077–2083.

35. Cunningham PJ, Hadley J. Expanding care versus expanding coverage: How to improve access to care. *Health Affairs* 2004;23(4):234–244.

36. Hadley J, Cunningham PJ. Availability of safety net providers and access to care of uninsured persons. *Health Serv Res* 2004;39(5):1527–1546.

37. Nampiaparampil D, Rising J. The National Health Service Corps: 25 years of success, an uncertain future. 2000. Available at: http://www.amsa.org/pdf/nhsc.pdf

38. Bureau of Health Professions. Shortage designation. 2004a. [Online]. Available at: http://bhpr.hrsa.gov/shortage

39. Bureau of Health Professions. National Health Service Corps Program Information. 2004b. [Online]. Available at: http://nhsc.bhpr.hrsa.gov/about

40. Cunningham PJ. (2002). *Mounting pressures: Physicians serving Medicaid patients and the uninsured, 1997–2001.* Center for Studying Health System Change Tracking Report, 2002.

41. Fairbrother G, Gusmano MK, Park HL, et al. Care for the uninsured in general internists' private offices. *Health Affairs* 2003;22(6):217–224.

42. O'Toole TP, Simms PM, Dixon BW. Primary care office policies regarding care of uninsured adult patients. *J Gen Int Med* 2001;16:693–696.

43. Bindman AB, Huen W, Vranizan K, et al. Physician Participation in Medi-Cal, 1996–1998. Medical Policy Institute. February 2002. [Online]. Available at: www.chcf.org

44. Komaromy M, Lurie N, Bindman AB. California physicians' willingness to care for the poor. *West J Med* 1995;162(2):127–132.

45. Mort EA, Edwards J, Emmonds DE, et al. Physician response to patient insurance status in ambulatory care clinical decision-making: Implications for quality of care. *Med Care* 1996;34(8):783–797.

46. O'Malley AS, Forrest CB, Politzer RM, et al. Health center trends, 1994–2001: What do they portend for the federal growth initiative? Health Affairs 2005;24(2):4 65–472.

47. Gusmano MK, Fairbrother G, Park H. Exploring the limits of the safety net: Community health centers and care for the uninsured. *Health Affairs* 2002;21(6):188–194.

48. Weissman JS, Moy E, Campbell EG, et al. Limits to the SafetyNet: Teaching hospital faculty report on their parents' access to care. *Health Affairs* 2003;22(6): 157–163.

Chapter 4

Legal Issues in the Care of Underserved Populations

Sara Rosenbaum, JD, and Sara E. Wilensky, JD, MPP

Objectives

- Summarize the basic elements of the legal environment for health care delivery in the United States, particularly for medically underserved populations.
- Identify the major laws and legal concepts that govern health care organization, financing, and health care delivery of health care for medically underserved populations.
- Describe the basic legal duties of health care providers toward individuals and patients.
- Review laws that prohibit discrimination in health care.
- Review concepts of health care quality and patient rights applicable to all patients regardless of economic or personal circumstances.

Understanding the laws and regulations governing the care of medically underserved populations is critical for clinicians serving these patients. Federal and state laws address barriers to health care and create a legal duty to furnish health care under limited circumstances. The law also shapes and drives the public and private health insurance arrangements that pay for most health care, including care delivered to low-income and vulnerable populations.

This chapter examines three major bodies of law that govern health care practice for medically underserved populations: (a) *access* to health care; (b) *payment for* health care, as well as some of the basic legal aspects of Medicaid, the nation's largest public health insurer; and (c) *health care quality* and *patient rights*.

ACCESS TO HEALTH CARE

John Pool is a person with human immunodeficiency virus (HIV). He is struck by a car and is brought by ambulance to the closest trauma center, bloodied and semiconscious. His partner, who accompanies him to the hospital, explains that John is HIV positive. Hospital personnel advise John's partner that John would be best served if, rather than receiving care at their facility, the partner were to drive John to the public hospital 20 minutes away, given its expertise in caring for persons with HIV.

HEALTH CARE AS A LEGAL RIGHT

A basic principle of US health law is that there is no legal right to health care and no corresponding legal duty to furnish care.[1] Most Americans have reasonable access to health care, and ethical principles of medical practice impose a moral obligation on professionals to act with respect for dignity and human rights. At the same time, the American Medical Association's (AMA) code of ethics specifically provides for virtually total autonomy in the selection of patients, specifying that "*a physician shall...except in emergencies, be free to choose whom to serve, with whom to associate, and the environment in which to provide medical care.*"[2]

Over the years, congress and most states have enacted laws aimed at prohibiting certain types of discrimination against certain groups of persons, including members of racial and ethnic minority groups and persons with conditions considered "disabling." Virtually no law, federal or state, prohibits discrimination against the poor.

Mr. Pool, the injured HIV-positive patient who was turned away from a hospital emergency department (ED), is based on an actual incident that came before a federal court in Ohio.[3] The US Supreme Court decided a case concerning a dentist in private practice who refused to fill a cavity for an HIV-positive patient unless she agreed to receive her care as a hospital outpatient, citing personal safety concerns.[4] Ruling in the patient's favor, the Court held that her HIV infection, even if asymptomatic, constitutes a disability under the Americans with Disabilities Act and that the dentist was obligated not to discriminate against her.

IMPACT OF RACE AND ETHNICITY

The Court's 1954 landmark decision in *Brown v. Board of Education*[5] permeated all aspects of public life, including the South's legally segregated health care systems. The decision in *Brown v Board of Education* struck down legal segregation and was subsequently interpreted to prohibit courts from enforcing contracts aimed at perpetuating segregation in private settings such as home sales.[6]

Although legally sanctioned segregation ended by the mid 20th century, significant health disparities based on race and ethnicity have persisted. Research suggests that vestiges of racial and ethnic discrimination are displayed in the attitudes and beliefs of health professionals and the culture of clinical practice.[7]

In a legal context, these attitudes and beliefs can result in practices that carry discriminatory effects. For example, institutions sometimes segregate Medicaid beneficiaries (who disproportionately are members of racial or ethnic minority groups) into separate hospital or nursing home wings, or separate managed care provider networks. The object of segregation is publicly insured persons, but the impact falls disproportionately on minority patients.

The refusal of health care providers to participate in Medicaid long served as a *de facto,* if not deliberate means of perpetuating racial discrimination in a clinical practice, because of the disproportionate enrollment of minority families.[8] Even though the refusal to participate in Medicaid may be the result of the program's very low payment levels,[9] the consequences are disproportionately serious for racial and ethnic minority patients.

IMPACT OF POVERTY

The example of Medicaid nonparticipation also illustrates the often-intertwined nature of race and poverty in segregation and exclusion. Poor persons, who are disproportionately members of racial and ethnic minority groups, are far more likely to be uninsured or publicly insured.[10] Yet federal law recognizes only the most limited protections against discrimination based on poverty.

Moreover, although federal civil rights laws protect patients who are members of racial or ethnic minority groups, these same laws afford nonparticipating health care providers a "business necessity" defense[11] to a claim of discriminatory practice. This defense precludes the imposition of remedies that otherwise might compel a provider's meaningful participation in such programs.

STATUTES GOVERNING HEALTH CARE ACCESS

THE EMERGENCY TREATMENT AND LABOR ACT

The Emergency Treatment and Labor Act (EMTALA), enacted in 1986,[12] creates a legally enforceable right of access to certain services furnished by hospitals with EDs. EMTALA rights apply at all Medicare-participating hospitals (the vast majority of US hospitals) and to all persons regardless of health insurance status, income, or other personal characteristics. Many states have laws that parallel EMTALA requirements, and that apply to all, or most, licensed hospitals, but EMTALA is the predominant federal statute governing emergency hospital access.

EMTALA was enacted to stop the practice of "patient dumping," that is, turning away medically indigent persons in need of hospital care.[1] The law is complex and nuanced. At the same time, EMTALA has certain fundamental requirements that together impose an unprecedented *legal and enforceable right to certain types of health care* on the part of individuals with emergency medical conditions, and a corresponding *legal duty of care* on the part of covered institutions. Consequently, EMTALA creates two basic hospital duties (Table 4-1).

Legal and Enforceable Right to Health Care

Hospitals must provide an "appropriate" examination to an individual who "comes to" a hospital's "dedicated ED" seeking care for an "emergency medical condition" (42 USC § 1395dd(e)(1)(A)). The concept of "comes to" can include persons who are not yet physically inside the ED but who are on the grounds of the hospital or in reasonable proximity and who are being transported to a facility by ambulance. A "dedicated ED" can include not only the actual ED but other parts

Table 4-1. EMTALA: COBRA Requirements

The Hospital
- Provide a medical screening examination to all patients who seek emergency care within 250 yards of the hospital's main buildings.
- Stabilize the patient's condition if necessary or arrange a medically appropriate transfer if the patient is unstable.
- The hospital must keep an accurate list of specialty physicians on call to stabilize emergency patients.
- Stabilized patients must be given a plan for appropriate follow-up care.
- Provide medically appropriate transfers of unstable patients.
—Complete transfer form, weighing risks and benefits of transfer.
—The patient may request transfer by written request.
—The patient must have an accepting physician.
—There must be written consent from the patient to transfer.
—The transfer must be by appropriate medical vehicle.
—There must be qualified transport personnel to meet the level of care needed by the patient.
—Copies of medical records and x-rays must be sent with patient.

Adapted from: Mantini SL. *What's EMTALA, and what are its implications?* ENA EMTALA Work Group. Emergency Nurses Association. Available at: http://www.ena.org/government/emtala/article1.asp

of a hospital which function as EDs a majority of the time (e.g., a hospital's off-campus outpatient facility). An "appropriate" examination means one that is nondiscriminatory and that adheres to the hospital's emergency examination protocols (42 CFR §489.24).

Under EMTALA, an "emergency medical condition" means a "medical condition manifesting itself by acute symptoms of sufficient severity (including severe pain) such that the absence of immediate medical attention could reasonably be expected to result in: (a) placing the health of the individual (or, with respect to a pregnant woman, the health of the woman or her unborn child) in serious jeopardy; (b) serious impairment to bodily functions; or (c) serious dysfunction of any bodily organ or part" (42 USC §1395dd(e)(1)). This definition explicitly includes psychiatric disturbances that present a risk of serious physical injury to either the patient or another person regardless of whether or not psychiatric services are provided by the transferring hospital.

Legal Duty of Care

The second EMTALA obligation is the duty to either stabilize an emergency condition or undertake a medically appropriate transfer in the case of an unstable patient. An appropriate transfer is one that is effectuated in a medically appropriate manner, a personal certification by a physician at the transferring facility that the benefits of the transfer outweigh its risks, and agreement on the part of the receiving institution to accept the transfer (42 USC §1395dd(b)). "Stabilized" is defined in the regulations as meaning "that no material deterioration of the [emergency medical] condition is likely, within reasonable medical probability, to result from or occur during the transfer of the individual from a facility." In the case of a pregnant woman having contractions the concept of medical emergency means "that there is inadequate time to effect a safe

transfer to another hospital before delivery, or that transfer may pose a threat to the health or safety of the woman or the unborn child" (USC §1395dd(e)(1)).

Potential Consequences of EMTALA Violation

Violation of EMTALA can result in a hospital's exclusion from Medicare, as well as serious financial sanctions imposed on both the hospital and its physicians. In addition, both individuals and hospitals that are "dumped on" have explicit rights under the law and can sue offending hospitals to vindicate those rights (42 USC §1395dd(d)). In the example of Mr. Pool, the hospital's effort to turn away an HIV-positive patient without furnishing a medical examination and either necessary stabilization or a medically appropriate transfer, raises a potential EMTALA claim. In addition, had his partner driven Mr. Pool to a public hospital that accepted the case, that hospital might have a claim against the "dumping" facility (Box 4-1).

CIVIL RIGHTS LAWS

Title VI of the Civil Rights Act of 1964

The Civil Rights Act, established civil rights protections in "places of public accommodation" such as restaurants, hotels, and public transportation systems, prohibits discrimination based on race or national origin by "recipients of federal assistance" (42 USC §2000d (2004)). "Federal assistance" covers grant programs such as Medicare, Medicaid, and grants under the Public Health Service Act (e.g., health professions training grants and health center grants). Physicians whose participation in federal assistance programs is limited to fee-for-service payments under Medicare Part B are not treated as federal financial recipients; the basis for this exemption is purely historical and exists nowhere in the statute.[8]

Box 4-1. Examples of Confirmed EMTALA Violations

Nature of Violation	Examples
Failure to provide appropriate transfer and keep log	• A bicycle accident victim was transferred without a screening exam or entry into the central log. The hospital told the rescue crew that the patient should go to another hospital because he met trauma criteria when he did not meet the criteria. The hospital also did not contact or send records to the receiving hospital.
Failure to screen, stabilize, and keep log	• A patient with end-stage renal disease was discharged without being stabilized and died 6 hours later. • A motor vehicle accident victim was not stabilized and became paralyzed in the emergency room. • An uninsured patient with suicidal symptoms was put into a taxi for transfer to another hospital without being examined. • An insured patient with a rash received screening while an uninsured patient with the same symptoms was sent to a clinic without screening. • A patient from a skilled nursing facility was diagnosed with pneumonia and medicated but sent back to the skilled nursing facility without a physician determination that he was stable; he returned later in worse condition and died.
Failure to meet receiving responsibilities, follow procedures, and provide appropriate transfer	• A hospital refused to accept transfer of an unstable patient with multiple traumas from a motor vehicle accident. • A possible sexual assault victim who arrived in an ambulance was sent to another hospital without screening, and there was no evidence in the record that the receiving hospital was notified or had agreed to accept the patient.

Adapted from: United States General Accounting Office Report to Congressional Committees. EMERGENCY CARE. EMTALA: Implementation and Enforcement Issues. Washington, DC: GAO-01-747, June 22, 2001.

Under Title VI, the concept of "discrimination" covers both acts of intentional segregation and exclusion, as well as practices that have *the effect* of subjecting persons to segregation and exclusion. As a result of a US Supreme Court decision issued in 2001, private individuals can sue to remedy intentional acts of discrimination, but only the federal government can enforce the *de facto* (i.e., effects) test.[13]

Conduct that might be considered as potentially in violation of the *de facto* test are segregating hospital or nursing home patients by source of payment (e.g., maintaining an "all-Medicaid" floor) or, in the case of a Health Maintenance Organization (HMO), which enrolls both privately insured and Medicaid insured persons, allowing network specialists to refuse to accept Medicaid referrals or referrals from primary care network providers in practice at health centers or other clinical care arrangements serving the poor.

The Department of Health and Human Service's (HHS) Office for Civil Rights has issued guidelines applicable to federal assistance recipients that require recipients to make their services accessible to patients with limited English-speaking abilities.[14] The guidelines offer a range of compliance approaches for providing both oral and written interpretation and translation services. Federal recipients decide which services to provide by using a four-factor test that weighs the number of limited English people served, the frequency they come into contact with a particular program or service, the nature and importance of the activity, and the resources available. In addition, the guidelines provide incentives for compliance by permitting affected organizations to secure certification of compliance. Facilities considered by HHS to be in compliance with the law have an additional and strong defense when individuals file complaints about the lack of services accessible to persons with limited English-speaking abilities.

James Geary, a pediatrician in private practice, decides to reduce his caseload as he approaches retirement. When deciding which patients he will continue to see, he first considers finances. He will no longer provide care to any Medicaid or uninsured children because they do not pay his full rate. In addition, he decides to eliminate several children with autism and Tourette's syndrome because he does not like to be around their outbursts and unusual movements.

The Americans with Disabilities Act

The Americans with Disabilities Act (ADA) and its companion, Section 504 of the Rehabilitation Act (29 USCA §794 (West 2004), prohibit discrimination against qualified persons with disabilities. As with Title VI, the ADA reaches both private and public conduct and both intentional discrimination and *de facto* conduct that result in discrimination. Unlike Title VI, however, the ADA reaches not only private conduct by entities that receive federal financial assistance (e.g., hospitals that accept Medicaid), but also private actors who receive no public funds. Thus, a dentist in private practice who takes no public funds of any sort is prohibited from discriminating against a qualified person with a disability just as would be a public hospital or health center.[4] Public programs of care are also covered by the ADA, as well as by its older legislative companion, Section 504.

Under the ADA, a disability is defined as a physical or mental impairment that significantly affects functioning in one or more areas of life activities (certain limitations apply, particularly in the employment context) (42 USCA §12101–12213).[15] A "qualified person with a disability" is a person who meets the requirements of the service or the program, with or without provision of any reasonable accommodations to make the program accessible. For example, a person who receives Supplemental Security Income (SSI) cash assistance for a disability is automatically qualified for Medicaid and thus is entitled to ADA protections against discriminatory treatment by Medicaid agencies. Similarly, an SSI recipient with a serious mental disability who lives in a health center's service area is considered to meet the center's eligibility rules and therefore can not be denied the center's services because she has a mental disability. A physician, hospital, or clinic dentist cannot arbitrarily refuse to treat a person who is HIV positive or has a mental illness, although a health provider may refuse treatment if there is a reasonable basis to deem a patient a public threat (which the provider would have to prove).[4] Similarly, states cannot administer Medicaid in ways that effectively confine persons with disabilities to medically unnecessary institutional settings as a condition for receiving covered services.[16] Dr. Geary, in the earlier example, is within his rights to refuse to take Medicaid or uninsured patients because there is no right to health care and discrimination based on poverty is legal. However, the ADA makes it illegal for him to arbitrarily refuse to care for the children who have autism or Tourette's syndrome (assuming he is qualified to care for them).

LEGAL OBLIGATIONS OF HILL BURTON FACILITIES

The Hill Burton Act (whose official title is the Hospital Survey and Construction Act of 1946) financed the construction and modernization of thousands of health care facilities. In exchange for their receipt of federal funds, facilities promised to provide a reasonable volume of uncompensated care to persons unable to pay (the uncompensated care obligation), as well as to serve the communities in which they were located (the community service obligation).[1] Hill Burton is the only US health law that ties its prohibitions to low socioeconomic status as opposed to race or disability.

The Hill Burton program's uncompensated care obligation was time-limited, and all such obligations have now expired. However, the community service obligation is perpetual; as a result, its provisions are still applicable. Under the community service obligation, facilities must furnish emergency care without regard to ability to pay (an obligation that parallels the later EMTALA legislation). More significantly, Hill Burton facilities are prohibited from discriminating in the provision of services on the basis of public insurance status. Therefore, facilities built with Hill Burton funds must make their services accessible to Medicaid beneficiaries.

LAWS THAT FINANCE HEALTH CARE FOR UNDERSERVED POPULATIONS

Federal and state governments have enacted laws to provide for investment in programs funding health care access. Laws that authorize expenditures for health care access also carry obligations for the entities that receive grant funds or payments. These obligations typically are enforceable by public oversight agencies but not individual patients. Examples of such laws are state and local laws authorizing the establishment and funding of public health agencies, state and local laws that create public hospitals and "health care districts," and federal laws authorizing the expenditure of funds to establish sources of health care. An example of a legal obligation connected to the receipt of grant funds is the obligation contained in most programs authorized under the Public Health Service (PHS) Act programs, which requires grantees to participate in Medicaid (Public Health Service Act, 42 USC §§254d-254c-18 (2004)). Medicaid participation is a requirement for health centers, as well as for Ryan White Care Act grantees, grant and loan recipients under the National Health Service Corps (Public Health Service Act, 42 USC §§254d–254t (2004)), and clinics funded under Title X (family planning clinics). Of course, PHS Act grantees are among the nation's most important sources of health care for Medicaid recipients. In 2002, for example, urban and rural health centers served over 4 million Medicaid beneficiaries, or approximately 10% of all Medicaid enrollees.[17]

Federal and state laws creating and financing the actual provision of health care typically share a number of common features, such as an obligation to serve certain populations or communities, an obligation to provide certain specific services as a condition of funding, and an obligation to serve low-income people free of charge or for a nominal fee. Federally funded health centers have a unique obligation to govern their operations using community boards with a majority of its members being actual patients of the health center.

MEDICAID: HEALTH CARE FINANCING FOR THE POOR

MEDICAID'S ROLE IN HEALTH CARE FINANCING FOR THE POOR

Medicaid is unique among US laws with respect to the rights that it confers on poor and underserved populations and the corresponding obligations it imposes on state Medicaid programs in exchange for the hundreds of billions of dollars it pays out annually. Thus, an understanding of the basic elements of Medicaid's eligibility and coverage requirements are critical to properly serving medically underserved and vulnerable populations.

Eligibility

Persons eligible for coverage are entitled to apply for coverage and to have their eligibility determined with reasonable promptness (42 CFR §435.930(a)(2001). In contrast, nonentitlement programs such as the State Children's Health Insurance Program (SCHIP) can set limits on the number of eligible people to be served. In this latter situation, individuals who meet eligibility criteria nonetheless can be turned away for coverage, with their names placed on a waiting list in states that maintain such lists (in a number of states, individuals simply would be told to reapply at some future date) (Box 4-2).[18]

Special vigilance is advisable in the case of patients who are Medicare beneficiaries. This is because millions of low-income Medicare beneficiaries (including all beneficiaries who receive SSI cash benefits) are also entitled to Medicaid and are known as "dual enrollees."[19] Medicaid covers many services that are not covered by Medicare. Also, Medicaid will pay the Medicare premium and deductible (and in some cases, the coinsurance). As of January 2006, when Medicare Part D prescription drug coverage took full effect, outpatient prescription drug coverage is no longer a Medicaid benefit for "dual enrollees," with very limited exceptions. Instead, these individuals are eligible for special subsidies that enable them to enroll in Medicare Part D plans; these special subsidies also cover Part D patient cost sharing and deductible responsibilities.

> Miriam Rodriguez has no legal US status and has been in the country for 4 years. She is pregnant. She has no health insurance and comes to your clinic for prenatal care. She has a number of health complications that will require that she receive specialty care during the pregnancy, and you already know that she will need a scheduled caesarean section delivery. You want her to enroll in Medicaid now in order to have a means to manage her specialty and inpatient care, including preregistration for delivery. You are deeply concerned about the quality of the care she will be able to receive from you in the absence of coverage.

Barriers to Medicaid Enrollment

State residency status is frequently cited as a barrier to Medicaid enrollment. It is important to remember that states cannot demand a permanent home address as a condition of eligibility, and thus cannot deny coverage to otherwise eligible homeless persons.[19] Similarly, migrant workers are considered to be residents of the state in which they are working or seeking work, and therefore can apply for coverage even as they travel.[19] A state with a large migrant population also can provide coverage on an out-of-state basis as families travel, just as private insurance can offer out-of-state coverage (see Chap. 25).

Legal status is one of the thorniest issues in Medicaid. The 1996 welfare reform legislation significantly restricted Medicaid eligibility for legal immigrants.[20] Persons who are otherwise eligible for benefits (e.g., low-income children and pregnant women), but who are

---

Box 4-2. Low-Income Patients Likely to Qualify for Medicaid

- Children under 18
- Women who are pregnant
- Working parents (particularly single mothers) of children
- Patients with very severe physical and mental disabilities
- Elderly patients

either undocumented persons or short-term (<5 years) legal residents are entitled to coverage only for emergency care.[19] Miriam, the undocumented immigrant who has been in the country less than 5 years, falls into this gap in Medicaid coverage. Even if Miriam would otherwise qualify for Medicaid as a poor pregnant resident, she is not eligible for full Medicaid benefits. Under the new law, the most Miriam may receive through Medicaid is emergency care, not the prenatal care to address her pregnancy complications or a prescheduled caesarean section. Once immigrants eligible for Medicaid attain long-term legal status, states may elect to provide federally assisted Medicaid coverage (nearly all have done so).[19] As of 2003, 19 states pay for prenatal care using state funds only for pregnant women who do not meet the legal status test applicable to full Medicaid coverage.

The problem of status as a *"public charge"* is a very serious one in immigration law, and has profound ramifications for eligibility in certain public assistance programs. The law defines a "public charge" as a person who is unable to support him- or herself and therefore depends on public cash assistance for income through programs such as Supplemental Security Income, Temporary Assistance to Needy Families, or General Assistance. Immigration officials consider whether people are likely to become a "public charge" when deciding whether they may enter the country or become permanent residents. In some instances, an immigrant may be deported if he or she becomes a "public charge" within 5 years of entry in the United States.

In an attempt to encourage Medicaid enrollment of eligible legally resident families,[21] guidelines issued by the Department of Justice in 1999 provide that receipt of Medicaid in a noninstitutional context does not constitute evidence of being a "public charge" for the purpose of determining who will be permitted to remain in the United States. Similarly, Department of Justice guidelines emphasize that the use of health centers and other public clinics by immigrants does not in any way affect their legal status, because such community services are not considered to be the type of means-tested public benefits that are barred to immigrants as a result of the 1996 welfare reform amendments.[21] Even so, as a result of fear and confusion about the law, many eligible immigrants do not seek health care because they do not want to risk being considered a "public charge."[22]

Persons who are found eligible for coverage must be furnished with their assistance with "reasonable promptness" and have the right to remain enrolled until they are no longer eligible for coverage (eligibility cannot be arbitrarily ended) (Furnishing Medicaid, in 42 CFR §435.930(b) 2001). In addition, when eligibility is denied or terminated, individuals have the right to a "fair hearing."

> You are managing the health care of Simon, a little boy born with cerebral palsy, who has both gross motor and speech delays. You want to order physical and speech therapy for him. He is insured by Medicaid. The Medicaid managed care organization of which he is a member denies your treatment request, telling you that because children with cerebral palsy cannot "recover" from their conditions, the company does not consider his care medically necessary. The company tells you that when the child enters school, "the school system will have to give him something."

Benefits and Coverage

Persons who are enrolled in the program are entitled to a defined set of benefits, known collectively as "medical assistance." In the case of children under 21, coverage is unusually broad, encompassing not only a wide array of preventive benefits (checkups, all recommended immunizations, vision, dental, and hearing care) but services and treatments needed to "ameliorate" mental and physical conditions. This special set of benefits is known as Early and Periodic Screening Diagnosis and Treatment (EPSDT) (Medical assistance, in 42 USC §1396d(a)(4)(B)). Simon, the boy with cerebral palsy, is entitled to coverage under EPSDT. Because EPSDT requires states to provide services to both cure and *ameliorate* children's medical conditions, a Medicaid agency is obligated to pay for full care for the child, even if its contract with the managed care organization allows the company to deny any services not needed to "cure" an illness or injury. Thus, a child enrolled in Medicaid remains entitled to all medically necessary EPSDT "ameliorative" care. Even if his or her managed care plan does not directly pay for the care, the Medicaid agency must do so. For this reason, appealing denials of necessary care for Medicaid beneficiaries, particularly children, is important.

In the case of adults, states may impose much stricter coverage limits and more stringent medical necessity definitions. Other than the "ameliorate" language of EPSDT, the Medicaid statute does not define "medical necessity" (42 CFR §440.230(d)). As a result, states have attempted to narrow coverage by adopting restrictive definitions of "medical necessity." Even though adult coverage is more limited, the breadth of benefits is substantial, and state agencies are prohibited from using unreasonable benefit limits or arbitrarily discriminating against persons with specific health conditions in the provision of required benefits (42 CFR §440.230 (1998)). Thus, for example, a state agency could not refuse to pay for medical care for psychiatric conditions while covering physician care for physical health problems.

The same fair hearing rules that apply to the denial of eligibility also apply to denials of specific types of coverage. As a consequence, health professionals working with medically underserved populations should be energetic in protesting denials of what they consider to involve medically necessary patient treatment. Advocacy for patients encompasses locating help in appealing coverage denials (e.g., legal services, or law firms in the community that take *pro bono* cases) and as importantly, providing expert written statements or, when necessary, oral testimony about the medical necessity of prescribed care (see Chap. 41). The right to appeal denials applies regardless of whether the denial comes from the state agency itself or from a managed care organization acting on the state's behalf.

Common Pitfalls in Understanding Legal Issues in Care of the Underserved

- With the exception of certain limited services related to medical emergencies, there is no legal right to health care in the United States.
- The government regulates health care in part through laws that set standards for federal programs such as Medicare, Medicaid, health centers, and the Ryan White Care Act. States may set standards through licensing and insurance laws.
- Physicians and other health professionals can legally choose not to treat patients who are poor (i.e., cannot pay or are covered by Medicaid or Medicare), but they cannot arbitrarily discriminate based on patient disability. Federal law does not prohibit physicians who participate in Medicare Part B only from selecting their patients based on race or national origin.
- Many immigrants mistakenly believe that use of public clinics or receipt of Medicaid may constitute evidence of being a "public charge" and undermine their bid for obtaining legal standing or citizenship.
- A health care provider may be liable for injuries caused by substandard health care that falls below the professional standard of care, even if the substandard care is the result in part of the poor quality coverage rules and decisions of a patient's HMO or managed care plan.

HEALTH CARE QUALITY

In general, health professionals have no legal obligation to furnish care to any person (known as no legal duty of care). Exceptions are hospital emergency care situations such as those described in the preceding, or

in which a provider is part of a managed care provider network and thus is contractually obligated to treat plan members. However, once a health professional accepts a patient into practice, he or she owes the patient a *duty to furnish health care of reasonable quality*. This duty sometimes is referred to as the "professional standard of care."

PROFESSIONAL STANDARD OF CARE

The *professional standard of care* guides the law of health care quality in all states. The professional standard of care is highly case-specific and factually intensive. In legal proceedings involving medical malpractice claims, whether or not a health professional has satisfied the professional standard of care (and even what that standard will be in any particular case) are questions of fact to be proved through the use of expert testimony as well as valid, relevant, and reliable evidence from studies and research. Failure to meet the standard of care can result in liability for injuries that are a reasonably foreseeable result of professional negligence.[1]

The law measures professional negligence under a *unitary standard* of conduct and without setting different standards of care for different populations based on the availability of resources.[23] Further, the failure of a health professional to "comply without protest" with a denial of coverage by a utilization review entity can result in provider liability if the provider acquiesces with a decision that he or she knows to be medically inappropriate.[24] Thus, for example, if a Medicaid HMO were to order the premature and medically inappropriate discharge of a hospitalized patient, and the physician were to acquiesce without an appeal and sign the discharge papers, it would be the physician (perhaps ironically) who could be sued for malpractice if the patient suffers injury or death. From the law's perspective, it is the physician who has the fiduciary medical relationship with the patient, and it is the physician who has broad powers over the patient's discharge.

LEGAL LIABILITY IN THE CONTEXT OF CARE FOR MEDICALLY UNDERSERVED POPULATIONS

Despite the apparent severity of these legal standards, the law is less harsh than would first appear. Courts have recognized that health professionals who understand the proper standard of care but are unable to meet it despite reasonable efforts consistent with the special nature of the physician–patient relationship, should not face liability.[25] In other words, the key to a defense in a professional liability action involving an indigent and vulnerable patient whose failure to receive proper care is the result of the larger problem of financing and access, would be the ability to demonstrate—through detailed medical records and notes and the written description of conduct—recognition of the proper standard of care, as well as an *active and energetic effort* to secure the proper level of care for the patient. Such efforts might include arranging assistance with a Medicaid application, protesting the denial of coverage and actively helping in an appeal, intervening with hospital administrators in opposition to pressure to discharge indigent patients, and other actions that demonstrate a real effort to "do the right thing."

In the case of patient self-determination over matters such as continued medical care in the face of futility, the right to refuse medical treatment, and the right to health information privacy, the law treats low-income persons as it would any other patient population. Correspondingly, physicians who care for medically underserved populations operate under the same legal obligations relating to these rights as they apply to any other of their patients.[1] These obligations may raise additional challenges where language is a barrier. Physicians must ensure that their patients' medical records properly document not only their communications with patients, but also their active effort to secure proper interpretation and translation services to ensure that communication is effective.

CONCLUSION

There is no legal right to health care under US law. At the same time, there is a set of statutes that enable access in medical emergencies and prohibit certain forms of health care discrimination. American law also creates important rights in health care financing. These rights are limited to certain defined categories of poor and medically indigent persons, and there is no federal law that creates coverage rights in all low-income persons. Health professionals should be familiar with the various statutory schemes not only because of their value to patients, but also because active efforts to pursue patient rights may be essential to avoiding claims of legal liability.

The law is so important to access and financing rights that some safety net providers have gone so far as to embed legal services into their programs. Other strategies might be the identification of community legal services programs and sources of *pro bono* legal assistance (a source of help in this regard may be local bar associations).

Where professional liability is concerned, health care safety net providers, like health providers generally, are extensively engaged in risk management. The more energetic the effort on the part of safety net providers to assist patients to secure access to care, the stronger the evidence that their practice is consistent with rigorous standards of patient care quality.

KEY CONCEPTS

- There is no legal right to health care in the United States.
- The federal government protects health through the court enforcement of laws and regulating programs supported by federal funding.
- Access to care issues, for example, are addressed through the following:
—EMTALA requires provision of medical care to everyone for emergency conditions by any institution receiving Medicare funding.
—Title VI of the Civil Rights Act of 1964 prohibits racial and ethnic discrimination by those who are recipients of governmental funding.
—HHS requires interpretive services for funded institutions seeing patients who speak little English.
—The Americans with Disabilities Act and Section 504 of the Rehabilitation Act prohibit both public and private discrimination of those with a disability.
—Medicaid, the major public program that helps address access to care issues, provides due process and antidiscrimination protections.
—Programs such as health centers and the Ryan White Care Act that fund health care for medically underserved or vulnerable persons as well as state and local laws establishing public hospitals.
- State government contributes to protecting the health and welfare of its citizens through the regulation of health care providers.
- Courts determine the meaning of laws, enforce legal rights, provide remedies to individuals, and have substantive law-making powers under the principles of common law.
- Health professionals have no legal duty to provide care in most situations.
- Providers owe their patients the accepted professional standard of care, even if that care is not covered.
- Providers must make an active effort to obtain the appropriate level of care for their patients or are potentially liable for the poor care their patients receive.

CORE COMPETENCY
Challenging Service Denials and Delayed Review Decisions

- Establish what the procedures are for the health care system or payer whose service denial you wish to challenge.
- Follow an *expedited* review procedure if you believe that the denial or the delay in service could have rapid and harmful effects on your patient.
- Use health care provider hotlines or other methods of direct contact when you are dealing with a delayed review decision.

Key tips:
  - ✓ Provide full, relevant clinical data to the agent denying the service.
  - ✓ Explain the reasons why alternatives will not work for your patient. Be specific as to whether the proposed alternative solutions have been tried and failed; or why they cannot be tried.
  - ✓ Describe the health consequences of denying the service. Use medical literature and/or expert opinion to support your claim.
  - ✓ Pay close attention to required forms and fill them out completely. Incomplete information can delay services for your patient.
  - ✓ Ascertain if you are dealing with a delayed review decision.
  - ✓ If your attempts to reverse a denial of service fail:
- Assist your patient in appealing the denial when possible (e.g., additional supporting information that might be needed for the appeal).
- If you do not believe that alternatives are reasonable
  - ✓ Document your efforts to challenge a denial of service in patient's chart.
  - ✓ Seek legal counsel and notify risk management at site of care.
  - ✓ Refuse to execute orders flowing from a denial (e.g., discharging a patient after additional hospital days have been refused) that you do not believe are clinically indicated.

DISCUSSION QUESTIONS

1. What role should the courts play? In what ways might the courts protect you as you serve vulnerable populations? For what reasons might the courts restrict or punish you?
2. Should there be a general right to health care in the United States? Should there be a general legal duty to provide care? How do your answers to these questions conflict or complement each other?
3. What, if anything, should providers do, legally and ethically, to improve access to care for vulnerable populations?

RESOURCES

http://www.kff.org
  Kaiser Family Foundation and the Kaiser Commission for Medicaid and the Uninsured

http://www.healthlaw.org
  National Health Law Program

http://www.hhs.gov
  United States Dept of Health and Human Services

http://www.urban.org
  The Urban Institute

REFERENCES

1. Rosenblatt R, Law S, Rosenbaum S. *Law and the American health care system.* Westbury, NY: Foundation Press, 1997.
2. American Medical Association. Principles of Medical Ethics. 2001. Accessed December 24, 2004. Available at: http://www.amaassn.org/ama/pub/category/2512.html
3. *Howe v Hull,* 874 F Supp 779 (ND Ohio 1994).
4. *Bragdon v Abbot,* 524 US 624 (1998).
5. *Brown v Board of Education,* 349 US 294 (1954).
6. *Shelly v Kraemer,* 334 US 1 (1948).
7. Smedley BD, Stith A, Nelson A, eds. *Unequal treatment: Confronting racial and ethnic disparities in health care.* National Academy Press: Washington, DC, 2003.
8. Smith DB. *Health care divided: Race and healing a nation.* Ann Arbor, MI: University of Michigan Press, 1999.
9. Schoenman J, Feldman J. *Results of the Medicare Payment Advisory Commission's 2002 survey of physicians.* Bethesda, MD: The Project HOPE Center for Health Affairs, 2002.
10. Institute of Medicine. Committee on Consequences of Uninsurance. *Coverage matters: Insurance and health care.* Washington, DC: National Academy Press, 2001.
11. Rosenbaum S, Teitelbaum J. Civil rights enforcement in the modern healthcare system: Reinvigorating the role of the federal government in the aftermath of Alexander v. Sandoval. *Yale J Health Policy Law Ethics* 2003;3: 215–252.
12. Emergency Medical Treatment and Labor Act of 1986 (renamed Examination and Treatment for Emergency Medical Conditions and Women in Labor Act in 1987), 42 USC §1395dd. 2004. (PL 99-272. The Omnibus Budget Reconciliation Act of 1989 deleted the word "active" from the title of EMTALA. Sec. 6211(h)(2)(c) of PL 101-239.
13. Alexander v. Sandoval, 532 US 275, 2001.
14. Guidance to Federal Financial Assistance Recipients Regarding Title VI Prohibition Against National Origin Discrimination Affecting Limited English Proficient Persons, in 68 Fed. Reg. 2003.47311–47323.
15. Americans with Disabilities Act (ADA) 42 USCA §§12101–12213 (West 2004).
16. Olmstead v. L.C., 527, US 581 (1999).
17. Rosenbaum S, Shin P, Darnell J. *Economic stress and the safety net: A Health Center Update, June 2004.* Kaiser Commission on Medicaid and the Uninsured. Accessed April 4, 2004. Available at: http://www.kff.org/uninsured/loader.cfm?url=/commonspot/security/getfile.cfm&PageID=42089

18. Kaiser Commission on Medicaid and the Uninsured. *Health Coverage for Low Income Children.* 2004. Accessed December 24, 2004. Available at: http://www.kff.org/uninsured/loader.cfm?url=/commonspot/security/getfile.cfm&PageID=46994

19. Schneider A, Elias R, Garfield E, et al. *The Medicaid resource book.* Washington, DC: Kaiser Commission on Medicaid and the Uninsured, 2002.

20. National Immigration Law Center. *Overview of immigrant eligibility for public programs.* Accessed December 24, 2004. Available at: http://www.nilc.org/immspbs/special/ovrvw_imm_ elig_fed_pgms_031904.pdf

21. National Immigration Law Center. *Administration clarifies public charge policy for immigrants who use health care and other safety net programs.* Accessed December 24, 2004. Available at: http://www.nilc.org/immspbs/bu/ebupdate994.htm#Highlights

22. Kaiser Commission on Medicaid and the Uninsured. *Immigrants' health care coverage and access.* August, 2004. Accessed April 1, 2005. Available at: http://www.kff.org/uninsured/loader.cfm?url=/commonspot/security/getfile.cfm&PageID=1551

23. Shilkret v. Annapolis Emergency Hospital, 349 A 2d.245, 249-250 (Md. 1975).

24. Wickline v. State, 239 Cal. Rptr. 810 (Cal. App. 1986).

25. Hall v. Hilbun, 466 So.2d.856 (Miss. 1985).

Chapter 5

Principles in the Ethical Care of Underserved Patients

Bernard Lo, MD

Objectives

- Identify the ethical dilemmas that commonly arise in the clinical care of medically underserved patients and populations.
- Review the ethical guidelines that should guide the physician's approach to such dilemmas and how to resolve them.
- Summarize what special responsibilities arise for physicians in the care of underserved patients

Eradicating the disparities in health and health care that exist between the world's rich and poor is medicine's biggest ethical challenge. As people advocate for the societal changes that this will require, they must also assure that the vulnerable patients actually cared for receive high-quality, ethical, and compassionate care. Providing this high-quality, ethical care can be challenging. Health care providers caring for underserved populations must act ethically in a health care system that has serious ethical shortcomings in access to and quality of care. Moreover, underserved patients frequently are members of ethnic and cultural groups whose decision-making customs may differ from those of white, middle class populations in the United States. In addition, underserved patients often have low health literacy or are educationally disadvantaged. Thus, to participate actively in their medical decisions and care they may need additional assistance to gain sufficient understanding of their medical situation. Mistrust of the health care system may be a potent, but unacknowledged, force in decision making.

FUNDAMENTAL ETHICAL GUIDELINES

Physicians should follow three fundamental but frequently conflicting ethical guidelines: justice, respect for persons, and acting in the patient's best interests.

JUSTICE

The term "justice" is used in a general sense to mean fairness: People should receive what they deserve. In addition, it is important to act consistently in cases that are similar in ethically relevant ways. Otherwise, decisions would be arbitrary, biased, and unfair. Justice forbids discrimination in health care based on race, religion, or gender and supports a moral right to health care, with access based on medical need rather than social or economic status.

Strong philosophical arguments support the idea that all persons should have access to a decent level of health care regardless of ability to pay; however, this is an aspiration rather than established public policy in the United States. Unlike most other countries, the United States does not recognize a legal right to health care (see Chap. 4). Clinicians face difficult dilemmas if patients with clear need for medical care cannot pay for medications, tests, or hospitalizations. In health care settings, justice often refers to the allocation of health care resources. Allocation decisions are unavoidable because resources are limited and could be spent on other social goods, such as education or affordable housing.

RESPECT FOR PERSONS

Treating patients with respect entails several ethical obligations. First, health care providers must accept the medical decisions of persons who are informed and acting freely. Individuals place different values on health, medical care, and risk. Hence, competent, informed patients have the power to reject their clinicians' recommendations about care; otherwise, their integrity and liberty are violated. More broadly, patients should have the right to choose among feasible options and share decision making with health care providers, because in most clinical settings different goals and approaches are possible, outcomes are uncertain, and an intervention may cause both benefits and harms.[1] Thus, allowing people to be active participants in decisions about their medical care respects their self-determination. In addition to respecting the decisions of autonomous patients, clinicians should take steps to promote patient autonomy, by disclosing information and helping patients deliberate.

A second meaning of respect pertains to patients whose decision-making capacity is impaired. Physicians should still treat them as persons with individual characteristics, preferences, and values. Decisions should follow their preferences and values, so far as they are known. In addition, all patients, whether autonomous or not, should be treated with compassion and dignity.

Respect also is related to other important ethical guidelines, such as avoiding misrepresentation, maintaining confidentiality, and keeping promises. Breaches of these other guidelines cause wrong or harm to patients and compromise their autonomy.

Informed Consent

Informed consent involves more than obtaining the patient's signature on consent forms. Clinicians must discuss with patients the nature of the proposed care, alternatives, risks and benefits of each, and likely consequences and obtain the patient's agreement to care.[2] Health care providers need to educate patients, answer their questions, make recommendations, and help them deliberate. Patients can be overwhelmed with medical jargon, needlessly complicated explanations, or too much information at once. Because underserved patients often have poor health literacy or may not speak English fluently, taking additional steps to help these patients make informed decisions (e.g., spending more time discussing unfamiliar medical terms and concepts and working with interpreters) is crucial (see Chaps. 9, 10, and 39).

The doctrine of informed consent means that adult patients may make decisions that differ from what health care providers recommend or what their families want them to do. Indeed, patients may refuse treatment that may save or prolong their lives, provided their decisions are informed and voluntary.

In many cultures, patients traditionally are not told of a diagnosis of cancer or other serious illness (see Chap. 22). In these cultures, disclosure of a grave diagnosis is believed to cause patients to suffer, whereas withholding information promotes serenity, security, and hope.[3] Being direct and explicit may be considered insensitive and cruel. Families and physicians may try to protect the patient by taking on decision-making responsibility.[4,5] Family members from such a cultural background may ask the provider not to tell the patient a serious diagnosis, or even to deceive the patient into believing that there is nothing seriously wrong. Patients should not be forced to receive information against their will, even in the name of promoting informed decisions. However, the crucial ethical issue is whether the individual patient wants to know his or her diagnosis, not what most people from that cultural heritage would want. Many individuals in these groups want to know their diagnosis and prognosis, even if they are terminally ill. Therefore, health care providers should ask patients how they want decisions to be made, saying that their usual practice is to provide information and make decisions together with patients, while offering patients the option not to be told information or turn over decision making to someone else. Respecting the choices of the patient regarding the decision-making process are important (see Core Competency).

Emergency Care

Informed consent is not required when patients cannot give consent and delay of treatment would place life or health in peril. People are presumed to want such emergency care unless they have previously indicated otherwise.

Futile Interventions

Autonomy does not entitle patients to insist on whatever care they want. Providers are not obligated to provide futile interventions that have no physiologic rationale or have already failed.[6,7] For example, cardiopulmonary resuscitation would be futile in a patient with progressive hypotension despite maximal therapy. However, clinicians should be wary of using the term "futile" in looser senses to justify unilateral decisions to forgo interventions when they believe that the probability of success is too low, no worthwhile goals can be achieved, the patient's quality of life is unacceptable, or the costs are too high. Such looser usages of the term are problematic because they may be inconsistent and mask inappropriate important value judgments.

Maintaining Confidentiality

Confidentiality respects patients' autonomy and privacy, encourages them to seek treatment and discuss their problems candidly, and prevents discrimination. However, maintaining confidentiality is not an absolute rule. Confidentiality may be overridden in certain situations to prevent serious harm to third parties or the patient.[8] The law may require physicians to override confidentiality in order to protect third parties, for example, public health reporting of tuberculosis and syphilis. In other situations, medical providers have a legal duty to report victims of elder abuse, child abuse, and domestic violence. These exceptions to confidentiality are justified because the risk is serious and probable, there are no less restrictive measures to avert risk, the adverse effects of overriding confidentiality are minimized, and these adverse effects are deemed acceptable by society.[33]

The recent Health Insurance Portability and Accountability Act (HIPAA) health privacy regulations have heightened awareness of the importance of confidentiality. The HIPAA regulations are not meant to inhibit transmission of information needed for patient treatment. Disclosure of patient information to other health care providers for the purposes of treatment without having the patient sign an authorization form is permissible.[34]

Avoiding Deception

Health care providers sometimes consider using lies or deception in order to protect the patient from bad news or obtain benefits for the patient. Lying refers to statements that the speaker knows are false and that are intended to mislead the listener. Deception, which is broader, may be defined as statements and actions that are intended to mislead the listener, whether or not they are literally true.[33] For example, the health care provider may tell a patient that she has a "small growth" so that she does not think she has cancer. Or the provider may complete and sign a form for a patient to get a bus pass, even though he does not meet the criteria for physical disability. Although deception under these circumstances may be motivated by a desire to help the patient, it is ethically problematic. Deception violates autonomy because the person who is deceived cannot make informed decisions if he or she receives misleading information. Furthermore, deception undermines social trust because people cannot trust that other statements by the speaker are truthful.[9] If clinicians are

known to use deception in some situations to help patients, they also may use it in other situations for other purposes, for instance, to deceive patients as well as third parties. It is especially problematic for them to lie or intentionally deceive others because the relationship between health care providers and patients and society depends on trust.

ACTING IN THE BEST INTERESTS OF PATIENTS

The guideline of beneficence requires clinicians to act for patients' benefit.[10] Lay people do not possess medical expertise and may be vulnerable because of their illness. They justifiably rely on medical providers to provide sound advice and promote their well-being. Medical professionals encourage such trust. Hence, clinicians have a fiduciary duty to act in the best interests of their patients. The interests of the patient should prevail over physicians', other providers', or third parties' (e.g., hospitals' or insurers') interests. These fiduciary obligations contrast sharply with business relationships, which are characterized by "let the buyer beware," not by trust and reliance.

The guideline of "do no harm" forbids physicians from providing ineffective interventions or acting without due care.[11] Although often cited, this precept often provides only limited guidance, because many beneficial interventions may have serious risks. The challenge is to provide interventions whose benefits outweigh the risks and whose risks are acceptable; both of these determinations need to be made from the perspective of the patient.

Unwise Patient Decisions

Patients' refusals of care may thwart their own goals or cause them serious harm. For example, a patient with shortness of breath caused by a severe asthma exacerbation may refuse treatment with bronchodilators and corticosteroids. Simple acceptance of such refusals, in the name of respecting patient autonomy, is ethically problematic. Acting in the patient's best interests requires eliciting patients' expectations and concerns, correcting misunderstandings, and trying to persuade them to accept highly beneficial therapies. If disagreements persist after discussions, the patient's informed choices and view of his or her best interests should prevail. Although refusing recommended, highly beneficial care does not render a patient incompetent, it may appropriately lead the physician to probe further to ensure that the patient is able to make informed decisions.

Helping Patients Gain Access to Care

Because health care resources for underserved patients are often constrained, health care providers may need to serve as advocates for their patients to help them get needed medical care (see Chap. 41). As advocates, providers intercede for or speak on behalf of their patients.[12] Advocacy should be based on sound clinical judgment and evidence. It is not doing whatever the patient requests or whatever the provider believes would be beneficial.

Advocating for a patient is fair only if it also would be appropriate for others to advocate for other patients in similar situations. For instance, patients may not be able to afford a prescribed medication, or they may be refused coverage for needed in-home services or physical therapy. Those who claim that their responsibility is only to order medically appropriate tests and treatments have a very restricted view of their professional responsibility. Indeed, patients receive little good if they face insurmountable barriers to obtaining ordered care. Thus, in addition to ordering tests and writing prescriptions, clinicians need to talk with patients about practical barriers to obtaining ordered care. Advocating for systems of care that eradicate these barriers is important to assuring all patients receive ethical care.

Furthermore, patients may lack shelter or other necessities. The concept of beneficence should be interpreted broadly to include not only medical tests and treatments, but also other goods, such as shelter, food, and clothing, the lack of which can adversely affect health. Referring patients to appropriate social service agencies and complete the administrative paperwork required to apply for social services or financial assistance is an important aspect of medical care.

Limits to Acting on Behalf of the Patient

The ethical obligation to act in the best interests of patients and be an advocate for them is not absolute or open ended.[13] Health care providers should be altruistic, but are not expected to be saints. Physicians cannot guarantee that they can obtain needed assistance for patients. Although often the point of contact for underserved patients with social institutions, it is unrealistic for clinicians to feel they are responsible for correcting all the injustices their patients encounter. Nor are they expected to use their personal resources to help patients fulfill their needs. Indeed to buy food for patients or to allow patients to share their homes would raise ethical problems by violating the boundaries of the doctor–patient relationship. Acting in the patient's interests means providing additional time and effort to a patient's care if such effort will have an important benefit for the patient and will not have undue personal burdens on the physician. It does not mean that physicians must make unreasonable sacrifices in their personal lives to serve their patients. Indeed, it would be counterproductive to try to do so (see Chap. 40).

Ethically Problematic Strategies Intended to Help Patients

In addition to helping individual patients obtain needed care, health care providers need to consider the larger social and political context that makes it difficult for patients to receive needed care.[14] To obtain benefits, such as disability, patients need providers to give information to third parties. Providers may consider, or patients may request, using lying or deception to help them gain such benefits. In one survey, 39% of physicians reported that during the past year they had exaggerated the severity of a patient's condition, changed a patient's billing diagnosis, or reported signs and symptoms the patient did not have in order to help the patient get needed care.[15] Such deception is more common when physicians believe that it is unfair for an insurance plan not to cover the intervention, when they believe that the insurer's appeals process is unwieldy, and when the patient's condition is more serious.[16] However, avoiding deception is a basic ethical guideline that serves to limit obligations to serve as patient advocates.[17] Those dealing with a specific case may not appreciate the impact of the practice of deception on the doctor–patient relationship and on the role of health care in society.

Another approach to helping low-income patients is not to collect the copayment required by insurers. Forgoing the income from such copayments is ethically praiseworthy because it makes medical care more affordable to patients with limited means. However, some insurers object to this practice, contending that if the physician is willing to accept a discounted rate for their services, then their usual fees are in fact lower than what they are charging the insurer. Insurers may then lower the reimbursement rate to the physician or even accuse the physician of fraud. Thus, the physician or clinic that wishes to give a discount to patients in need is wise to seek legal counsel to make sure it is being done in a manner than avoids legal liability.

BEDSIDE RATIONING: CONFLICTING ETHICAL GUIDELINES

Mrs. Diaz is a 76-year-old woman with severe dementia. She recognizes her family only occasionally and does not respond to questions or requests by health care workers. She develops chronic renal failure and symptoms of uremia. While competent, she had never expressed her preferences regarding renal dialysis. Although her primary physician and the nephrologist strongly recommend that renal dialysis not be performed, her family insists on it; they believe that as long as she recognizes them and smiles, her life is meaningful and should be prolonged. They understand that dialysis would not improve her mental functioning or mobility.

> At the time, the public hospital in the community is considering closing obstetric and substance abuse services because of budget deficits. The physicians feel they are accomplices with an unjust health care system if they use resources on this patient when more pressing health needs are unmet. A vascular surgery consultant writes in the medical record, "In the current climate of out-of-control medical costs, it is unconscionable to provide expensive care for this patient."[33]

In accordance with the guideline of beneficence, the family is acting as surrogate for a patient who lacks decision-making capacity. In this case, the family believes that dialysis is in Mrs. Diaz's best interests, according to their assessment of her quality of life. However, the physicians believe that Mrs. Diaz's quality of life is so poor that the cost of dialysis is not justified. They claim that the guideline of justice requires them to allocate resources fairly among the population as a whole and act as responsible stewards of scarce medical resources. Physicians should support enlightened public policies about allocation. However, in most circumstances, attempts by physicians to redistribute health care resources at the level of the individual patient, although well intentioned, generally are both unjustified and ineffective.

ARGUMENTS AGAINST BEDSIDE RATIONING

Traditionally, bedside rationing by physicians has been considered unethical.[18,19] At the bedside, physicians generally should act as patient advocates within constraints set by society, reasonable insurance coverage, and sound clinical practice. One eminent physician wrote, "Physicians are required to do everything that they believe may benefit each patient without regard to costs or other societal considerations. In caring for an individual patient, the doctor must act solely as the patient's advocate, against the apparent interests of society as a whole."[20]

There are several strong ethical reasons against bedside rationing in the case of Mrs. Diaz. First, no public policy authorizes physicians to carry out such rationing. The physicians caring for Mrs. Diaz felt partly responsible for the soaring cost of health care. However, no public policy authorizes physicians to limit the care of patients on renal dialysis to save resources for other patients. On the contrary, US public policy pays for dialysis to all patients with end-stage renal failure through the Medicare program. Second, bedside rationing would be inconsistent and unfair. Physicians at one hospital might withhold dialysis from Mrs. Diaz, whereas physicians at another hospital might provide it. Treating similar patients unequally violates the ethical guideline of justice. Whether Mrs. Diaz receives dialysis or not should not be based on the physician or hospital that provides her care, particularly, because underserved populations often have little choice of providers. Bedside rationing also may be unfair if certain patients or interventions are singled out for review. It makes little sense to limit one health care intervention as not cost effective without scrutinizing the cost effectiveness of other interventions, such as intensive care for patients with extremely poor prognoses. Unfairness also may result from unilateral quality of life judgments made by physicians. Empiric studies show that physicians tend to rate a patient's quality of life lower than do patients or their families. This may be particularly true if patients and physicians come from different backgrounds. Physicians believed that Mrs. Diaz's quality of life fell below a threshold of acceptability. However, the family, who seem loving and well-intentioned, believe that her life still has meaning and value. In the US culture, which prizes respect for the beliefs and values of individual patients or their surrogates, there is no societal warrant for physicians to impose their own evaluations of quality of life to override the family's assessment in this situation.

Third, money saved by rationing usually cannot be reallocated. Physicians in the United States who save money on the care of an individual patient generally cannot redirect those resources to patients or projects that have higher priority.[21] If physicians terminated dialysis on Mrs. Diaz, they could not redirect funds to more pressing medical or social needs, such as prenatal care or childhood immunizations. In the absence of broader health care reform, attempts to limit health care costs at the bedside are ineffective gestures that could lead to disparities in health care.

RECOMMENDATIONS ABOUT BEDSIDE RATIONING

Limiting care for one patient in order to have resources available to patients who would benefit more from them can be justified in some situations if several conditions are met.[22] First, saved resources would be reallocated to interventions that provide greater benefits for the population of patients receiving care. Second, the physicians would not benefit personally from saving resources. Third, the limitations in care would be applied to all similar patients, with no exceptions on the basis of privileged social status. Keeping in mind these conditions, physicians who are considering rationing care at the bedside should take several actions. First, physicians should try to obtain more resources for the services that they believe will meaningfully benefit a patient's health. Second, physicians should make bedside rationing decisions openly. In particular, physicians should notify other members of the health care team, as well as patients or surrogates when they are considering rationing care. Discussing rationing dilemmas explicitly may identify unquestioned assumptions and hidden value judgments. When people must make their arguments and values explicit, others can present rebuttals or disagreements. A second opinion from another attending physician, or from a hospital ethics committee or consultant, may improve decision making. For example, such review may clarify the prognosis of the patients or point out unwarranted value judgments.

In several situations, bedside rationing can be justified. An example is when the intensive care unit (ICU) is full and a patient in the hospital develops a crisis that is unlikely to respond well without ICU care. In this situation, it would be appropriate to transfer a more stable patient with less urgent need of intensive care out of the unit to a general ward bed.

In these situations where rationing is permissible, clinicians may be reluctant to ration interventions to patients who are already receiving care because of loyalty or fidelity. That is, doctors may believe that they have implicitly promised to provide ongoing care and not to curtail it to benefit other patients. The emotional appeal of this position is clear, and keeping promises is an important ethical guideline. However, maintaining fidelity should refer to appropriate ongoing care, not to unlimited care regardless of the benefits to the patient or the harm to others.

Common Pitfalls in Ethical Care of Underserved Patients

- Often more than one ethical guideline is at play in a case; these different guidelines may direct providers to act in opposite ways. There may be strong reasons both for and against a particular course of action.
- Stakeholders may have different values and approaches to decision making. Physicians, nurses, family members, and the patient may not agree on the risks and benefits of an intervention, the patient's quality of life, or the process of decision making.
- In determining the ethically appropriate course of action, providers need to articulate the reasoning that led them to their recommendation or position.

PATIENTS WHO LACK DECISION-MAKING CAPACITY

Patients may not be able to make informed decisions because of unconsciousness, dementia, delirium, or other medical conditions. The highly publicized case of Terri Schiavo, a young woman in a persistent vegetative state, illustrated how difficult and contentious decisions can be for such patients.[23,24] In this case, the husband and parents disagreed sharply over whether her feeding tube should be discontinued. In a lengthy legal process, the state and federal courts, the Florida state legislature, congress, and the president were involved in the case. In cases involving patients who lack decision-making capacity, physicians need to ask two questions: Who is the appropriate surrogate? What would the patient want done?

ASSESSING CAPACITY TO MAKE MEDICAL DECISIONS

All adults are considered legally competent unless declared incompetent by a court. In practice, physicians usually determine that patients lack the capacity to make health care decisions and arrange for surrogates to make them, without involving the courts. By definition, competent patients can express a choice and appreciate the medical situation, nature of the proposed care, and alternatives, as well as the risks, benefits, and consequences of each.[25] Their choices should be consistent with their values and not result from delusions or hallucinations.

Patients who carry a diagnosis such as dementia, schizophrenia, or substance abuse should not be automatically considered to lack decision-making capacity. Although such diagnoses may raise the question of decision-making capacity, the physician needs to evaluate each patient as an individual.[25] Psychiatrists may help in evaluating difficult cases because they are skilled at interviewing mentally impaired patients and can identify treatable depression or psychosis. When impairments are fluctuating or reversible, decisions should be postponed if possible until the patient recovers decision-making capacity.

CHOICE OF SURROGATE

If a patient lacks decision-making capacity, physicians generally ask family members to serve as surrogates. This approach is appropriate because most patients want their family members to be surrogates, and family members generally know the patient's preferences and have the patient's best interests at heart. Patients may designate a particular individual to serve as proxy; such choices should be respected. Some states have established a prioritized list of which relative may serve as surrogate if the patient has not designated a proxy.

STANDARDS FOR SURROGATE DECISION MAKING

Advance Directives

These are statements by competent patients to direct care if they later lose decision-making capacity. They may indicate: (a) what interventions they would refuse or accept; or (b) who should serve as surrogate. Following advance directives respects patients' autonomy.[26]

Physicians can encourage patients to provide advance directives, to indicate both what they would want and who should be surrogate. In addition, physicians should discuss with patients the scenarios that are likely to occur and the options for each. These discussions help ensure that advance directives are informed and up-to-date. Furthermore, doctors should encourage patients to discuss their preferences with their proxy. The federal Patient Self-Determination Act requires hospitals and health maintenance organizations to inform patients of their right to make health care decisions and to provide advance directives.

Substituted Judgment

In the absence of clear advance directives, surrogates and physicians should try to decide as the patient would under the circumstances, using all information that they know about the patient. Although such substituted judgments try to respect the patient's values, they may be speculative or inaccurate. Commonly, surrogates may be mistaken about the patient's preferences, particularly when they have not been discussed explicitly.

Best Interests

When the patient's preferences are unclear or unknown, decisions should be based on the patient's best interests. Patients generally take into account the quality of life as well as the duration of life when making decisions for themselves. It is understandable that surrogates would also consider quality of life of patients who lack decision-making capacity. Judgments about quality of life are appropriate if they reflect the patient's own values. Bias or discrimination may occur, however, if others project their values onto the patient or weigh the perceived social worth of the patient.

LEGAL ISSUES

Physicians need to know pertinent state laws about patients who lack decision-making capacity.[27] A few state courts allow doctors to forgo life-sustaining interventions only if patients have provided written advance directives or very specific oral ones.

CULTURAL ISSUES

Advance directives are supported in the United States by court rulings, professional ethics, and common clinical practice. However, in many cultures, decisions for patients who lack decision-making capacity are made quite differently.[28] First, in some other cultures, planning in advance for serious illness is considered inappropriate. It is viewed as impolite and insensitive to talk explicitly about serious illness and death. Second, the individual may be regarded as a member of an extended family unit. Thus, patients expect their children to take care of them and make appropriate decisions for them. To complete a written advance directive telling them what to do may seem unnecessary or mistrustful. To name one person as decision maker also may seem inappropriate because it devalues the role of other family members and the importance of family consensus. Third, families from some cultural or ethnic backgrounds may mistrust the health care system and believe that doctors discuss advance directives because they do not want to provide care that patients need. Such mistrust is understandable in light of the history of discrimination, segregation, and unequal access to medical care that, for example, African Americans have experienced.[29] Physicians need to understand such concerns and views.

Open-ended questions can elicit the patient's and family's preferences for decision making and their concerns and values. Physicians need to spend sufficient time listening attentively to understand the patient's and family's perspective.[30] If patients and families feel that the physician understands them, they are likely to be more willing in turn to listen to the physician's recommendations. It is helpful to ask specifically about lack of trust in the medical system and to acknowledge that this is an understandable reaction.

DISAGREEMENTS

Disagreements may occur among potential surrogates or between the physician and surrogate. Physicians can remind everyone to base decisions on what the patient would want, not what they would want for themselves. Consultation with the hospital ethics committee or another physician often helps resolve disputes.[31,32] Such consultation is also helpful when patients have no surrogate and no advance directives. The courts should be used only as a last resort when disagreements cannot be resolved in the clinical setting.

CONCLUSION

Ethical dilemmas are inevitable in clinical medicine because individual health care workers, patients, and families have different preferences and priorities. Patients, family members, and other health care workers may have different religious or cultural backgrounds than the physician. Furthermore, health care resources for underserved populations do not meet their clinical needs.

Clinical ethics can indicate which actions are clearly right or wrong and which are controversial. Some positions on specific ethical issues can be shown to be untenable because they are internally inconsistent or do not take into account countervailing arguments. In other situations, people can be persuaded to reach agreement in a particular case, even though they hold different world views.

Although analysis of ethical issues is essential, few dilemmas in clinical ethics are resolved solely by philosophical arguments. Good communication and interpersonal skills are also needed. Physicians need to identify and address common factors such as emotions, misunderstandings, interpersonal conflicts, and time pressures that often complicate clinical dilemmas. Indeed, many "ethical" dilemmas are settled by addressing these issues directly through showing respect for others, concern, and compassion.

Physicians confronting ethical dilemmas can get help from other members of the health care team, colleagues, or the hospital ethics committee. Such discussions often can clarify the ethical issues and suggest ways to improve communication and deal with strong emotions. When struggling with difficult ethical issues, physicians may need to reevaluate their basic convictions, tolerate uncertainty, and maintain their integrity while respecting the opinions of others.

KEY CONCEPTS

- In the care of any patient, ethical dilemmas may arise. Patients may disagree with providers' recommendations. People may disagree over how to weigh the benefits and risks of an intervention. The well-being of the individual patient may conflict with the well-being of other persons.
- In caring for underserved patients, providers have additional responsibilities to:
  ✓ Overcome barriers to informed consent.
  ✓ Obtain access to care and social services.
  ✓ Understand and respond to the cultural framework of the patient.
  ✓ Advocate for change in public policies that contribute to health disparities.
- Physician responsibilities to underserved patients are not absolute or unlimited. Advocacy needs to be balanced with physician well-being. Physicians need time to carry out personal and family activities.

CORE COMPETENCY

Responding to Family Requests Not to Tell the Patient a Diagnosis of Cancer

A 70-year-old Cantonese-speaking man is found to have a carcinoma of the lung. The children ask the physician not to tell their father he has cancer. They say that if he is told, he will lose hope. (This situation can occur with patients from any cultural background.)

- *Determine what the patient wants.* Individual patients may wish to know they have cancer, even if this is not customary in their culture. This conversation is best done before embarking on a diagnosis and confirmed before delivering results.
  ✓ ASK patients for THEIR preferences
    Example: "Many patients want to know their test results, whereas other patients want the doctor to tell a family member. I will do whatever you prefer. Do you want me to tell you the test results?"
  ✓ Respect the patient's preferences.
- *Elicit the family's concerns.*
  ✓ Ask about fears
    Example: "What do you fear most about telling your father he has cancer?"
  ✓ Validate feelings as the natural reactions of loving relatives
  ✓ Explore steps be taken to address concerns and to help family and patient cope.
  ✓ Offer compassion and empathy, and help to mobilize support for family and patient.
- *Plan for future contingencies if withholding information.* If the diagnosis is withheld, physicians need to anticipate future issues that might arise.
  ✓ Ask regularly if patients have questions or want to discuss anything else about their condition. Patients who do not want to be told their diagnosis may change their minds.
  ✓ Do not promise family members that the patient will not learn a serious diagnosis. (It may be disclosed inadvertently.)
  ✓ Communicate patient's desires to other health care team members.

DISCUSSION QUESTIONS

1. A 34-year-old primary school teacher is diagnosed with active tuberculosis. The patient is afraid that she will lose her job if her case is reported. She will start treatment immediately and notes that summer vacation has just started. She is willing to come to the office to take her medicine or take tests to prove she is taking her drugs. Should she be reported to public health officials? What ethical considerations support your position?

2. A 62-year-old woman is diagnosed with localized stage I breast cancer, which usually can be cured with lumpectomy plus radiation or mastectomy. The patient is Cantonese speaking, and her daughters request that you not tell her she has cancer. "In her generation, people aren't told they have cancer. She would just give up hope. It would be disrespectful to make her suffer, rather than have the family bear the burden of her illness. Just tell her she needs an operation, and she'll agree to it." Do you agree to the daughters' request? Give the ethical considerations for your decision.

RESOURCES

Beauchamp TL, Childress JF. Principles of biomedical ethics, 5th ed. New York: Oxford University Press, 2001.

Lo B. Resolving ethical dilemmas: A guide for clinicians, 3rd ed. Baltimore: Williams & Wilkins, 2005.

Meisel A. The right to die, 2nd ed. New York: John Wiley & Sons, 1995.

Snyder L, Leffler C, Ethics and Humans Rights Committee of the American College of Physicians. Ethics manual, 5th ed. Ann Intern Med 2005;142:560–582.

REFERENCES

1. Shultz MM. From informed consent to patient choice: A new protected interest. Yale Law J 1985;95:219–299.
2. Berg JW, Lidz CW, Appelbaum PS. Informed consent: Legal theory and clinical practice, 2nd ed. New York: Oxford University Press, 2001.
3. Gordon DB, Paci E. Disclosure practices and cultural narratives: Understanding concealment and silence around cancer in Tuscany, Italy. Soc Sci Med 1997;46: 1433–1452.
4. Surbone A. Truth telling to the patient. JAMA 1992;268: 1661–1662.
5. Blackhall LJ, Murphy ST, Frank G, et al. Ethnicity and attitudes toward patient autonomy. JAMA 1995;274: 820–825.
6. Helft PR, Siegler M, Lantos J. The rise and fall of the futility movement. N Engl J Med 2000;343(4):293–296.
7. Kite S, Wilkinson S. Beyond futility: To what extent is the concept of futility useful in clinical decision-making about CPR? Lancet 2002;3:638–642.
8. Gostin LO. Public health law: Power, duty, restraint. Berkeley, CA: University of California Press, 2000.
9. Bok S. Lying: Moral choices in public and private life. New York: Pantheon Books, 1978.
10. Hall MA, Berenson RA. Ethical practice in managed care: A dose of realism. Ann Intern Med 1998;128:395–402.
11. Beauchamp TL, Childress JF. Principles of biomedical ethics. New York: Oxford University Press, 2001.
12. Povar GJ, Blumen H, Daniel J, et al. Ethics in practice: managed care and the changing health care environment:

13. Jonsen AR. Watching the doctor. N Engl J Med 1983;308: 1531–1535.
14. Putsch RW, Pololi L. Distributive justice in American healthcare: Institutions, power, and the equitable care of patients. Am J Manag Care 2004;10(Spec No):SP45–53.
15. Wynia MK, Cummins DS, VanGeest JB, et al. Physician manipulation of reimbursement rules for patients: between a rock and a hard place. JAMA 2000;283(14):1858–1865.
16. Werner RM, Alexander GC, Fagerlin A, et al. The "hassle factor": What motivates physicians to manipulate reimbursement rules? Arch Intern Med 2002;162(10):1134–1139.
17. Morreim EH. Gaming the system: Dodging the rules, ruling the dodgers. Arch Intern Med 1991;151:443-447.
18. Pellegrino ED, Thomasma DG. For the patient's good: The restoration of beneficence in health care. New York: Oxford University Press, 1988.
19. Kassirer JP. Managing care: Should we adopt a new ethic? N Engl J Med 1998;339:397–398.
20. Levinsky NG. The doctor's master. N Engl J Med 1984;311:1573–1575.
21. Daniels N. Why saying no to patients in the United States is so hard. N Engl J Med 1986;314:1380–1383.
22. Pearson SD. Caring and cost: The challenge for physician advocacy. Ann Intern Med 2000;133(2):148–153.
23. Quill TE. Terri Schiavo: A tragedy compounded. N Engl J Med 2005;352(16):1630–1633.
24. Annas GJ. "Culture of life" politics at the bedside: The case of Terri Schiavo. N Engl J Med 2005;352(16): 1710–1715.
25. Grisso T, Appelbaum P. Assessing competence to consent to treatment: A guide for physicians and other health professionals. New York: Oxford University Press, 1998.
26. Lo B, Steinbrook RL. Resuscitating advance directives. Arch Intern Med 2004;164(14):1501–1506.
27. Sabatino CS. The legal and functional status of the medical proxy: Suggestions for statutory reform. J Law Med Ethics 1999;(27)1:46–51.
28. Kagawa-Singer M, Blackhall LJ. Negotiating cross-cultural issues at the end of life: "You got to go where he lives." JAMA 2001;286(23):2993–3001.
29. Crawley LM, Marshall PA, Lo B, et al., Strategies for culturally effective end-of-life care. Ann Intern Med 2002; 136(9):673–679.
30. Lo B, Quill T, Tulsky J. Discussing palliative care with patients. Ann Intern Med 1999;130:744–749.
31. Schneiderman LJ, Gilmer T, Teetzel HD, et al. Effect of ethics consultations on non-beneficial life-sustaining treatments in the intensive care setting: A multi-center, prospective, randomized, controlled trial. JAMA 2003; 290:1166–1172.
32. Lo B. Answers and questions about ethics consultations. JAMA 2003;290:298–299.
33. Lo B. Resolving ethical dilemmas: A guide for clinicians. Philadelphia: Lippincott Williams & Wilkins, 2005.
34. Lo B, Dornbrand L, Dubler NN. HIPAA and patient care: The role for professional judgment. JAMA 2005;293: 1766–1771.

PART 2

Practice

Alicia Fernandez, MD and Dean Schillinger, MD, editors

CHAPTERS

Chapter 6

Creating a Context for Effective Intervention in the Clinical Care of Vulnerable Patients

Dean Schillinger, MD, Teresa J. Villela, MD, and George William Saba, PhD

Objectives

- Describe building a therapeutic alliance, eliciting the patient's narrative, and assessing the patient's vulnerabilities and strengths.

- Explore the critical components of therapeutic alliance: building trust, conveying empathy, and collaboration.

- Describe the relevance of the therapeutic alliance to the effective care of vulnerable patients.

- List the benefits of eliciting the patient's narrative.

- Review common psychosocial vulnerabilities and illustrate how identifying them can help create a patient-centered clinical encounter.

Ms. Sviridov is a 67-year-old woman with chronic arthritis pain, hypertension, prior stroke, diastolic dysfunction and diabetes. Despite a sizable, guideline-based medication regimen and frequent visits to both a primary care physician and a cardiologist, she has recalcitrant heart failure, requiring multiple hospital admissions. An extensive cardiac work-up has been unrevealing.

Vulnerable patients experience a triple jeopardy when it comes to health care: They are more likely to be ill, and more likely to have difficulty accessing care. When they do, the care they receive is more likely to be suboptimal. This reflects a mismatch between the psychosocial vulnerabilities that patients bring to the clinical encounter and the knowledge, attitudes, skills, and beliefs of the clinicians caring for them. This chapter focuses on the centrality of strong provider–patient relationships to all efforts to improve the patient's health. Three essential strategies are recommended to promote a context for effective care for vulnerable patients: building a therapeutic alliance, eliciting the patient's story or "narrative," and assessing for the patient's psychosocial vulnerabilities and strengths. Clinicians can use a combination of these approaches to create more productive and effective interactions and relationships with vulnerable patients (Fig. 6-1).

VULNERABILITY AND THERAPEUTIC ALLIANCE

Psychosocial vulnerabilities can affect health and health care through three pathways either alone or in concert (Fig. 6-2). The first is a direct path, in which the vulnerability in and of itself leads to poor health. Concrete examples of this mechanism might be intravenous drug

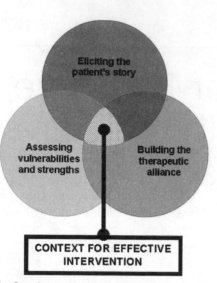

Figure 6-1. Creating a context for effective intervention in the clinical care of vulnerable patients.

abuse and skin abscesses, or intimate partner violence and head trauma. A second path is an indirect one, where the vulnerability attenuates the benefits of medical treatment on coexisting medical conditions (e.g., the vulnerability presents a barrier to optimal acute, chronic, and/or preventive care), thereby accelerating disease course. Examples of this include the effects of depression on nonadherence to medications among patients with heart disease; or inability to pay for medications and poor diabetes control. The third mechanism, also an indirect one, is mediated entirely through the therapeutic alliance. In this path, the vulnerability affects components of the relationship or therapeutic

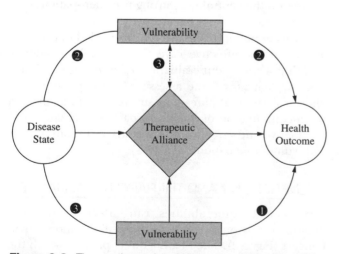

Figure 6-2. Three pathways by which psychosocial vulnerabilities affect health and health care in the clinical encounter (see text for details).

alliance with the provider (e.g., open disclosure, mutual trust, caring, and engagement), thereby limiting the benefits of a collaborative relationship on care. Examples of this include a patient with an undisclosed illness that is inconsistent with a prescribed treatment plan; a physician whose belief systems about addiction impedes true engagement with a patient with a substance use disorder; or a patient with limited literacy that impedes follow-through with prescribed treatment plan, thereby leading to mutual frustration and blame.[1]

WHAT IS THE THERAPEUTIC ALLIANCE?

The term "therapeutic alliance" derives from a combination of the Greek *therapeuein* (to serve) and the Latin *alligare* (to bind) and was initially developed in the field of psychotherapy to describe a trusting, respectful, collaborative, and caring relationship between therapist and patient. Studies demonstrated that, regardless of the theoretical model of therapy, the presence of a therapeutic alliance was associated with positive treatment outcomes.[2]

In the field of medicine, a therapeutic alliance exists when patient and provider develop mutual trusting, caring, and respectful bonds that allow collaboration in care and treatment.[3-5] "Patient-" and "relationship-centered" care models build on the notion of the therapeutic alliance, and research reveals that patients reporting greater trust, increased satisfaction, and more collaborative relationships with clinicians have increased adherence to medication and treatment regimens and better health outcomes.[6-8]

Trust

Mutuality, particularly in trust, is crucial. Patients need to trust in their clinicians' integrity and competence as healers. Clinicians need to trust that patients enter the relationship trying to do their best.

Empathy

Empathy too is necessary to form a strong therapeutic alliance. Demonstrating empathy, or recognizing and understanding the beliefs and emotions of another without injecting one's own, allows the clinician to connect emotionally with the patient without pity or overidentification, enriching the encounter for both. Feeling understood, particularly by your medical provider, can be profoundly comforting. Providing comfort is a reward in itself. Understanding a patient also imbues a provider's efforts—even the mundane filling out of forms—with meaning.

Respect

Expressing respect for patients and treating them with dignity are also important to creating therapeutic bonds. Respect requires a willingness to take the time to understand and explain, creating a context in which communication can occur as equals.

Agreement and Collaboration

Clinicians and patients both need to feel comfortable articulating and agreeing on the goals of treatment. An honest dialogue may naturally lead to disagreement about these goals or how best to achieve them. Collaboration requires a meaningful partnership in which clinician and patient perceive that they are working together toward a common goal and committed to resolving inevitable conflicts.

Broadening the Alliance

Initially the fields of psychotherapy and health care envisioned the therapeutic alliance as a one-to-one relationship between clinician and patient. With the influence of systems theory, this alliance broadened to include other important people involved in the care (e.g., family; consulting clinicians).[9,10] Recent work by Wagner and our own group.[11,12] has further highlighted the important role that health systems play in either fostering or eroding the therapeutic alliance based on the policies they promote.

THERAPEUTIC ALLIANCE AND VULNERABLE PATIENTS

A growing body of evidence suggests that it is precisely with vulnerable patients that the therapeutic alliance can have its most profound benefits. In the therapeutic alliance, clinicians offer a professional relationship aimed at helping patients feel comfortable to be as open and honest as is necessary to receive the best care. Clinicians are permitted access to the interior of patients' lives that few other people are allowed. Because of their privileged position, they can build an alliance that empowers patients and reduces barriers to their care.

Empowerment

Vulnerable patients often experience human relationships as broken or disrupted (e.g., because of violence, immigration, mental illness, homelessness, illness). Through the therapeutic alliance, clinicians can offer a reliable, dependable, and continuous presence that is supportive, accepting, and nonjudgmental. They can provide safety, thus allowing patients to tell the stories of their lives and illness and disclose their vulnerabilities. By examining the patients' strengths and resources, clinicians can provide a sense of dignity and hope. Through validating their experiences, clinicians can help patients feel less marginalized. In supporting patients as competent and strong, clinicians can help empower them to become actively involved in their care.

Access to Care and Related Resources

Vulnerable patients often face limited access to health care and social services. They are often unaware of what is available and may not have the facility to negotiate complex, bureaucratic systems. Clinicians are in a position to remedy both of these barriers. Through the therapeutic alliance, clinicians can help patients feel safe enough to reveal concerns or problems beyond the presenting problem, which they might not otherwise have done. For example, a patient seeking care for their diabetes may disclose that they live with an abusive partner, drink alcohol regularly, or are only sporadically housed. The clinician has the ability both to collaborate on treatment plans, as well as facilitate entry into the various health and social systems that can address those vulnerabilities. The therapeutic alliance can help patients feel assured that clinicians will not abuse the disclosure of information (e.g., leading to rejection or legal action) but will help them access resources critical for their health.

WHAT CAN HAPPEN WHEN THE THERAPEUTIC ALLIANCE IS ABSENT?

The absence of a therapeutic alliance can result in serious consequences for the health of vulnerable patients.

Trust

Clinicians often enter into relationships with patients assuming they share the same goals and will trust each other to do their best to attain them. However, many patients enter into the relationship with a degree of mistrust. This may result from their personal experiences with institutions in which they have felt betrayed or unwelcome or be rooted in broader, historical experiences of their community. Clinicians should not automatically assume that they have patients' immediate, total trust; rather, they often must earn it by demonstrating trustworthiness.

Caring

Poor and minority patients frequently receive care in teaching hospitals and community health centers where the turnover of providers is high. Patients may question provider's motivation and commitment, fearing that they are educational fodder for trainees who will go on to care for the privileged. When clinicians do not offer certain treatments, they may be suspicious about the clinicians' willingness to expend resources for them. When clinicians persuasively argue for unwanted treatments, they may fear being used as experimental "guinea pigs." Rather than raising concerns or disagreements with a clinician whose motives they question, they may choose not to follow through on recommended treatment or simply not return for care.

Respect

Perceived disrespect and discrimination because of race or socioeconomic status has been associated with lower satisfaction with the health care system and worse health outcomes among patients with chronic illness.[13] Significant proportions of blacks, Latinos, and Asians and those with lower educational attainment have reported that they were treated with disrespect, were treated unfairly, or received worse care because of their position in society.[14] These perceptions influenced whether patients followed recommended advice or delayed needed care for chronic illness. Communicating respect is essential to convincing vulnerable patients that clinicians are willing to enter into a relationship based on equality and dignity.

Mutual Agreement and Collaboration

In the absence of a trusting relationship, true collaboration may be difficult to achieve. Fear of being punished or treated unfairly for speaking truthfully can lead patients to withhold their beliefs and values about a suggested treatment or be unwilling to follow through on a recommendation. Clinicians, in turn, feel frustrated and mistrustful when they wonder if they are being misled or if the patients really care about their health.

Shared decision making is often promoted as a model for mutual agreement and collaboration. However, research with diverse populations suggests that clinicians and patients apparently engaging in the cardinal behaviors of shared decision making may still not perceive that a collaborative partnership exists between them.[1] Indeed, being treated with respect and dignity may be more important than engaging in shared decision making, and lead to positive outcomes (i.e., higher satisfaction, adherence, receipt of optimal preventive care).[15]

BUILDING A THERAPEUTIC ALLIANCE WITH VULNERABLE PATIENTS

There are no simple, protocol-like statements or behaviors that can be employed to make another human being feel cared about or respected. However, if a practitioner consciously strives to transmit a sense of trust, caring, and respect along with a desire to enter into true partnership, the likelihood of forming productive relationships with patients is increased. Some guidelines to consider in this process include the following.

Demonstrate Commitment to the Relationship

It is important to state clearly the desire to be available to patients within the scope of practice (e.g., *"I will be your regular doctor. Here is my telephone number with a voice mail; I check it daily and will get back to you as soon as possible."*); be clear about between-visit expectations (e.g., *"I will check*

into support groups and tell you at our next appointment."); and follow through on promises.

Allow for the Humanity of the Patient and Clinician to Emerge

The humanity of the health care worker and patient should be expressed and elicited. This may include the sharing of beliefs, values, and feelings as they relate to the clinical issues facing them (e.g., express concern about suffering, *"I am sorry you have to deal with this pain;"* self-disclosure to identify a shared history or common interests with the patient, *"As a parent, I can't imagine how incredibly strong you had to be to escape with your children."*).

Elicit Patients' Stories or Health "Narratives"

This interviewing approach can provide critical insights into a patient's illness model, allow for expression of the patient's humanity, and uncover important psychosocial vulnerabilities (see Core Competency).

Search Actively for Patients' Strengths and Resources

Health care workers commonly focus on what is wrong or dysfunctional in the patient's life. An added search, and one just as vigorous as the search for deficits, is to identify and validate each patient's strengths and resilience (e.g., *"You have been through a lot of suffering in your life, how have you been able to survive?" "Who gives you the strength to deal with difficult things?"*). Reflecting on how the patient has used these resources in previously difficult times can provide a positive starting point for healing (e.g., *"You have talked about turning to God when dealing with other major crises in your life; have you thought of doing that now?"*). The power for healing does not rest solely with the clinician, but must involve an empowered patient and family (e.g., *"Your sister has helped you with your reading problem in other parts of your life; can she help now in dealing with your diabetes?"*).

Express Caring Overtly

Health care workers need to clearly state that they care about their patients as people, and not assume they know. When hearing patients describe difficult or painful experiences, they can acknowledge the patient's perspective (e.g., *"I can't imagine how difficult your life has been;" "What you have lived through sounds so frightening;" "I know you're afraid going through these tests and treatments; is there anything I can do to make it less scary?"*). A number of nonverbal behaviors and verbal statements also can overtly express caring: (a) body language (e.g., sitting in proximity; a focused, unhurried posture); (b) active listening and reframing (e.g., *"It sounds to me that you felt betrayed by the people you trusted most; am I right with that?"*); (c) support (e.g., *"I know you are trying very hard to live on your own now; I think you are doing great, and I want to do whatever I can to support you."*); and (d) validation (e.g., *"You are right to feel that you do not deserve to be abused."*). Caring also can be communicated a number of indirect ways, such as making an unexpected phone call to follow-up with a patient in crisis (e.g., *"I know you had your colonoscopy yesterday, and I wanted to see how you are doing."*). Not all patients (or clinicians) are comfortable with touch. However, some patients believe clinicians are afraid to touch them. Maintaining physical contact during painful or uplifting moments can activate a mutual human connection.

Create a Context for Conflict to Emerge and Get Addressed

Health care workers need to inform patients that they are happy to discuss different beliefs and feelings. Clinicians must allay any fears that voicing disagreement will incur displeasure or even punishment from the provider. A corollary to this is that patients need to know that they can change their minds about treatment plans and decisions at any time. Patients need repeated reassurance and reminders that disagreement will not cost them the provider's regard and care (e.g., *"I will not be angry or upset if you disagree; it would be very helpful to know how you really feel, because together we can figure out the best thing to do"*). Building a therapeutic alliance does not require practitioners to deny an educated viewpoint, but rather to adopt nonthreatening ways of communicating this difference with patients.

Clarify Boundaries

Vulnerable patients often may experience considerable intrusion into their personal lives by government institutions or social service agencies. They may be required to disclose more information than others, and find it shared across agencies without their knowledge or permission. Health care workers should clarify why they are inquiring about certain information (e.g., *"I want to ask more specifically about your family because they seem important in your care, and I want to understand how they help you."*) and what is confidential or required to be shared (e.g., *"I will keep whatever you tell me confidential unless I think you may harm yourself or someone else; then I must tell others to protect you from any harm."*). They should also clarify their own boundaries; it is not uncommon for a relationship between a clinician and a patient to evolve into one of unhealthy dependence or unrealistic expectations.

ADDRESS THE THERAPEUTIC ALLIANCE DIRECTLY

When caring for a patient who is doing poorly clinically but receiving optimal "medical" management, health care workers should consider if the therapeutic alliance needs attention. They can directly state their desire to have a strong relationship and a real sense of partnership. They can ask if the patient would want any changes in the relationship, reassuring them that speaking honestly is not only acceptable, but essential to working together.

ELICITING THE PATIENT'S STORY, OR "NARRATIVE"

> Ms. Sviridov's new primary care physician asks about her life. She describes an active singing career in the past, a rich family life, and the importance of her church. She acknowledges that profound depression and concern over the welfare of her drug-abusing son interfere with her caring for herself.

WHAT IS THE PATIENT'S PERSPECTIVE?

Many factors (individual, familial, societal, spiritual, cultural) shape a person's concepts and experiences of health and illness. These inform an individual's sense of responsibility as a patient, expectations of health care providers and family members, and the meaning of healing and recovery. Personal concepts of health determine what preventive and self-care behaviors are considered appropriate, which symptoms seem worrisome, and when to seek help from health care professionals. These explanatory models encompass the meaning of the illness, the presumed cause, its proposed trajectory, the degree of hope of cure, and how treatment should be conducted.[16]

The same factors that influence how a person thinks about health and illness obviously affect other aspects of his or her life, and eliciting information about these influences can unveil perspectives important to health care. For example, how an individual makes decisions about health care may resemble how he or she makes decisions about parenting or work; the process for how a family decided to immigrate to the United States may be very similar to how they will approach a difficult treatment decision; one's explanation of life difficulties and the narrative of how one has prevailed over them may illustrate how one will face challenging health problems as well. For example, illness may be framed hopefully or pessimistically; patients identify themselves as efficacious, victimized, independent, isolated, or strengthened by support from others.

IMPORTANCE OF ELICITING THE PATIENT'S PERSPECTIVE

Patients' perspectives—a complex mixture of very personal beliefs, values, and assumptions reflecting multiple influences—can determine how they develop a relationship with their clinician, and whether they feel understood and respected or misunderstood and discounted. Clinicians, in turn, have their own individual perspectives on health and illness, and ascribe specific meaning to their role as healers. Assuming a shared understanding and not exploring the differences may lead to greater distance and misunderstanding. Eliciting patients' perspectives allows for empathy and also can uncover interests or experiences common to both patient and clinician, thereby reducing the social distance that often confounds the development of a therapeutic alliance.

Eliciting the patient's story can improve patient trust, satisfaction, and adherence (see Core Competency). In a meta-analysis of the effect of physician communication on health, Stewart[8] found that effective communication within the history-taking section of the visit consistently correlated with improved health outcomes, including emotional health, symptom resolution, function, physiologic measures (e.g., blood pressure and blood glucose), and pain control. In his studies of patient trust, Thom[17] found that receptive communication behaviors, such as "letting the whole story be told" was associated with patient trust, satisfaction, and adherence. Clinicians too benefit from understanding their patients' stories. This enriches and brings meaning to interactions and allows providers to be both more effective and engaged.

Furthermore, sometimes the way people frame their illnesses can cause suffering. Within the context of a strong therapeutic alliance it is even possible to recast some narratives as part of the healing process. For example, a patient who feels incompetent, through learning to control his or her illness, might grow to feel capable and empowered in realms beyond the medical.

ASSESSING AND ACKNOWLEDGING PSYCHOSOCIAL VULNERABILITIES

Ms. Sviridov's physician suggests he make a home visit. Exploring her initial refusal, he learns that her son deals drugs from her apartment. Eventually, with the support of her physician and adult protective services, she is able to demand that her son leave. She receives support and assistance from home health services and her church group. Her conditions stabilize and she is not rehospitalized.

Much of clinical training and guideline development focuses on pathophysiology, disease, diagnosis, and treatment. However, seasoned clinicians are acutely aware of the gap between the outcomes that are expected (e.g., from reading textbooks or following guidelines) and the outcomes that are actually achieved in practice. Although there are many reasons for the observed variation in quality and health outcomes, one of the most important and frequently least appreciated factors is the patient's social context. A wide range of psychosocial vulnerabilities can impinge on a patient's ability to carry out the treatment plan and interfere with the therapeutic alliance (see Box 6-1).

When faced with a patient who is doing poorly from a clinical standpoint, many clinicians do not reflect on the psychosocial factors that may be influencing the patient's course. Some clinicians simply throw up their arms and attribute a patient's clinical decline to his or her social milieu in a global or at times derogatory fashion, referring to such a patient as "nonadherent," a "difficult patient," or a "social nightmare," without digging deeper. Such clinicians often believe that addressing psychosocial problems is "not my job," stating, *"I can't fix his social problems."* Still others may not have the communication skills to uncover underlying psychosocial problems, or to address them and integrate this knowledge to forge more appropriate treatment plans and a more genuine, engaged therapeutic alliance.

Assessing psychosocial vulnerabilities is central to caring for patients in any setting and at many points during the process of care, particularly when treatments appear to be failing. Some vulnerabilities are apparent from the first encounter, whereas others may be hidden. For some patients and problems, it is not until a positive relationship has been established that a patient feels comfortable enough to disclose sensitive information. Similarly, patients may perceive a problem to be

Box 6-1. Generating a Differential Diagnosis of Psychosocial Vulnerabilities

Violence
Uninsured
Literacy and language
Neglect
Economic hardship
Race/ethnic discordance, discrimination
Addiction
Brain disorders (e.g., depression, dementia, personality disorder)
Immigrant status
Legal status
Isolation/informal caregiving burden
Transportation problems
Illness model
Eyes and ears
Shelter

irrelevant to their health and neglect to discuss it. When assessing for areas of vulnerability, the clinician should be nonjudgmental, allowing the patient to respond at his or her own pace. Using open-ended questions and responding to patient cues may enable a patient to reveal the important nonclinical factors that may be impeding progress.

Brief screening instruments, many of which have been validated cross-culturally and in non-English languages, also can be useful. They exist for many problems and are discussed extensively in other chapters in this textbook.

Common Pitfalls in Assessing for Vulnerability

- Failure to recognize the contribution of psychosocial vulnerabilities to the patient's illness
- Failure to acknowledge vulnerability and explore how the vulnerability may be affecting care
- Failure to address the vulnerability
- Failure to integrate knowledge of the vulnerability into treatment plans
- Failure to recognize the shame and stigma associated with vulnerabilities
- Failure to identify and acknowledge strengths, resilience, and range of resources

---

It is important to raise four important *caveats* about assessing for psychosocial vulnerability. The first is that in the pursuit of identifying vulnerability, the clinician should be reminded of the importance of simultaneously identifying and acknowledging an individual's *strengths, resilience,* and range of *resources,* such as one's belief in a higher power or support from a religious community; or the love and support provided by a spouse, friend, or pet. Reflecting back to patients' examples of how they have overcome difficulty in the past and identifying patterns of success is critical to building self-efficacy and developing a therapeutic alliance in the face of vulnerability.

Second, vulnerability is *context-dependent.* For example, in countries with universal health care coverage, lack of insurance is simply not a liability. Conversely, absence of interpretation services may exacerbate the effects of limited English proficiency when compared to settings with interpretation; presence of a methadone treatment program or a mobile treatment van in one's clinic may mitigate the untoward health effects of heroin addiction and housing instability, respectively. As such, the effects of vulnerability on health care can be influenced by altering the context in which caregiving takes place, which most frequently means adapting the clinical encounter. This suggests

that when caring for vulnerable populations, clinicians and systems also should perform *self-assessments,* and carefully explore the ways in which the caregiving context can be adapted to best attenuate (or even eliminate) the health effects of vulnerability.

Third, in the process of assessment, the clinician should be sensitive to the concerns of patients with respect to shame and stigma.[18] It is clear that a number of factors listed in Box 6-1 may elicit feelings of shame, such as having limited literacy, being marginally housed, having mental illness, or being addicted.

Fourth, after identifying vulnerability, the clinician should not forget the important step of exploring with the patient, in a supportive and nonjudgmental manner, how the vulnerability may be affecting both health and care and how to mitigate these effects. Only by doing so can the clinicians develop a more effective treatment plan while enhancing the therapeutic alliance.

CONCLUSION

Depending on the skills, attitudes, and orientation of clinicians and the systems in which they work, the clinical encounter can increase social distance and exacerbate the effects of vulnerability on health, or productively engage with patients to mitigate or even eliminate the effects of vulnerability on health. Fostering the therapeutic alliance requires developing trust, conveying empathy, and collaborating around treatment goals. Building a therapeutic alliance, eliciting the patient's narrative, and assessing for vulnerabilities and strengths are critical to creating a context for more effective care.

KEY CONCEPTS

- Vulnerable patients often experience fragmentation and disconnection in their lives and health care.
- The therapeutic alliance is an important means to reduce the effects of vulnerability on health outcomes.
- Eliciting the patient's story or perspective is an effective means to uncover health beliefs, develop shared meaning, enable empathy, foster the therapeutic alliance, uncover patient vulnerabilities, and reveal patient resilience.
- Clinicians are better equipped to develop effective treatment plans by identifying vulnerabilities and acknowledging to the patient and other clinicians involved in the patient's care how such factors might influence the effectiveness of treatment.

CORE COMPETENCY
Eliciting the Patient's Perspective

- Let patients know that hearing their perspective is important to you.
- Explain why you think discussing family, coping styles, and the like is important to their health.
- Take the time necessary, and use the time well.
- Set a climate of interest, concern, and calm.
- Use an inquiry style that fosters more, not less, information.
—Maintain a high degree of curiosity; be aware of patient's verbal or emotional cues.
—Follow-up on cues, such as, *"It seemed that talking about that brought up some feelings for you. Why is that?"*
- Use open-ended questions and reflective statements.
- Discover the patient's explanatory model.
—Ask the Kleinman questions:
  What do you call the problem? What do you think has caused the problem? Why do you think it started when it did? What do you think the sickness does? How does it work? How severe is the sickness? Will it have a short or long course? What kind of treatment do you think you should receive? What are the most important results you hope to receive from this treatment? What are the chief problems the sickness has caused you? What do you fear most about the sickness?[16]
- Consider the interpersonal context of patients' general health care framework (see Chap 19).
- Focus on the meaning of what patients are saying.
- Avoid using technical, medical jargon (see Chap 10).
- Do not try to gather the entire perspective in one appointment, but try to gain some insight every time.

DISCUSSION QUESTIONS

1. Discuss clinical experiences you have had with vulnerable patients in which the presence or absence of strategies such as building a therapeutic alliance, eliciting patients' narratives, and assessing for vulnerabilities and strengths influenced the process and perhaps the outcome of their health care.
2. Consider what structural and health policy changes would need to be made to better incorporate the strategies of building a therapeutic alliance, eliciting patients' narratives, and assessing for vulnerabilities and strengths into the day to day clinical care of vulnerable patients.
3. What are some of the most surprising or fascinating nonmedical pieces of information you learned about the last patient you cared for and how did it influence either the treatment plan or your relationship with the patient and his or her family?
4. Discuss how personal beliefs, values, and assumptions about vulnerable patients affects the ability to create a

context for effective care using strategies such as building a therapeutic alliance, eliciting patients' narratives, and assessing for vulnerabilities and strengths.

RESOURCES

American Academy of Communication in Healthcare (AACH) website: http://www.aachonline.org [formerly known as the American Academy of Physician and Patient (AAPP)].

Lipkin M Jr, Putnam SM, Lazare A, eds. *The medical interview: Clinical care, education, and research.* New York: Springer, 1995.

Young RK, ed. *A piece of my mind: A new collection of essays from JAMA, the Journal of the American Medical Association.* Chicago: AMA Press, c2000.

REFERENCES

1. Saba GW, et al. Shared decision making and experience of partnership in primary care. *Ann Fam Med* 2006;(1):54–62.
2. Freedheim DK. *History of psychotherapy: A century of change.* Washington, DC: American Psychological Association, 1992.
3. Balint M. *The doctor, his patient and the illness.* New York: International University Press, 1957.
4. Bordin ES. The generalizability of the psychoanalytic concept of the working alliance. *Psychother Theory Res Pract* 1979;16:252–260.
5. Bordin ES. Theory and research on the therapeutic working alliance: new directions. In: Horvath AO, Greenberg LS, eds. *The working alliance: Theory, research and practice.* New York: Wiley, 1994.
6. Kaplan SH, Greenfield S, Ware JE Jr. Assessing the effects of physician-patient interactions on the outcomes of chronic disease. *Med Care* 1989;27(3 Suppl):S110–127.
7. Kaplan SH, et al. Patient and visit characteristics related to physicians' participatory decision-making style. Results from the Medical Outcomes Study. *Med Care* 1995; 33(12):1176–1187.
8. Stewart M, et al. The impact of patient-centered care on outcomes. *J Fam Pract* 2000;49(9):796–804.
9. McDaniel S, Campbell T, Seaburn DB. *Family-oriented primary care.* New York: Springer-Verlag, 1990.
10. Pinsof W. An integrative systems perspective on the therapeutic alliance: Theoretical, clinical and research implications. In: Horvath AO, Greenberg LS, eds. *The working alliance: Theory, research and practice.* New York: Wiley, 1994.
11. Wagner EH. Chronic disease management: What will it take to improve care for chronic illness? *Eff Clin Pract* 1998;1(1):2–4.
12. Schillinger D. Improving chronic disease care for populations with limited health literacy. In: Nielsen-Bohlman LEA, ed. *Health literacy: A prescription to end confusion.* Washington, DC: National Academies Press, 2004.
13. Piette JD, Bibbins-Domingo K, Schillinger D. Health care discrimination, processes of care, and diabetes patients' health status. *Patient Ed Coun* 2006;60(1):41–48.

14. Blanchard J, Lurie N. R-E-S-P-E-C-T: Patient reports of disrespect in the health care setting and its impact on care. *J Fam Pract* 2004;53(9):721–730.

15. Beach MC, et al. Do patients treated with dignity report higher satisfaction, adherence, and receipt of preventive care? *Ann Fam Med* 2005;3(4):331–338.

16. Kleinman A. *The illness narratives: Suffering, healing and the human condition.* New York: Basic Books, 1988.

17. Thom DH, Hall MA, Pawlson LG. Measuring patients' trust in physicians when assessing quality of care. *Health Aff (Millwood)* 2004;23(4):124–132.

18. Lazare A. Shame and humiliation in the medical encounter. *Arch Intern Med* 1987;147(9):1653–1658.

Chapter 7

Promoting Behavior Change

Daniel S. Lessler, MD, MHA, and Christopher Dunn, PhD

Objectives

- Identify the importance and effectiveness of health behavior change counseling.
- Describe the theoretical basis for modern approaches to behavior change counseling.
- Review an evidence-based and practical approach to behavior change counseling.
- Discuss the limitations of this approach when applied in a cross-cultural context.
- Describe how systems of care can be designed to support health behavior change on the part of patients.

> Mr. Abera is a 52-year-old Ethiopian man; he is conversant in English and works as a short-order cook. Mr. Abera's medical problems include hypertension, obesity, and osteoarthritis of his knees. Mr. Abera smokes one pack of cigarettes daily.

Disparities in health among poor and underserved populations are at least in part explained by differences in health behavior.[1] Sedentary lifestyle, obesity, and smoking are more prevalent in people of lower socioeconomic position, and among racial and ethnic minorities.[2-4] Moreover, physicians are less likely to initiate conversations about health behavior change with lower-income patients.[5] This is the case even though low-income patients are more likely to report acting on these physician recommendations than are middle- and higher-income patients.[6]

This chapter reviews the theoretical underpinnings of modern approaches to behavior change counseling, and describes how physicians and health care systems can collaborate with their patients to support sustained changes in health behavior.

PROMOTING BEHAVIOR CHANGE: IMPORTANT BUT CHALLENGING

> Mr. Abera's primary care provider has told him on numerous occasions to quit smoking. Mr. Abera has tried to quit, but has not yet succeeded. Mr. Abera's primary care provider is skeptical that Mr. Abera will ever change his ways.

Health care providers (and especially physicians) often view discussions about health behavior change as futile and frustrating endeavors.[7,8] To make matters worse, pessimism about behavior change, unspoken but implied, can be transmitted from senior physicians to residents. Although junior physicians would emulate their seniors practicing successful behavioral counseling with patients, such role models can be scarce in training environments.

Physicians are not alone in their frustration. For most patients, adopting and continually practicing behaviors that enhance health and reduce the risks of chronic disease is difficult. Health behavior change may be even more difficult for medically underserved and vulnerable populations, whose communities lack important resources that enable behavior change, such as accessible and safe environments in which to exercise, or stores that provide fresh fruit and vegetables at a reasonable price.

Fortunately, during the last quarter century or more, the understanding of why, when, and how patients adopt and maintain healthy behaviors has matured into an evidence-based approach to promoting behavior change. For example, it is now known that only a small proportion of patients who currently recognize the importance of adopting a given healthy behavior are actually ready, willing, and able to do so immediately. Nonetheless, most of these patients are actively involved in making the requisite cognitive and incremental behavior changes that are a vital part of a process ultimately leading to behavior change. Clinician recognition and understanding of the preparative groundwork that precedes more definitive behavior change can enable clinicians to serve their patients better by first focusing on helping patients prepare for change, rather than trying to persuade them to launch into immediate action. On the other hand, exhorting less ready patients to take immediate action actually can disrupt and slow down the delicate process of "thought rearrangement" that must precede definitive behavior change.

Two decades of behavioral research indicate that physicians can successfully promote health behavior change in their patients.[9,10] Health care providers who understand behavior change theory and who practice a patient-centered approach to behavior change counseling achieve the best outcomes.

Common Pitfalls

- Failing to understand that behavior change is the end result of a process that begins with the patient thinking about making a change
- Creating a dialectic where the clinician argues for change while the patient argues against it
- Viewing behavior change counseling as taking more time than is available in a 20-minute patient encounter
- Failing to create systems of care that assist patients to follow through on their behavior change goals

BEHAVIOR CHANGE THEORY

Mr. Abera is actively thinking about getting more exercise; but he is not sure that he really could exercise more often.

HOW DOES CHANGE OCCUR?

The Stages of Change Model describes a universal pattern of change discovered in people who had quit smoking "naturally," without professional help.[11] The Stages of Change Model, which has been validated across multiple unhealthy lifestyle behaviors, describes a sequence of internal and external events that unfolds as people progress toward the goal of maintaining healthy behavior change. At first, they deny or are unaware that a problem exists (e.g., being overweight), but as their concerns accrue (e.g., chronic knee pain), change becomes more important. They may begin to experiment with new behaviors that are interspersed with relapses. Finally, healthy change is maintained. As discussed in this chapter, a key to the thought rearrangement that begins early in this change process is the emergence and blossoming of perceived *importance*.

The Stages of Change Model implies that premature focus on action with patients who are not yet ready to change only diverts their attention from the task of thought rearrangement. This provokes resistance. The flavor of this resistance varies with patients' cultures (e.g., arguing against the need for change, passive smiling, silence, changing the topic, passive compliance), but the authors' clinical experience is that the outcome is universally unpleasant: Rapport is damaged and patients resist.

There are five sequential stages in the Stages of Change Model, each demanding different practitioner skills: precontemplation, contemplation, preparation, action, and maintenance (see Box 33-1). Patients in the three final stages of change, *preparation* (is committing to and planning to change), *action* (has recently made a behavior change), and *maintenance* (is sustaining it), are less challenging for health care providers. These patients proactively ask for advice or willingly accept it. However, patients in *precontemplation* (not even considering change soon) and *contemplation* (considering change but very ambivalent about it) force health care providers to be more skillful. For precontemplators, the cons of changing far outweigh the pros. In other words, the *importance* of change is low, challenging providers to help increase it. For patients in contemplation, the importance of change is blooming, yet they are pulled in two directions simultaneously: *On one hand, I would like to exercise more and on the other hand, I truly enjoy my nap after work.*

Both precontemplators and contemplators resist exhortation by providers to take action with "yes, but" statements. The Stages of Change Model reminds practitioners not to outstrip their patients' readiness levels. It takes time for patients to navigate the earlier cognitive stages of the change process. Many have experienced patients who finally take action after years of thinking and talking about change. Their thinking and talking was indispensable preparation.

WHY DOES CHANGE OCCUR?

> Mr. Abera knows that getting more exercise is important for his health. But the only time he has to exercise is evenings, and he lives in an unsafe area of the city.

The Stages of Change Model describes the topography of the change process (the "how" of change), other theories address the "why" of change (Table 7-1). Counseling methods that exploit the unique insights of these theories are most effective in enhancing the behavior change in patients. These theories are described now, because they have shaped Motivational Interviewing, the foundation for the evidence-based counseling approach presented later in this chapter.[12]

Humanistic theory is at the core of Motivational Interviewing, because the spirit of motivational interviewing is patient-centered; it is a way of being with patients. *Humanistic theory* asserts that people are naturally driven to seek health and happiness. Three conditions in helping relationships are necessary to enhance this powerful inner drive toward health: warmth, accurate understanding of the person by the helper, and unconditional positive regard.[13]

As mentioned, successful change requires that patients perceive change as important. The Health Belief Model identifies two important sources that influence the chances that a patient will adopt a healthy behavior: a sense of personal vulnerability to a given risk, and a belief that the benefits of the new behavior outweigh the costs.[14] By providing medical information to patients in a clear and straightforward manner (e.g., jargon-free), physicians can increase the importance their patients attach to changing their health behavior.

The other vital ingredient for successful behavior change is *confidence. Self-efficacy theory* posits that people must be confident in their ability to perform a given behavior change before they will undertake it.[15] For example, many patients are discouraged about eating better or quitting smoking because they have tried to change but experienced relapses that they perceive to be "failures." Providers might raise confidence by helping patients identify barriers to sustained change, and brainstorming strategies for overcoming these barriers. Providers also should inform patients that relapsing is not a failure but rather a natural part of successful change.

STYLE IS EVERYTHING

Behavioral theory not only identifies importance and confidence as fruitful targets for counseling; it also guides the *style* of offering advice and information to patients. *Reactance theory* warns that people will resist even good advice if they perceive it as limiting their personal freedom.[16] In the Motivational Interviewing model, the style of giving advice is to first elicit from patients what they think they should do, before offering medical advice. *Self-Determination Theory* postulates

Table 7-1. Behavioral Theory and Its Implications for Promoting Behavior Change

	Theory	Implications
Humanistic Theory	People are most likely to change in presence of a person who accepts them as they are.	Listen, understand, and accept the patient as he or she is before the change.
Stages of Change Model	Change occurs in a sequence of stages.	Assist with thought rearrangement early on; remember that relapse is not failure.
Self-Efficacy Theory	People will try to change if they believe they are able to do it.	Tell the patient that change is possible; underline the patient's strengths that might help him or her to succeed.
Health Beliefs Model	Change is important to people if they believe they are vulnerable to risk and change will pay off.	Offer medical information to establish risk and benefits.
Self-Determination Theory	Change is more lasting if it results from internal reasons rather than external pressure.	Find the patient's internal reasons for change. (What is important to this patient?)
Reactance Theory	People resist good advice if they perceive it to limit their freedom.	Offer the patient a menu of behavioral topics and a menu of change plan options.
Self Perception Theory	What people hear themselves say or see themselves doing about any given issue influences their position on that issue.	"Change talk" is a barometer of how well an interview is going.

Box 7-1. Elements of Effective Behavior Change Counselling

- Encourages the patient to describe symptoms and feelings in his or her own words and without frequent interruptions
- Offers periodic reflections (short summaries) that acknowledge the patient's feelings and point of view and show the patient that she or he is being properly understood

- Provides medical information and advice that is jargon-free and tailored to the patient's comprehension of the problem.
- Promotes shared decision making about the care plan, conveying that the patient has a degree of control over his or her health care decisions

---

that people are more likely to sustain a behavior change if it is initiated from internal reasons rather than external pressure.[17] Therefore, the style of Motivational Interviewing is to learn from patients their internal reasons for change, before offering advice. For example, a provider who learns from a patient that the patient dearly wants to remain involved in his granddaughter's life for as long as possible might suggest to the patient that quitting smoking would increase the chances of this happening.

Finally, *Self-Perception Theory* reminds the practitioner of the mutual causality between self-perceptions and behavior. In other words, people not only change their behavior to make it more consistent with their beliefs. (*"I am a person who believes in good health; therefore, I should substitute teriyaki tofu for hamburger."*) They also change their beliefs to make them more consistent with their perceived behavior. (*"I notice myself substituting tofu for burger; therefore, I must be a person who believes in good health."*) According to self-perception theory, "acting as if" kindles lasting change.[18] Therefore, the Motivational Interviewing practitioner helps patients make small incremental changes that kindle larger change. (*"I see myself eating better, so I must value good health; maybe I will start exercising more, as well . . ."*)

This chapter has been describing the theoretical basis for a particular patient-centered style of behavioral counseling known as Motivational Interviewing.[12] The medical version of Motivational Interviewing was developed by Rollnick and called simply *Behavior Change Counseling*.[19] Although Behavior Change Counseling manifests the same patient-centered style as Motivational Interviewing, it is designed for practitioners without psychotherapy backgrounds, operating in short encounters in medical settings. Motivational interviewing is effective in the treatment of patients with substance abuse, and Behavior Change Counseling based on Motivational Interviewing principles has shown promise in medical settings.[20–22]

The style of Behavior Change Counseling flows naturally from the theory and spirit of Motivational Interviewing. This style is characterized by open-ended questions and supportive dialogue (Box 7-1).[23]

THE CLINICIAN'S BAROMETER

How well a behavioral discussion is going is indicated by *how the patient talks about change:* Is the patient in favor of change? Neutral? Against it? "Change talk" is a term that refers to patient statements made in favor of change. When "change talk" occurs, the interview is going well. If the patient is taking the "no change" side of the argument, it is a signal to the clinician to refocus on the patient's reasons for wanting to change.

Categories of "change talk" include a *desire* to change, the *rationale* for change, and the *ability* to change. However, the ultimate in "change talk" is "commitment language," which is a strong signal that behavior change will soon occur.[24] The practitioner should listen for change talk (Box 7-2) so as to let the patient guide him or her through the sequence of Behavior Change Counseling methods described in the following section.

Box 7-2. Categories of "Change Talk"

Categories	Examples
Desire	"I really want to get my blood sugars under control."
Rationale	"If I don't take better care of myself, I won't be able to attend my grandson's graduation this spring."
Ability	"I know that I can change if I just put my mind to it."
Commitment language	"I am definitely going to take this medicine," and, "Just tell me what I have to do and I'll do it."

BEHAVIOR CHANGE COUNSELING

> At his recent clinic visit, Mr. Abera's primary care provider showed him a menu of behaviors that could improve Mr. Abera's health. Mr. Abera told his primary care provider that he was not ready to quit smoking, but that he did want to try to get more exercise.

Behavior Change Counseling has been distilled into a sequence of three clinical tasks: getting started, boosting importance and confidence, and discussing action options.[19] Following a simple checklist protects practitioners from getting ahead of the patient's readiness level (Box 7-3).

TASK 1: GETTING STARTED

The goal of Task 1 is for the clinician and patient to agree on a behavioral topic for discussion. At the outset of the visit, ask the patient for permission to spend the last few minutes discussing lifestyle changes that the patient might be contemplating to improve his or her health (of course, sometimes an entire visit is devoted to discussing behavior change, such as a visit that focuses on smoking cessation).

To begin discussing behavior change, it is helpful to provide patients with a visual menu of health behavior topics. Figure 7-1 provides an example of such a menu that focuses on behavior change options for patients with diabetes.[25] The menu gives patients the freedom to identify those lifestyle topics of greatest importance to them (and for which they are at least in the contemplation stage of readiness). The menu also may help patients not yet contemplating health behavior change to choose a topic they can at least discuss in a hypothetical way. (*"If you were to someday make a healthy change, in which area might that be?"*) Finally, the menu provides the provider with an opportunity to identify any behavior change(s) that might afford the patient the greatest medical advantage. (*"As long as you know that quitting smoking would give you the greatest health advantage, because you aren't ready to discuss it, let's talk about what you are most ready to discuss today . . ."*) Including a blank circle on the menu of topics reminds the provider and patient that the patient may have a topic in mind to discuss that he or she considers more important than the other domains on the card.[19]

TASK 2: BOOSTING IMPORTANCE AND CONFIDENCE

Once a behavioral topic is chosen from the menu, Task 2 is to use a scripted set of three questions that explore importance and confidence, and is effective in eliciting "change talk." This includes discussion of the patient's reasons for wanting to change and perceived barriers to change (Table 7-2). The same three questions are used for both importance and confidence.[19]

1. *"I'd like to understand how important it is to you personally to (make the change under discussion). If 0 is not important and 10 is very important, what number would you give yourself today?"* Higher numbers mean the patient is more ready to change.
2. *"Why did you give it a (number the patient gave) and not a (lower number than the patient gave)?"* This elicits change talk. (*"I gave it a 7 and not a 3, because I'm afraid of cancer."*)
3. *"What would it take for you to give it a (higher number than the patient gave)?"* The answer to this question tells the provider what specific medical information might serve to increase the patient's importance, either by increasing her or his concern or removing barriers.

The same three questions can be used for exploring confidence.

1. *"If you were to decide to (make the change under discussion), how confident are you that you would be successful, if 0 is not at all confident and 10 is very confident?"* This tells the provider the patient's confidence level relative to importance. Some providers then try to raise whichever is lower.
2. *"Why did you give it a (number the patient gave it) and not a (lower number than the patient gave)?"* The answer to this question promotes "change talk" and may help identify the patient's strengths. (*"I know I can quit drinking if I put my mind to it, because I have already quit smoking."*)
3. *"What would it take for you to give it a (higher number than the patient gave it)?"* This identifies barriers to change that both people can now collaboratively address.

Box 7-3. Checklist of the Patient's Readiness Level for Behavior Change

1. Did my patient agree to discuss the topic of change?
2. Is change important to him or her?

3. If so, is she confident that he or she can change?
4. If so, how much is he or she ready to do?

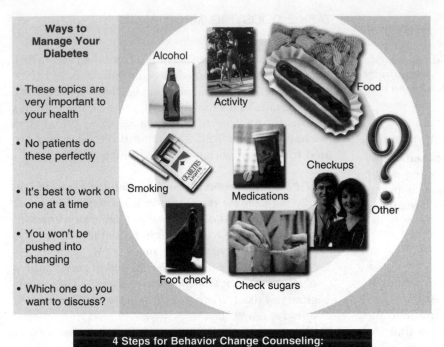

Ways to Manage Your Diabetes

- These topics are very important to your health

- No patients do these perfectly

- It's best to work on one at a time

- You won't be pushed into changing

- Which one do you want to discuss?

Alcohol

Activity

Food

Smoking

Medications

Checkups

Other

Foot check

Check sugars

4 Steps for Behavior Change Counseling:

1. **Select one topic collaboratively.**

2. **Elicit patient's view on this topic:**
   - How **important** is it to change (1–10)?
   - Why didn't you give yourself a lower number?
   - What would it take to give yourself a higher number?
   - How **confident** are you in your ability to change?
   - Why didn't you give yourself a higher number?
   - What would it take to give yourself a higher number?

3. **Summarize your patient's view**

4. **Exchange information or advice (using Elicit-Provide-Elicit method):**
   - **Elicit** patient's ideas first
   - **Provide** your information/advice next
   - **Elicit** patient's reaction/commitment

Close on good terms

Figure 7-1. Menu of behavior change options for patients with diabetes. (From: Stott NC, Rollnick S, Rees MR, et al. Innovation in clinical method: Diabetes care and negotiating skills. Fam Pract 1995;12:413–418.)

Table 7-2. The Importance and Confidence Profile Guides Counseling Strategy

	Low Confidence	**High Confidence**
High importance	Boost confidence by addressing barriers, modifying goals, or offering hope.	Go for it! Identify specific, attainable goals and collaboratively form an action plan.
Low importance	Boost importance with medical information of interest to the patient, or consider choosing a different behavioral topic.	Boost importance with medical information of interest to the patient.

The most powerful tools for boosting importance and confidence are medical information, advice, and hope. Here is where style is perhaps more important than ever. The authors suggest using the "elicit-provide-elicit" sequence of advice or information giving (Box 7-4).[19]

Consider the following two styles of giving information to raise the importance of medication adherence for a patient with severe asthma.

Provider: *"Instead of your rescue inhaler, you would be better off using a preventive medicine, long term."*

Patient: *"But I've heard that steroids are dangerous to take all the time."*

In the preceding exchange, the patient was diverted from the requisite thought rearrangement about preventive medication. Using the elicit-provide-elicit

Box 7-4. Elicit-Provide-Elicit Sequence

Step 1. *Elicit* what the patient knows (information) or thinks he or she should do (advice).

Step 2. *Provide* your information or advice, tailored to what the patient said when you previously elicited his or her view.

Step 3. *Elicit* again your patient's reaction (or commitment if the patient is more ready).

---

sequence, the exchange might have gone like this instead.

Provider elicits: *"Can you tell me a little about what you already know about rescue versus long-term asthma medicines?"*

Patient: *"Well, I've been told that steroids are really bad for you in the long run."*

Provider provides information: *"Yes, it's true that for a very small number of people, steroids can have harmful side-effects. It's also true that the number of people with severe asthma like you, who get permanent damage to their lungs from repeated asthma attacks, is much larger than the number who experience serious side effects from the steroid."*

Provider elicits reaction: *"What do you make of that?"*

Patient: *"Really? I didn't know that. I thought it was just discomfort. I mean, am I really harming my lungs when I get an attack?"* (The importance of taking corticosteroids is again raised.)

Confidence can be more daunting for providers to address than importance, because information or advice may not as readily boost confidence. Providers can lend the patient their own hope. Often, it is as simple as saying, *"I believe you can do it."*

TASK 3: DISCUSSING ACTION OPTIONS

Once the patient's importance and confidence levels are established, Task 3 is to develop with the patient a plan that matches her readiness level. With less ready patients, this might be simply to think more about the topic. With more ready patients, the plan might be to experiment with a small incremental change in behavior. Providers can be effective in helping patients become specific and realistic about their goals. She wants to lose weight; but does she want to reduce fats and sweets in her diet, or only sweets? He wants to change his drinking, but does he want to cut down or quit drinking altogether? Also, if patients choose extremely difficult goals (e.g., lose 30 pounds in 1 month), providers should help them modify their goals to be specific and attainable.

The session is now at a juncture: It can either be closed on good terms, thus paving the way for open discussion at a later date, or move ahead to discussing a plan. To determine which it will be, the provider might ask the patient, *"Where does all this leave you now?"*[12] The strength of the patient's commitment language in response to this question is informative.

- *"I'm determined to do it."* (strong commitment)
- *"Well, I don't know. It's high time I did something about this, I'm just not sure when."* (less strong commitment)
- *"I'm not the kind of person who likes to set goals."* (weak commitment)

For patients with strong commitment language, mental rehearsal greatly improves follow-through. To do this, ask patients to form a simple plan: "Whenever situation X arises, I will perform action Y." Situation X can be any event already occurring regularly in that patient's life, such as going outside for the morning paper. Action Y is the new behavior to be linked to this regular event. (*"Every time I go outside for the morning paper, I will first walk fast around the block."*) Linking a new behavior to a daily, automatic one puts the new behavior on "autopilot," greatly increasing follow-through.[26] This strategy has been found to improve numerous health behaviors, among them receiving cervical cancer screening,[27] and exercising regularly.[28]

The clinician should acknowledge the ambivalence of patients with less strong commitment. It may help to normalize the patient's ambivalence and describe how other patients have approached the initial hurdle of getting started. For example, the clinician might say, *"I find that many of my patients feel the same way you do when they begin thinking about making a change. Sometimes it helps to begin by trying out new behaviors on a few occasions to see how it goes. What do you think?"*

For patients with weak commitment, the goal should be to close the conversation on good terms. The clinician might say, *"It sounds like you're not feeling ready to make this change right now. Would it be okay if I checked in with you at our next visit to see where you're at with it?"* (Box 7-5).

Box 7-5. Helping Patients with Decision Making

1. Acknowledge that change is hard.
2. Help patients identify what has led them to make changes in the past.
3. Do not rush patients into decision making.

4. If you find yourself arguing with the patient, refocus the discussion on the patient's own interpretation of the pros and cons of change.
5. Recognize that failure to reach a decision is not a failed consultation.

BEHAVIOR CHANGE IN A CROSS-CULTURAL CONTEXT

> Mr. Abera was born in Ethiopia and he came to the United States 10 years ago.

The theoretical models that underlie the approach to promoting behavior change, as well as the explicit counseling method described in the preceding, have not been comprehensively evaluated in socioeconomically disadvantaged, non-white, or non-Western peoples.[29] This said, in the United States, the Stages of Change Model has been validated in at least one clinic that cares for predominantly poor and underserved populations.[30] Moreover, there is evidence that behavior change counseling based on motivational interviewing can be effective in non-white and non-Western peoples. Motivational Interviewing appears to be a promising strategy for modifying dietary behavior among African Americans.[21] A similar approach recently was found to be effective in promoting the use of household-level water disinfection and safe storage in Zambia in order to prevent diarrheal illness.[31,32]

Many providers are apprehensive about how best to interact with a patient from a culture different from their own. (*Should I speak with more or less authority? Should I be discussing this with or without the family present?*) The overarching principle for interacting with all patients is to "seek first to understand." Given that culturally matched techniques for promoting behavior change have not been comprehensively evaluated in non-Western populations, the authors believe that a patient-centered style of communication (as described) transcends cultural differences and is essential to successfully promoting behavior change.[33,34]

Educating oneself about the customs and mores of peoples from outside the United States can be very helpful to clinicians who practice cross-cultural medicine (www.ethnomed.org). However, gleaning generalities of other cultures, although generating useful hypotheses, risks perpetuating stereotypes and may be inaccurate.[35] Clinicians rarely misstep by following the axiom, "When in doubt, ask your patient." As well, clinicians should trust their perceptions of how patients feel. Despite some individual, age, and cultural differences among people, Ekman's work on facial expressions suggests that certain facial expressions—including joy, disgust, and pain—can be reliably interpreted across cultures.[36]

THE IMPORTANCE OF CONTINUITY AND CLINICAL SYSTEMS

> Mr. Abera and his primary care provider develop an action plan: Mr. Abera will walk to work in the mornings, rather than take the bus. A week later, the clinic nurse calls Mr. Abera to ask how things are going.

Promoting behavior change in patients takes time, and is probably best accomplished in the context of an ongoing provider–patient relationship. Most patients need months or even years to successfully adopt and sustain the practice of a new health behavior. Brief interventions are well suited to an ongoing change process.

A SYSTEMS-BASED APPROACH

Although physicians can promote health behavior change in the context of their one-on-one interactions with patients, promoting health behavior change is optimally accomplished using a systems approach to care.[37]

Prior to a visit, patients can be prompted to think about and encouraged to discuss with their provider behavioral changes they have made or are thinking about making, or are having difficulty in making. Such "patient activation" strategies have proved effective at improving clinical outcomes in patients with chronic illness.[38,39]

Clinic systems also can assist patients in following through on behavioral action plans. Documenting behavior counseling discussions and action plans makes other members of the health care team aware of a patient's behavioral goals. Team members then can support patients in achieving their goals; for example, by proactively following up with patients by phone to assess patient progress and help troubleshoot barriers to implementing an action plan.[40] Feedback and coaching that are relatively immediate and ongoing have the greatest efficacy.[41] Role modeling and peer support can further increase a patient's ability to sustain healthy behaviors.

Patients pursue behavioral changes in the communities in which they live, not in physician offices. Clinics should attempt to identify, catalogue, and link patients to community-based and Internet resources that can help patients to achieve their behavioral goals.[37] Examples of community-based resources include toll-free "quit smoking" lines; exercise programs sponsored by departments of public parks and recreation; and other programs sponsored by nonprofit organizations such as the YMCA and disease-specific advocacy groups (e.g., local chapters of the American Diabetes Association).

KEY CONCEPTS

- Behavior change begins with thinking about change and proceeds through a series of cognitive stages.
- A nonjudgmental and patient-centered style of communicating with patients increases the clinician's effectiveness in promoting behavior change.
- Conversations about behavior change should be tailored to the patient's stage of readiness for change.
- Assessing the importance a patient attaches to changing a behavior, and the patient's confidence in his or her ability to make a change, should guide behavior change discussions and goal setting.
- Patients are more likely to change when cared for by clinics that implement systems to assist patients in achieving their behavioral goals.

CONCLUSION

Health behavior profoundly affects health outcomes. People who are free of disease, those who exercise regularly, maintain ideal body weight, do not smoke, undergo cancer screening at recommended intervals and so on, on average will be less likely to develop chronic disease and live longer. Among people who have one or more chronic illness, those who not only adopt healthy behaviors, but also self-manage their illness with regular monitoring and adjusting their behavior minimize complications and have a better quality of life.

Clinicians must take the long view on promoting behavior change, and recognize that by using a patient-centered style and evidence-based techniques they can effectively assist patients to adopt healthier behaviors, as well as reduce the burden of suffering for those who contend with chronic illness.

CORE COMPETENCY
Behavior Change Counseling

- Select one topic collaboratively
  Don't focus prematurely on a problem or an action with which the patient does not agree.
- Elicit patient's views on the topic:
  How important is it to change (on a scale of 1-10)?
  Why didn't you give yourself a lower number?
  What would it take to give yourself a higher number?
  How confident are you in your ability to change (on a scale of 1-10)?
  Why didn't you give yourself a higher number?
  What would it take to give yourself a higher number?
- Summarize your patient's view.
  Make supportive statements to build confidence ("It is so great that you are thinking about making this change..."
  Don't push patients into denying that they have something to change.
- Exchange information or advice using the elicit-provide-elicit method.
  Elicit you patient's ideas first
  Provide information/advice next
  Elicit your patient's reaction/commitment

Adapted from: Miller WR, Rollnick S. Motivational interviewing: Preparing people to change addictive behavior. New York: Guilford Press, 1991.

DISCUSSION QUESTIONS

1. "Dancing versus wrestling" can be a useful metaphor for behavior change counseling. "Wrestling" ends with a winner and a loser (or two losers!). "Dancing" means the patient is doing most of the talking. Think back to a recent patient with whom you danced and another with whom you wrestled. What do you think you may have done that led you to dance with one and wrestle with the other?
2. Think back on a healthy behavior change that you yourself made some time in the past. Did you perceive making the change as important for your health? Why? What were the circumstances that led you to make this change?
3. Imagine that Mr. Abera is your patient. What kinds of barriers might he face in making lifestyle changes, such as getting more exercise or eating fewer calories? In what ways could you and your clinic help Mr. Abera to achieve his goal of getting more exercise?

RESOURCES

Rollnick S, Mason P, Butler C. Health behavior change: A guide for practitioners. London: Churchill Livingstone, 1999.
http://www.bayerinstitute.org
http://www.ethnomed.org
http://www.improvingchroniccare.org

REFERENCES

1. Lantz PM, House JS, Lepkowski JM, et al. Socioeconomic factors, health behaviors, and mortality: Results from a nationally representative prospective study of US adults. *JAMA* 1998;279:1703–1708.
2. Ribisl KM, Winkleby MA, Fortmann SP, et al. The interplay of socioeconomic status and ethnicity on Hispanic and white men's cardiovascular disease risk and health communication patterns. *Health Educ Res* 1998;13:407–417.
3. Winkleby MA, Kraemer HC, Ahn DK, et al. Ethnic and socioeconomic differences in cardiovascular disease risk factors: Findings for women from the Third National Health and Nutrition Examination Survey, 1988–1994. *JAMA* 1998;280:356–362.
4. Crespo CJ, Smit E, Andersen RE, et al. Race/ethnicity, social class and their relation to physical inactivity during leisure time: Results from the Third National Health and Nutrition Examination Survey, 1988–1994. *Am J Prev Med* 2000;18:46–53.
5. Komaromy M, Lurie N, Bindman AB. California physicians' willingness to care for the poor. *West J Med* 1995;162:127–132.
6. Taira DA, Safran DG, Seto TB, et al. The relationship between patient income and physician discussion of health risk behaviors. *JAMA* 1997;278:1412–1417.
7. Butler C, Rollnick S, Stott N. The practitioner, the patient and resistance to change: Recent ideas on compliance. *CMAJ* 1996;154:1357–1362.
8. Levinson W, Cohen MS, Brady D, et al. To change or not to change: "Sounds like you have a dilemma." *Ann Intern Med* 2001;135(5):386–391.
9. Kahan M, Wilson L, Becker L. Effectiveness of physician-based interventions with problem drinkers: A review. *CMAJ* 1995;152:851–859.
10. Mojica WA, Suttorp MJ, Sherman SE, et al. Smoking-cessation interventions by type of provider: A meta-analysis. *Am J Prev Med* 2004;26:391–401.
11. Prochaska J, Diclemente C. Toward a comprehensive model of change. In: Miller WR, Heather N, eds. *Treating addictive behaviors*. New York: Plenum Press, 1986:3–27.
12. Miller WR, Rollnick S. *Motivational interviewing: Preparing people for change*, 2nd ed. New York: Guilford Press, 2002.
13. Rogers CR. *On becoming a person*. New York: Houghton Mifflin, 1961.
14. Janz NK, Becker MH. The health belief model: A decade later. *Health Educ Quart* 1984;11:1–47.
15. Bandura A. Self-efficacy mechanism in human agency. *Amer Psychol* 1982;37:122–147.
16. Brehm J. *A theory of psychological reactance*. New York: Academic Press, 1966.
17. Deci EL, Ryan RM. *Intrinsic motivation and self-determination in human behavior*. New York: Plenum, 1985.
18. Bem DJ. Self-perception theory. In: Berkowitz L, ed. *Advances in experimental social psychology*, vol. 6. New York: Academic Press, 1972:1–62.
19. Rollnick S, Mason P, Butler C. *Health behavior change: A guide for practitioners*. London: Churchill Livingstone, 1999.
20. Dunn C, Deroo L, Rivara FP. The use of brief interventions adapted from motivational interviewing across behavioral domains: A systematic review. *Addiction* 2001;96:1725–1742.
21. Resnicow K, Jackson A, Wang T, et al. A motivational interviewing intervention to increase fruit and vegetable intake through Black churches: Results of the Eat for Life trial. *Am J Public Health* 2001;91:1686–1693.
22. Britt E, Hudson SM, Blampied NM. Motivational interviewing in health settings: A review. *Patient Educ Couns* 2004;53:147–155.
23. Mead N, Bower P. Patient-centered consultations and outcomes in primary care: A review of the literature. *Patient Educ Couns* 2002;48:51–61.
24. Amrhein PC, Miller WR, Yahne CE, et al. Client commitment language during motivational interviewing predicts drug use outcomes. *J Consult Clin Psychol* 2003;71:862–878.
25. Stott NC, Rollnick S, Rees MR, et al. Innovation in clinical method: Diabetes care and negotiating skills. *Fam Pract* 1995;12:413–418.
26. Gollwitzer PM, Schaal B. Metacognition in action: the importance of implementation intentions. *Pers Soc Psychol Rev* 1998;2:124–136.
27. Sheeran P, Orbell S. Using implementation intentions to increase attendance for cervical cancer screening. *Health Psychol* 2000;19:283–289.
28. Milne S, Orbell S, Sheeran P. Combining motivational and volitional interventions to promote exercise participation: Protection motivation theory and implementation intentions. *Br J Health Psychol* 2002;7(Pt 2):163–184.
29. Emmons KM, Rollnick S. Motivational interviewing in health care settings. Opportunities and limitations. *Am J Prev Med* 2001;20:68–74.
30. Gil KM, Schrop SL, Kline SC, et al. Stages of change analysis of smokers attending clinics for the medically underserved. *J Fam Pract* 2002;51:1018.
31. Thevos AK, Kaona FA, Siajunza MT, et al. Adoption of safe water behaviors in Zambia: Comparing educational and motivational approaches. *Educ Health (Abingdon)* 2000;13:366–376.
32. Quick RE, Kimura A, Thevos A, et al. Diarrhea prevention through household-level water disinfection and safe storage in Zambia. *Am J Trop Med Hyg* 2002;66:584–589.
33. Tucker CM, Herman KC, Pedersen TR, et al. Cultural sensitivity in physician-patient relationships: Perspectives of an ethnically diverse sample of low-income primary care patients. *Med Care* 2003;41:859–870.
34. Piette JD, Schillinger D, Potter MB, et al. Dimensions of patient-provider communication and diabetes self-care in an ethnically diverse population. *J Gen Intern Med* 2003;18:624–633.

35. Kreuter MW, Lukwago SN, Bucholtz RD, et al. Achieving cultural appropriateness in health promotion programs: Targeted and tailored approaches. *Health Educ Behav* 2003;30:133–146.

36. Ekman P, Sorenson ER, Friesen WV. Pan-cultural elements of facial displays of emotions. *Science* 1969;164:86–88.

37. Wagner EH, Austin BT, Davis C, et al. Improving chronic illness care: Translating evidence into action. *Health Aff (Millwood)* 2001;20:64–78.

38. Greenfield S, Kaplan SH, Ware JE Jr, et al. Patients' participation in medical care: Effects on blood sugar control and quality of life in diabetes. *J Gen Intern Med* 1988;3: 448–457.

39. Glasgow RE, La Chance PA, Toobert DJ, et al. Long-term effects and costs of brief behavioural dietary intervention for patients with diabetes delivered from the medical office. *Patient Educ Couns* 1997;32:175–184.

40. Von Korff M, Gruman J, Schaefer J, et al. Collaborative management of chronic illness. *Ann Intern Med* 1997;127: 1097–1102.

41. Clark NM. Management of chronic disease by patients. *Annu Rev Public Health* 2003;24:289–313.

Chapter 8

Assessing and Promoting Medication Adherence

Kirsten Bibbins-Domingo, PhD, MD, and M. Robin DiMatteo, PhD

Objectives

- Define medication adherence.
- Describe the scope and consequences of medication nonadherence.
- Summarize the patient, clinician, and system factors that contribute to medication nonadherence.
- Describe clinician–patient communication strategies to assess and promote medication adherence.
- Identify interventions to promote medication adherence.

Mr. Bradley is a 52-year-old postal carrier who left his job 1 year ago because of worsening heart failure and diabetes. Despite regular outpatient care from both a cardiologist and general internist, he has been hospitalized four times over the past year for management of heart failure. During each hospitalization, physicians suspected that the patient had not adhered with his medication regimen.

Adherence is defined by the World Health Organization as "the extent to which a person's behavior—taking medications, following a diet, and/or executing lifestyle changes—corresponds to agreed recommendations from a health care provider."[1] Although patients often are labeled nonadherent if they fail to follow medical recommendations, nonadherence may signify a breakdown of the collaborative partnership between clinicians and patients, or may be evidence of health system deficiencies that fail to support their efforts. Therefore, strategies to improve adherence should strengthen the collaboration between patients and clinicians and mitigate patient, clinician, and system barriers.

This chapter describes the problem of medication nonadherence, and explores patient, clinician, and system factors that contribute to nonadherence. It provides communication strategies designed to identify nonadherence, clarify the causes of nonadherence, and promote higher levels of adherence.

SCOPE OF THE PROBLEM

Mr. Bradley's clinical picture is complex and his responses to treatment are unexpectedly poor. He has had frequent hospitalizations for his multiple chronic illnesses, and few of his medications seem to be working as predicted.

Studies suggest that as many as half of medical patients do not completely follow the treatment recommendations of their clinicians.[1,2] Nonadherence is of particular concern among those with multiple chronic medical problems, such as hypertension and diabetes,[3,4] as well as among lower income patients who may face many barriers to adherence, including rising medication costs.[5]

The consequence of nonadherence can be devastating. Over 100,000 deaths annually have been attributed to nonadherence with medication regimens.[6] Medication nonadherence also leads to higher rates of hospitalizations, emergency room visits, and outpatient visits, as well as worsening health status.[2,7] In addition to adverse health consequences and potential financial waste, nonadherence can lead to frustration for both patients and clinicians and thus may contribute to breakdown in this relationship.

FACTORS ASSOCIATED WITH NONADHERENCE

ISSUES AT THE INTERFACE OF PATIENT AND TREATMENT

> Mr. Bradley takes nine different medications: six for management of a heart disease and three medications for his diabetes. Since leaving his job, he has experienced severe financial strain and now suffers from depression.

Nonadherence usually is viewed from the perspective of the health care provider, for whom the patient's behavior may appear to be irrational. However, there are multiple reasons that patients choose not to follow the advice of their health care providers, particularly when complex medication regimens or their side-effects conflict with the patient's personal identity or goals.[8] Understanding the elements at the interface of patient and treatment may contribute to better assessment and management of nonadherence.

Medication Effects and Side-Effects

All medications have potential side-effects, and the number of side-effects increases with the complexity of the regimen. Although clinicians may be vigilant for serious side-effects, they may be less conscious of those that are not life threatening, but nevertheless significantly interfere with a patient's functioning. In addition, the desired effect of the medication may be misperceived by the patient as an adverse effect. For example, patients inadvertently may be taking diuretic medications at night, leading to disrupted sleep. Switching diuretics to morning dosing may relieve this problem. However, such changes in the dosing schedule may prove challenging for individuals who do not have ready access to bathroom facilities in the work place.

The seriousness of side-effects is often idiosyncratic, and must be assessed for patients individually. In addition, patients may have different levels of tolerance for medication side-effects. For example, although the cough associated with the use of angiotensin converting enzyme (ACE) inhibitors is inconsequential for many patients, it may prompt avoidance in others. Patients may be reluctant to discuss certain side-effects with their clinicians (e.g., loss of libido associated with some medications).

In addition to the actual effects and side-effects of medications, unrelated new or recurrent symptoms may be attributed to a new medication by some patients and thus may contribute to nonadherence.

Regimen Complexity

The average older patient with two or more chronic illnesses is treated with more than six daily medications. Although many of these may be taken once daily, others may require multiple daily doses. Patients may experience scheduling conflicts associated with their medication regimens, particularly when their medication schedules change frequently, such as with warfarin, insulin, and diuretics. Some medications must be taken with food and others require an empty stomach. This complexity is further compounded by the fact that certain medications must not be taken at the same time as others. Coordinating a complex regimen with the normal activities of daily living is challenging. Many work environments do not permit scheduled breaks to take medications or monitor effects of medications (e.g., blood sugar check for diabetes). Those with marginal living situations may not have proper storage facilities (e.g., refrigeration).

Confusion

Even if a patient chooses to follow recommendations, misunderstanding, uncertainty, and confusion about the actual recommendation can lead to nonadherence. Patients may recall and comprehend as little as 50% of what is conveyed to them in a medical visit,[9–12] and often do not have a clear understanding of the doses and indications for each of their medications. Additionally, patients may not appreciate that treatment of chronic conditions such as hypertension and diabetes requires the ongoing use of medications, and consequently may fail to obtain refills once their prescription is completed.

Cognitive Impairments

Patients with cognitive impairments that result from aging or complications of underlying diseases (e.g., cerebrovascular disease) may be at particular risk for confusion with their medication regimens.[13]

Language and Low Functional Health Literacy

Language barriers and low functional health literacy[14] have been recognized as important contributors to confusion with medication regimens. Health literacy refers to patients' ability to "obtain, process, and understand the basic health information and services they need to make appropriate health decisions."[15] Patients who may be particularly vulnerable to low functional health literacy include older patients, members of racial/ethnic minorities, and those with limited English proficiency. As many as 50% of patients cared for at public hospitals may have low functional health literacy.[16]

Health Beliefs

Patients' beliefs about health, health care, or their particular medical conditions may differ substantially from those of their health care providers. These beliefs may range from use of complementary and alternative medicines, to religious beliefs and the conviction that there is no need to take medications if one is asymptomatic (often encountered in the treatment of hypertension).[17] Such health beliefs on the part of patients do not invariably lead to nonadherence if the beliefs are acknowledged and integrated into the patient's overall treatment plan. Clinicians who engage patients in nonjudgmental discussions of their use of complementary and alternative medicines, for example, may be better able to establish the rapport necessary to enable improved adherence, as well as identify potential serious interactions among treatments.

Social Support

Social support plays an important role in overall health and well-being, and appears to be instrumental in insuring medication adherence.[18] Social support encompasses emotional (love, affirmation), as well as practical support (food, shelter, money, transportation). Lack of social support likely increases nonadherence because of stress and diversion of patient time and energy.

Depression

Depression is common in the outpatient setting and particularly prevalent among those with multiple health problems.[19] Depressed patients are less likely to follow through on medical recommendations,[20] possibly because of hopelessness and lack of confidence in the effectiveness or worth of the treatment. Depressed patients also are likely to be isolated, lacking the social support necessary for adherence.

Substance Use

Dependence on alcohol or illicit drugs is an important independent factor contributing to nonadherence, and may be more prevalent in patients challenged by depression or social isolation, which also affect adherence. Patients actively using illicit drugs or alcohol may be prone to erratic use of prescribed medications. In addition, use of these illicit drugs or alcohol may worsen the conditions that their medications were prescribed to treat (e.g., hypertension, depression). The advent of effective pharmacologic-based treatments for addictions has led to efforts aimed at improving adherence among patients with dependence on illicit drugs or alcohol.[21]

Cost

The cost of medications is recognized as a common reason for medication nonadherence.[3,5,22,23] An increasing number of patients are uninsured, or may have insurance that does not cover the cost of medications. Even those with prescription drug benefits are often charged high copayments for each medication, which may represent a significant portion of a low-income patient's monthly budget. Some health plans and systems impose a prior authorization process, which requires patients to self-advocate, complete complex forms, and successfully negotiate alternatives with their clinician. Patients taking medications for chronic conditions may try to make their medications last longer (e.g., skipping doses, taking daily medications every other day), or fail to fill prescriptions when they are experiencing acute financial constraints.

Studies have shown that although clinicians understand that the cost of medications may affect adherence, they rarely initiate conversations about this barrier. Paradoxically, when they do, discussions frequently are not targeted at those patients most likely to have financial problems. Additionally, physicians often lack adequate knowledge of insurance and formulary restrictions to change their prescribing patterns, which could alleviate some cost burdens.[24-26]

HEALTH SYSTEM FACTORS

> After leaving his job, Mr. Bradley lost his private health insurance. Mr. Bradley began receiving his care at the public hospital, and because of formulary differences had to switch from one type of beta-blocker, which is taken once a day, to another type of beta-blocker, which is taken twice a day. Further, his outpatient medications have been changed during each of his four hospitalizations.

The environment in which patients and clinicians discuss health care recommendations can either support adherence or undermine it. The following are factors within the health care system that may contribute to nonadherence.

Fragmented Care

Patients with multiple chronic illnesses often are treated by more than one clinician, each of whom may be prescribing or adjusting medications. Recent technological advances have facilitated communication among physicians caring for the same patient (e.g., increasing use of electronic medical records), yet faulty or lapsed communication systems still contribute to confusion over care, as well as overt medical errors. These lapses are particularly likely to occur at the time of hospital discharge, when adjustments to the outpatient medication regimen are implemented, often without adequate patient education or communication with outpatient physicians.

Time Constraints

When arriving at their treatment recommendations, clinicians often do not have sufficient time to offer clear explanations or assess whether patients understand them. Unfortunately, very few health systems provide standardized education tools that clinicians can employ with patients who have been prescribed a new medication. Additionally, clinicians often feel that they do not have adequate time to explore differing health beliefs or any of the other patient factors that may contribute to nonadherence.

Pharmacists and pharmacy staff may feel pressured by similar time constraints that limit their potential as resources in the realm of patient education, and for the reinforcement they can offer about proper medication use.

Refill Restrictions

Many insurance plans impose restrictions on quantities of medications and the timing of medication refills. Such restrictions include limiting each prescription to a 30-day supply, allowing refills only when there are 2 to 3 days of medications left, and requiring physician approval for more than six total medications in a month. These restrictions can pose significant challenges for patients who need to fill prescriptions around complex work or family schedules, have difficulties navigating the bureaucratic processes, or have multiple chronic conditions whose medications may need to be filled on different days of the month.

Formulary Restrictions

Within a given class of medications, there are often multiple options with equivalent efficacy. Frequently payers reimburse for only one or two of the medications within a particular class, and require higher copayments or complete payments for other medications within the class. Clinicians usually treat a panel of patients with a variety of different insurance plans; therefore, they may be unaware of formulary restrictions and may fail to choose those with the lowest cost (and equivalent efficacy). Within a given plan, formularies often change (reflecting the availability of generic medications or negotiation of a lower price for a particular brand), requiring the patient to request another prescription from the clinician, or leading to confusion about pills of a different color or shape. Patients switch or lose jobs necessitating changes in, or loss of, their health insurance and subsequent formulary changes.

New medications within a given class, simply substituted in accordance with the formulary rules of the insurer, will likely appear different, and may be given on a different dosing schedule and have a different side-effect profile or interactions with other chronic medications. All of these can result in considerable confusion for patients.

THE HEALTH CARE PROVIDER'S ROLE IN ASSESSING AND PROMOTING ADHERENCE

The clinician, within the context of the patient–clinician relationship, can play an important role in promoting adherence by: (a) recognizing nonadherence; (b) identifying the factors that may be contributing to nonadherence; and (c) pursuing strategies that enhance the partnership with the patient (see Key Concepts).

PATIENT–CLINICIAN COMMUNICATION

Effective communication is critical to ensuring adherence, and is a hallmark of strong patient–clinician partnerships. Clear explanations of health recommendations minimize patient confusion. An environment that encourages bidirectional communication establishes rapport, conveys compassion, and makes it more likely that factors impeding adherence will be elicited. It increases patient satisfaction and trust in medical care, and contributes to a shared process of decision making about medical recommendations.

Patients who are poor, are members of race/ethnic minority groups, or have limited health literacy or English proficiency are likely to report less effective patient–clinician communication.[14] Increasing clinician awareness of the sociocultural context of their patients' health may improve patient–clinician communication, adherence, and overall health care.

IDENTIFYING PATIENTS WITH ADHERENCE DIFFICULTIES

Mr. Bradley returns to his general internist after his last two hospitalizations. She expresses concern for his frequent admissions, and asks Mr. Bradley to speculate about the factors that might be leading to his worsening heart failure. She also states that sometimes it is difficult for patients to take a lot of medications every day, and wonders whether Mr. Bradley has ever experienced any difficulties taking his medications.

Adherence must be reassessed at regular intervals for all patients, particularly when new medications are started or existing medications are changed.

Patients may be reluctant or embarrassed to admit that they are having difficulty with adherence. Patients may be unwilling to reveal their confusion, difficulty reading or understanding instructions, financial problems, or lack of the social supports necessary to maintain their regimens. They may feel that their health beliefs will

Table 8-1. Strategies for Assessing Adherence

- Use introductory statements that acknowledge the difficulty with adherence.
  "Taking pills every day can be hard. Most people have problems taking their pills at some point. I am going to ask you about problems you may have had taking your pills. I'm asking because I want to find a way to make it easier for you to take them. Can you tell me or show me how you take your medications?"
- Confirm an understanding of the regimen.
  Have patients bring in their pill bottles or make use of visual aids. If patients are confused, use strategies for increasing recall and comprehension of regimen.
- Ask about their medication schedule over the past 3 days, one day at a time.
  Start with the day prior to the visit and go through the entire day, asking how medications were taken or about missed doses. Then proceed with the day 2 days before the visit. If no doses were missed in the preceding 3 days, ask about the last time a dose was missed. Again make use of visual aids or pill bottles.
- Ask about reasons for missed doses.
  Begin with open-ended questions and then prompt if unable to elicit a response, suggesting common reasons why adherence may be difficult—forgot, too busy with other things, too many side-effects, feeling sick or depressed, ran out of pills, difficulty paying for medications, etc.
- Ask about effects that are particular to the medication regimen.
  Again, prompts may be necessary—nausea, headaches, depression, sexual side effects, difficulty swallowing pills, lack of access to refrigeration, difficulty obtaining pills from pharmacy.

Source: Machtinger E, Bangsberg DR. Adherence to HIV antiretroviral therapy. Accessed September 27, 2005. Available at: http://hivinsite.ucsf.edu/InSite.jsp/InSite?page=kb-03-02-09

not be understood or respected by their physicians. Some clinicians may make patients feel that their difficulty with adherence is unusual, further inhibiting discussion.

There are a number of ways to initiate discussions of adherence with outpatients (Table 8-1). These conversations should acknowledge that adherence can be difficult. Ideally such conversations use open-ended questions to engage patients and allow them to reveal the barriers that are most important to them, as well as more probing questions to discern the contribution of specific barriers.

Clearly, detailed adherence assessment is a time-consuming process. However, many experts have suggested that for certain high-risk patients (e.g., the elderly, those with multiple chronic conditions, those with cognitive impairment or communication barriers, those on medications with a narrow therapeutic window), visits solely for the purpose of medication review may be necessary. Such visits can be conducted by physicians, nurses, or clinical pharmacists[27] who can focus on a review of the medications, their proper administration (e.g., metered dose inhalers, insulin), and potential side-effects.

IDENTIFYING FACTORS CONTRIBUTING TO NONADHERENCE

Mr. Bradley states, "the doctors in the hospital keep changing my meds around." He admits to being confused about what medications he is supposed to be taking. In addition, Mr. Bradley acknowledges sometimes missing doses of medications, especially at the end of the month when "money is tight." Finally, Mr. Bradley expresses increasing hopelessness at the loss of his job and his worsening medical condition. "I just didn't think my life would turn out this way."

Adherence first requires that patients have a clear understanding of their health care providers' recommendations. Clinicians directly contribute to nonadherence when they fail to deliver clear explanations and assess patients' understanding of these recommendations. Comprehension can increase by techniques that ask patients to restate information to assure that it was understood,[12,28,29] such as with the "teach-back method" (Fig. 8-1). This interactive communication loop is useful for gauging the extent to which recommendations are understood by patients and for initiating the dialogue between clinicians and patients about other specific challenges to adherence. The "teach-back"

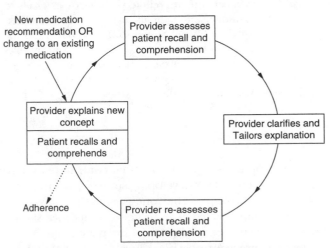

Figure 8-1. Interactive communication loop for educating patients regarding a change in their medication regimen. (Adapted from Schillinger D, et al. Closing the loop: Physician communication with diabetic patients who have low health literacy. Arch Intern Med 2003;163(1):83–90.)

method may help to uncover cognitive impairments or literacy limitations and prompt the clinician to refocus educational efforts to accommodate these challenges. This dialogue also may uncover differing patient perceptions or health beliefs about their medications and serve as an entry point for further exploration of these beliefs.

Clinicians must explore factors unique to particular patients or to the environment in which the clinician practices. Awareness should include accurate and up-to-date knowledge regarding medication side-effects, costs, prescriptions from other clinicians, and restrictions to formularies.

Common Pitfalls in the Identification of Patients with Adherence Difficulties

- Failing to recognize that difficulty with medication adherence is common
- Failing to recognize the importance of effective patient–provider communication in assessing and promoting medication adherence among all patients
- Failing to accurately identify patients who have difficulty with medication adherence
- Failing to identify the patient, clinician, and systems factors that may pose barriers to medication adherence
- Failing to target specific interventions that are appropriate to particular medication adherence barriers

---

INTERVENTIONS TO PROMOTE MEDICATION ADHERENCE

Mr. Bradley and his general internist review his medication regimen together. She asks him to return the following week to meet with the clinic pharmacist in order to reinforce his understanding of his current regimen, and asks that he bring all of his pill bottles so that outdated medications and those not indicated could be culled. She arranges for Mr. Bradley to see a social worker to review services he might qualify for to alleviate his financial crisis. Finally, she discusses Mr. Bradley's depressive symptoms with him, including options for treatment.

Identifying the specific factors that contribute to nonadherence is crucial for developing strategies to effectively address nonadherence. The "one-size-fits-all" approach is not appropriate; strategies to promote adherence should be tailored to the specific needs of the patient.

Several interventions have been studied that have the potential to promote adherence. These interventions, in concert with a clinician's recommendations, may help to enhance adherence.

Simplified Treatment Regimens

Single daily dosing of medications, reduced numbers of medications, and coordination of doses should be used, as appropriate. This strategy has been shown to be consistently effective in a variety of chronic conditions.[30,31]

Collaborative Planning

Patients and clinicians should collaborate to develop dosing schedules that accommodate the patient's daily schedule. Side-effects should be discussed whenever new therapies are initiated. Follow-up visits should readdress side-effects and dosing schedules; plans should be redesigned as these change. Collaborative planning also may include discussion of financial barriers to the initiation of medications and may include referrals to social workers or in-home support services to facilitate adherence.

Patient Education

Patients should be educated about their disease and the ways in which adherence to their medication regimens can alter the course of their disease. Educational interventions of this type are particularly important for chronic illnesses that require ongoing medications. Pharmacists, nurses, and health educators may all effectively describe disease processes (for chronic diseases such as diabetes, asthma, human immunodeficiency virus [HIV]) or the proper use of difficult to administer medications (e.g., insulin, metered dose inhalers). Education efforts should be readdressed at regular intervals because repetition is the key to learning.

Medication Review Visits

Patients may benefit from a visit devoted exclusively to a review of their medications. Pharmacists are particularly well suited to conduct such visits, as they are able to focus exclusively on medications, their proper administration, and potential side-effects. It has been shown that the inclusion of pharmacists on a multidisciplinary care team increases adherence and reduces adverse events.[27,32]

Review of medications is important not only at the initiation of a new medication regimen, but also for patients whose medications may not have changed substantially. Such reviews should address whether treatment for a particular condition is still indicated and consistent with the latest evidence, as well as whether a regimen can be simplified.

Case Management

For many patients the complexity of their disease (e.g., heart failure, HIV), their comorbid illnesses (e.g., psychiatric illness, substance use), or their social situation (e.g., homelessness) may pose additional challenges to adherence that can be most effectively addressed with intensive, multidisciplinary interventions. In these interventions, clinicians may partner with nurses, social workers, health educators, pharmacists, dieticians, and others to provide follow-up to support and identify ongoing barriers to adherence.[33,34]

System Reminders

Integrated health systems and large-chain pharmacies have employed automated reminder systems to enhance adherence with chronic medications. Patients may receive reminders to refill their medications several days prior to finishing their current prescription and may be reminded again if they fail to fill prescriptions in a timely manner.[35] Some systems identify patients that persistently underfill their prescriptions for a particular chronic disease and may use this information to target referrals for case management or other more intensive interventions.[36]

Some disease management programs incorporate regular automated telephone contact with patients to screen for a variety of potential difficulties with disease management, including medication adherence. These systems permit timely identification of adherence difficulties as well as targeted use of nurse, health educator, pharmacists, and physician time to focus on particular patients with adherence difficulties.[37]

Directly Observed Therapy

In this approach, patients receive their medications each day from a health provider (or reliable surrogate) and are observed taking them. It has been used successfully to address nonadherence in the treatment of tuberculosis,[38] and has been suggested for treatment of HIV and substance use.[39,40]

Medication Adherence Devices

The following devices are particularly useful for patients who are confused or have complicated medication regimens.

Medication Organizer Pillboxes, medi-sets, and other versions of medication organizers are readily available in clinics and pharmacies. Pharmacists, case managers, or nurses can help to facilitate filling the organizer correctly. Pharmacies may pre-fill pillboxes or bubble packs that may further enhance use of these devices.

Visual Medication Schedules Visual medication schedules are tools in which pictures of the prescribed medications are placed on a weekly calendar in the corresponding doses. One such visual medication schedule designed, developed and piloted by Drs Edward Machtinger and Dean Schillinger and produced by Tim Peters and Company, a health product software company, is displayed below (Fig. 8-2). Such schedules are now available through some computer programs and from drug manufacturers. Many clinicians create these schedules by simply affixing the actual pill to a paper calendar.

Reminders Reminder devices such as alarms on watches or beepers can be sufficient to enhance adherence. This is particularly true of regimens that require frequent daily dosing and regimens in which doses must be taken on a tightly timed schedule. This strategy has been used effectively in the treatment of HIV.[41]

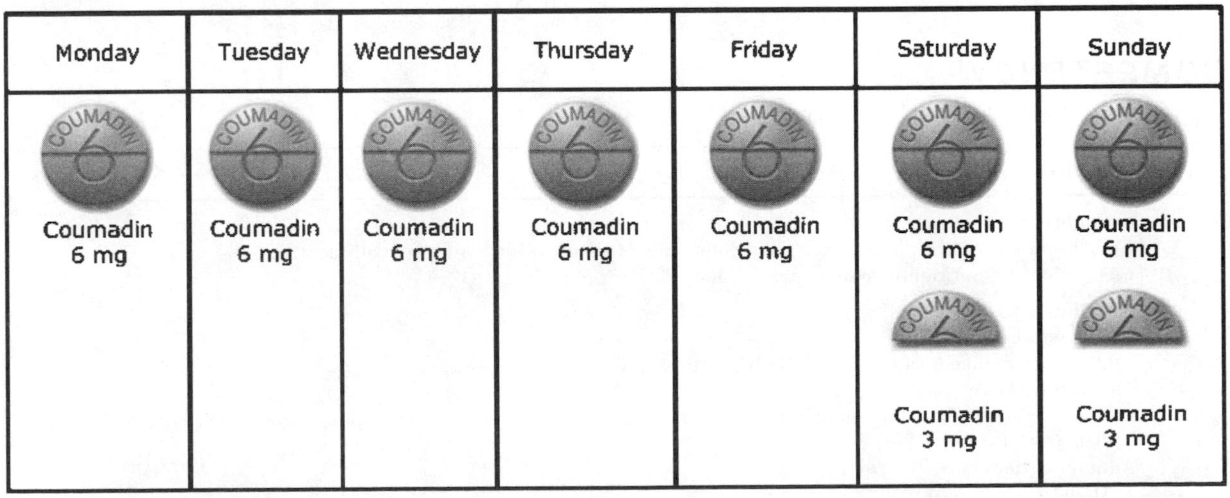

Monday	Tuesday	Wednesday	Thursday	Friday	Saturday	Sunday
Coumadin 6 mg	Coumadin 6 mg	Coumadin 6 mg	Coumadin 6 mg	Coumadin 6 mg	Coumadin 6 mg	Coumadin 6 mg
					Coumadin 3 mg	Coumadin 3 mg

Remember: Take these pills correctly and you can prevent strokes and bleeding!

Figure 8-2. Visual medical schedule for warfarin therapy. (Copyright Tim Peters and Company.)

Nonclinician Factors

It is important to note that a number of the interventions described in the preceding would be most effective were they to be implemented systematically, but have not been for a variety of reasons, and are often out of the control of the individual clinician. As such, advocacy efforts also should occur outside of clinicians' offices for substantive reform to occur. Reduction in pill burden by combining preparations into a single pill (e.g., HIV) could greatly simplify the regimens of patients with chronic diseases. Innovative packaging (e.g., oral contraceptives) and labeling of pharmaceutical products could enhance understanding for patients with linguistic or literacy barriers, and widespread use of assertive technology by pharmacy systems could enhance refill adherence.

CONCLUSION

Vulnerable patient populations may be more at risk of medication nonadherence. Strong patient–clinician relationships, effective communication, and health system improvements can identify contributing factors and facilitate the development of targeted strategies to promote adherence.

DISCUSSION QUESTIONS

1. What factors identified in this case study posed challenges for medication adherence in Mr. Bradley's case?
2. How might you initiate a discussion about medication adherence with Mr. Bradley? How might follow-up discussions assess and promote adherence?

KEY CONCEPTS IN ASSESSING AND PROMOTING MEDICATION ADHERENCE

- Establish an effective patient–provider partnership.
- Recognize that medication adherence is a major challenge and identify nonjudgmental ways to assess adherence.
- Develop interactive communication techniques to assess recall and comprehension about medications to minimize confusion and elicit patient concerns.
- Know the various patient, clinician, and system factors that may make medication adherence a challenge and develop strategies to identify these.
- Tailor specific interventions designed to enhance medication adherence to the needs of your patient.

3. What additional interventions are you aware of for promoting medication adherence and how have they been used?

RESOURCES

http://www.talkaboutrx.org
http://www.nlm.nih.gov/medlineplus/druginformation.html
http://www.safemedication.com
http://www.atdn.org/sf.html
http://www.rxassist.org
http://www.medpin.org

CORE COMPETENCY

Summary of Barriers to Adherence and Potential Solutions

Barrier	Potential Intervention
Side-effects	Simplified treatment regimen Collaborative planning discuss effects and potential side effects within context of daily activities) Medication review (inquire about common side-effects)
Complexity	Simplified treatment regimen Collaborative planning Additional patient education (particularly for chronic diseases such as asthma, diabetes, heart failure, HIV) Medication review visits Case management (multidisciplinary teams that may be particularly effective for chronic diseases such as heart failure, diabetes, HIV) Adherence devices • Medication organizers • Visual medication schedule: may be particularly useful for regimens with changing daily doses (e.g., warfarin) • Reminder devices: particularly if doses must be taken on strict time schedule • System refill reminder

Confusion	Simplified treatment regimen
	Collaborative planning
	Medication review visits; encourage patients to bring pill bottles and demonstrate how medications are taken
	Adherence devices
	• Medication organizers: consider prefilled pill boxes
	• Visual medication schedule: may be useful even for regimens that do not change daily
	• System refill reminders
Health beliefs	Collaborative planning explore health beliefs and possible integration of medication regimen into these beliefs (readdress at subsequent visits as well)
Social support	Collaborative planning: include family members in education about disease and proper medication use
	Case management may be particularly useful in patients lacking adequate social supports
Depression and substance use	Treat underlying depression and/or substance use
	Case management programs that target individuals with psychiatric or substance use problems
Cost	Simplified treatment regimen: be aware of formulary restrictions and financial consequences of the introduction of a new medication
	Collaborative planning: address financial barriers to medication use directly; elicit help from social worker, for questions about insurance and social services
	Medication review: consider discussion of essential versus nonessential medications, and the consequence of restricting different classes of medications
Fragmented care	Enhance communication among clinicians, particularly during hospitalizations
	Medication review visits: encourage patients to bring pill bottles and review medications changed or initiated by other clinicians
Time constraints	Multidisciplinary health care team
	• Collaborative planning: identify financial problems and elicit assistance of social workers, in-home support, etc.
	• Medication review visits: pharmacists
	• Additional patient education: nurses, pharmacists, health educators
	• Case management: integrated approach that may be appropriate for particular disease management or high-risk populations
Refill restrictions	Be aware of refill restrictions when choosing medications
	Collaborative planning: explicit discussion of how to fill medications
	System refill reminders
Formulary	Be aware of formulary restriction when choosing medications

REFERENCES

1. Sabaté E. *Adherence to long-term therapies. Evidence for action.* Geneva: World Health Organization, 2003.
2. DiMatteo MR, et al. Patient adherence and medical treatment outcomes: A meta-analysis. *Med Care* 2002;40:794–811.
3. Goldman DP, et al. Pharmacy benefits and the use of drugs by the chronically ill. *JAMA* 2004;291(19):2344–2350.
4. DiMatteo MR. Variations in patients' adherence to medical recommendations: A quantitative review of 50 years of research. *Med Care* 2004;42:200–209.
5. Mojtabai R, Olfson M. Medication costs, adherence, and health outcomes among Medicare beneficiaries. *Health Aff (Millwood)* 2003;22(4):220–229.
6. Peterson AM, Takiya L, Finley R. Meta-analysis of trials of interventions to improve medication adherence. *Am J Health Syst Pharm* 2003;60(7):657–665.
7. Balkrishnan R, et al. Predictors of medication adherence and associated health care costs in an older population with type 2 diabetes mellitus: A longitudinal cohort study. *Clin Ther* 2003;25:2958–2971.
8. Sieber WJ, Kaplan RM. Informed adherence: The need for shared medical decision making. *Control Clin Trials* 2000;21(5 Suppl):233S–240S.
9. Roter DL. The outpatient medical encounter and elderly patients. *Clin Geriatr Med* 2000;16(1):95–107.
10. Rost K, Roter D. Predictors of recall of medication regimens and recommendations for lifestyle change in elderly patients. *Gerontologist* 1987;27(4):510–515.
11. Crane JA. Patient comprehension of doctor-patient communication on discharge from the emergency department. *J Emerg Med* 1997;15:1–7.
12. Bertakis KD. The communication of information from physician to patient: A method for increasing patient retention and satisfaction. *J Fam Pract* 1977;5:217–222.
13. Salas M, et al. Impaired cognitive function and compliance with antihypertensive drugs in elderly: The Rotterdam Study. *Clin Pharmacol Ther* 2001;70(6):561–566.
14. Schillinger D, et al. Functional health literacy and the quality of physician-patient communication among diabetes patients. *Patient Educ Counsel* 2004;52(3):315–323.
15. Institute of Medicine. *Health literacy: A prescription to end confusion.* Washington, DC: National Academies Press, 2004.
16. Gazmararian JA, et al. Health literacy among Medicare enrollees in a managed care organization. *JAMA* 1999;281:545–551.
17. Sharkness CM, Snow DA. The patient's view of hypertension and compliance. *Am J Prev Med* 1992;8(3):141–146.

18. DiMatteo MR. Social support and patient adherence to medical treatment: A meta-analysis. *Health Psychol* 2004; 23:207–218.

19. Wells KB, et al. How the medical comorbidity of depressed patients differs across health care settings: Results from the Medical Outcomes Study. *Amer J Psychiatry* 1991; 148 (12): 1688–1696.

20. DiMatteo MR, Lepper HS, Croghan TW. Depression is a risk factor for noncompliance with medical treatment: Meta-analysis of the effects of anxiety and depression on patient adherence. *Arch Intern Med* 2000;160:2101–2107.

21. Weiss RD. Adherence to pharmacotherapy in patients with alcohol and opioid dependence. *Addiction* 2004; 99(11):382–392.

22. Piette JD, et al. Health insurance status, cost-related medication underuse, and outcomes among diabetes patients in three systems of care. *Med Care* 2004;42(2):102–109.

23. Steinman MA, Sands LP, Covinsky KE. Self-restriction of medications due to cost in seniors without prescription coverage. *J Gen Intern Med* 2001;16(12):793–799.

24. Heisler M, Wagner TH, Piette JD. Clinician identification of chronically ill patients who have problems paying for prescription medications. *Am J Med* 2004;116(11):753–738.

25. Reichert S, Simon T, Halm EA. Physicians' attitudes about prescribing and knowledge of the costs of common medications. *Arch Intern Med* 2000;160(18):2799–2803.

26. Alexander GC, Casalino LP, Meltzer DO. Patient-physician communication about out-of-pocket costs. *JAMA* 2003; 290:953–958.

27. Zermansky AG, et al. Randomised controlled trial of clinical medication review by a pharmacist of elderly patients receiving repeat prescriptions in general practice. *BMJ* 2001;323(7325):1340–1343.

28. Ong LM, et al. Doctor-patient communication: A review of the literature. *Soc Sci Med* 1995;40(7):903–918.

29. Schillinger D, et al. Closing the loop: Physician communication with diabetic patients who have low health literacy. *Arch Intern Med* 2003;163(1):83–90.

30. Stone VE, et al. Perspectives on adherence and simplicity for HIV-infected patients on antiretroviral therapy: Self-report of the relative importance of multiple attributes of highly active antiretroviral therapy (HAART) regimens in predicting adherence. *J Acquir Immune Def Syndr* 2004; 36(3):808–816.

31. Schroeder K, Fahey T, Ebrahim S. Interventions for improving adherence to treatment in patients with high blood pressure in ambulatory settings. *Cochrane Database Syst Rev* 2004;2:CD004804.

32. Gattis WA, et al. Reduction in heart failure events by the addition of a clinical pharmacist to the heart failure management team: Results of the Pharmacist in Heart Failure Assessment Recommendation and Monitoring (PHARM) Study. *Arch Intern Med* 1999;159(16):1939–1945.

33. Rich MW, et al. A multidisciplinary intervention to prevent the readmission of elderly patients with congestive heart failure. *N Engl J Med* 1995;333(18):1190–1195.

34. Renders CM, et al. Interventions to improve the management of diabetes mellitus in primary care, outpatient and community settings. *Cochrane Database Syst Rev*, 2001;1.

35. Krueger KP, Felkey BG, Berger BA. Improving adherence and persistence: A review and assessment of interventions and description of steps toward a national adherence initiative. *J Am Pharm Assoc* 2003;43(6):668–678.

36. Karter AJ, et al. Missed appointments and poor glycemic control: An opportunity to identify high-risk diabetic patients. *Med Care* 2004;42(2):110–115.

37. Piette JD, Weinberger M, McPhee SJ. The effect of automated calls with telephone nurse follow-up on patient-centered outcomes of diabetes care: A randomized, controlled trial. *Med Care* 2000;38(2):218–230.

38. WHO. *Treatment of tuberculosis: Guidelines for national programmes.* Geneva, Switzerland: World Health Organization, 1997.

39. Conway B, et al. Directly observed therapy for the management of HIV-infected patients in a methadone program. *Clin Infect Dis* 2004;38(Suppl 5):S402–408.

40. Foisy MM, Akai PS. Pharmaceutical care for HIV patients on directly observed therapy. *Ann Pharmacother* 2004; 38(4):550–556.

41. Chesney MA, et al. Self-reported adherence to antiretroviral medications among participants in HIV clinical trials: The AACTG adherence instruments. Patient Care Committee & Adherence Working Group of the Outcomes Committee of the Adult AIDS Clinical Trials Group (AACTG). *AIDS Care* 2000;12:255–266.

42. Machtinger E, Bangsberg DR. Adherence to HIV antiretroviral therapy. Accessed September 27, 2005. Available at: http://hivinsite.ucsf.edu/InSite.jsp/InSite? page = kb-03-02-09

Chapter 9

Navigating Cross-Cultural Communication

JudyAnn Bigby, MD

Objectives

- Define cross-cultural communication.
- Review evidence for the need to improve cross-cultural communication.
- Describe challenges to effective cross-cultural communication and how they impact clinical care.
- Describe strategies for effective cross-cultural communication.

Ms. Jones is a 56-year-old African-American classroom assistant who was hospitalized with a stroke. Her course rapidly deteriorated and her physicians determined that aggressive treatment would be futile. They approached her family with the recommendation that life support be removed. The doctors explained that Ms. Jones had multiorgan failure and little hope of recovery. Her family, a daughter and two sisters, were shocked by this recommendation and accused the physicians, all of whom were white, of substandard care.

When patients and physicians interact, cross-cultural communication is a common occurrence as patients and clinicians differ in many important ways. Patients from vulnerable populations (including persons from racial and ethnic minority populations, low-income persons, and persons with low educational attainment) and health care providers face unique challenges to effective communication. These challenges are borne of the differences in life experiences, cultural norms, assumptions, expectations, and barriers inherent in a health care system in which the biomedical model of health predominates.

Culture is a coherent system of beliefs, values, and lifestyles held by individuals, their communities, and the larger sociopolitical structure in which they live. Culture is a dynamic entity and is responsive to changes such as socioeconomic position, immigration, and other factors (Fig. 9-1). Cross-cultural communication in the context of health care is both complicated and complex because of these multiple determinants of culture and the inherent complexities of medical management. Effective cross-cultural communication acknowledges the interplay of race, ethnicity, cultural norms, religion, socioeconomic position, and education to achieve a common understanding or aim. Effective cross-cultural communication also results in sharing of key information and demonstration of caring. This chapter discusses common barriers to effective cross-cultural communication and how to overcome them. (For a discussion of the effective use of interpreters see Chap. 26.)

EXTENT OF THE PROBLEM

There is abundant evidence that patients are concerned about the lack of effective communication with their physicians and other health care providers. Communication with physicians is a problem among English-speaking patients. Physicians give more

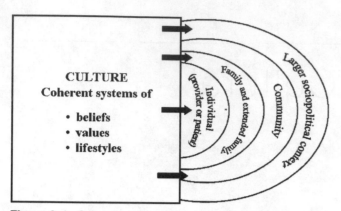

Figure 9-1. Culture is a coherent system of beliefs, values, and lifestyles. Individuals' culture is influenced not only by their personal circumstances but also that of their families and extended families cultures, the culture of their communities, and the culture of the larger social political environment. Individuals, families, communities, and societal cultural systems are dynamic and responsive to multiple forces such as socioeconomic conditions.

information and offer more support and encouragement to patients who ask questions and express concerns. Creating an obvious feedback loop, patients ask more questions when physicians engage in partnership-building behaviors, but physicians engage in more partnership-building behaviors when the patient is more educated.[1] African Americans are less likely than whites to report that their doctors include them in decision making, especially when the patient and doctor are of different races.[2] Physicians are more verbally dominant and engage in less patient-centered communication with African-American patients than with white patients, and African Americans report that their doctors do not explain test results, medical conditions, and treatments.[3]

The Commonwealth Fund reported results of a national survey in which 39% of Latinos, 27% of Asian Americans, 23% of African Americans, and 16% of whites reported problems with communication, specifically that their doctor did not listen to everything they had to say, they were not able to understand their doctors, and they were not able to ask questions during their visits.[4] Latinos and Asian Americans also report that physicians do not adequately involve them in decision making.[5]

Ineffective cross-cultural communication is of particular concern in the management of chronic disease and the context of end-of-life care. African Americans report that they would like to discuss preferences for resuscitation in the event of a cardiopulmonary arrest, but they are more likely than whites not to have done so.[6] African Americans are more likely to want family

members to make decisions for them at the end of life compared with others, but believe that physicians would not involve families in collaborative decision making.[7]

Despite the recent attention to cultural competence in medical school curricula, several studies document persistent deficits in cross-cultural communication among medical students. One study showed that medical students display poorer interviewing skills when interviewing English-speaking Latinos than when interviewing whites. They demonstrated less empathy and rapport-building skills with Latinos and provided more and better explanations to whites than to Latinos.[8]

CHALLENGES IN CROSS-CULTURAL COMMUNICATION

Ms. Jones' family is not concerned about the medical evidence that suggests that further treatment is futile. Their life experience has taught them that life is precious, withstanding suffering is a sign of faith, and that African Americans have often beaten the odds and defied death. They do not completely trust the health care system to do the best for Ms. Jones.

Multiple barriers at the patient, provider, and health care system levels interact, and all contribute to the patient's assessment of the effectiveness of communication. Clear disagreement has arisen between Ms. Jones' family and her medical team about appropriate care. Interactions between the family and the health care providers are strained. The health care providers do not understand the family's reaction; they believe the family does not understand the limits of medical technology in this clinical situation. The family believes the physicians are acting out of prejudice or bias and are not offering Ms. Jones the same care she would receive were she white. The physicians did not involve the family in their decision making, but simply presented them with their recommendation about withdrawing life support. They have failed to consider that racial discordance and/or other potential differences (e.g., religion, spirituality, and social context) may have led to this communication breakdown.

PATIENT-LEVEL BARRIERS

Assertiveness Training

Researchers have demonstrated that patients can learn assertiveness skills that result in more participatory clinical interactions. Although this suggests that patient assertiveness training is one approach to ensuring that patients receive better and more information,[8] some cultures consider it inappropriate for patients to ask questions of the health care provider.[9]

Trust

Lack of trust of the health care provider may be a significant barrier to effective communication. One strategy that some patients may use to protect against stereotyping by providers is to withhold information that they perceive would be viewed negatively by providers. Trust is particularly relevant for groups that have historically experienced bias in the health care system, as reflected in denial of service, segregated service, or blatantly inferior service.[10] The legacy of past abuses such as the US Public Health Service Syphilis Experiment continues to influence some African Americans' ability to trust the system.[11]

Fund of Knowledge

Health care providers may not appreciate that some patients are unfamiliar with key concepts in care, including prevention, self-management, and chronic disease processes. This discordance significantly impacts the patient's and provider's expectations of the goals of the health care visit. It is important for providers to develop skills that permit them to ascertain the extent of patients' understanding of their clinical condition, and to work with them to establish appropriate, mutually acceptable strategies for addressing these issues.

PROVIDER-LEVEL BARRIERS

Lack of Cultural Competence

Provider deficiencies are the most frequently described contributors to poor cross-cultural communication, likely because they have been the most thoroughly researched. Physicians are less satisfied with their interactions with patients who are racially, ethnically, and linguistically diverse. They perceive that patients from these groups are less interested in prevention, managing their illnesses, and engaging in healthy behaviors.[12,13] Frustration may stem from the provider's lack of awareness as to the influence of their own cultural norms. Attitudes about and personal response to difference are telegraphed negatively to patients, as are ignorance of the health beliefs and behaviors of unfamiliar cultures. Physicians and patients often do not discuss "cultural rules" until there is a problem.

Stereotyping

Stereotyping is a particularly important challenge when caring for vulnerable patients. Providers are eager to learn about specific health beliefs of distinct cultural groups. However, knowledge about general cultural beliefs in specific populations is insufficient for effective cross-cultural communication. Persons from racial and ethnic minority groups represent a wide range of cultures, beliefs, and attitudes depending on place of birth, educational attainment, socioeconomic position, acculturation, and other factors. However, knowledge of general health beliefs and attitudes of a group of people can be used to generate hypotheses that can be tested with individual patients.

The unconscious (and certainly the conscious) use of appearance or some other personal characteristic to stereotype patients is a routine occurrence. Studies demonstrate that physicians, residents, and medical students appear to exhibit bias against African Americans and Latinos, for example, in clinical decision making related to cardiac procedures, cardiac rehabilitation, and use of analgesics for fractures. In recent studies African Americans were judged more likely to be substance abusers compared with whites, and were rated as less intelligent and less educated than whites.[8,14]

INTERSECTION OF PATIENT AND PROVIDER BARRIERS

Patients and providers each enter interactions with assumptions about the other party, and cultural factors influence their predetermined expectations about how the encounter will proceed (Fig. 9-2).[15] If they are conscious of how these assumptions are developed they may reexamine them and develop new or different assumptions based on clues provided by the individual.

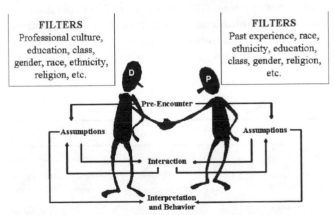

Figure 9-2. Both the doctor (D) and patient (P) use filters that influence assumptions made about each other and each understanding of the interaction. These assumptions influence the interpretation of what happened in the interaction and subsequent behavior. When the doctor and/or patient are aware of how they use their filters, they may reexamine their assumptions and thus influence the interaction and interpretation of the interaction.

Box 9-1. Systems-Level Challenges to Effective Cross-Cultural Communication

- Growing diversity of the US population without concurrent diversification of health care professional staffs
- Increasing emphasis on technology and use of electronic medical records, which may underemphasize the need to talk to patients face to face
- Pressure on health care providers to care for more and sicker patients in shorter clinical encounters

- Inequitable distribution of resources among the safety net providers who provide a disproportionate amount of the care for vulnerable populations
- Growing number of uninsured and inadequate reimbursement by Medicaid jeopardizes resources necessary for effective communication (e.g., interpreters and appropriately designed patient information materials)

Common Pitfalls

- Failing to appreciate culture differences, rendering one's own values dominant, and dismissing the value systems held by others.
- Making the medical model the only or dominant paradigm
- Stereotyping groups as a short cut to understanding whether and how the patient values cultural norms.
- Bias and lack of personal awareness of bias.
- Using medical jargon and technical language.
- Failing to check for meaning and understanding with patient.
- Failing to inquire about patient preferences about decision making.

SYSTEMS-LEVEL BARRIERS

Historically, health care professionals have received little or no training in cross-cultural communication. In addition, many system-level forces obstruct improvements in effective communication (see Box 9-1). Furthermore, the physical limitations of clinical sites often do not facilitate the unique decision-making styles of some groups.

In cultures in which family decision making is valued above the individual one-on-one interactions, examination rooms may be too small, whereas conference rooms to hold family meetings are frequently nonexistent, and the hours of operation do not accommodate work and care-taking schedules of extended families.

SOLUTIONS TO EFFECTIVE CROSS-CULTURAL COMMUNICATION

Ms. Jones' family ask permission to include their pastor in the next discussion about her care. They want reassurance from her caretakers that she will be treated with dignity and that her needs will not be ignored. They also want the opportunity to make sure that a family member who is arriving from out of town has an opportunity to see her before she dies. The providers are able to accommodate this request.

Effective cross-cultural communication requires the health care provider to integrate his or her personal awareness of cultural beliefs and attitudes with clinical expertise, and use knowledge of the patient's specific cultural and social context, as well as the broader social context to accomplish mutually determined goals of care (see Chap. 22). Table 9-1 shows a model developed

Table 9-1. Respect Model

Action	Comment
Respect	Show a demonstrable attitude involving both verbal and nonverbal communications.
Explanatory model	What is the patient's point of view about his or her illness? How does it compare to the provider's point of view? Both points of view should be elicited and reconciled.
Sociocultural context	How do class, race, ethnicity, gender, education, sexual orientation, immigrant status, and family and gender roles impact care?
Power	Acknowledge the power differential between patients and physicians.
Empathy	Put into words the significance of the patient's concerns so that the patient feels understood.
Concerns and fears	Elicit the patient's emotions and underlying concerns.
Therapeutic alliance/trust	Provide a measurable outcome that enhances adherence and engagement in health care.

Model developed by the Boston University Residency Program in Internal Medicine Diversity Curriculum Taskforce and adapted from: Bigby J. Beyond culture. Strategies for caring for patients from diverse racial, ethnic, and cultural groups. In Bigby J, ed. Cross-cultural medicine. Philadelphia: American College of Physicians, 2003.

by the Boston University Residency Program in Internal Medicine Diversity Curriculum Taskforce for caring for patients from diverse racial, ethnic, and cultural groups.[16]

PERSONAL AWARENESS

For the clinician, exploring one's personal identity is an important first step in developing effective cross-cultural communication. Understanding how one's own race, ethnicity, culture, socioeconomic position, and other characteristics influence one's practice as a physician can help to expose sources of one's own beliefs and biases (see Fig. 9-1).

Assessing personal awareness is an ongoing process of self-reflection throughout one's career. Individual providers also may become more aware of the assumptions they make about others based on their group identity in medicine. A set of questions designed to assess and enhance personal awareness is shown in Table 9-2.

CULTURAL ASSESSMENT

"You've got to find out the identity of a person to even get to know them."

(Patient, as quoted in Kagawa-Singer)[6]

Discovering a patient's identity is enormously rewarding, and is the first step toward effective cross-cultural communication. Prior to the clinical encounter, providers may collect general information about specific cultural groups with whom they are unfamiliar. General knowledge about different cultural groups may be helpful for understanding general cultural values and beliefs and

may uncover health beliefs and attitudes generally held by a specific cultural group. Several web sites contain information about specific groups (see Resources).

General cultural information should be considered a foundation for understanding cultural norms. This information can be used to generate hypotheses about the potential health beliefs of a particular patient. These hypotheses then can be directly tested with an individual patient or family. For example, persons of Chinese origin commonly do not want to be directly informed about grave diagnoses. To test whether a particular patient's beliefs are congruent with this hypothesis a provider might say, "In general I give patients as much information as possible about their medical conditions. I understand that in some cultures, in some families, knowing these details is not always seen as helpful. Can you tell me your thoughts about this?" Using a narrative, open-ended style, as opposed to asking specific questions, may be effective. With the cultural context in place, the specifics of a patient's life experience gain greater meaning (Box 9-2).

CREATE AN ENVIRONMENT THAT BUILDS TRUST

Building trust is a key component of effective cross-cultural communication. Patients view trust-building behaviors as a sign that providers are invested in them as individuals and that they want to help patients, and articulate behaviors that they would like physicians to exhibit (Table 9-3). Trust-building behaviors display respect and build rapport. Small actions such as asking a patient how she prefers to be addressed go a long way to demonstrate respect. Providers often are unaware that there is a power differential in their relationships

Table 9-2. Assessing Personal Self-Awareness

1. How do you define your own racial or ethnic identity?
2. What did you learn to value while you were growing up?
3. Which features of your own racial or ethnic group do you view positively?
4. Which features of your own racial or ethnic group do you view negatively?
5. What are some characteristics that are important to your identity?
6. While you were growing up, were the schools and neighborhoods homogenous, or racially and/or ethnically mixed? What about socioeconomically? At what point in your life did you have the opportunity to interact with people who were different from you?
7. Are there culturally distinct groups with which you feel comfortable?
8. Are there culturally distinct groups with which you feel uncomfortable?
9. What is the racial/ethnic or sociocultural characteristic of the patients with whom you feel most competent in establishing rapport and a treatment plan?
10. What is the racial/ethnic or sociocultural characteristic of patients with whom you have the most difficulty establishing rapport and establishing a treatment plan?
11. How do factors related to your racial or ethnic identity and/or from your life experience affect how you interact with patients from backgrounds that are different from your own?

Adapted from: Goldman R, Monroe AD, Dube C. Ann Behav Sci Med Educ 1996;3:37–46.

Box 9-2. Key Information in the Cultural Assessment

- Level of formal education
- Generational status (e.g., first-generation American)
- Level of encapsulation within ethnic and family social network (e.g., living in a community with a large concentration of a cultural group)
- Age at immigration (if applicable)

- Degree of migration back and forth to country of origin (if applicable)
- Area of origin in native country (if applicable)
- Occupation currently (and before migration, if applicable)
- Religion
- Personal or family experience in the health care system

with patients. The difference in power may stem from personal characteristics such as educational attainment and class and is reinforced by the hierarchic relationships in health care that result from differential knowledge, information, and status. Empathy and demonstration of empathy are meaningful ways to improve patient satisfaction while demonstrating concern. Empathic behavior requires active listening (nodding, encouraging), picking up on patients' concerns ("Sounds like you . . ."), identifying the factual content of the patient's statement (What I heard you say . . ."), asking about affective responses, and requesting clarification.[17] Eliciting the patient's concerns is also an effective partnership-building tool. The end result of these behaviors should be a meaningful therapeutic alliance.

Some aspects of a patient's cultural values and beliefs are relevant to clinical situations and some are not. Let the patient provide advice and guidance. For example, ask about interactional norms (how younger clinicians show respect for elders; how older clinicians allow young patients to ask questions or express an opinion; how gender roles translate to clinical situations). Providers must be able to assess patients' (or an individual patient's) values and beliefs, and incorporate this

information into clinical assessments and decision making. Identify strategies taken from the patient's cultural orientation that can be used to enhance the therapeutic alliance; acknowledge those that seem counterproductive. These behaviors are consistent with behaviors and attitudes that others have described as being important for improving cross-cultural communication[13] and that exhibit patient-centered approaches.[1] It is important to remember that, as illustrated in Figure 9-2, the absence of these provider behaviors may be interpreted as disrespectful and biased, based on the patient's past experience of racial, ethnic, or cultural biases.

IDENTIFY THE PATIENT'S EXPLANATORY MODEL OF ILLNESS

"The patient needs to open up to tell you these things."
(Patient as quoted in Kagawa-Singer)[6]

Identifying the patient's explanatory model of his or her illness is a fundamental aspect of cross-cultural communication. Kleinman and colleagues[18] have developed an anthropologic approach to eliciting a comprehensive understanding (Box 9-3). When asked in a

Table 9-3. Trust-Building Behaviors

Actions	Attitudes
Introduce yourself by name, title, and role.	Do not make assumptions.
Ask the patient what she or he prefers to be called.	Pay attention to cultural beliefs.
Make an effort to make the person comfortable.	Acknowledge and respect different perspectives.
Do not appear to be rushed.	Distinguish the person as an individual.
Ask personal questions. (How is your daughter doing now? Is school any better for her?)	Display genuine concern.
Use plain language.	
Listen for the patient's style of telling about symptoms.	
Listen to questions.	
Be responsive.	
Hold patient information as confidential.	
Ask patient if they are satisfied with the appointment.	
Apologize when there is a problem.	

Box 9-3. Anthropologic Approach to Eliciting a Comprehensive Understanding

- What do you call your problem?
- What name do you give it?
- Why do you think your illness started?
- When did it begin?
- How severe is it?
- What do you fear most about your illness?

- What are the major problems your illness has caused?
- Do you have any ideas about what treatment you should receive or others who would be helpful?

From: Kleinman A, Eisenberg L, Good B. Culture, illness, and care: Clinical lessons from anthropologic and cross-cultural research. *Ann Intern Med* 1978;88:251–258.

respectful, caring manner these questions can facilitate an understanding of the patient's expectations and provide important information that a traditional medical interview would miss. Preface these questions with a respectful introduction, such as, "I know that patients and doctors sometimes have different ideas about what causes certain symptoms or illnesses. I'd like to know more about your ideas about your problem."

Acknowledge what the patient has shared by summarizing what you have heard. Describe to the patient your assessment of the problem and acknowledge any discrepancies between your interpretation and the patient's. Avoid medical jargon or technical language. Explain how your assessment addresses the concerns identified by the patient. Check to see if the patient has heard and understood what you said. "Do you have any questions about what I have just said? Is there anything that you need me to explain in more detail?"

It may be useful to summarize the understanding of the patient's major concerns. From this process, the patient and provider can develop a problem list that reflects their negotiation. If the patient is hesitant to agree, explore the source of hesitation and begin to negotiate again.

NEGOTIATE A PLAN FOR FURTHER EVALUATION AND TREATMENT

Once the problem list and possible diagnosis are identified, the provider can begin to make recommendations for next steps. Ask the patient about whom he or she would like to involve in the process and then accommodate the patient's request by agreeing to meet with important family members or others. Address the patient confidentiality up front and ask for clear guidance about how much information the patient would like to share with his or her family.

The process of developing a diagnostic and treatment plan affords an opportunity to ask about the patient's use of alternative and complementary therapies and about the patient's expectations for treatment. As the provider outlines possible strategies for further diagnostic evaluation or appropriate treatments, the provider should allow the patient to stop and ask questions. Confirm the patient's comprehension by asking him or her to describe his or her understanding of the next steps. Provide language and literacy-level–appropriate written instructions for patients that identify the problem, tests, and relevant instructions for undergoing the tests, and any prescribed medications. The information also should outline any self-management instructions for the patient. Ask the patient how well he or she thinks she can adhere to the plan. If an expensive test or medication is part of the strategy, ask in a respectful way if the patient plans to follow through. "This medication is very expensive. I notice that you don't have insurance for medication. Many people would not be able to buy this medicine. Do you think you will have a problem?"

Patients often wait until the end of the encounter to raise concerns and fears. Budget time accordingly, and use empathic statements to build rapport.[17] Sometimes patients rely on nonverbal cues to convey these concerns. They also may use indirect questions to inquire about issues about which they are uncomfortable. They may pose hypothetical situations or talk about what happened to a family member or friend. Providers may answer indirectly or if they feel it is appropriate, ask the patient about how the hypothetical applies to him or her.

NEGOTIATING THROUGH DISAGREEMENT

When there is a disagreement between the provider and patient it is important to acknowledge it. Identify the patient's most pressing concern and begin to outline what you can do to address this concern. If the patient rejects your concerns or diagnosis, break the problem down into smaller parts to identify whether there are any elements that the patient accepts and for which he or she can agree to seek further evaluation or treatment (see Core Competency).

IDENTIFY DESIRED OUTCOMES

Effective cross-cultural communication can improve clinical outcomes from both the patient and provider perspective.[19] Effective communication is associated with increased satisfaction for the patient and provider.[5] Patient adherence and an enhanced understanding of the disease process and treatment also may improve with effective cross-cultural communication.[21]

CONCLUSION

Cross-cultural communication is a critical skill for today's medical providers. Effective communication in the context of significant cultural differences requires concerted efforts to ensure open exchange. Because a single medical encounter with one provider is often the gateway to an array of health care services for vulnerable populations, the quality of the encounter may be an important determinant of access to care for an entire family. Fortunately, the skills required for effective communication are attainable by most health care providers.

KEY CONCEPTS IN NAVIGATING CROSS-CULTURAL COMMUNICATION

- Assess your own cultural beliefs and attitudes.
  - —Acknowledge your major cultural identity.
  - —Identify possible areas of discomfort.
  - —Identify possible areas of bias.
  - —Examine your assumptions when dealing with individual patients.
- Perform a cultural assessment on the patient.
  - —Identify the patient's major cultural identity by asking.
  - —Identify generational status.
  - —Assess level of formal education, employment history, immigration status, role of religion and spirituality, and past experience in the health care system.
  - —Test hypotheses about health beliefs and attitudes using general information about specific cultural groups.
- Create an environment that builds trust.
  - —Employ trust-building behaviors in interactions with all patients.
  - —Identify the patient's explanatory model of illness and the patient's desired outcomes.
  - —Negotiate a diagnostic and treatment plan that incorporates the patient's model.
  - —Acknowledge the patient's concerns with empathy.
  - —Identify patient preferences for family or other key individuals' involvement.
  - —Encourage the patient to ask questions.
  - —Summarize and ask if you have it right.

CORE COMPETENCY
Negotiating Conflicts

Patients and providers do not always agree on a plan of action, even when the provider has tried to be sensitive to the cultural perspective of the patient. When the patient and provider disagree about the course of action in a clinical situation it is important for them to recognize that there are effective strategies for resolving the conflict. The conflict rarely should lead to patients seeking care elsewhere, although sometimes that is the solution to the problem.

Define the problem.
Make sure the provider and patient agree on the conflict.
Provider: *"Mr. Smith I think that we have come to a point where we don't agree on the next course of action. I understand that you want to be admitted to the hospital, but I believe your problem does not require hospitalization. I think that with appropriate antibiotics your infection will resolve and we can provide close follow-up for you as an outpatient."*
Mr. Smith: *"Dr. Jones, I know my body and I don't feel well. The last time a doctor sent me home when I thought I should be admitted I had a heart attack at home."*
Examine your own motivations.
Have any other factors influenced your decisions?
Does the patient have unique social or other circumstances that warrant consideration? If you are not sure, ask.
Acknowledge the patient's concerns.
Demonstrate trust-building behavior. (Make an effort to make the patient comfortable. Do not appear to be rushed.)
Be responsive to the patient's statement. (*"I heard you say you have been sent home inappropriately before."*)
Demonstrate empathy. (*"That must have been scary for you. I am sorry that you had to go through that experience."*)
Ask questions to identify the patient's specific concerns. (*"Sometimes, some people have not been treated fairly in our health care system. Do you think that is a problem in your case?"* or *"What do you think will happen to you if you go home today?"*)
Be responsive to patients' concerns. (*"I understand your feelings that you were mistreated in the past."*)
Identify opportunities for a compromise.
Ask whether the patient thinks there are alternatives.
Ask if he or she has other family members or someone else with whom he or she is close who should be involved in the discussion.
Devise a list of possible compromises between the two positions.
Ask if patient is comfortable with one of the alternative plans.
Restate the compromise you have reached and ask if patient has same understanding.
Assess the patient's satisfaction with the outcome.
Acknowledge the patient's willingness to share his or her thoughts.
Apologize about the disagreement.
Ask if he or she is satisfied with the resolution.
Ask what can be done to avoid conflicts in the future.

DISCUSSION QUESTIONS

1. Discuss some of the barriers to effective cross-cultural communication at the patient, provider, and health systems level. What are some strategies for addressing systems level barriers?
2. Think back to a time when you needed health care. What was your experience like? Did you have a good relationship with your provider? What made the relationship work? How was it problematic? What role did your race or ethnicity play?
3. What are key places for training providers in effective cross-cultural communication? How would you design such opportunities?
4. Return to the case of Ms. Jones. Write a role play that illustrates how you think her providers could approach her family with news of Ms. Jones' poor prognosis. How would you ask the family about end-of-life care for Ms. Jones?

RESOURCES

http://www.diversityrx.org
Provides a summary of the wide spectrum of strategies available to overcome linguistic and cultural barriers to care, and describes their application in model programs around the country.

http://www.ethnomed.org
The EthnoMed site contains information about cultural beliefs, medical issues, and other related issues pertinent to the health care of recent immigrants to Seattle or the United States, many of whom are refugees fleeing war-torn parts of the world.

http://gucchd.georgetown.edu/nccc/index.html
The mission of the National Center for Cultural Competence (NCCC) is to increase the capacity of health and mental health programs to design implement, and evaluate culturally and linguistically competent service delivery systems.
Bigby J. *Cross-cultural medicine.* Philadelphia: American College of Physicians; 2003.

REFERENCES

1. Street RL Jr. Gender differences in health care provider-patient communication: Are they due to style, stereotypes, or accommodation? *Patient Educ Counsel* 2002;48:201–206.
2. Cooper-Patrick L, Gallo JJ, Gonzales JJ, et al. Race, gender, and partnership in the patient-physician relationship. *JAMA* 1999;282:583–589.
3. Johnson RL, Roter D, Powe NR, et al. Patient race/ethnicity and quality of patient-physician communication during medical visits. *Am J Public Health* 2004;94: 2084–2090.
4. Collins KS, Hughes DL, Doty MM, et al. Diverse communities, common concerns: Assessing health care quality for minority Americans. New York: The Commonwealth Fund, 2002. Accessed on August 21, 2005. Available at: http://www.cmwf.org/publications/publications_show.htm?doc_id=221257
5. Saha S, Arbelaez JJ, Cooper LA. Patient-physician relationships and racial disparities in the quality of health care. *Am J Public Health* 2003;93:1713–1719.
6. Kagawa-Singer M, Blackhall LJ. Negotiating cross-cultural issues at the end of life. "You got to go where he lives." *JAMA* 2001;286:2993–3001.
7. Degenholtz HB, Thomas SB, Miller MJ. Race and intensive care unit: Disparities and preferences for end-of-life care. *Crit Care Med* 2003;31:S373–378.
8. Ferguson WJ, Candib LM. Culture, language, and the doctor-patient relationship. *Fam Med* 2002;34:53–61.
9. Skelton JR, Kai J, Loudon RF. Cross-cultural communication in medicine: Questions for educators. *Med Educ* 200135:257–261.
10. Boulware LE, Cooper LA, Ratner LE, et al. Race and trust in the health care system. *Public Health Rep* 2003;118: 358–365.
11. Corbie-Smith G. The continuing legacy of the Tuskegee Syphilis Study: Considerations for clinical investigation. *Am J Med Sci* 1999;317:5–8.
12. Kamath CC, O'Fallon M, Offord KP, et al. Provider satisfaction in clinical encounters with ethnic immigrant populations. *Mayo Clinic Proc* 2003;78:1353–1360.
13. Shapiro J, Hollingshead J, Morrison E. Resident, faculty, and patient views of cultural competence. *Med Educ* 2002;36:749–759.
14. Smedley BD, Stith AY, Nelson AR, eds. *Unequal treatment. Confronting racial and ethnic disparities in health care.* Washington, DC: National Academies Press, 2003:162–167.
15. Kagawa-Singer M, Kassim-Lakha S. A strategy to reduce cross-cultural miscommunication and increase the likelihood of improving health outcomes. *Acad Med* 2003;78: 577–587.
16. Bigby J. Beyond culture. Strategies for caring for patients from diverse racial, ethnic, and cultural groups. In: Bigby J, ed. *Cross-cultural medicine.* Philadelphia: American College of Physicians, 2002:1–28.
17. Coulehan JL, Platt FW, Egener B, et al. "Let me see if I have this right . . .": Words that help build empathy. *Ann Intern Med* 2001;135:221–227.
18. Kleinman A, Eisenberg L, Good B. Culture, illness, and care: Clinical lessons from anthropologic and cross-cultural research. *Ann Intern Med* 1978;88:251–258.
19. Horner RD, Salazar W, Geiger J, et al. Changing health care professionals' behaviors to eliminate disparities in healthcare: What do we know? How might we proceed? *Am J Manag Care* 2004:10:S12–S19.
20. Goldman R, Monroe AD, Dube C. Cultural self-awareness: A component of culturally responsive care. *Ann Behav Sci Med Educ* 1996;3:37–46.
21. Taylor SL, Lurie N. The role of culturally competent communication in reducing ethnic and racial healthcare disparities. Am J Manang Care. 2004 Sep;10 Spec No:SP1-4.

Chapter 10

Improving the Effectiveness of Patient Education: A Focus on Limited Health Literacy

Michael K. Paasche-Orlow, MD, MA, MPH, and Ruth M. Parker MD

Objectives

- Review the complexity of health care and the evidence that many patients do not have adequate health literacy.
- Demonstrate that clarity is essential.
- Describe the importance of being specific.
- Review how to reinforce ideas through multiple channels of communication.
- Discuss how to help patients to ask questions.
- Illustrate how to confirm comprehension, so that patients and providers share a common understanding about what patients need to do to take care of themselves.

Ms. Shales is a 78-year-old patient who has received her care at the same clinic for 25 years. She has hypertension, diabetes, hypercholesterolemia, breast cancer treated with lumpectomy/radiation, gastroesophageal reflux, and osteoarthritis. Her medications include hydrochlorothiazide, lisinopril, atorvastatin, omeprazole, acetaminophen, insulin, and capsaicin cream. She completed high school but does not feel she can understand all the information provided about her illness. Although generally happy with the care she has received, Ms. Shales complains that her doctors spend little time explaining things to her and that she is embarrassed to ask questions. She has noticed that it is much more difficult for her to remember things and she finds that it is difficult to read and understand the labels on her medication bottles. She has been hospitalized twice in the last 18 months for management of her diabetes.

Patients must have an adequate understanding of their prescribed health and self-care regimen in order to be able to take care of their health. Health literacy is "the degree to which individuals have the capacity to obtain, process, and understand basic health information and services needed to make appropriate health decisions."[1] Many factors affect an individual's ability to comprehend, and in turn use or act on, health information and communication. Basic literacy skills (proficiency in reading, writing, listening, interpreting images, interacting with documents, facility with numerical concepts, and basic computation) are central to the broader concept of health literacy. These include oral communication, evaluating risk, and health system navigation.

Health literacy, together with self-management, has been highlighted by the Institute of Medicine as one of the 20 national priority areas in which quality improvement could transform health care in America.[2] The modern US health system relies on a variety of interpersonal, textual, and electronic media to present health information.[3] Too often people with the greatest health burdens have limited access to relevant health information. In part, this results from the complex and cumbersome ways health information is presented. Additionally, many people, particularly those with limited literacy skills, have difficulty understanding health terminology and instructions.

This chapter discusses critical insights and communication techniques clinicians can use to promote high-quality health care with patients who have limited health literacy. Topics reviewed are the complexity of the health care system, challenges faced by patients, barriers presented by clinicians, role of shame and stigma, use of multiple channels of communication to promote comprehension, and importance of reviewing information to crystallize key ideas and actions plans. Although this chapter is oriented to the care of those with limited health literacy, most studies demonstrate that such techniques also benefit those with adequate health literacy.

SCOPE OF THE PROBLEM

Over the past 50 years, basic literacy has improved in the United States. However, over 90 million American adults struggle to read and understand basic materials.[3,4] Thus, given the high literacy demands required to function successfully as a patient,[5] it is no wonder that approximately one in four American adults has limited health literacy and an additional 20% of patients have marginal health literacy.[6] This problem is not uniformly distributed in society. The prevalence of limited health literacy is higher among patients who are older and are from ethnic and racial minorities. It has been estimated that as many as 50% of patients cared for at public hospitals may have low functional health literacy.[7,8]

People with limited health literacy, compared with those with adequate health literacy, have higher rates of hospitalization,[9,10] worse health status,[11] receive fewer preventive services,[12] may have more poorly controlled disease (e.g., diabetes mellitus[13] or HIV[14]), and overall, have less knowledge about their medical conditions.[15] Furthermore, although physicians and patients often have a concordant impression about the quality of their clinical interactions, discordance may be more likely to occur with patients who have limited health literacy.[16,17]

BARRIERS TO OPTIMAL CARE FOR THOSE WITH LIMITED HEALTH LITERACY

There are multiple reasons why people with limited health literacy have worse health status. In the health care context, these include increasing complexity of

health care, difficulties with health care access and use, limitations of patient–physician communication, and failure of clinicians to consistently promote patient self-management skills or recognize other barriers to health literacy.[18,19]

INCREASING COMPLEXITY OF HEALTH CARE

The central problem is not just the limited health literacy skills of patients, but the complexity of the tasks needed to function successfully as a patient.[20] For example, successful management of diabetes requires that the patient learn many different things: new concepts about diet and nutrition, how to recognize the warning signs of hypoglycemia and hyperglycemia, how to use a glucometer, as well as how to manage a complicated and often changing drug regimen. Clinical screening for limited health literacy is not enough to overcome the difficulties these individuals might face in successfully managing such a complex problem. In fact, additional systemwide support for patients and clinicians is needed to improve patient outcomes.[21]

DIFFICULTIES WITH HEALTH CARE ACCESS AND USE

Most studies of patients with limited health literacy have been conducted among people with medical problems who are currently receiving care. However, patients with limited health literacy may have difficulty accessing and appropriately using the health system. For example, insurance companies or government programs often introduce hurdles that may be insurmountable to people with limited health literacy; consequently, people may not seek care and may present for health care in worse health status.

Furthermore, the safeguards that have been developed to protect patients' rights ironically may make it more difficult for them to understand these rights. Informed consent is undermined by the development of forms that cannot be read and understood by many patients.[22] Similar examples can be found in Patients' Bill of Rights documents and the Federal Health Insurance Portability and Accessibility Act, which, in the name of protecting patients' rights and privacy, have promulgated documents that are indiscernible by the majority of patients.[23,24]

LIMITATIONS IN PATIENT–PHYSICIAN COMMUNICATION

Attempts to establish a clinical environment that is sensitive to the needs of patients with limited health literacy must appreciate how hard it is to be a patient. Health care practitioners often assume that their patients are functionally literate.[25–27] Consequently many clinicians have no idea that some of their patients do not have even basic literacy skills, no less the capacity to navigate complex and technologically sophisticated health care systems.

Patients often have a hard time understanding and remembering what to do. In addition, health care settings are difficult places for a person to say, "I do not know." Some clinicians may make patients feel that their difficulty with understanding and adherence is unusual, further inhibiting discussion. Therefore, many patients conceal their poor understanding because of shame or assumptions that the clinician is too busy and does not want to be bothered with their questions.[28] Instead of requesting further explanation, many patients prefer to stay quiet and avoid the potential embarrassment of having their low literacy or poor comprehension revealed.[28,29]

Importantly, most patients with limited health literacy can learn and remember the information they need to manage their medical care if presented in a clear and careful manner, with the appropriate reinforcements.[30] Thus, clinicians must be active listeners and collaborate with patients to identify important gaps in understanding, and promote skill-building to assist them in the care of their disease (see Chap. 12).

LANGUAGE AND CULTURE

Differences in language and culture contribute to poor understanding for many, but in the United States the majority of those with limited literacy are native born, white Americans.[31–33] Nevertheless, there is a growing population of adults in America for whom English is not their first language.[33] As such, in many instances, the appropriate response to poor understanding is to provide language-appropriate and culturally competent services (see Chap. 26). Interpreters are crucial and should be readily available. However, quality interpretation services are not a panacea, as patients may have limited health literacy in any language.

OTHER BARRIERS TO OPTIMAL CARE

Studies suggest that as many as half of medical patients do not completely follow the treatment recommendations of their clinicians (see Chap. X). Barriers other than limited health literacy can contribute to this poor adherence. Elderly patients who develop poor vision may not tell clinicians that they are no longer able to read.[34] Poor memory because of undiagnosed or subclinical progressive dementia or other causes is another reason why elderly or chronically ill patients might have limited health literacy. Patients with cognitive limitations may be less likely to benefit from educational interventions designed to ameliorate reading barriers.

A small proportion of patients with limited health literacy may have learning disabilities (previously diagnosed or undiagnosed). A learning disability is a "disorder in one or more of the basic psychological processes involved in understanding or in using spoken or written language, which may manifest itself in an imperfect ability to listen, think, speak, read, write, spell or do mathematical calculations" (the regulations for Public Law (PL) 101-476, the Individuals with Disabilities Education Act). Actual educational attainment, as opposed to how long a person stayed in school, can help clinicians understand a patient's skills. Similarly, understanding sensory, neural, or cognitive challenges that may compound a patient's functional limitations are also keys to developing an individually tailored approach to patient education to support patients with concurrent limitations.

Common Pitfalls in the Care of Patients with Limited Health Literacy

- Assuming your explanation is simple. Remember: What is easy for you is easy for you!
- Using jargon to obfuscate the fact that we do not know what we are talking about or assert our authority
- Failing to be specific
- Overwhelming patients with too much information
- Relying on words alone
- Training patients to be ashamed of not understanding
- Failing to assess patient understanding and/or explore their beliefs about their illness
- Believing that "screening" for limited health literacy, in the absence of additional interventions, will improve patient outcomes

---

APPROACHES TO IMPROVING HEALTH OUTCOMES FOR PATIENTS WITH LIMITED HEALTH LITERACY

Ms. Shales recently presented to the emergency department (ED) complaining of "weakness," and laboratory evaluation revealed a potassium level of 3.0 mmol/L (normal range 3.5 to 5.1). The ED physician instructed her to continue taking her regular medicines, but also to eat a banana daily. Her primary care physician saw her a week later for a regularly scheduled appointment, and repeat potassium was 3.1 mmol/L. Her clinic physician gave her refills for her medications, and reinforced the instructions to eat bananas. One week after this, she had an appointment with her oncologist, who told her to continue eating bananas. Because of ongoing weakness, she subsequently presented to the walk-in clinic with a complaint of "feeling tired" for weeks, and "being tired of eating so many bananas." When asked for her current medications, Ms. S. pulled out six pill bottles, including two containing hydrochlorothiazide. Ms. Shales revealed that she takes both, explaining: "The labels on the two are different, and one is a capsule and the other a tablet, so they must be different." Examination revealed that one bottle was labeled "hydrochlorothiazide 25 mg" and other bottle was labeled "hydrochlorothiazidecap 12.5 mg."

INTERPRETIVE FRAMING

It can be easy to forget how something that is ordinary for a clinician can be difficult for a patient. A technique to help patients understand what clinicians mean is *interpretive framing*. If you tell a patient that she has a "mass," you should also interpret what this means. A very common clinical challenge occurs when health care providers attempt to communicate about the risks of different outcomes or even when numerical concepts are used to convey ideas.[35] By telling a patient "the goal for the top number of your blood pressure is 135 and today it is 148" you are giving a simple, somewhat useful frame.[36] However, many patients will not know how to understand the meaning or importance of being 13 points above the goal.[37] Unless the clinician provides explicit interpretation, the patient will be left to discern the relevance of the comments based on affective signals. In Ms. Shales case, her physician never explained the risks of her medications and when she changed the dose of her diuretic, it was not made clear that her original prescription should be discontinued. Consequently, it is understandable that Ms. Shales might fail to understand that two drugs that look different, with different names and doses, may actually be the same drug, and if taken together might be dangerous. Asking to see a patient's actual medications and inquiring as to how they take them is an important practice for clinicians to perform.

KEEP COMMUNICATION SIMPLE

Explain everything using clear and simple words. The most important skill to advance this practice is for the teacher to have a full and clear understanding of what he or she is trying to teach. Unfortunately, clinicians may not have insight into the fact that they are using jargon or lay words that have dual or specialized meanings.[38,39] Furthermore, clinicians who use jargon despite having a clear understanding of the material may be using language to assert their authority over patients. This practice can compromise patient comprehension, and may make it more difficult to engage your patient as an active learner.

Regrettably, many of the terms that seem common enough to clinicians are not at all clear to patients. Although clinicians often use the word "diet" to indicate all of what a person eats, patients often think the word "diet" indicates a moderation of the normal eating pattern to lose weight. A recent study demonstrated that patients' understanding of jargon did not increase when the physician provided an explanation, suggesting that the best strategy may simply be to avoid jargon altogether.[40]

BE SPECIFIC

When establishing a sensitive clinical environment it is important to be specific. If you tell a patient, "take two pills twice a day," how is he or she supposed to know what time of day to do that? If you give a patient a suppository, how are you going to make certain that it is not swallowed? If you instruct a parent to "give two teaspoons every 4 hours," will she or he know what a teaspoon is (Fig. 10-1)? The key is to think through the things you are asking patients to do, break down each activity into discrete actions, and then specifically instruct patients about completing these specific actions. A final check that patient and provider share a common understanding is crucial.

FOCUS ON A SHORT SET OF SPECIFIC ACTION ITEMS

It is important to avoid information overload when working with a patient. When confronted with too much information and too many options, patients do not learn or retain as much information and are more likely to make poor decisions; that is, they choose options that are not concordant with their values.[41] Select a discrete set of skill or action items. Focus clinical encounters on discussion of a few topics and shift

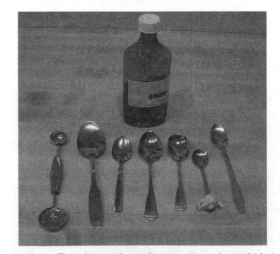

Figure 10-1. The picture shows items patients brought in to show how they measured their children's medications.

the learning paradigm from teaching about a diagnosis to discussion of what needs to be done.

MAINTAIN MULTIPLE CHANNELS OF COMMUNICATION

It is useful to employ multiple channels of communication. Reinforcement through several teaching modalities improves comprehension and retention. Although not a cure-all for all misunderstandings, diagrams, videos, interactive media, audiotapes, telephone help lines, and community-based health education programs can help reinforce, clarify, and remind patients of important health information.[42] Critical self-care activities can be supported by additional points of contact with the patient in the patient's home or via telephone, and may be conducted by a coordinated team of care providers.[43–45] Even providing a patient with a simple list of instructions to reinforce what was agreed on verbally in the clinic visit can be very useful.

Most people can benefit from the use of multiple channels of communication. However, people with defined learning disabilities may be accommodated with a specific educational plan. Through neuropsychological testing, an Individualized Educational Plan (IEP) is developed to optimize the educational experience for the patient. IEP programs have been available throughout the United States for decades; however, many clinicians are unfamiliar with learning disability, do not know that IEPs include information on the best way for such patients to learn, and that clinical teaching can be adapted accordingly. For example, people who have a limited active working memory may have difficulty with auditory processing and learn better with written instructions.[46]

ESTABLISH A COLLABORATIVE LEARNING ENVIRONMENT

Establishing a collaborative learning environment in which patients are not embarrassed to ask questions can improve outcomes. Clinicians use many cues to indicate that they are rushed and cannot wait for their questions. If you ask, "Do you have any questions?" as you stand up to leave the examination room, you are teaching your patient that the correct answer is "no." When you ask your patients if they have any questions, they must believe you really care to listen and will not shame them because of their confusion. Patients are more likely to ask questions if the interactional dynamics already have established that the clinician will allow the patient to assert him- or herself. If patients are not asking questions, it may be time to examine your interviewing technique. However, asking patients, "Do you understand?" is not an effective way to uncover miscommunication.

EXPLORE PATIENTS' BELIEFS AND CONFIRM UNDERSTANDING

Another step in establishing a clinical environment that is sensitive to the needs of patients with limited health literacy is to explore patients beliefs and confirm understanding.[42] This can be done by having the patient teach the information back to you, a process known as "teach back" or the "show-me" approach (see Fig. 8-1).

If you want to be certain that the patient understands and is not simply parroting your statements, ask the patient to state in his or her own words the information you have given. This technique also enables the clinician to elicit patients' perspectives on management changes as well as their understanding of the issues at hand. The teach-back method, as well as several other communication techniques described in the preceding, requires practice, for example, through role-playing with colleagues. Clinicians also can evaluate and hone their interviewing skills by reviewing videotaped patient encounters.

KEY CONCEPTS

- Assess patient understanding and elicit beliefs.
- Use multiple channels to reinforce your message.
- Focus on a short set of action items.
- Be specific.
- Do not just ask, "Do you understand?" Create a question-asking atmosphere.
- Make certain you understand what you need to say.
- Confirm comprehension.

As a way to integrate the ideas presented in this chapter and exhibit the objectives, consider the following encounter.

Catherine, a 35-year-old woman with asthma, presented to the outpatient center 2 weeks after a brief hospitalization for an asthma exacerbation. Although she has never been intubated, this was her third hospitalization for asthma. She stopped smoking cigarettes 20 days ago when she began coughing and wheezing, but is now back to smoking one pack per day. Catherine agrees to participate in a smoking cessation group in which she will be given nicotine replacement. It is unclear whether she is able to differentiate her steroid inhaler (which is to be taken two puffs every morning and evening), from her rescue medication (which is to be taken two puffs every 4 to 6 hours as needed for wheezing) and it unclear if she was using her spacer.

To help correct this problem she was given a marker and two stickers on which she wrote "STEROIDS" and "Wheezy," which she pasted to the correct inhalers. When asked, "What do you think about this one?" (pointing at the steroid inhaler), she admitted that she was not certain if it helped her asthma, and when asked, "Well, what do you think about it?" she said, "I don't like it because steroids make me hold water, you know, fat." The fact that inhaled steroids do not have the same untoward effects as steroid pills was reviewed and the teach-back method was employed to further elicit any fears or concerns about steroids (there were none). The hope that the steroid inhaler might help her breathing if she took it every day (2 puffs in the morning and 2 puffs in the evening) was then discussed. She agreed to take it every day until the next visit, when the topic would be discussed again.

Then an empty inhaler device and spacer were taken to review their proper use, because a high proportion of patients do not use their inhalers correctly. It was explained that knowing how to use an inhaler is not obvious. Then the following six steps were described and demonstrated: (1) Shaking the inhaler, (2) Exhaling prior to actuation, (3) Closing lips tightly around the mouthpiece, (4) Pressing down once on the canister, (5) Taking a full/deep breath without triggering the auditory "whistle" indicator of the spacer, and (6) Holding the breath for at least 5 seconds. After explaining that you go through this whole process twice in order to take the two puffs, the patient tried it. It was observed that she forgot to shake her inhaler and actuated the inhaler twice in rapid succession. After providing encouragement about the fact that she had performed four of the six tasks correctly, how to perform the two steps she had missed was demonstrated again. The patient was asked to demonstrate inhaler technique again until she was able to perform the entire activity correctly ("teach-to-goal" approach).[30] At the end of the encounter she received a handout with diagrams as a reminder.

CONCLUSION

During the last decade, there has been growing attention to the challenges of limited health literacy and the extent to which basic understanding of disease processes and treatments relates to health care quality.[3] Health literacy can be thought of as currency for navigating a very complex health system that places extraordinary literacy demands on its users.[1] Health care providers have the opportunity to make the health care system easier for patients to use so that they can derive maximum benefit from it.

Millions of Americans have inadequate health literacy skills. Printed materials written in clear, plain language alone will not adequately bridge the health literacy gap. Providers of health care must assess what patients understand about their health and help them gain the skills and motivation to take care of themselves. When this "mutual" understanding is reached, everyone can then work together to ensure that patients have the information they need to manage their acute and chronic health needs. A culture of care that encourages patients to ask questions and strives for mutual "meaning" with patients about their understanding of how they can take better care of themselves must be created.

CORE COMPETENCY

Provide interpretive framing. Elicit and translate medical data into meaningful information. For example:

TESTS: *"The echocardiogram will show how well your heart is squeezing. It doesn't hurt. They put some jelly on your chest and use a special camera to get a movie of your heart pumping."*

MEDICATIONS

- Have patients bring in their medications every visit and demonstrate how they take them.
- Use computer programs to check what medications look like and look up those you do not recognize.
- Use pictures, graphics, pills taped to a box, prefilled syringes to assist in and promote adherence.

ELICIT patient beliefs and listen to how they make meaning of their condition. EXPLAIN diagnoses and diagnostic tests using the patient"s own words; draw pictures; provide simple step by step instructions.

EXPLAIN the concept of chronic disease.

"X is a problem we do not know how to cure. We DO know how to prevent the problems that come with having X, but it means that you will need to see me on a regular basis and may need to take some medications for the rest of your life."

Keep communication simple: Use plain words and uncomplicated sentences.

AVOID medical jargon and abbreviations: Say "heart attack," not "MI."

"We need to see if the cancer has spread," not "metastasized."

Be specific: Provide all the detail needed to complete critical tasks. Discuss *individual steps* in each task and barriers that the patient may have to each one.

For example: Explain the steps required to obtain fecal occult blood tests: How to open the cards, collect stool, wipe on the cards, close, and send in.

Focus on specific action steps:

- Slow down.
- Negotiate priorities.
- Limit the goals for each encounter.

Create short- and long-term goals:

- Assess the steps required to reach them.

  For example, a short-term goal may be to teach a patient to know his or her medications and their purpose. A long-term goal may be to control the blood pressure. Short-term goals may be the steps required to attain long-term goals.

Determine what patients understand and believe:

- Explore attitudes and beliefs.

  For example, ask about attitudes toward taking medications, the cause of illness, and the treatments the patient should be receiving. Ask what the patient thinks the consequences of having this illness are and if he or she knows anyone with this illness.

Confirm comprehension:

  Ask patients to repeat back to you how they are to take their medications or why you are ordering a certain test. *"To be sure I explained it to you well enough, would you mind telling me what the new medication is and how you will take it?"*

Extend the reach of communication:

- Use local patient education and web-based resources.
- Engage multiple members of the health care team in patient education.
- Write or draw simple instructions to take home.

Encourage questions and collaboration:

  Ask, *"What questions do you have?"* not *"Do you have questions?"*
  Negotiate steps and goals; use action plans.

DISCUSSION QUESTIONS

1. Describe ways to help patients ask questions or admit that they do not understand something.
2. Imagine that you are with a person who knows nothing about the US health system. Choose an activity related to patient care (e.g., getting a prescription). Can you explain how to complete the activity correctly?
3. How can you tell if a patient understands what he or she needs to do for a particular self-care regimen?
4. Practice a teach-back through role-play. Use the example of self-management of diabetes for a chronic condition. What information do both clinician and patient need to understand in order for the patient to take care of his or her health? Can you teach this so your patient understands what he or she needs to do?

RESOURCES

http://www.foundation.acponline.org
  The American College of Physicians provides information on conferences and a video about health literacy and medical errors.

http://www.ama-assn.org/ama/pub/category/8115.html
  The American Medical Association has developed a Health Literacy tool kit and video.

http://www.aelweb.vcu.edu/publications/healthlit/
  This website provides resources to help adult education instructors understand the problem of health literacy and the needs of adult learners.

http://www.cahealthliteracy.org/
  The California Health Literacy Initiative hosts the Health Literacy Resource Center, which is a resource for health literacy information and training.

http://www.healthyroadsmedia.org/
  Healthy Roads Media. This site contains free audio, written, and multimedia health education materials for a number of chronic conditions in a number of languages, and targeting lower literacy populations.

http://www.iha4health.org/index.cfm?CFID=11738999&CFTOKEN=4521560&MenuItemID=112&MenuSubID=41&MenuGroup=Home
  The Institute for Healthcare Advancement has presented an advance health care directive developed for patients with low literacy.

http://www.nap.edu/catalog/10883.html
  The National Academies Press provides electronic access to the Institute of Medicine report, Health Literacy: A Prescription to End Confusion.

http://www.ohri.ca/decisionaid
  This website, maintained by the International Patient Decision Aid Standards Collaboration, has close to 500 patient decision aids in English in various stages of development.

http://www.hsph.harvard.edu/healthliteracy/curricula.html
  The National Center for the Study of Adult Learning and Literacy website has a broad range of resources.

http://www.worlded.org/us/health/lincs/
  World Education maintains a collection on Health and Literacy for the National Institute for Literacy.

http://www.nlm.nih.gov/pubs/cbm/healthliteracybarriers.html
  The National Library of Medicine maintains a bibliography on health literacy.

http://www.sis.nlm.nih.gov/outreach/rhin.html
  Refugee Health Information Network, Supported by the National Library of Medicine. This website is a source of multilingual, multicultural health information for refugees and their care providers. One of its objectives of the network is to identify and make accessible culturally and linguistically appropriate health and medical information in order to improve health services for refugees.

http://www.med.unc.edu/medicine/generalm/decisionmaking/
  This University of North Carolina Web site provides material to assist patient-provider communication and promote shared decision-making in health care settings.

http://www.healthsystem.virginia.edu/internet/som-hlc/home.cfm
  This University of Virginia Health System website describes steps for building a health literacy curriculum

REFERENCES

1. Ratzan SC, Parker RM. Introduction. In: Selden CR, Zorn M, Ratzan SC, et al, eds. *National Library of Medicine Current Bibliographies in Medicine: Health literacy.* [Available at: http://www.nlm.nih.gov/pubs/cbm/hliteracy.html]. Vol. NLM Pub. No. CBM 2000-1. Bethesda, MD: National Institutes of Health, U.S. Department of Health and Human Services, 2000.

2. Institute of Medicine. Committee on Identifying Priority Areas for Quality Improvement. *Priority areas for national action: Transforming health care quality.* Washington, DC: National Academies Press, 2003.

3. Nielsen-Bohlman LT, et al. Institute of Medicine. *Health Literacy: A prescription to end confusion. Committee on Health Literacy, Board on Neuroscience and Behavioral Health.* Washington DC: National Academies Press, 2004.

4. Weiss BD. Epidemiology of low health literacy. In: Schwartzberg JG, VanGeest JB, Wang CC, eds. *Understanding health literacy: Implications for medicine and public health.* Chicago: American Medical Association Press, 2005.

5. Kirsch I. *The International Adult Literacy Survey (IALS): Understanding what was measured.* Princeton, NJ: Educational Testing Service, 2001.

6. Paasche-Orlow MK. The challenges of informed consent for low-literate populations. In: Schwartzberg JG, VanGeest JB, Wang CC, eds. *Understanding health literacy: Implications for medicine and public health.* Chicago: American Medical Association Press, 2005.

7. Paasche-Orlow MK. The prevalence of limited health literacy. *J Gen Intern Med* 2005;20(2):175–184.

8. Baker DW, et al. The association between age and health literacy among elderly persons. *J Gerontol B Psychol Sci Soc Sci* 2000;55(6):S368–S374.

9. Baker DW, et al. Health literacy and the risk of hospital admission. *J Gen Intern Med* 1998;13(12):791–798.

10. Baker DW, et al. Functional health literacy and the risk of hospital admission among Medicare managed care enrollees. *Am J Public Health* 2002;92(8):1278–1283.

11. Gazmararian J, et al. A multivariate analysis of factors associated with depression: Evaluating the role of health literacy as a potential contributor. *Arch Intern Med* 2000; 160(21):3307–3314.

12. Scott TL, et al. Health literacy and preventive health care use among medicare enrollees in a managed care organization. *Med Care* 2002;40(5):395–404.

13. Schillinger D, et al. Association of health literacy with diabetes outcomes. *JAMA* 2002;288(4):475–482.

14. Kalichman SC, Rompa D. Functional health literacy is associated with health status and health-related knowledge in people living with HIV-AIDS. *J Acquir Immune Defic Syndr* 2004;25(4):337–344.

15. DeWalt DA, et al. Literacy and health outcomes: A systematic review of the literature. *J Gen Intern Med* 2004a; 19(12):1228–1239.

16. Roter D. Health literacy and the patient-provider relationship. In: Schwartzberg JG, VanGeest JB, Wang CC, eds. *Understanding health literacy: Implications for medicine and public health.* Chicago: American Medical Association Press, 2005.

17. Schillinger D, et al. Functional health literacy and the quality of physician-patient communication among diabetes patients. *Patient Educ Couns* 2004;52(3):315–323.

18. Baker DW. Reading between the lines: Deciphering the connections between literacy and health. *J Gen Intern Med* 1999;14(5):315–317.

19. Schillinger D, Davis T. A conceptual framework for the relationship between health literacy and health care outcomes: The chronic disease exemplar. In: Schwartzberg JG, VanGeest JB, Wang CC, eds. *Understanding health literacy: Implications for medicine and public health.* Chicago: American Medical Association Press, 2005.

20. Rudd RR, Renzulli D, Pereira A, et al. Literacy demands in health care settings: The patient perspective. In: Schwartzberg JG, VanGeest JB, Wang CC, eds. Understanding health literacy: Implications for medicine and public health. Chicago: American Medical Association Press, 2005.

21. Seligman H, et al. Physician notification of their diabetes patients with limited health literacy. A randomized, controlled trial. *J Gen Intern Med* 2005;20(11):1001–1007.

22. Paasche-Orlow MK, Taylor HA, Brancati FL. Readability standards for informed-consent forms as compared with actual readability. *N Engl J Med* 2003a;348(8):721–726.

23. Paasche-Orlow MK, Jacob DM, Powell JN. Notices of privacy practices: A survey of the Health Insurance Portability and Accountability Act of 1996 documents presented to patients at U.S. hospitals. *Med Care* 2005;43(6): 558–564.

24. Hochhauser M. Informed consent and patient's rights documents: A right, a rite, or a rewrite? *Ethics Behav* 1999; 9(1):1–20.

25. Bass PF III, et al. Residents' ability to identify patients with poor literacy skills. *Acad Med* 2002;77(10): 1039–1041.

26. Horowitz CR, et al. Low health literacy is common and unhealthy: Do we recognize it in our own patients? *J Gen Intern Med* 2004;19(Suppl 1):176.

27. Lindau ST, et al. The association of health literacy with cervical cancer prevention knowledge and health behaviors in a multiethnic cohort of women. *Am J Obstet Gynecol* 2002;186(5):938–943.

28. Parikh NS, et al. Shame and health literacy: The unspoken connection. *Patient Educ Couns* 1996;27(1):33–39.

29. Baker DW, et al. The health care experience of patients with low literacy. Arch Fam Med 1996;5(6):329–334.

30. Paasche-Orlow MK, et al. Tailored education may reduce health literacy disparities in asthma self-management. *Am J Respir Crit Care Med* 2005;172(8):980–986.

31. Ad Hoc Committee on Health Literacy for the Council on Scientific Affairs AMA. Health literacy: Report of the Council on Scientific Affairs. *JAMA* 1999;281(6):552–557.

32. Kirsch I, et al. *Adult literacy in America: A first look at the findings of the national adult literacy survey.* Washington, DC: National Center for Education Statistics, U.S. Department of Education, 1993.

33. Shin HB, Bruno R. U.S. Census 2000: Language use and English-speaking ability. 2003. Available at: http:// www. census.gov/prod/2003pubs/c2kbr-29.pdf

34. Friedman SM, et al. Characteristics of discrepancies between self-reported visual function and measured reading speed. Salisbury Eye Evaluation Project Team. *Invest Ophthalmol Vis Sci* 1999;40(5):858–864.

35. Schwartz LM, et al. The role of numeracy in understanding the benefit of screening mammography. *Ann Intern Med* 1997:127(11):966–972.

36. Zikmund-Fisher BJ, Fagerlin A, Ubel PA. "Is 28% good or bad?" Evaluability and preference reversals in health care decisions. *Med Decis Making* 2004;24(2):142–148.

37. Adelsward V, Sachs L. The meaning of 6.8: Numeracy and normality in health information talks. *Soc Sci Med* 1996;43(8):1179–1187.

38. Waggoner WC, Sherman BB. Who understands? II: A survey of 27 words, phrases, or symbols used in proposed clinical research consent forms. *IRB* 1996;18(3):8–10.

39. Waggoner WC, Mayo DM. Who understands? A survey of 25 words or phrases commonly used in proposed clinical research consent forms. *IRB* 1995;17(1):6–9.

40. Castro CM, Wilson C, Schillinger D. Babel babble: Physicians' use of jargon with diabetes patients. *J Gen Intern Med* 2004;19(S1):124.

41. Ubel PA. Is information always a good thing? Helping patients make "good" decisions. *Med Care* 2002;40(9 Suppl): V39–V44.

42. Schillinger D, et al. Closing the loop: Physician communication with diabetic patients who have low health literacy. *Arch Intern Med* 2003;163(1):83–90.

43. DeWalt DA, et al. Development and pilot testing of a disease management program for low literacy patients with heart failure. *Patient Educ Couns* 2004b;55(1):78–86.

44. Rothman R, et al. The relationship between literacy and glycemic control in a diabetes disease-management program. *Diabetes Educ* 2004a;30(2):263–273.

45. Rothman RL, et al. Influence of patient literacy on the effectiveness of a primary care-based diabetes disease management program. *JAMA* 2004b;292(14):1711–1716.

46. Committee on Children with Disabilities of the American Academy of Pediatrics. The pediatrician's role in development and implementation of an Individual Education Plan (IEP) and/or an Individual Family Service Plan (IFSP). *Pediatrics* 1999;104(1 Pt 1):124–127.

Chapter 11

The Home Visit: Mobile Outreach

Dan Wlodarczyk, MD, and Margaret B. Wheeler, MS, MD

Objectives

- Review the development and evidence for benefit of home care and mobile outreach programs.
- Review the pros and cons of home visits to vulnerable patients.
- Identify patients best suited for targeted home visits.
- Identify populations and situations best suited for mobile outreach.
- Discuss the rationale for mobile services to homeless individuals.
- Summarize the limitations of mobile outreach services and the need to make these services a linkage to ongoing primary care.

Dr. Jones sees some of her patients in their homes, works closely with a home health agency, and rides a homeless van once a week. When she offers to see a patient at home, the usual response is, "I didn't know anyone did that any more!"

Dr. Jones and the van workers have noticed a young woman who watches them from an abandoned warehouse. Over months they gain her trust. It becomes clear that she is developmentally delayed and has a severe trauma history.

Eliminating barriers and providing patient-centered care are at the core of most attempts to improve the quality and equity of health care in the United States. Placing the patient's convenience above that of the health care provider by providing care where they live is so patient-centered that it changes the dynamics of the encounter. Patients who might otherwise never come to medical attention can be seen before their condition reaches a crisis.[1,2] Those who find it difficult or frightening to go to the doctor are particularly well served by medical care that comes to them. This chapter discusses health care delivered in the home or

through mobile outreach. It reviews the rationale, evidence, and practical suggestions for these forms of health care delivery. It concentrates in particular on home visits, because few providers receive explicit training about making them and on mobile services for the homeless (Box 11-1).

HOME CARE

Until the last century, most doctors made house calls and many medical practitioners were itinerants. In 1930, house calls represented 40% of all patient–physician interactions. By 1950, the number had dropped to 10% and by 1980 to 0.6%.[3] A recent study showed that <1% of elderly Medicare beneficiaries over the age of 65 received house calls from physicians.[3]

As medicine has become more technological, requiring diagnostic testing and treatment that is not portable, patients have traveled to see the doctor rather than the other way around. Most mobile medicine has been in the form of ambulances, which assure expeditious transport to the technological haven of the hospital. Technological advances are now making mobile and home care more possible again. Moreover, with pressures

> ## Box 11-1. Common Pitfalls in Caring for Patients with Significant Barriers to Care
>
> - Homebound patients may not get important medical care.
> - Not all barriers to care are physical. Patients who fear legal reprisal—such as prostitutes, substance users, or undocumented immigrants—may hesitate to access necessary medical services.
>
> - Often patients at highest risk for medical illness are most likely not to receive appropriate care.
> - Patients in rural areas may have virtually no access to needed medical care.
> - Many physicians have little to no training in conducting home visits or working as part of a case management team.

to shorten hospital stays and contain costs, care has shifted back into the home. In fact, during the 1990s home care became big business. Medicare's home care expenditures were growing so rapidly that policy makers reduced reimbursements for some equipment and interventions.

Nurses and other health professionals deliver most home care as it is now practiced. Indeed, rather than going to the patient's home, physicians are now much more likely to be consultants to a team of health care professionals who are the ones actually making the house calls. Nevertheless, understanding the role and value of home visits and working as a member of a home care team is important for all medical providers.

Research on the efficacy of home care has not always been of the highest quality and many different models of home care have been evaluated. Nevertheless, studies of interdisciplinary home care, post-hospitalization interventions, and geriatric assessment models have shown these delay functional decline and reduce permanent nursing home placement;[4] reduce hospitalizations; and improve the quality of life. A metaanalysis of home care studies indicates that deaths of younger, healthier patients may be decreased with home care interventions.[5]

HOME VISIT TO VULNERABLE PATIENTS

> Ms. Powers, a 78-year African-American old woman, lives alone. She has congestive heart failure, hypertension, obesity, and a nonhealing lower leg ulcer. Her children, except for one son, have moved away. Ms. Powers misses two appointments in a row with Dr. Jones.

Home visits, whether performed by doctors, nurses, or other health professionals, can make care more convenient for the patient. Understanding the conditions in which their patients' live gives providers critical insight into interventions necessary to provide effective health care. Home visits uncover problems that either

would never have become known in the office or whose discovery would have been delayed. Home visits have been documented to expose and allow intervention for new or worsening medical problems, confusion about medications,[6] and home environments that increase risk for falls in the elderly,[7] or asthma exacerbations in children.[8] Another benefit of home visits is the strengthening effect it can have on the therapeutic alliance between providers and patients.

Because it is impossible to visit all of the patients a provider cares for, some criteria are needed to select those most likely to benefit. High-priority patients include those who are very ill, who have little support, or are failing current care (Box 11-2).

GOALS OF HOME VISITS

> Dr. Jones calls Ms. Powers. She says she cannot get to the clinic. Her son lives in an apartment in the garage, but he has a problem with alcohol and drugs and does not help her. Dr. Jones asks her permission to make a home visit later in the week.

Home visits can be highly enlightening. They allow the provider not only to see patients who have difficulty coming to the clinic, but to better understand how and where the person lives, the degree of social support, who is available to help, and how he or she organizes medications, and make a general determination of the patient's physical safety in the home. The home visit embodies the cliché that when it comes to understanding how someone lives, one look is worth a thousand words.

In general, the goal of home visits is to intervene so that patients may remain safely at home and have their medical problems effectively treated. Occasionally a home visit is undertaken mainly to cement and deepen the patient–provider relationship. More often, the goal is to target patient's specific needs and the result is an increase in health care services. Some examples of the types of services that may be mobilized include nursing

Box 11-2. Indications for a Home Visit

Homebound patient

- Unable to leave home except in an ambulance
- Recent or severe disabilities, difficulty getting out of home to car, etc.
- Terminally ill, wishing to die at home
- Refuse to be seen in the office
- Recent hospitalization

Inpatients/outpatients

- Recent falls
- Unexplained difficulties in management
- Repeated hospitalizations

- Little social support
- Multiple comorbidities
- Recent disability
- Unexplained missed appointments

Frail elders

- Suspected abuse
- Assess caregiver abilities and burnout
- Family and support assessment
- Environmental assessment
- Geriatric assessment
- Considering institutionalization

---

services; physical and occupational therapy; pharmacy delivery of prefilled medi-sets; social services, such as meal delivery; increase social contact through community-based senior citizen organizations; outreach from religious groups or community clubs; and more coordinated care from family and friends. In addition, the home visit may provide support and reassurance for the caregivers at home who may feel under stress and ill prepared for their responsibilities.[9] Government programs such as Medicare and Medicaid pay for some types of in-home health care services. Community or faith-based organization often provide social services and social support free of charge (see Core Competency).

MEDICAL VISIT ADAPTED TO HOME

The etiquette and dynamics of visiting a patient at home are quite complex. The rules that govern conversation between guest and host predominate, although visiting health care providers are allowed greater access to the house and personal information. As both a guest (usually an honored one) and a medical professional, special license is granted to ask personal questions, and look in the liquor cabinet, bedroom, and bath. Being in the patient's house also may likely heighten the sense of intimacy between the provider and patient. Patients may be less inhibited socially and emotionally, and the rules of the office visit are modified. Patients may feel freer to ask questions, or reveal their ignorance or personal woes, for example. Visiting someone's home can reveal the full spectrum of a patient's identity and make it easier to discuss religious beliefs, cultural background, and the structure and interaction of family. Occasionally, a patient misunderstands this increased intimacy and the provider feels unsafe. If this

is a possibility, it is prudent to go with another member of the home care team.

> Ms. Powers' house is dark and needs repair. Ms. Powers drops a key out the window to let Dr. Jones in. The stairs are dark and the handrail is loose. Ms. Powers' bedroom is piled with boxes and the carpeting smells of urine. Ms. Powers apologizes for the condition of her home. She has been sleeping in a chair because of her shortness of breath, and it has been hard for her to get to the bathroom. She does not feel she could make it back up the stairs if she went down. She used to enjoy going to church, but has not been able to attend for months. She is sad and lonely and worries about her son.
>
> Dr. Jones diagnoses decompensated heart failure and urges hospitalization, but Ms. Power's refuses, fearing that she will never get back home. She agrees to allow Dr. Jones to have her medicines delivered and have a home health nurse visit. With the help of a social worker, Dr. Jones arranges for in-home support and "meals on wheels" delivery, and contacts Ms. Powers' daughter and pastor. Medicare pays for a hospital bed that allows her to elevate her head and legs and a bedside commode to facilitate hygiene. Physical therapists help make the home safer and her stronger.

The home visit, as the case of Ms. Powers illustrates, reveals rich information about a patient that is very difficult to obtain in any other way. Ms. Powers' physical surroundings are isolating and hazardous. She has become homebound and isolated. Her heart failure has become worse, and she has been without medications for some time. Although she refused hospitalization—a common occurrence among the frail elderly—Dr. Jones, with the help of a health care team, was able to mobilize resources to meet her needs, and for the moment, she can remain safely at home.

Box 11-3. Pros and Cons of Home Visits

Pros	Cons
See first-hand the patient's living conditions and understand some of his or her vulnerabilities	Time intensive
Access the need for in-home support services	Usually not performed by primary care provider (though nurses etc. may be more skillfull)
Establish or strengthen the patient–provider relationship.	Limited in scope of examination and ancillary services
Spend uninterrupted, more focused time with your patient	May lead to patient's removal from the home for safety reasons
Meet involved family members and friends	May not be able to bill for a home visit
Professionally satisfying experience for the provider	The area may not be safe
Linkage to comprehensive home assessment and services	May lack the necessary experience and feel uncomfortable in making a home visit
Even in resource-poor areas, some resources usually are available; they may be faith or community based	Comprehensive services may not be available in certain areas

Home visits are also very useful in special situations, such as assessing suspected elder abuse (see Chap. 20) and child abuse, or at the beginning or end of life. Health workers who enter the home to help new mothers nurse and learn to care for their babies have been very successful. Helping families support a patient die peacefully at home is another rewarding and thriving use of home care (see Core Competency) (Box 11-3).

MOBILE VAN OUTREACH SERVICES

Mobile medical units can be as elaborate as advanced field hospitals used in war and disasters or as humble as the practitioner who arrives with a backpack (Figs. 11-1 and 11-2). Home care and mobile van outreach services have much in common, most importantly that they address barriers to care by bringing care directly to patients. Generally, what distinguishes mobile medical vans from home care is that mobile vans are often equipped to deliver slightly more technological care—take x-rays or provide dental care, for example. Mobile vans also target populations of high-risk patients in whom barriers to care may go beyond being homebound—homeless patients, migrant workers, or prostitutes, for example. Patients who are homebound usually have had some contact with the medical system before home care is instituted. Medical outreach vans have the capability of reaching people who might not

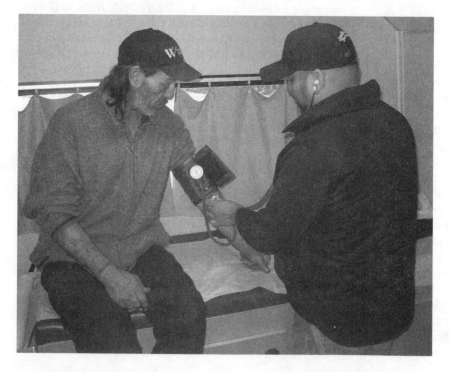

Figure 11-1. The Street Outreach Services van has a confidential examination space for evaluation and treatment of problems. Here an outreach worker checks vital signs.

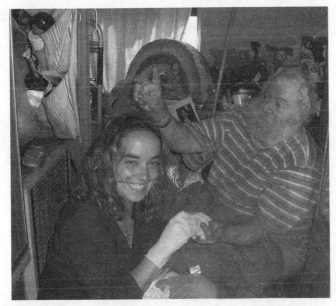

Figure 11-2. The street outreach van visits a man living in a camper on the streets of San Francisco.

otherwise have access to care. Mobile outreach services can be a powerful means of delivering the full spectrum of care from emergency room–level care to preventive medicine.[10]

Studies of mobile care are few. Those that do exist show that these services reach patients who might not otherwise come to medical attention and those who are at particularly high risk.[11] For example, intravenous drug users who use mobile needle exchanges engage in riskier behavior than do those who frequent fixed site exchanges.[12] Mobile HIV counseling treatment and even directly observed therapy reach especially vulnerable patients.[13] A review of mobile outreach services provided to 4587 homeless people in 18 communities in the United States showed that homeless people contacted by street outreach were homeless for longer periods of time and were more likely to have psychotic disorders than homeless people contacted in shelters or social service agencies. Although these patients were more severely impaired and less motivated to seek out services than those in shelters, the outreach services were able to successfully engage the most troubled among this group, and substantial improvements did occur.[14]

Mobile vans also make sense when resources and populations are sparse.[15] Dental outreach in rural areas has demonstrated efficacy.[16] Moreover, when there is particular community resistance to establishing a clinic for stigmatized groups (i.e., methadone users, prostitutes, or undocumented or homeless people), a mobile service also has a role to play. Mobile mental health services effectively target crisis situations as well as marginalized

mentally ill populations; those who are homeless or live in underserved rural or minority communities.[17,18]

MOBILE OUTREACH SERVICE TO HOMELESS PEOPLE

> Mr. Swanson is hospitalized for 2 months after severe head trauma and seizures. He leaves the hospital against medical advice (AMA) and has no follow-up appointments or medications. He approaches the outreach van and asks for snacks.

Homeless populations are a perfect target for mobile outreach services. Homeless people suffer disproportionately from illness and early mortality and have decreased access to medical care. Medical treatment can decrease morbidity and mortality and link patients to important services. Homeless patients are stigmatized and growing in numbers.

Although there are no exact numbers, it is estimated that 3.5 million people in the United States experience homelessness each year.[19] Persistent and abject poverty is the unifying thread in this demographic tapestry, which includes people of all ages, sexes, regions of the country, and racial or ethnic backgrounds.[20] The United States Conference of Mayors 2004 Hunger and Homelessness survey of 27 cities showed that all but one were documenting increased requests for emergency food, and that 20% of those requests were unmet.[21] In response to this crisis, federal and national organizations have collaborated with cities to tackle the issue of homelessness and care for homeless people. As part of these efforts, cities with widely spread out homeless encampments have implemented the use of outreach vans. Other communities with areas of high homeless density support free clinics or have created systems that link mobile and fixed services; inpatient and emergency room care with outreach.[22] Today there are health care for the homeless programs in every state and hundreds of programs in major cities (see Chap. 24).

In San Francisco, as in other major cities, there are several mobile outreach vans that are funded by public and nonprofit organizations. The vans are often "specialized" and target specific populations (e.g., youth at high risk for HIV, substance users, public inebriants) or provide specific services such as mobile delivery of tuberculosis medications to single-room occupancy (SRO) hotels and shelters. Vans also deliver both acute medical and preventative services. Like mobile medical services in other big cities, San Francisco's SOS (Street Outreach Services) van is a well-respected service upon which the many homeless people trust and depend. Each day of the week, it cruises a designated area of the city; the exact route changes because of the movement of encampments by police enforcement of vagrancy laws, or when van workers are notified that a particular individual is in need of service. Two outreach workers (one of whom is an Americorp volunteer, or a registered nurse), an attending physician, and a medical resident staff the van. The van has an examination room with an examination table, a sink, and a wall-mounted oto-ophthalmoscope. The van carries prescription medications primarily for infections and asthma, over-the-counter medications, toiletries, hygiene supplies, supplies to permit incision and drainage of abscess and facilitate wound care, and splinting materials. Additionally, the van carries some clothing and snacks. Once a month a pet van, staffed by a volunteer veterinarian, cares for the pets of homeless people. (Pets provide companionship and safety to homeless people. They are so important that people will neglect their own health problems and not go to the hospital until their pet's safety is ensured.)

The goal of all these efforts is to provide a positive medical experience to homeless patients. Slowly, the mobile outreach workers can build a bridge that will get the homeless person needed care and services. A British study of bringing a "mobile surgery" to people sleeping in the "rough" found that within a month of seeing a physician in the mobile surgery over one-third of the patients attended a drop-in clinic for homeless people.[23] This demonstrates that outreach services can be a first step in linking homeless patients with more comprehensive services. In some systems, providing comprehensive services includes helping patients obtain important entitlements such as public assistance. In San Francisco, the street homeless similarly have high rates of physical and mental health problems, and often many visits are needed to gain their trust and engage them in services. Meaningful improvements in the person's life can occur with persistence on the part of the outreach team and a little good luck. These may include obtaining permanent housing, benefits such as social security disability, sobriety, treatment for physical and mental problems, and rebuilding important personal relationships.

Medical students and residents gain important insight into the lives and needs of homeless patients by riding the homeless vans. It is one of the most highly rated experiences at the authors' institution. Moreover, those who are exposed to patients in this way are more likely to seek out similar experiences in the future.

> Mr. Swanson lives in the "field," a large area with mounds of broken concrete densely overgrown with weeds that shields many homeless encampments. Signs on the fence warn about toxic contamination. Before his hospitalization, Mr. Swanson was found unconscious after being severely beaten while he slept in the "field." When he leaves AMA from the hospital, this is where he returns.

> Despite neurosurgery, his brain is damaged, his speech is slow, and he has arm weakness. Mr. Swanson had not kept any follow-up appointments or taken any of his medicines.

Mr. Swanson approaches the medical van not for help with his problems, but for some snacks and clothing. This is common and the reason why these are important components of the van's supplies. Like many homeless people, Mr. Swanson places a higher priority on obtaining food and clothing than on receiving medical services. Obtaining shelter and guarding physical safety also trumps addressing medical concerns. These are not unreasonable priorities: Physical violence is a significant cause of morbidity and mortality in the homeless.

Homeless patients are at higher risk for health problems than people who are housed. A cohort of homeless people in Philadelphia were found to have a fourfold increase in mortality compared with the general population.[24] Homeless women have very high rates of sexual assault as well.[27] In San Francisco, most homeless deaths are related to substance use or trauma.[25] In Toronto, homeless women >45 years of age had 10 times the mortality rate of the general population.[26] Homeless women have very high rates of sexual assault as well. Following up on medical care also is not easy for homeless patients. Keeping track of appointments or storing medications is difficult. Without an address or telephone, and with the cognitive and physical impairments common in homeless patients, reminders may not work. Mobile outreach may work to mitigate some of these barriers to care, either by providing the care directly or helping to connect patients with needed resources.

> Mr. Swanson lives by panhandling and working on cars. His own pickup truck and all his possessions, including his identification and tools, were towed when he was hospitalized.

It is not uncommon for homeless people to lose all of their possessions if they are hospitalized or incarcerated. Their unattended possessions are taken by others or thrown out. The police may impound vehicles. Lacking money or identification, the costs associated with these losses can be immense for a homeless person. Fears of these losses may spur patients to leave the hospital AMA. Other reasons that homeless people leave the hospital AMA may include disagreements over pain medication or food; perceived disrespectful treatment; and the need to take care of personal business, like getting their check or prevent withdrawal from addictions not being treated in the hospital; or the need to care for their friends, pets, or vehicles.

Box 11-4. Strengths and Limitations of Mobile Outreach Services

Strengths	Limitations
Meet clients on their terms	Can identify untreated chronic illnesses
Develop trust	May not be seeing those in greatest need
Link to site of comprehensive care and other resources	May take several visits to dispel mistrust
Address immediate needs	Limited resources in the van
Begin to formulate a treatment plan including applying for entitlements	Insufficient resources to address even basic needs
	Without a plan, the van may be providing "band-aid care"
Can make appointments and assess hospital or clinic records through internet or phone	Not all vans are connected to the hospital or clinic network
	Chronic disease management may be impossible

Through a combined effort of the outreach staff and the county hospital, Mr. Swanson's discharge medicines are filled and he receives help in applying for Social Security disability. The van takes him to appointments. Psychometric testing documents his loss of cognitive function and a psychiatrist sees him. He is awarded SSI and Medicaid, and moves back home with his parents.

The van may be an initial point of contact for a snack, but the real objective is to provide a link to more comprehensive care that addresses the multiple needs of homeless patients. The needs may range from the mundane, such as obtaining an identification card (which is essential to applying for entitlements), to obtaining specialized psychometric testing, to quantifying and documenting the level of cognitive impairment, which is useful in supporting the SSI application. It often takes a team effort to provide these complicated patients with the level of care that they need (Box 11-4).

CONCLUSION

Patient-centered care is particularly important for patients at high risk for morbidity and mortality who have concomitant barriers to accessing appropriate care. Home care and mobile outreach services are two models of providing care to vulnerable and marginalized patients. Targeted home visits can provide first-hand information about how and where the patient lives and about support systems. It allows for assessment of health status and mobilization of appropriate resources and services. Mobile outreach services also allow providers to reduce or eradicate barriers to care and connect patients with needed services and resources. Mobile outreach to homeless persons can be an effective way to extend the safety net to this vulnerable population. The key is linkage to more comprehensive services that can meet these persons' needs and provide ongoing care. Mobile outreach can help make this linkage by dispelling mistrust, addressing immediate needs, and providing personalized assistance and attention.

KEY CONCEPTS ON MOBILE OUTREACH SERVICES

- Mobile outreach services effectively target high-risk marginalized populations.
- Mobile outreach services decrease barriers to appropriate care for the highest-risk populations.
- Mobile outreach services can provide the full gamut of care, from acute medical care to preventive services.
- Mobile outreach is effective in rural areas with few medical resources.
- Mortality rates are increased in homeless people; identification and intensive outreach to those at highest risk may reduce excessive mortality.
- Mobile services can extend but not replace the safety net.
- Outreach services should have a plan to link persons with the services they need.

DISCUSSION QUESTIONS

1. Imagine that Ms. P. is your patient. What services are available in your community to a homebound senior? Who would you ask if you did not know?
2. What types of patients do you think would benefit from a targeted home visit by you or a referral to a public health nurse or home care agency?
3. How would you approach a homeless person rehospitalized for osteomyelitis who needs 6 weeks of IV antibiotics, and who has a history of signing out AMA?
4. What barriers do homeless people face in obtaining ongoing medical care?

CORE COMPETENCY
Making a Home Visit

Who qualifies for home care services?

- People with Medicare/Medicaid and insured patients.
- Homebound patients or those with great difficulty leaving home.
- Skilled need, home PT, nursing needs; may qualify for multiple services.
- May also qualify for a home health aide to help shop, bathe, etc.
- Through home care you can order hospital beds, O_2, walkers, railings, etc.
- People without insurance may be referred to other systems, such as mobile care and public health nurse systems.

Preparing for the home visit
Identify your goals

- Evaluate safety.
- Assess social support.
- Review medication.
- Reinforce therapeutic alliance: more time, more intimate, different power dynamic.
- Provide social support for patient and family.
- Evaluate barriers to medical compliance.
- Evaluate elder abuse.
- Evaluate medical condition.
- Coordinate with other health care providers.

Before leaving

- Review medical records.
- Get billing forms, paperwork, or other assessment forms (DPOA, lab slips, etc.).
- Consider special supplies and equipment.
- Call patient and caregivers for directions and advise them you are coming.
- Arrange with other health care providers if you want to coordinate a visit.
- Invite a colleague to join you if you have safety concerns.

Terminally ill patients

- Focus on both the family and the patient.
- Maximize patient comfort and minimize caregiver burnout, fear, panic, guilt, and confusion.
- Involve hospice organizations.
- Discuss prehospital DNR form and DPOA.
- Reassure and model use of pain medications.
- Review the discomfort of eating in the final days.
- Review expected scenarios for death.
- Provide contact numbers for emergency help and reassurance.
- Hospice workers pronounce death, and contact the coroner and mortuary.

Tips on What to Take Along on Home Visits	Tips on What to Look for During the Visit	Functional Assessment
Stethoscope and blood pressure cuff	Surrounding neighborhood for safety, availability of stores. Accessibility to public transportation	What is patient able to do in the home?
Examination gloves	Condition of the entrance, a bell, can door be opened	What ADLs do they need help doing?
Flashlight	Condition of stairs, hand rails, lighting	
Gauze and other wound care supplies	Available support of family and friends in the building; general condition of living space	Assess emergency contacts. Assess expectations of long-term care. Clues for caretaker stress: disturbed sleep, incontinence(?), financial stress
Plastic bag to dispose of gloves, gauze	Safety of floors, extension cords, rugs that can slide	Safety of medication/ cleaning agents if children
Durable Power of Attorney for Health forms	Kitchen: Is there food, are conditions sanitary? Where do they shop?	Heating; paint condition; asthma exacerbators? Stove safety? Stove used for heat?
Prehospital DNR forms	Bedroom: Is bed adequate; is a hospital bed needed?	Bedside commode needed?
Progress note: Paper to record the visit and pertinent telephone and contact information	Bathroom: Is it safe; how do they get in the tub, bath mat, grab bars?	Evidence of smoking? Smoking in bed? Liquor supplies? Other smells (urine, pets, etc.)
Disposable tape measure	How and who organizes the medications. Check for old pill bottles. What do they take? Evaluate for medi-sets or home delivery of medicines.	Safety devices: Smoke alarm; telephone accessibility, etc.
List of community resources, important telephone numbers	Evaluate for in-home support, in-home nursing, adult protective services, adult day health care	Mobilize community agencies; social work consultation

RESOURCES

O'Connell JJ, ed. The health care of homeless persons: A manual of communicable diseases and common problems in shelters and on the streets. Available free online at: www.bhchp.ord

Eighner L. *Travels with Lizabeth: Three years on the road and streets.* New York: Ballantine Books, 1993. A book about a homeless man and his dog. It gives you insights into how a homeless person might feel during a hospitalization.

National Alliance to End Homelessness. 2002. A nonprofit organization whose mission is to mobilize an alliance to end homelessness. Available at: http://www.endhomelessness.org/

National Coalition for the Homeless. Available at: http://www.nationalhomeless.org/

National Health Care for the Homeless Council. Available free online at: www.nhchc.org

REFERENCES

1. Campion EW. Home alone, and in danger. *N Engl J Med* 1996;334:1738–1739.
2. Gurley RJ, Lum N, Sande M, et al. Persons found in their homes helpless or dead. *N Engl J Med* 1996;334:1710–1716.
3. Meyer GS, Gibbons RV. House calls to the elderly: A vanishing practice among physicians. *N Engl J Med* 1997;337:1815–1820.
4. Stuck AE, Aronow HU, Steiner A, et al. A trial of annual in-home comprehensive geriatric assessments for elderly people living in the community. *N Engl J Med* 1995;333:1184–1189.
5. Stuck AE, Egger M, Hammer A, et al. Home visits to prevent nursing home admission and functional decline in elderly people: Systematic review and meta-regression analysis. *JAMA* 2002;287:1022–1028.
6. Hsia Der E, Rubenstein LZ, Choy GS. The benefits of in-home pharmacy evaluation for older persons. *J Am Geriatr Soc* 1997;45:211–214.
7. Nikolaus T, Bach M. Preventing falls in community-dwelling frail older people using a home intervention team (HIT): results from the randomized Falls-HIT trial. *J Am Geriatr Soc* 2003;51:300–305.
8. Butz AM, Syron L, Johnson B, et al. Home-based asthma self-management education for inner city children. *Public Health Nurs* 2005;22:189–199.
9. Campion EW. Can house calls survive? *N Engl J Med* 1997;337:1840–1841.
10. Nuttbrock L, McQuistion H, Rosenblum A, et al. Broadening perspectives on mobile medical outreach to homeless people. *J Health Care Poor Underserved* 2003;14:5–16.
11. Cameron K, Hansen E. Health planning for immigrants. *Health Prog* 2005;86:26–29, 60.
12. Miller CL, Tyndall M, Spittal P, et al. Risk-taking behaviors among injecting drug users who obtain syringes from pharmacies, fixed sites, and mobile van needle exchanges. *J Urban Health* 2002;79:257–265.
13. Bell DN, Martinez J, Botwinick G, et al. Case finding for HIV-positive youth: A special type of hidden population. *J Adolesc Health* 2003;33:10–22.
14. Lam JA, Rosenheck R. Street outreach for homeless persons with serious mental illness: Is it effective? *Med Care* 1999;37:894–907.
15. Hayward KS. Facilitating interdisciplinary practice through mobile service provision to the rural older adult. *Geriatr Nurs* 2005;26:29–33.
16. Douglass JM. Mobile dental vans: planning considerations and productivity. *J Public Health Dent* 2005;65:110–113.
17. Cornelius LJ, Simpson GM, Ting L, et al. Reach out and I'll be there: mental health crisis intervention and mobile outreach services to Urban African Americans. *Health Soc Work* 2003;28:74–78.
18. Morris DW, Warnock JK. Effectiveness of a mobile outreach and crisis services unit in reducing psychiatric symptoms in a population of homeless persons with severe mental illness. *J Okla State Med Assoc* 2001;94:343–346.
19. National Coalition for the Homeless. 2002. Accessed at: http://www.nationalhomeless.org/
20. Levy BD, O'Connell JJ. Health care for homeless persons. *N Engl J Med* 2004;350:2329–2332.
21. Lowe ET, Slater A, Welfley J, Moye T. Hunger and Homelessness Survey. A status report on hunger and homelessness in America's cities. A 27-city survey. December 2004. Available at: http://www.usmayors.org/uscm/hungersurvey/2004/onlinereport/HungerAndHomelessnessReport2004.pdf
22. Nakonezny PA, Ojeda M. Health services utilization between older and younger homeless adults. *Gerontologist* 2005;45:249–254.
23. Ramsden SS, Nyiri P, Bridgewater J, et al. A mobile surgery for single homeless people in London. *BMJ* 1989;298:372–374.
24. Hibbs JR, Benner L, Klugman L, et al. Mortality in a cohort of homeless adults in Philadelphia. *N Engl J Med* 1994;331:304–309.
25. Deaths among homeless persons: San Francisco, 1985–1990. *MMWR Morb Mortal Wkly Rep* 1991;40:877–880.
26. Cheung AM, Hwang SW. Risk of death among homeless women: a cohort study and review of the literature. *CMAJ* 2004;170:1243–1247.
27. Kushel MB, Evans JL, Perry S, Robertson MJ, Moss AR. No door to lock: victimization among homeless and marginally housed persons. *Arch Intern Med.* 2003 Nov 10; 163(20): 2492–9.

Chapter 12

Group Medical Visits for Underserved Populations

Hali Hammer, MD

Objectives

- Define the group medical visit.
- Review the most common group medical visit models.
- Discuss the advantages of group medical visits, particularly for underserved populations.
- Describe some of the obstacles to establishing group-based models of care in safety net health settings.

Liu Su Chen is a 72-year-old woman with type 2 diabetes, hypertension, and osteoarthritis. She and her husband emigrated from mainland China 20 years ago. Although her husband is fluent in written and spoken English, Mrs. Chen neither speaks nor reads English.

In the last 2 years, Mrs. Chen's diabetes, which had been very well controlled, is now poorly controlled and she has become increasingly disabled by arthritis in both knees. Mrs. Chen's doctor has referred her to a nutritionist and diabetes educator to help her learn to control her blood sugar. Now on maximum doses of the three diabetes medicines that she can tolerate, as well as multiple medications for other chronic problems, Mrs. Chen is resistant when her doctor begins to discuss starting her on insulin therapy. She says, "I only know one person who has taken insulin for her diabetes, and she died within a year of starting the shots!"

A colleague of Mrs. Chen's physician recently began offering diabetes care to groups of 8 to 15 patients at a time in Cantonese and English.

Efforts to reform ambulatory care have focused on optimizing access to care while making efficient use of limited resources. This chapter describes a new model of care delivery, the group medical visit (GMV), an innovative approach that is gaining widespread acceptance, and has been studied in diverse health care settings and patient populations. The discussion presents both the advantages of providing group-based care and its challenges, particularly among underserved populations.

WHAT IS A GROUP MEDICAL VISIT?

Mrs. Chen's doctor convinces her to attend one of the new group visits by pointing out that she may meet other people who are taking insulin, and that everything will be presented in her language.

The group medical visit, sometimes called a "cluster visit,"[1] "chronic care clinic,"[2] "shared medical appointment,"[3] and "cooperative health care clinic,"[4,5] has been proposed and studied as a means of increasing access while improving the care provided in relation to the traditional brief, one-on-one clinical encounter. Many different models of group-based care have been developed, each tailored to the specific population served.

Box 12-1. Goals of Group-Based Care

- Peer support during the clinical encounter
- Point-of-care collaboration by an interdisciplinary team
- Interactive group education

Most of the current models were developed in response to demands to improve quality of care, increase access to limited provider resources, and optimize patient satisfaction in an increasingly competitive health care environment. Many of the existing models of group-based care were developed in managed care or academic practice settings and have been implemented with predominantly insured and higher socioeconomic patients.[4,6] However, group models employed in low socioeconomic or uninsured populations show similar benefits (Box 12-1).

A group medical visit is a clinical encounter between one or more clinicians and a group of patients. Most GMVs target patients with a common health concern (e.g., age >65, a particular chronic illness, or pregnancy). Group visits offer routine care, group support, and education. The GMVs typically occur more frequently than usual individual visits (monthly to quarterly), involve a stable set of 8 to 25 patients, and last from 90 minutes to 3 hours, depending on the model.

Table 12-1 presents a typical GMV format. In most models, the meeting begins with group time, usually a "check-in" structured on individual goals. Group education and discussion are also typically built into the group time, and focused on topics that are applicable to many patients with the targeted condition. Sessions include time for group facilitators to interact individually with participants, and time is set aside before or after the group meeting for private consultations and examinations with the clinicians.

MODELS OF GROUP MEDICAL VISITS

COOPERATIVE HEALTH CARE CLINICS

Developed by John Scott and colleagues at Colorado Kaiser Permanente Medical Group, cooperative health care clinics (CHCC) originally targeted high-utilizing elderly patients, with the primary goal of decreasing unnecessary emergency department and urgent care use.[4,5,7] These are monthly GMVs cofacilitated by a physician and nurse for a targeted group of 20 to 25 patients. Each CHCC includes group education, social time, one-on-one contact with the physician and/or nurse, and an opportunity for questions and answers. CHCCs also have been used in specialty settings (diabetes GMVs in endocrinology clinics, stroke GMVs offered by a neurology practice). Typically CHCCs replace the individual encounter or decrease the frequency of one-on-one visits.

Table 12-1. Sample Group Medical Visit Format

Time (min)	Activity	Content
15	Check-in	Blood pressure and other vital signs are checked during the group discussion. Each participant's check-in is structured by the individual goals that were set at the prior session.
30	Group learning	Group facilitators lead a discussion on a topic decided on by the group at the previous visit. Handouts and other visual aids may be used.
30	One-on-one	Group facilitators move around the room, meeting with each participant briefly and doing the following: • Addressing issues that were not raised in the group • Performing focused physical examinations • Refilling prescriptions • Ordering referrals, laboratory tests, and treatments as indicated • Establishing whether the patient needs a private examination after the GMV • Following up on individual issues raised during the check-in period Group members mingle with each other during this one-on-one time, often with refreshments.
15	Question and answer/planning	Patients ask questions related to their health and choose a group learning topic for the next session.
30	Optional private examinations (10 min per exam)	Providers offer a maximum of three private examinations per GMV session. Other GMV members either socialize or leave the clinic.

Adapted from: Miller D, et al. Group medical visits for low-income women with chronic disease: A feasibility study. *J Womens Health (Larchmont)* 2004;13(2):217–225.

DROP-IN GROUP MEDICAL APPOINTMENT

Unlike CHCCs, drop-in group medical appointments (DIGMAs) target all patients in a busy physician's panel rather than patients who share a common medical problem or characteristic. Developed by Edward Noffsinger at Kaiser Permanente in San Jose, CA, DIGMAs increase patients' access to their physician by opening up extended appointments that they can use as often as they choose.[6] Usually cofacilitated by a behavioral health professional (psychologist, social worker, health educator, or therapist) and the physician, they provide the opportunity for more holistic, "mind–body" medicine than usually is possible in an individual clinic visit. DIGMAs are group medical appointments with the added support group component fostered by the involvement of the behavioralist. DIGMAs have been successful in easing time constraints commonly imposed on both primary and specialty care practices.

CHRONIC CARE CLINICS

Chronic care clinics (CCC) are planned clinical encounters for targeted patients with a specific medical condition in a primary care practice.[2] Based on the "mini-clinic" developed in general practices in the United Kingdom, the CCC is a half-day–long session during which 8 to 12 patients have brief one-on-one visits with a primary care physician and other providers (pharmacist, nutritionist), and also group education and discussion. These differ from the other GMV models in that the physician encounter with the patient is individual, but it is linked to group education on the same day. These usually occur three to four times per year and supplement the regular individual visit.

CLUSTER VISITS

Cluster visits are directed at patients with a particular chronic illness, most commonly diabetes.[1] These are monthly GMVs of 10 to 18 patients for a finite period of time, usually 6 months. They are led by a specially trained nurse educator, and supported by physicians who are readily available for consultation. There is also judicious use of referrals to nutritionists, behavioralists, pharmacists, and social workers. The cluster visit model, which also was developed at Kaiser Permanente, incorporates nurse care management, including frequent telephone follow-up between visits, coordination of needed ancillary services, and intensive medication management. In contrast to the models discussed above, cluster visits replace usual primary and specialty care for the targeted chronic illness during the intervention period.

GROUP PRENATAL VISITS

Group-based prenatal care has been offered in a number of different settings.[8,9] Much of routine prenatal care involves repeating similar pregnancy-related health information to each woman at frequent periodic checks. The repetition inherent in prenatal care and the benefit for pregnant women of sharing the experience of pregnancy and parenting with other women makes pregnancy an ideal time for group-based care.

The most widely practiced and studied model of group prenatal care, CenteringPregnancy, was conceived by Sharon Schindler Rising. In this model, a cohort of 8 to 12 pregnant women at a similar gestational stage meets together for the duration of prenatal care. Groups are cofacilitated by an obstetric care provider (physician, certified nurse midwife, or nurse practitioner) and a registered nurse or other prenatal services team member. During each of the 2-hour group sessions, women and their support people (partners, friends) participate in self-care activities, facilitated group discussions on topics related to childbearing and parenting, community-building activities, and physical assessment by the obstetric provider. Unlike the other GMV models described in the preceding, CenteringPregnancy originally was developed for socioeconomically diverse patient populations, and although it has been used in managed care, private, and academic practice settings, it has been primarily employed in underserved populations.

GROUP WELL-CHILD VISITS

Group well-child care was one of the first models of GMVs in the United States.[10,11] In most settings, the GMV replaces the usual periodic well-baby visits in the first year of life (newborn, 2, 4, 6, 9, and 12 months) with primary care visits in a group setting. With an emphasis on age-specific anticipatory guidance and group support for parents of infants of the same age, these GMVs minimize the repetition inherent in well-child care and also are an efficient way for clinicians to provide routine primary care.

CHALLENGES IN IMPLEMENTING GROUP MEDICAL VISITS FOR UNDERSERVED POPULATIONS

SPACE

Ambulatory care practices, which are designed for individual visits, are challenged by the practical changes required to accommodate group-based care. The main obstacle for many practices planning GMVs is the lack of available rooms large enough to accommodate 8 to

20 people. Although space is limited in many ambulatory care settings, public health clinics may have even more severe space constraints.

ATTENDANCE

There is the perception among patients that anything that happens in groups is education or a "class." Thus, it may be perceived as different from medical care, and consequently undervalued. As a result, it is often difficult to get all patients to come to GMVs consistently; sporadic attendance detracts from the group's ability to gel into a cohesive, supportive unit. Many groups have reported low recruitment rates for group interventions in socioeconomically disadvantaged populations.[12-14] In contrast to the older, privately insured patients originally targeted by GMVs, uninsured or underinsured patients are more likely to be employed and/or caring for children. Because of time constraints and other factors, these individuals may be harder to engage in groups. In an effort to address this problem, GMVs often have built incentives into the plan: most commonly healthy snacks, but also on-site child care, transportation vouchers, and health-related "giveaways," such as exercise bands, pedometers, and recipe books.

TRAINING

Minimal training in group facilitation and participatory learning is essential to the success of GMVs. However, many health centers, especially publicly funded clinics, lack resources for additional training for staff that would enable them to perform outside of their normal scope of practice. Furthermore, if the GMV is seen only as "extra care," it may not be prioritized when making staffing decisions and there may be resistance to obtaining special training.

Published and online training guides are available for the various GMV models. One example is the Group Visit Facilitators Training Manual and Protocol of the Improving Diabetes Efforts Across Language and Literacy (IDEALL) project at San Francisco General Hospital.

PERSONNEL

It is often difficult for safety net health centers to put together a functioning team of providers to work on any new endeavor. To make a GMV work, there must be explicit articulation of the role of each member of the team. The scheduling clerk, for example, is integrally important to the success of any group because it may be his or her success at getting patients to attend that determines a group's success or failure.

SCHEDULING

GMVs are hard to incorporate into traditional clinic schedules. Because the benefits of group-based care are often not apparent to frontline clinic staff, there is often resistance to making the necessary changes to existing schedules.

COST

Few studies to date have shown that group-based care is cost effective.[1,4,5] Moreover, there is a great deal of uncertainty about reimbursement from publicly funded payers, which varies from state to state. Reimbursement for group-based prenatal care may be more consistent than for chronic illness groups because of the precedent in prenatal care for payment for ancillary medical services. There is no CPT (Medicare billing) code specifically for group-based care. Most practices that have successfully billed for group-based care have done so by using visit codes for the face-to-face time spent directly with the provider. However, it is notable that most of the GMV models were developed and continue to be most widely used in closed health maintenance organizations (e.g., Kaiser Permanente) where there is little outside billing for clinical services.

CONFIDENTIALITY

Maintaining confidentiality is one of the main concerns expressed when group-based care is first introduced to health care professionals. The fear is that patients will not disclose important health information because of the lack of privacy. Interestingly, when this has been studied in qualitative analysis of the experience of GMVs participants, very few patients report this as a barrier to participation.[14] The Health Insurance Portability and Accountability Act of 1996 (HIPAA) protects involuntary disclosure of medical information without the written permission of the patient. Many GMV facilitators now ask participants to sign a confidentiality statement at the onset of the GMV, and to date the authors are unaware of challenges to GMVs on the basis of HIPAA.

VARIED LEVELS OF MEDICAL FLUENCY, EDUCATION, AND COGNITION

Patients cared for in public health centers are diverse. The wide variation in health literacy and education, and the prevalence of cognitive dysfunction, make designing an intervention suitable for a group of patients, rather than for an individual, a challenge. There are now ongoing trials of GMV models tailored to the education, language, and health literacy needs of the subpopulations served in public health settings. Nevertheless, when so much of the GMV is spent on group learning and verbal interactions, it is harder to meet the needs of a broadly diverse patient population. To ensure that all participants are as active as possible, it is important to monitor the extent of patient participation and engagement in the GMV. A useful set of measures for cofacilitators to complete after each GMV is presented in Table 12-2. Answering these assessment questions enables the cofacilitators to identify those patients who are less involved and develop a plan to engage them in future GMVs.

COEXISTING PSYCHIATRIC PROBLEMS

Psychiatric comorbidities are more common among those with chronic illness. Among diabetics alone, depression is three times as common as it is in the general population. Most chronic illness groups address psychological problems related to the illness and other psychosocial issues. In some public health settings cognitive-behavioral GMVs are being offered for patients living with chronic illness.

The psychological aspects of pregnancy and parenting also are addressed in most group-based prenatal care and parenting groups.

Common Pitfalls

- Many public health clinics lack a room to accommodate a group of patients.
- Many clinics resist investing staff resources and training required for group facilitation.
- It is difficult to make a business case for group visits because there is conflicting evidence of their cost effectiveness.
- Facilitating a group of individuals with diverse cultural, linguistic, educational, and psychological issues can be particularly challenging.
- There are often concerns about patient confidentiality when initiating group medical visits.
- It is challenging to get patients to engage in care in a group setting.

Table 12-2. Facilitator Self-Evaluation Form

1. How well did you think this group session went today?

1	2	3	4	5	6	7
Not at all		Some		Mostly		Completely

2. Do you think you and your cofacilitator worked well together as a team?

1	2	3	4	5	6	7
Not at all		Some		Mostly		Completely

3. Did you meet your goals and objectives for this group visit?

1	2	3	4	5	6	7
Not at all		Some		Mostly		Completely

4. Were you able to engage group members to participate?

1	2	3	4	5	6	7
Not at all		Some		Mostly		Completely

5. Did patients seem to engage in the group visit (i.e., asked questions, stayed till the end, learned from each other)?

1	2	3	4	5	6	7
Not at all		Some		Mostly		Completely

6. General impressions (i.e., notable events/elements)

_____

_____

7. What problems can you identify that are preventing the group from functioning optimally?

_____

_____

8. What do you need to do before the next session to improve the next group visit?

_____

From: Improving Diabetes Efforts Across Language and Literacy (IDEALL) Project. Group visit facilitators training manual and protocol. San Francisco General Hospital, San Francisco, CA. Available at: www.cmwf.org/tools/tools_show.htm?doc_id=228393

BENEFITS OF GROUP MEDICAL VISITS IN UNDERSERVED POPULATIONS

> Mrs. Chen has few friends or family members who have diabetes, and no close acquaintances who have to use insulin injections. At the first group appointment, she is interested to hear another woman talk about her experience of initiating insulin therapy, and how much better she felt after she had learned to give herself injections and her sugar went down.

Although most of the existing GMV models were developed in managed care settings, more recent applications (i.e., prenatal and well-child GMVs) have proved effective in public health settings (Box 12-2).

SUPPORT GROUP ASPECT

Support groups for patients with chronic illness have been studied in a number of different settings. Group support has been shown to improve patient satisfaction and psychosocial outcomes.[15,16] Moreover, support groups are effective in diverse patient populations. Individuals with chronic illness express satisfaction and show improved self-management practices when they interact with others living with the same condition. There is also the opportunity to discuss psychosocial sequelae of their illness (sexual dysfunction, social isolation, disability, depression, changes in body image), which is less likely to occur in the brief individual visit with a health care provider who has not experienced similar problems and who is not a peer. The simple process of identifying oneself with another individual in the group can have a powerful effect, especially in the setting of isolation and confusion. In addition, GMV participants have a sense of accountability to other members of the group, which may promote positive behavior change and healthy practices.

JUDICIOUS USE OF HEALTH CARE RESOURCES

> Mr. and Mrs. Chen have noticed that their doctor seems increasingly rushed, and the clinic more busy. They usually get about 10 minutes of her time, much of which is spent working through an interpreter, and it often takes months to get a follow-up appointment. Previously, this was not such a problem because Mrs. Chen could always see the Diabetes Nurse Case Manager when she had a diabetes-related problem and could not get into see her doctor. Now, the clinic has no nurse assigned specifically to diabetes care.

GMVs have the potential to lead to more efficient use of limited health care resources. Studies that target high users of health care show decreased hospitalizations and emergency department use after GMV attendance.[1,4,5] Included in the group education provided during chronic illness, prenatal, and well-child group visits are clear guidelines to help patients understand the indications for urgent medical attention. They also include self-management skills to address medical problems before they become urgent. For example, most chronic illness groups employ patient education materials based on "stop signs," color-coded guides for patients with asthma, diabetes, and congestive heart failure. These materials use objective (blood sugar, peak flow) and subjective (nonhealing foot sore, poor response to nebulizer therapy) measures to tell patients when to seek professional attention. Instruction in the use of such tools, as well as guiding parents and pregnant women about when to go to the hospital or emergency room, can be done as easily and perhaps more effectively in a group setting than in individual visits.

LANGUAGE AND LITERACY

> The Chens' primary care provider is a monolingual English speaking family physician. Mrs. Chen relies primarily on her 78-year-old husband, and occasionally a hospital interpreter, to translate all of her medical interactions. Mrs. Chen now finds herself engaged during her group appointments in a way she has not been before because she can understand everything that is being said by the doctor and health educator, and does not need to rely on translation. She also finds that she learns a lot about her diabetes from her peers because they use expressions she understands.

Box 12-2. Advantages of Group-Based Care for Socioeconomically Disadvantaged Patients

- GMVs attempt to address the problems of limited access to physicians and other medical providers.
- GMVs are better designed to minimize barriers of language and literacy.
- GMVs may more effectively promote disease self-management and positive behavior change.

- GMVs provide social support, which may be a significant factor in improving the health status of underserved individuals.

Language barriers and low functional health literacy are associated with poor quality of care for patients with chronic illness.[17,18] Non–English speaking patients have poor access to language-concordant health education materials and health care providers, lower satisfaction with care, lower knowledge of their medication regimen, poor self-management, and worse health status (see Chaps. 10 and 26). In addition, language discordance between primary care providers and patients is associated with poor self-reported interpersonal processes of care.[19] Through GMVs, language concordance can be achieved much more efficiently either through the use of a bilingual cofacilitator or a single interpreter to translate for eight or more patients at one time. Patients with low health literacy report difficulties with many aspects of communication in the health care setting, including worse comprehension of both written and oral communication. Group-based care has the potential to diminish these barriers through tailoring educational approaches to the literacy needs of a group of patients. There is some evidence that when GMVs are tailored to the language and literacy needs of patients, there are significantly higher levels of engagement among traditionally hard-to-reach patients.[20]

SELF-MANAGEMENT TRAINING

> Mrs. Chen always leaves her doctor's appointments with a clear understanding of what medications she should take and what her doctor thinks she should be doing to keep her sugar under control, such as not eating sweets or starches and exercising regularly. She usually keeps those things in mind for the first day or two after the visit, but loses track of them during the months that elapse between appointments.

Problem-focused one-on-one consultations with a clinician, occasionally supplemented by noncontiguous educational sessions with ancillary providers (nurse educators, pharmacists, nutritionists, pharmacists), are the mainstay of traditional ambulatory care. This often is an ineffective and inefficient model for implementing the lifestyle changes so important for management of chronic medical problems. Practitioners have only recently begun to realize that successful chronic illness management relies as much on having an active patient "self-manager" as it does on an "active provider" choosing the right medication or other treatment.[21–23] The traditional practice of imparting medical information and imploring the patient to make significant lifestyle changes is often so clearly in conflict with normal daily living that it is ignored or forgotten. Moreover, traditional health education usually does not take into account cultural or environmental influences on health behaviors.

There is a movement in health education toward a participatory approach to patient education.[24] This involves patient-directed discussion of what is possible, in terms of lifestyle changes, followed by patient-determined goal setting.[21] Ideally, goal setting is done in the context of a continuity relationship with a physician or other health professional so that the discussion of goals for lifestyle change is ongoing and dynamic. By bringing this discussion into the group session, it is enriched by the contributions of others with the same condition. Unfortunately, most doctors are not trained in self-management education or the participatory learning approach; the group setting affords the opportunity to engage health educators and others to participate in the care of a cohort of patients in an ongoing manner.

EXPANDED ROLE OF FAMILY MEMBERS AND OTHER SUPPORT PEOPLE

> Mr. Chen has never fully understood his role in helping his wife live with diabetes. He feels useful when he serves as her translator, but does not feel like he can ask his own questions of the doctor. He enjoys the group visits because there are other family members without diabetes who come to the groups and he has now identified ways to best help his wife, such as supporting her self-management goals and drawing up her insulin syringes.

Usual ambulatory medical practice has little role for close family members in the care of pregnant women or individuals with chronic illness. Except in the case of parents of children with asthma and other chronic disease, spouses and other primary caregivers are rarely actively engaged in treatment plans. GMVs, which in many settings are open to support people of the target patients, provide a unique opportunity to make explicit this role in the course of a medical visit. Most group facilitators encourage the active participation of family members, even engaging them to work on their own health-related goals.

CONCLUSION

> Six months after she started attending the GMVs, Liu Su Chen is using insulin to control her diabetes. She enjoys the social interaction so much that she has joined an exercise group at her neighborhood senior center. She is even considering undergoing training so that she can be a peer leader for a "Living with Chronic Illness" support and education group starting at her church.

Group-based ambulatory care is a feasible and effective alternative to the traditional one-on-one encounter. Participation in GMVs leads to improved clinical outcomes and is also associated with high levels of satisfaction for both patients and providers. In this era of increasingly limited health care resources and providers with less time and more demands constraining their clinical encounters, GMVs are an exciting example of redesigning ambulatory practice to meet the unique needs of diverse patient populations.

KEY CONCEPTS

- Group medical visits are an innovative approach to providing care.
- Many different group medical visit models exist.
- All group medical visit models incorporate health education, self-management, peer support, and medical care.

CORE COMPETENCY
Guidelines for Empowerment-Based Facilitation

When you facilitate, you are balancing the ideas and opinions of the various members so the conversation will flow and the discussion will be productive. Awareness of the following issues and how you address them during your groups will lead to greater patient empowerment.

1. Create a psychologically safe (accepting, uncritical) environment for personal reflection and sharing.
2. Communicate effectively. Clarify ideas within the group to foster dialogue, learning, and decision making.
   - Repeat remarks made by various speakers.
   - Define ambiguous words or ask the group to define them.
   - When it is not necessary for you to answer a question asked, throw it back at the group.
   - Ask participants for suggestions on how the discussion should continue, and present a few ideas based on observations of how the dialogue is progressing.
   - Keep the conversation on track by asking "why" and "how" questions.
   - Summarize the ideas mentioned.
3. Accept your role as a provider, educator, or facilitator, not group therapist. You are there to guide the groups and encourage participants, not to solve every participant's problems.

4. Balance the needs of verbal and reticent group members. Ensure that every participant has an opportunity to speak. Balance the needs of verbal and nonverbal group members by asking open-ended questions.
5. Foster understanding. In spite of disagreements within the group, you must encourage participants to understand (not necessarily agree with) differing points of view; highlight agreements made, and point out differences. This is the only way a productive discussion can take place.
6. Provide an opportunity for significant others and family members to express opinions or concerns.
7. Guide discussions to stay focused on course objective. To increase the exchange of ideas and communication within the group, in addition to personal experiences, suggest other methods of discussion, such as brainstorming, small group–large group discussions, writing, performing, flip chart, or silent reflection. The goal is to increase participants' self-awareness, foster skills such as goal setting, and enable them to plan and carry out self-directed behavior changes.

Adapted from: Arnold MS, et al. Guidelines for facilitating a patient empowerment program. *Diabetes Educ* 1995;21(4): 308–312.

DISCUSSION QUESTIONS

1. Considering what you know about Mrs. Chen and her medical problems, make a list of some possible topics for group discussion for a GMV in which she is enrolled.
2. Describe a patient whom you have encountered who would benefit from group-based care.
3. If Mrs. Chen were your patient, how would you talk to her about the GMVs in such a way to convince her to give it a try?
4. Discuss some of the potential challenges to instituting group-based prenatal care in some of the ambulatory care settings with which you are familiar.
5. Do you think group-based care is a replacement for usual care, or an adjunct? Discuss the circumstances in which you might feel one way or another.

RESOURCES

Action Plan Project of the UCSF Collaborative Research Network: www.action-plans.org

Improving Chronic Illness Care. Group visit starter kit. Available at: www.improvingchroniccare.org/improvement/docs/startkit.doc

Improving Diabetes Efforts Across Language and Literacy (IDEALL) Project. Group visit facilitators training manual and protocol. San Francisco General Hospital, San Francisco, CA. Available at: www.cmwf.org/tools/tools_show.htm?doc_id=228393

Institute for Healthcare Improvement. Continuing care clinic handbook. Available at:www.ihi.org

Lorig K, Holman HR, Sobel D, et al. *Living a healthy life with chronic conditions*, 2nd ed. Palo Alto, CA: Bull Publications, 2000.

REFERENCES

1. Sadur CN, et al. Diabetes management in a health maintenance organization. Efficacy of care management using cluster visits. *Diabetes Care* 1999;22(12):2011–2017.

2. Wagner EH, et al. Chronic care clinics for diabetes in primary care: A system-wide randomized trial. *Diabetes Care* 2001;24(4):695–700.

3. Noffsinger EB. Working smarter: Group visits save time. *Physicians Practice* 2002 Spring.

4. Beck A, et al. A randomized trial of group outpatient visits for chronically ill older HMO members: The Cooperative Health Care Clinic. *J Am Geriatr Soc* 1997; 45(5):543–549.

5. Scott JC, et al. Effectiveness of a group outpatient visit model for chronically ill older health maintenance organization members: A 2-year randomized trial of the cooperative health care clinic. *J Am Geriatr Soc* 2004; 52(9):1463–14670.

6. Noffsinger EB, Scott JC. Understanding today's group visit models. *Group Pract J* 2000;48(2):46–58.

7. Coleman EA, et al. Reducing emergency visits in older adults with chronic illness. A randomized, controlled trial of group visits. *Effect Clin Pract* 2001;4(2):49–57.

8. Novick G. CenteringPregnancy and the current state of prenatal care. *J Midwif Wom Health* 2004;49(5):405–411.

9. Rising SS. Centering pregnancy. An interdisciplinary model of empowerment. *J Nurse Midwifery* 1998;43(1): 46–54.

10. Osborn LM, Woolley FR. Use of groups in well child care. *Pediatrics* 1981;67(5):701–706.

11. Taylor JA, Davis RL, Kemper KJ. Health care utilization and health status in high-risk children randomized to receive group or individual well child care. *Pediatrics* 1997;100(3):E1.

12. Auslander W, et al. A controlled evaluation of staging dietary patterns to reduce the risk of diabetes in African-American women. *Diabetes Care* 2002;25(5):809–814.

13. Brown SA, et al. Culturally competent diabetes self-management education for Mexican Americans: The Starr County border health initiative. *Diabetes Care* 2002;25(2):259–268.

14. Miller D, et al. Group medical visits for low-income women with chronic disease: A feasibility study. *J Womens Health (Larchmont)* 2004;13(2):217–225.

15. Lorig KR, et al. Chronic disease self-management program: 2-year health status and health care utilization outcomes. *Med Care* 2001;39(11):1217–1223.

16. Messmer Uccelli M, et al. Peer support groups in multiple sclerosis: Current effectiveness and future directions. *Multiple Sclerosis* 2004;10(1):80–84.

17. Bierman AS, Clancy CM. Health disparities among older women: Identifying opportunities to improve quality of care and functional health outcomes. *J Am Med Womens Assoc* 2001;56(4):155–159, 188.

18. Schillinger D, et al. Association of health literacy with diabetes outcomes. *JAMA* 2002;288(4):475–482.

19. Fernandez A, et al. Physician language ability and cultural competence. An exploratory study of communication with Spanish-speaking patients. *J Gen Intern Med* 2004;19(2):167–174.

20. Schillinger D, et al. Can disease management interventions engage hard-to-reach patients in primary care? *J Gen Intern Med* 2004;19(Suppl):103.

21. Bodenheimer T, et al. Patient self-management of chronic disease in primary care. *JAMA* 2002;288(19): 2469–2475.

22. Norris SL, Engelgau MM, Narayan KM. Effectiveness of self-management training in type 2 diabetes: A systematic review of randomized controlled trials. *Diabetes Care* 2001;24(3):561–587.

23. Thoonen BP, et al. Self-management of asthma in general practice, asthma control and quality of life: A randomised controlled trial. *Thorax* 2003;58(1):30–36.

24. Roter DL, Stashefsky-Margalit R, Rudd R. Current perspectives on patient education in the US. *Patient Educ Couns* 2001;44(1):79–86.

25. Arnold MS, et al. Guidelines for facilitating a patient empowerment program. *Diabetes Educ* 1995;21(4):308–312.

Chapter 13

Applying Interactive Health Technologies for Vulnerable Populations

John D. Piette, PhD, and Dean Schillinger, MD

Objectives

- Describe the rationale for using interactive health technologies (IHTs) as an adjunct to the care of socioeconomically vulnerable patients.

- Review potential uses of IHTs in chronic illness care.

- Review the evidence for the effectiveness of IHTs in chronic illness care.

- Describe the characteristics of patients best suited to use IHTs as part of their care.

- Review the use of IHT as a method of improving communication between providers of health care (inpatient and outpatient; community and health system).

Jason, a patient with active human immunodeficiency virus (HIV) disease and occasional cocaine use, has difficulty adhering to the multipill HIV regimen. He enrolled in a novel web-based program in which he was equipped with a text pager that reminded him when and how to take his medications and prompted him to enter simple adherence data. If he did not respond or reported poor adherence, his case manager attempted to connect with him either in person or by phone. Several months after enrollment in the program, his viral load dropped to the undetectable level.

Innovative methods to educate patients and providers, promote adherence, and enhance communication both between patients and providers and among providers across different settings have become available through the growth of computer-based technologies. Interactive web-based programs that help count calories, assess risk of disease, remind patients to take medications, or assist them by promoting more informed decision making are a few examples of how these technologies are being adapted to improve patient care. Innovations such as these may indeed have the greatest impact on improving the care of vulnerable patients, for whom the greatest barriers to effective care often exist.

Access to the Internet is becoming commonplace. However, use of interactive health technologies (IHTs) in the care of socioeconomically vulnerable patients has been limited. Many low-income patients lack computers in their home; or when computers are available, patients may not have the consistent, reliable access to the Internet that some IHT communication platforms require, or they may have low-speed (e.g., "dial-up") access that makes web-based graphics, audio, and video frustrating.

In addition, socioeconomically vulnerable patients often have limited health literacy,[1] limited English proficiency, or other communication challenges that serve as formidable barriers to the use of most standard Internet-based IHT services. Consequently, these patients may have difficulty accessing "off-the-shelf" IHTs, even when those technologies have proved beneficial for other patient groups. Despite these potential barriers, safety net health systems striving to improve treatment access and quality can use IHTs successfully if careful attention is given to how those services are designed.

This chapter discusses those principles relevant to IHT use for most types of patient care. However, the focus is primarily on the use of IHTs to promote more effective communication and disease management among patients with chronic health problems, such as diabetes, heart failure, or depression. These patients represent the majority of visits and uncompensated health care costs within safety net heath systems. Such patients often lack the resources required to manage their condition successfully, and access barriers significantly add to the difficulty of meeting the demands of their illness. Rather than focus on specific types of IHT technology, the chapter focuses on concepts that are relevant for most currently available (and soon-to-be-developed) technologic platforms. E-mail, automated telephone calls, clinic-based multimedia supports, and even the Internet can address many gaps in care.

THE FUNCTIONS OF INTERACTIVE HEALTH TECHNOLOGIES IN CHRONIC ILLNESS CARE

In general, IHTs can assist patients by enhancing their ability to communicate effectively with others who may help them manage their chronic conditions. Despite the obvious importance of clinician-patient communication, health care providers often are unaware of patients' self-management goals[2] or the financial pressures they struggle with because of their treatment.[3,4] In addition to financial access barriers; geographic distance, language barriers, long waiting times, and restrictive work schedules all conspire to make typical face-to-face communication within outpatient settings especially difficult for socioeconomically vulnerable patients.[5] Some chronically ill patients may need weekly or even daily support for their self-care; however, such demands strain even the most effective care management systems and are impossible to meet by most safety net providers. Despite their limitations, IHTs may be ideally suited to redress the difficulties faced by safety net health care systems and the patients they serve.

Many IHT-based disease management interventions (particularly those developed in the early 1990s) attempted to address multiple self-management problems simultaneously. Earlier enthusiasts of these new technologies often operated based on the expectation that (because they were so novel and exciting) technology-based interventions *per se* would have a therapeutic benefit, and therefore that careful consideration of intervention goals was less important. However, like all clinical services, IHT-based services are most effective when they are designed with specific, targeted goals in mind. For chronically ill patients treated in safety net health systems, IHTs may be used to address the following needs: (a) assisting patients with administrative tasks (e.g., remembering when follow-up visits are scheduled); (b) ongoing patient monitoring and surveillance to identify health and behavioral problems; (c) delivering patient education or other information to assist in disease self-management; or (d) facilitating informal support (e.g., peer support) for coping with illness.

USING INTERACTIVE HEALTH TECHNOLOGIES TO SUPPORT ADMINISTRATIVE PROCESSES OF CARE

Ms. Sepulveda, a 53-year-old uninsured Spanish-speaking woman has diabetes and hypertension, with persistently elevated hemoglobin A1cs and blood pressure. As a participant in a program that uses an automated telephone outreach system, she responds that she is not checking her blood sugar and not taking one of her blood pressure medications. Her prescriptions for a glucometer and a new blood pressure medication had been denied at the pharmacy and she does not have a follow-up appointment with her primary care provider. She has lost her job and her health insurance and thinks that she could no longer receive care. A glucometer and supplies are obtained via the hospital pharmacy, the prescription for the new blood pressure medication is changed to a medication on the hospital formulary, and she is given appointments with her primary care provider, a diabetes educator, and the ophthalmologist.

Chronically ill patients face a daunting task when managing their health problems: handling numerous medications, coordinating repeated visits to different clinicians, and navigating the continually changing requirements for insurance or benefits. Even those with insurance can be financially strained by the costs of treatments and medications. Studies indicate that chronically ill patients have difficulty meeting these administrative challenges, particularly if they have little education or limited English proficiency. Patients often miss scheduled appointments, and no-show rates are often highest among individuals with the greatest need for clinical care.[6] In a recent study, more than one-third of diabetes patients with either no health insurance or Medicaid coverage reported forgoing prescription drug use in the prior year because of cost concerns, despite the fact that those patients were almost universally eligible for first-dollar medication coverage through state and regional financial assistance programs.[4]

IHTs can assist patients managing the complexity of their formal health care use as well as their self-care. Automated reminder calls delivered via an "interactive voice response" (IVR) telephone system to patients undergoing medication treatment for tuberculosis increased visit attendance rates relative to controls.[7] Even though patients were not aware that IVR reminders would be coming to their homes, the calls were effective for patients with a variety of primary languages, including Mandarin, Vietnamese, Tagalog, and Spanish. Other studies have found that automated reminders can increase attendance rates for routine vaccinations[8] and can assist patients in taking their medications as prescribed.[9] Importantly, "low-tech" alternatives to automated telephone calls also improve attendance rates,[10] but that IVR reminders are cost effective even in the context of these more labor-intensive alternatives. The technology used to deliver IVR reminders is relatively simple and inexpensive, and the research in this area is sufficiently definitive that safety net providers should consider incorporating such reminders into usual outpatient care. Other forms of IHTs, such as e-mail[11] or text messaging to cell phones, may be effective in assisting vulnerable patients with the administrative functions of their disease management. However, the reach of these interventions will almost certainly be less than systems requiring only that patients have access to standard telephones.[12]

USING INTERACTIVE HEALTH TECHNOLOGIES FOR ONGOING PATIENT MONITORING

> Mr. Yu, a 65-year-old Cantonese speaking man with diabetes is a participant in a diabetes program that uses an automated telephone outreach system. His response triggers a nurse callback about a foot problem, and he describes blisters on his right foot. He had recently increased his walking in shoes that no longer fit well. Mr Yu had continued to walk despite the discomfort because "his doctor told him how important walking was for controlling diabetes." The nurse scheduled Mr. Yu to see the podiatrist to reassess shoe fit, and he was fully evaluated and given new shoes within 3 weeks.

Most patient monitoring occurs during face-to-face outpatient visits. Few health systems have the information systems needed to trigger a comprehensive assessment when patients seek care through different entry points (e.g., an emergency department), and many patients have difficulty keeping scheduled office visits.[13] Consequently, chronic disease treatment plans often reflect patients' historical problems more than their current needs, opportunities to prevent health crises are missed, and educational efforts lack the timeliness needed to be effective.

IHTs can assist clinicians in gathering up-to-date information about patients' health status and behavioral needs. For example, low-income diabetes patients can and will complete brief IVR assessments of their glucose self-monitoring values and self-management behaviors.[14,15] IVR data appear reliable even when reported by individuals with psychiatric disorders.[16] Such assessments can accurately triage patients into groups with high-, medium-, and low-risk for adverse outcomes.

Careful consideration must be given to the ways in which health systems respond to IVR-reported this information. Clinic-based "case finding" or screening with feedback to providers can have little impact on patient outcomes,[17,18] often because providers have limited ability to change practice patterns or because treatment changes are not tightly linked with health outcomes. Providers who are pressed for time or treat patients with multiple urgent complaints often lack the resources required to follow-up effectively on serious, but chronic patient needs (e.g., dysthymia, functional limitations, or self-management problems). Moreover, IHT-based patient monitoring with limited clinical specificity may generate unnecessary outpatient visits, straining scarce resources in public clinics and indirectly denying access to other patients with acute health concerns. *Given the state of the science in IHT patient monitoring, safety net providers should carefully consider the frequency and content of IHT assessments, and the implications of both erroneously identifying patients as having serious health problems versus missing problems because of "false-negative"assessment reports.*

USING INTERACTIVE HEALTH TECHNOLOGIES FOR PATIENT EDUCATION AND SELF-MANAGEMENT SUPPORT

> Mrs. Miller is a 78-year-old widow who lives alone and only rarely attends her appointments. She has never followed through with referrals for diabetes education. As a participant in a program that uses an automated telephone outreach system she responds that she is drinking cranberry juice and sodas daily. She is not aware that this makes her diabetes control more difficult. After receiving tailored health education messages from the phone system, and a reinforcing phone discussion with the nurse about the importance of trying to avoid sugary foods and drinks, Mrs. Miller makes a behavioral action plan and begins diluting her juice with water, and drinking diet soda. Her diabetes control improves.

Patients with chronic illnesses require enormous amounts of health information that change with the disease course. Unfortunately, providers infrequently engage in the types of communication behaviors that are associated with greater patient retention and understanding,[19] and many are unaware of their patients' self-management goals.[2] When patients face language barriers or health literacy deficits, many lack even rudimentary information about their disease or its self-care.[20]

IHTs can provide patients with the information they need at a time when they are best able to assimilate it. Unlike written patient education material, IHTs such as web-based patient education resources can be multimodal (i.e., including graphics, video, and audio) and provide information at a pace that is comfortable for users.[21] Importantly, the information provided by IHTs can be tailored to patients' unique sociodemographic, clinical, and psychological characteristics; and studies show that such tailoring can be important in prompting behavior changes.[22] For example, diabetes patients are interested in receiving health education via IHT,[23] and non–English speakers treated in public clinics may be especially interested in accessing IVR health education with practical information or inspiring messages about self-management, such as how to cope with medication side-effects and cook healthy meals.[24]

Most patients remember only a small proportion of the educational messages provided during typical outpatient encounters.[25] *Given that many patients spend a significant amount of time waiting to be seen by clinicians, safety net health systems should consider making interactive educational kiosks available within outpatient settings.* Models for such services are available,[26] and research shows that they can assist patients in identifying self-management goals and barriers, and ultimately improving their self-care. In the context of busy primary care practices,[27] such services can address patients' need for self-management education without adding tasks to the schedules of primary care providers.

USING INTERACTIVE HEALTH TECHNOLOGIES TO FACILITATE INFORMAL SUPPORT

Safety net health systems are often poorly positioned to address patients' need for assistance in coping emotionally with their illness, and mental health insurance benefits are typically inadequate to meet patients' need for counseling. Chronic illness can present an enormous drain on patients' emotional resources. Depression is common among patients with diseases such as diabetes and heart failure,[28,29] and patients with comorbid psychiatric problems often have worse outcomes[30,31] and

increased rates of service use. Many socioeconomically vulnerable patients lack effective social support, and low social support is a risk factor for poor self-care and increased morbidity and mortality.[32,33]

Patients who provide support to others may achieve health benefits themselves; for example, less depression,[34] heightened self-esteem and self-efficacy,[35] improved quality of life (even after adjusting for potential confounders),[36] improved health behaviors,[37] decreased mortality risk,[38,39] and improved health outcomes and function.[40,41] Peer support (i.e., support between individuals living with the same illness or self-management challenges) can be especially effective in reducing problematic health behaviors[42,43] and mental health symptoms.[44] Most models of providing chronic disease peer support require patients to attend frequent outpatient visits. Given the constraints on safety net providers and their patients, these intervention models often are unrealistic. Unfortunately, studies evaluating IHT-facilitated opportunities for peer support have shown mixed results.[45,46] Importantly, IHT-facilitated informal support services are feasible; however, there is currently little evidence for or against these interventions' impact on patients' self-management or health outcomes.

Common Pitfalls in Using Interactive Health Technologies

- Poorly supported IHT programs can lead to increased resource use devoted to clinically insignificant problems.
- IHTs are no panacea: They cannot eradicate all barriers to care.
- IHTs that address simple problems, such as reminders, monitoring, and self-management information, may be the most effective.
- Not all patients benefit from IHT interventions. Some do not need additional support; others are not successfully targeted.
- To be effective for marginalized patients, such as the homeless or severely mentally ill, IHTs require special adaptations and require personalized professional interpersonal support.
- Developing an IHT without active involvement of the end users (both patients and providers) is unlikely to work.
- IHTs that do not involve interactions with clinicians and are not integrated into primary care have limited benefit and actually may lead to confusion.
- IHTs are an adjunct, not a replacement or alternative, to personalized care.

THE CHARACTERISTICS OF PATIENTS WHO CAN BENEFIT FROM INTERACTIVE HEALTH TECHNOLOGIES

Patients with a variety of sociodemographic and clinical characteristics, including those with limited functional health literacy or English proficiency,[23] can and will use IHT as part of their usual outpatient care. In fact, among patients with poorly controlled diabetes, those with limited functional health literacy or English proficiency were *more* likely than those with adequate health literacy and English speakers to engage with the system (Fig. 13-1). Consequently, if designed with the end-users in mind, IVR and other IHTs may have the greatest uptake among patients with communication barriers.

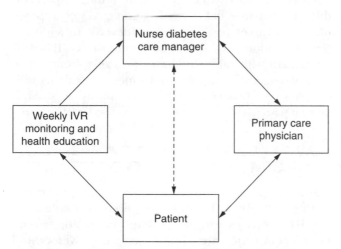

Figure 13-1. The Interactive Voice Response (IVR) System of the IDEALL Project. With extensive input from patients, the authors designed an IVR system sensitive to the literacy and language requirements of the target population. Each week, patients receive a rotating set of questions about diabetes self-care, psychosocial aspects of diabetes care, as well as receipt of preventive services. Patients who answer out of range on an item (based on predetermined thresholds) receive an immediate automated health education message in the form of a narrative to encourage them to reflect on their self-care behavior and consider setting goals and developing an action plan around self-care. Patients who answer out of range also receive a call back from a bilingual nurse care manager to encourage them to set goals and develop an action plan to improve their overall health. The nurse care manager is trained to perform motivational interviewing, assess and overcome barriers to successful diabetes care and health communication, and suggest changes in medical management. Guided by a clinical protocol, the care manager communicates with patients' primary care physicians to implement such changes. The IDEALL Project system is designed in such a way as to promote the efficiency of the nurse care manager by having her only perform those outreach phone calls to patients who, by virtue of their responses to the system, report a need for further support. The IDEALL system requires about 10 minutes to complete per week, and runs for 39 weeks (9 months).

Nevertheless, the potential benefits of these technologies probably are not equally distributed across patients. Many patients, including some treated in safety net health systems, already have the resources they need to manage their illness effectively. As a result, they may receive little additional benefit from the types of support (e.g., reminders, ongoing monitoring, patient education, and informal support) that are possible through IHT.[47,48] At the opposite extreme, some patients treated by safety net providers lack the basic necessities that would be essential to take advantage of the support available through IHT. In particular, patients with serious psychiatric disorders, unstable residences, or inconsistent telephone access may not benefit from the types of services even the most creative IHTs can provide.

Safety net providers should carefully consider which patients could benefit from IHT-based self management supports. Often, patients with the poorest health status (e.g., diabetes patients with the worst glycemic control or heart failure patients with repeated acute exacerbations) are targeted for these additional services; however, these may not be the patients who can benefit the most. Rather IHTs may be of greatest benefit to patients who fall between the two extremes of adequate self-management support and intractable social or psychiatric need; that is, the large number of patients who simply need additional reminders, monitoring, self-management information, and other services that they cannot access through usual outpatient sources of care.

LINKING INTERACTIVE HEALTH TECHNOLOGIES WITH USUAL PROCESSES OF CARE

Studies suggest that the outcomes of IHT services are proportional to the extent that they support "live" clinician resources and are integrated with usual processes of outpatient care (Fig. 13-2). When IHT programs are not linked to clinical responses, improvement in knowledge and perceived social support may occur, but only slight benefit in the more important realms of self-efficacy, health behavior, or health outcomes can be demonstrated.[49] In addition, IHTs that are closely linked with patients' usual outpatient services are used more consistently over time and may improve important outcomes such as cholesterol levels,

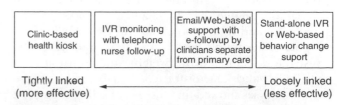

Figure 13-2. Relationship between IHT linkage to patients' usual clinical care and evidence of intervention effectiveness.

symptom burden, and rates of preventable hospitalizations. Furthermore, having a centralized, guideline-driven system for out-of-range IHT responses, for example, through a nurse care manager may ensure more consistent and effective treatment plans.

"STAND-ALONE" INTERACTIVE HEALTH TECHNOLOGY INTERVENTIONS

In general, interventions designed to operate as stand-alone services (i.e., interventions that are completely automated, with no follow-up by clinicians), often are seen by patients as superfluous and are used with decreasing frequency over time.[50] For example, Pinto and colleagues developed a call-in IVR program to assist patients with increasing their physical activity levels.[51] Although the recorded messages were tailored and based on sound health behavior change theory, the investigators found that as many as one in four study participants never called the toll-free number to receive behavior-change messages, and fewer than half were using the system after 3 months. Not surprisingly, the intervention had no significant impact on patients' behavior.

INTERACTIVE HEALTH TECHNOLOGY INTERVENTIONS WITH WEAK LINKS TO CLINICIAN FOLLOW-UP

IHT-delivered interventions with weak linkage between clinicians and patients' usual care yield modest intervention outcomes.[52–54] Even with elaborately structured web sites and multiple opportunities for e-counseling, there are often no discernible differences among the interventions and control groups.[52] In addition, patient log-ons progressively decreased over time. In two important studies,[53,54] patients were randomized to either a basic Internet educational program focused on weight management or to an enhanced "e-counseling" condition. The enhanced condition consisted of a theoretically based series of e-mail counseling sessions by a behavioral therapist, in which patients' progress toward behavioral goals was monitored and they received regular feedback. The e-counseling patients had no face-to-face or telephone contact with their counselor, nor did counselors consult with patients' other health care providers. The first study found that the e-counseling group lost more weight and had a greater change in waist circumference than the standard Internet education group, and more participants in e-counseling met the goal of 5% weight loss.[53,54] In the second trial,[54] the investigators evaluated overweight adults with at least one additional risk factor for type 2 diabetes. Intention-to-treat analyses showed that the e-counseling group lost more weight, had greater decreases in percentage of initial body weight, and had a greater reduction in waist circumference. In both studies, patients' log-ons were consistently greater in the group receiving e-counseling than in the group receiving standard Internet services; however, log-ons decreased precipitously over time in both studies regardless of experimental condition.[50]

INTERACTIVE HEALTH TECHNOLOGY INTERVENTIONS TIGHTLY LINKED WITH CLINICIAN FOLLOW-UP

IHT services most closely identified with patients' outpatient primary care can improve behavioral and health outcomes. For example, rigorous randomized trials have investigated clinic based behavioral assessments delivered via a multimedia kiosk in order to identify barriers to self-management and structure behavioral interactions between patients and their clinicians.[26,48] Such systems have shown consistent, lasting impacts on difficult-to-change behaviors (e.g., diet) as well as physiologic outcomes (e.g., cholesterol levels). In addition, several randomized trials have demonstrated that IVR assessment with rapid follow-up by a telephone nurse care manager can improve outcomes for patients with diabetes or hypertension[47,55–57] or improve survival among patients with advanced congestive heart failure.[45]

HOW SHOULD SAFETY NET PROVIDERS DELIVER INTERACTIVE HEALTH TECHNOLOGY SERVICES?

Numerous private companies produce generic versions of the hardware and software required for implementing IHT services within a safety net health system. Other companies are clinical service providers and offer IHT-supported care management services by charging health systems on a per-patient-per-month basis or other capitated model. The choice of whether to provide IHT services "in-house" or through a contracted service agency is important, and both options have their advantages.

One advantage of in-house IHT delivery is that the health care organization can have more control over the intervention process and content. For example, in-house IHTs provide greater opportunity to add or remove patients from lists of individuals receiving the service, modify the patient messages, or design and change clinician reports. One issue to explore when considering outsourced IHT supports is that making changes in patients' communication protocol could be more difficult and costly because of distance barriers and the company's financial incentives.

A disadvantage of in-house IHT is that the responsibility for managing the technical aspects of the system falls on the health care organization. Most IHT systems require the use of specialized programming languages and equipment; health systems need to consider whether they have the resources to fund this infrastructure over time. Although it is not clear whether in-house or subcontracted IHT is less costly in the long term, equipment purchase for in-house IHT may represent a significant initial investment, whereas subcontracted costs can be more constant and predictable.

An important issue to address when using subcontracted IHT services is that these services may complicate care coordination, especially if the vendor includes its own set of educators and others who will provide some follow-up when a patient problem is identified. Those clinicians often do not have access to patients' medical records and could make inappropriate changes to treatment plans if clear lines of communication are not established. Without clear protocols for information exchange, even appropriate advice or medication adjustments by outside staff may not be communicated to patients' primary care team or documented in patients' charts. Because many patients receive care from multiple providers, clear and consistent lines of communication between IHT services and others involved in patients' care are critical so that patients do not become confused as to where they should turn for help when they have a clinical or technical problem using the IHT system.

EVALUATING INTERACTIVE HEALTH TECHNOLOGIES

IHTs can improve the disease management and health outcomes for patients treated by safety net providers, assuming careful thought is given to the intervention's function, the patients and clinicians it is designed to serve, and how it relates to patients' usual care. Evaluations of new IHT services should reflect the intervention's goals. For example, an intervention designed to increase rates of ophthalmologic examinations among patients with diabetes may not save an organization money in the short term, and decision makers should be clear about desired evaluation criteria up front. As described in previous sections, IHT interventions can play multiple roles in chronic illness care; it may be difficult to implement an intervention that addresses all of these goals simultaneously. Priorities should be set to select the optimal role of the system in the context of other available services.

Traditionally, the gold standard for determining the potential benefits of novel services such as IHTs has been evaluation within the context of a tightly controlled randomized trial. However, many services that have proved efficacious in a research context have shown disappointing results in more "real-world" settings or have not been translated into services that can benefit patients in typical outpatient practices. As a consequence, policy makers and clinicians have begun to conceptualize program evaluation more broadly, including a range of program characteristics in addition to efficacy in randomized trials. The RE-AIM (Reach, Efficacy, Adoption, Implementation, and Maintenance) framework is one tool for

evaluating IHTs. This framework suggests that these services (particularly clinic-based multimedia educational systems and IVR) may be useful despite only modest impacts on patient outcomes, because of their low marginal cost, ease of use, and ready availability to patients facing access barriers.[12] Safety net providers may find that IHTs can benefit their patients by using perspectives such as that provided by RE-AIM.

CONCLUSION

New IHT applications are continually developing along with the constantly changing backdrop of devices used by chronically ill patients to communicate with one another and their clinicians. As traditional health care resources evolve, IHTs may be able to fill the gaps that arise in care within safety net health systems because of cuts in funding or decreases in the number of available clinicians. With careful attention to how IHT services address longstanding clinical challenges, these tools may alleviate some of the stresses on safety net clinicians and provide the support for patients between outpatient visits that is crucial to effective self-management and often impossible to deliver through traditional practice models.

KEY CONCEPTS

- IHTs can serve four goals in chronic illness care:
  - —Assisting patients with administrative tasks
  - —Providing ongoing patient monitoring
  - —Delivering patient education and supporting self-management
  - —Facilitating informal support
- Carefully consider the goals an IHT service is addressing.
- Interactive voice response (IVR) systems are simple and inexpensive tools that should be considered by safety net providers.
- If carefully designed with input from end users, IHTs have great potential to alleviate some of the barriers experienced by vulnerable populations (e.g., social isolation, poor access, communication barriers).
- Patients can provide reliable information via IHT between outpatient encounters.
- Interactive educational kiosks used in outpatient settings can assist patients in self-management and behavior change efforts.
- IHT-facilitated informal (peer) support services are feasible, but their impact on patients' self-management or health outcomes is not known.
- IHT is most effective when closely linked with usual outpatient care.

CORE COMPETENCY

Interactive Health Technologies: Assessing Your Practice Setting and Clinical Challenges

> Could an interactive health technology help?
>
> - Define a problem that you would like to address
> - What traditional methods have you employed to address the problem?
> - Why have these approaches failed or only partially succeeded?
> - What types of IHT technologies do you think might help address the problem?
> - What are clinician attitudes toward integrating IHT applications?
> - What are the characteristics of patients and which adaptations might your IHT need to have the greatest reach and effectiveness?
>
> Review "off-the-shelf" programs
>
> - Will they work for your setting and your patients?
> - Can you adapt them to suit your needs?
> - Do they allow for integration with clinic personnel and workflow?
> - Do you have resources and staff to support the IHT or develop and implement your own?

DISCUSSION QUESTIONS

1. IHT services (e.g., regular IVR assessment calls) may identify important health or self-management problems between outpatient visits. However, such systems also may provide ambiguous clinical data that require additional follow-up by clinicians. Given that most safety net health systems are already burdened with pressing patient care problems, what are the benefits and costs of "trolling" for additional problems via IHTs? For what types of patients and health problems may IHT monitoring be most useful?

2. Should public health systems develop web-based educational supports for their patients, even though not all patients could use them? How should clinicians and administrators assess such services, so that scarce resources are used effectively without investing excessive time and money in evaluating intervention effects?

3. Clinicians need accurate and timely information to make decisions, but IHTs can add enormous amounts of data (e.g., guidelines, clinician reminders, patient functional status information) to the process of care. How much information is too much? How should clinicians and health systems decide what IHT information is helpful in patient care and what is simply a distraction?

4. Should safety net health systems develop the infrastructure for delivering IHT services "in-house" or contract such services with an outside vendor?

RESOURCES

For information on evaluating IHT's within the RE-AIM framework, see: http://www.RE-AIM.org

For information regarding the IDEALL Project at San Francisco General Hospital, see: http://www.cmwf.org

For information on the use of telephone care in chronic disease management, see: http://www.chcf.org/topics/chronicdisease/index.cfm

REFERENCES

1. Ad Hoc Committee on Health Literacy for the Council on Scientific Affairs. Health literacy: Report of the Council on Scientific Affairs. *JAMA* 1999;281(6):552–557.

2. Heisler M, et al. When do patients and their physicians agree on diabetes treatment goals and strategies, and what difference does it make? *J Gen Intern Med* 2003; 18(11):893–902.

3. Alexander GC, Casalino LP, Meltzer DO. Patient-physician communication about out-of-pocket costs. *JAMA* 2003; 290(7):953–958.

4. Piette JD, et al. Health insurance status, cost-related medication underuse, and outcomes among diabetes patients in three systems of care. *Med Care* 2004;42(2):102–109.

5. Smedley BD, Stith AY, Nelson AR, eds. *Unequal treatment: Confronting racial and ethnic disparities in health care: A report of the Institute of Medicine.* Washington, DC: National Academy Press, 2002.

6. Karter AJ, et al. Missed appointments and poor glycemic control: An opportunity to identify high-risk diabetic patients. *Med Care* 2004;42(2):110–115.

7. Tanke ED, Leirer VO. Automated telephone reminders in tuberculosis care. *Med Care* 1994;32(4):380–389.

8. Stehr-Green PA, et al. Evaluation of telephoned computer-generated reminders to improve immunization coverage at inner-city clinics. *Public Health Rep* 1993;108(4): 426–430.

9. Leirer VO, et al. Elders' nonadherence: Its assessment and medication reminding by voice mail. *Gerontologist* 1991;31(4):514–520.

10. Lieu TA, et al. Effectiveness and cost-effectiveness of letters, automated telephone messages, or both for underimmunized children in a health maintenance organization. *Pediatrics* 1998;101(4):E3.

11. Moyer CA, et al. Bridging the electronic divide: Patient and provider perspectives on e-mail communication in primary care. *Am J Manag Care* 2002;8(5):427–433.

12. Glasgow RE, et al. Interactive behavior change technology. A partial solution to the competing demands of primary care. *Am J Prev Med* 2004;27(2 Suppl):80–87.

13. Moore CG, Wilson-Witherspoon P, Probst JC. Time and money: Effects of no-shows at a family practice residency clinic. *Fam Med* 2001;33(7):522–527.

14. Piette JD, et al. Use of automated telephone disease management calls in an ethnically diverse sample of low-income patients with diabetes. *Diabetes Care* 1999; 22(8):1302–1309.

15. Piette JD, Weinberger M, McPhee SJ. The effect of automated calls with telephone nurse follow-up on patient-centered outcomes of diabetes care: A randomized, controlled trial. *Med Care* 2000;38(2):218–230.

16. Kobak KA, et al. Computerized screening for psychiatric disorders in an outpatient community mental health clinic. *Psychiatr Serv* 1997;48(8):1048–1057.

17. Rubenstein LV, et al. Improving patient function: A randomized trial of functional disability screening. *Ann Intern Med* 1989;111(10):836–842.

18. Reiber GE, et al. Diabetes quality improvement in Department of Veterans Affairs Ambulatory Care Clinics: A group-randomized clinical trial. *Diabetes Care* 2004;27 (Suppl 2):B61–68.

19. Schillinger D, et al. Closing the loop: Physician communication with diabetic patients who have low health literacy. *Arch Intern Med* 2003;163(1):83–90.

20. Williams MV, et al. Relationship of functional health literacy to patients' knowledge of their chronic disease. A study of patients with hypertension and diabetes. *Arch Intern Med* 1998;158(2):166–172.

21. Street RL, Gold WR, Manning T. *Health promotion and interactive technology: Theoretical applications and future directions.* Mahwah, NJ: Lawrence Erlbaum Associates, 1997.

22. Kreuter MW, Strecher VJ, Glassman B. One size does not fit all: The case for tailoring print materials. *Ann Behav Med* 1999;21(4):276–283.

23. Piette JD Patient education via automated calls: A study of English and Spanish speakers with diabetes. *Am J Prev Med* 1999;17(2):138–141.

24. Zrebiec JF, Jacobson AM. What attracts patients with diabetes to an internet support group? A 21-month longitudinal website study. *Diabet Med* 2001;18(2):154–158.

25. Rost K, Carter W, Inui T. Introduction of information during the initial medical visit: Consequences for patient follow-through with physician recommendations for medication. *Soc Sci Med* 1989;28(4):315–321.

26. Glasgow RE, Toobert DJ, Hampson SE. Effects of a brief office-based intervention to facilitate diabetes dietary self-management. *Diabetes Care* 1996;19(8):835–842.

27. Stange KC, Woolf SH, Gjeltema K. One minute for prevention: The power of leveraging to fulfill the promise of health behavior counseling. *Am J Prev Med* 2002;22(4):320–323.

28. Piette JD, Richardson C, Valenstein M. Addressing the needs of patients with multiple chronic illnesses: The case of diabetes and depression. *Am J Manag Care* 2004; 10(2 Pt 2):152–162.

29. Guck TP, et al. Depression and congestive heart failure. *Congest Heart Fail* 2003;9(3):163–169.

30. Lustman PJ, et al. Depression and poor glycemic control: A meta-analytic review of the literature. *Diabetes Care* 2000;23(7):934–942.

31. Rumsfeld JS, et al. Depressive symptoms are the strongest predictors of short-term declines in health status in patients with heart failure. *J Am Coll Cardiol* 2003; 42(10):1811–1817.

32. House JS, Landis KR, Umberson D. Social relationships and health. *Science* 1988;241(4865):540–545.

33. Glasgow RE, Toobert DJ. Social environment and regimen adherence among type II diabetic patients. *Diabetes Care* 1988;11(5):377–386.

34. Musick MA, Wilson J. Volunteering and depression: The role of psychological and social resources in different age groups. *Soc Sci Med* 2003;56(2):259–269.

35. Wheeler JA, Gorey KM, Greenblatt B. The beneficial effects of volunteering for older volunteers and the people they serve: A meta-analysis. *Int J Aging Hum Dev* 1998;47(1):69–79.

36. West DA, Kellner R, Moore-West M. The effects of loneliness: A review of the literature. *Compr Psychiatry* 1986;27(4):351–363.

37. Schwartz CE, Sendor M. Helping others helps oneself: Response shift effects in peer support. *Soc Sci Med* 1999;48(11):1563–1575.

38. Musick MA, Herzog AR, House JS. Volunteering and mortality among older adults: Findings from a national sample. *J Gerontol B Psychol Sci Soc Sci* 1999;54(3):S173–180.

39. Brown SL, et al. Providing social support may be more beneficial than receiving it: Results from a prospective study of mortality. *Psychol Sci* 2003;14(4):320–327.

40. Van Willigen M. Differential benefits of volunteering across the life course. *J Gerontol B Psychol Soc Sci* 2000;55(5):S308–318.

41. Davis C, et al. Benefits to volunteers in a community-based health promotion and chronic illness self-management program for the elderly. *J Gerontol Nurs* 1998;24(10):16–23.

42. Arnstein P, et al. From chronic pain patient to peer: Benefits and risks of volunteering. *Pain Manag Nurs* 2002;3(3):94–103.

43. Keyserling TC, et al. A randomized trial of an intervention to improve self-care behaviors of African-American women with type 2 diabetes: Impact on physical activity. *Diabetes Care* 2002;25(9):1576–1583.

44. Winzelberg AJ, et al. Evaluation of an internet support group for women with primary breast cancer. *Cancer* 2003;97(5):1164–1173.

45. Goldberg LR, et al. Randomized trial of a daily electronic home monitoring system in patients with advanced heart failure: The Weight Monitoring in Heart Failure (WHARF) trial. *Am Heart J* 2003;146(4):705–712.

46. Lorig KR, et al. Can a back pain e-mail discussion group improve health status and lower health care costs? A randomized study. *Arch Intern Med* 2002;162(7):792–796.

47. Piette JD, et al. Impact of automated calls with nurse follow-up on diabetes treatment outcomes in a Department of Veterans Affairs Health Care System: A randomized controlled trial. *Diabetes Care* 2001; 24(2):202–208.

48. Glasgow RE, Toobert DJ. Brief, computer-assisted diabetes dietary self-management counseling: Effects on behavior, physiologic outcomes, and quality of life. *Med Care* 2000;38(11):1062–1073.

49. Murray E, et al. Interactive health communication applications for people with chronic disease. *Cochrane Database Syst Rev,* 20044:CD004274.

50. Piette JD. *Using interactive health technologies to support diabetes self-care.* Hauppauge, NY: Nova Science Publishers, 2005.

51. Piette JD, et al. Do automated calls with nurse follow-up improve self-care and glycemic control among vulnerable patients with diabetes? *Am J Med* 2000;108(1):20–27.

52. McKay HG, et al. The diabetes network internet-based physical activity intervention: A randomized pilot study. *Diabetes Care* 2001;24(8):1328–1334.

53. Tate DF, Wing RR, Winett RA. Using Internet technology to deliver a behavioral weight loss program. *JAMA* 2001;285(9):1172–1177.

54. Tate DF, Jackvony EH, Wing RR. Effects of Internet behavioral counseling on weight loss in adults at risk for type 2 diabetes: A randomized trial. *JAMA* 2003; 289(14): 1833–1836.

55. Piette JD. Interactive voice response systems in the diagnosis and management of chronic disease. *Am J Manag Care* 2000;6(7):817–827.

56. Pinto BM, et al. Effects of a computer-based, telephone-counseling system on physical activity. *Am J Prev Med* 2002;23(2):113–120.

57. Friedman RH, et al. A telecommunications system for monitoring and counseling patients with hypertension. Impact on medication adherence and blood pressure control. *Am J Hypertens* 1996;9(4 Pt 1):285–292.

Chapter 14

Applying Principles and Practice of Quality Improvement to Better Care for the Underserved

Gordon D. Schiff, MD, and Seijeoung Kim, RN, PhD

Objectives

- Illustrate the structure–process–outcome paradigm, and demonstrate how it is relevant to quality measurement and improvement in community clinics.

- Review six key activity areas in which quality improvement can be applied by health care institutions to deliver better services for the medically underserved population.

- Describe five quality tools that have become staples in the toolkit of modern quality professionals.

- Articulate dilemmas of designing services and programs to optimize improvement and patient safety culture.

- Summarize factors that will inspire readers to incorporate quality improvement activities into their daily practice, as well as to become quality leaders in their organizations.

You have just completed your first week working at a neighborhood health center serving underserved populations. You are struck by the overwhelming nature of the problems patients bring to the clinic. Many have no telephones, are homeless, cannot afford bus fare to the clinic, are using illegal drugs, or speak little English. In addition to the patients' troubles, the clinic itself has problems. There is not enough staff to answer phones; patients wait months for appointments and hours in the waiting room; medical records and laboratory results are often missing; patients rarely see the same provider twice; medications often are not available, and medication mix-ups are frequent. Worse yet, both patients and staff seem resigned to these conditions.

What can be done about this? How can quality health care be provided within these constraints? How can these problems help in understanding underlying health care system issues and openings for improvement?

This chapter outlines approaches to improving quality. It introduces the structure–process–outcome framework, and then discusses six areas of quality-enhancing activities (Fig. 14-1). It uses these to introduce ideas from the quality improvement literature and practice that are particularly relevant to the care of vulnerable populations. Finally, it describes modern tools that help accomplish these activities.

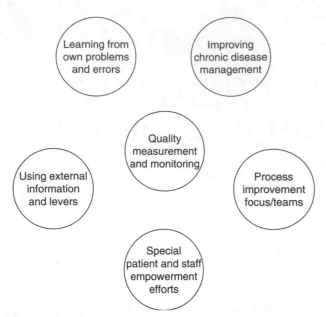

Figure 14-1. Quality improvement activity areas.

MEASURING AND IMPROVING QUALITY

Think back to the excitement and challenge of when you first began learning your field: the thrill of figuring out the structure and function of a human anatomical body part or organ; the tremendous satisfaction you felt in actually helping a patient by treating an infection with an antibiotic, or reducing the risk of future suffering by helping a patient change his or her diet or stop smoking. Just as clinical medicine is based on understanding anatomy, physiology (or pathophysiology), human behavior, and evidence-based treatment outcomes or effectiveness, caring for the ailing health care institutions and systems is based on a science of quality improvement. However, while clinical medicine traditionally helps patients one at a time, quality improvement activities touch the entire community of patients by re-engineering encounters delivered by the clinician.

STRUCTURE–PROCESS–OUTCOME TRIAD MODEL

One of the most useful ways to understand and ultimately improve health care quality is the simple but powerful *structure–process–outcome* triad model formulated by Avedis Donabedian.[1]

To assess the quality of a community clinic, for example, one might examine indicators of quality related to its *structure*. Does it have the material (building, equipment), human, and organizational requisites in place to deliver safe, high-quality care? The second element of Donabedian's triad considers the degree to which the clinic *processes* conform to high-quality practices. Do women receive regular mammograms? Is the HbA1c of diabetic patients being checked? The third way to make inferences about quality is through health *outcomes,* changes in health that can reasonably be attributed to the clinic's health services. What is the mortality or stroke rate for hypertensive patients? What percentage of diabetic patients have drug reactions or require admission to the hospital?

There is considerable debate about which types of quality indicators are the most important and useful.[2] Some combination is needed to provide a complete picture. Some argue that outcomes are the bottom line, and are therefore all that really matter. Others insist that fair comparisons of outcomes require very complex adjustments for case-mix differences.[3,4] Others argue that when you "adjust for" race and socioeconomic status, you are thereby "adjusting away" inadequacies in health care and socioeconomic and/or racial disparities in quality.[5,6]

Process measures can avoid many of these dilemmas. However, the validity of a process measure depends on the evidence linking a particular practice to improved outcomes. One special advantage of process measures is that they are better than outcomes at directing what to do when rates are suboptimal, and can offer insight as to where to target corrective efforts. Hence, although outcome measures may indicate that patients' stroke mortality rates are high, process data on rates of increasing antihypertensive medications when blood pressure exceeds target levels, for example, might actually suggest how to change practice to reduce this mortality rate (see Core Competency).

QUALITY ACTIVITY #1: MEASUREMENT FOR LEARNING AND CHANGE

How can these seemingly abstract quality concepts help to examine and improve the clinic? Just as collecting subjective (symptoms) and objective (physical examination and laboratory) data is the key to clinical assessment and interventions for the ailing patient, assessing quality measures is also a key tool for quality improvement.

In a clinical environment, the following five perspectives should guide quality measurement.

1. *Quality measures are not fundamentally about technique or statistics.* Rather, they are about deciding what is important—important to the clinic's mission and direction, and important to the clinic's patients. Deciding whether, how, and what to measure is a reflection of an organization's commitment to accountability and learning.[7]

Accountability implies a willingness to expose the effectiveness of one's practices to scrutiny (internal or external), and to hear from a variety of one's customers (i.e., staff, patients, the community, and regulatory agencies) about problems, successes, and areas for improvement. Having in-depth knowledge of these "customers" allows one to identify appropriate target needs. Organizations that are unwilling or unable to honestly analyze their practices inevitably will be less accountable and learn less than an organization with a culture that is supportive of data-driven decentralized self-examination, in which claims about services or service improvement can be objectively and openly scrutinized and implemented.

2. *Measurement is the secret to innovation.* Measurement allows clinicians and quality improvement practitioners to experiment with new approaches and learn from successes and failures. The literature and the clinic itself (suggestions from staff, patients, and quality improvement teams) are full of good *change ideas*—promising ideas that are worth assessing and testing locally to determine whether they lead to sustainable improvement. These local tests of process changes should be based on validated statistical methods such as statistical process control (discussed below).[8] Rather than implementing full-scale changes that may or may not be improvements, measurement allows one to test changes in care delivery on a smaller scale.

3. To the greatest extent possible, *data collection should be integrated into the daily workflow* rather than as an added (and usually retrospective) task. Capturing data in real time is more efficient, timely, credible, and empowering. Examples of real-time data that are increasingly automatically recorded and available are laboratory and pharmacy data that can be relatively easily downloaded, and even linked together.

4. *Front line staff should be maximally involved in data collection decisions,* and should be responsible for recording the data as well. Electronic tools make this self-monitoring approach easier and more powerful. As clinics become more computerized, capturing data in real time will occur more automatically. A fundamental issue in implementing such participatory and automated data collection systems is how the data will be used. Will they be used in a threatening way as surveillance to judge practitioners? Or instead will they be used as a tool to better understand how the clinic works, and how its day-to-day processes can be improved (Box 14-1)?[9]

5. Although cross-sectional data, collected at a single point in time, can be useful, *modern quality improvement practice is based on repeated looks.* By collecting a series of data points over time, a clinical site can determine whether a process is stable and whether it is getting better or worse, particularly in response to interventions. Such time series data are plotted on *statistical process control* charts (Fig. 14-2).By looking at how the data points behave, the chart can help pinpoint where to target interventions. It can identify where the problems are more likely fixable by system redesign (*common cause* variations) versus those that are likely the result of a particular event or person's practice (*special cause* variations).

Figure 14-3 illustrates how the common cause variation changes in response to systemwide process interventions. For example, if trying to improve patient waiting time, the first change might be redesign of practitioners' schedules; the second change a new registration system, and so on. The merits of this type of study design are increasingly being recognized by medical journals.[10]

Box 14-1. Measurement for Judgment and Punishment versus Learning and Improvement

You have just collected and analyzed patient satisfaction data on your clinic's 30 primary care physicians. The data were obtained from questionnaires from a sample of 600 patients (20 patients from each physician) asking about the care patients received from their physicians. The results show a normal distribution of scores, with some physicians with extremely high ratings and others falling on the lower end of the curve.

The same day you get these results, a growing budget shortfall comes to a crisis. As a medical director, you are informed that a 10% cut in the physician budget is necessary. Which physicians should you let go?

The obvious answer (and the one most often chosen when this case is presented as a quality exercise) is to select the three outlier doctors with the lowest quality scores. Using the data in this way, however, is not a wise answer.

As explained by Dr. Brent James, a quality leader at LDS Hospital who presented this true case example: If you use this questionnaire as a punitive judgment tool rather than for feedback and learning, you destroy its value. By using the data to keep score and judge the practitioners, you have made the doctors defensive instead of receptive to data that can show ways to better serve their patients. Although the manager might wish otherwise, this tool should not be used for this purpose.[9]

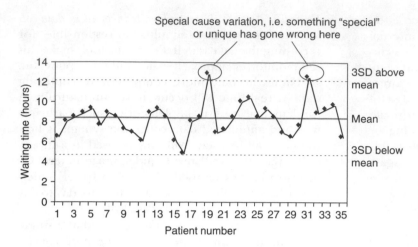

Special cause variation, i.e. something "special"
or unique has gone wrong here

Figure 14-2. Signs of special cause variation (Adapted from Statistical Process Control. Rachel Harvey, NHS Modernisation Agency, at: http://www.modern.nhs.uk/esc/8237/SPC_General_RH.ppt

QUALITY ACTIVITY #2: WHERE QUALITY FALLS SHORT: LEARNING FROM PROBLEMS AND ERROR

The Institute of Medicine has published two historic monographs grappling with the problem of health care quality. The first report, *To Err Is Human,*[11] focused on the problem of medical errors—mistakes that must be eliminated or minimized if there is to be safer health care. The report created a flurry of attention and debate around its controversial calculation of 48,000 to 98,000 annual deaths from errors. Although it received less attention, the report's most important contribution was a series of error prevention recommendations. Box 14-2 summarizes these principles and recommendations. They convey lessons from leading international safety experts, and capture what can be learned from studying errors.

A second IOM report, *Crossing the Quality Chasm,*[12] examines ways that health care quality fails more broadly. The IOM defines six key attributes of good quality care (safe, effective, patient centered, timely, efficient, equitable) and documents the myriad ways the US health system falls short in meeting these aims,

including tens of thousands of deaths and untold suffering from poor quality each year.

Although the data from these two reports may perversely reassure one that your clinic is not the only place where there are quality problems, it should also challenge you to commit yourself to overcoming the needless suffering and waste of resources associated with poor quality.

Learning from Your Institution's Problems

Health care organizations can learn from self-investigation of adverse events, and by establishing non-punitive mechanisms to ensure that this is an ongoing and systematic process. The reporting of problems should be welcomed. They should be routinely and reliably followed up without reflex denial, defensiveness, prejudice, or preconceived conclusions. Sometimes learning from near-miss events can be even more rewarding than investigating those resulting in more serious adverse outcomes, because they are less personally or legally threatening.

A good problem-reporting and tracking system directs multiple streams of data through preestablished channels. Such a system can integrate information from such disparate sources as malpractice allegations, staff

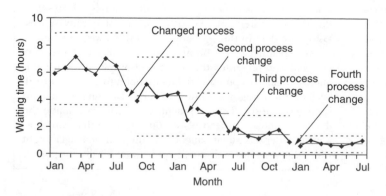

Figure 14-3. Changing the process. Adapted from Statistical Process Control. Rachel Harvey, NHS Modernisation Agency, at: http://www.modern.nhs.uk/esc/8237/SPC_General_RH.ppt

---

Box 14-2. Creating Safety Systems in Health Care Organizations

Creating Safety Systems in Health Care Organizations

Principle 1. Provide leadership

Principle 2. Redesign processes to respect human limits

Principle 3. Promote effective teamwork

Principle 4. Anticipate the unexpected

Principle 5. Create a learning environment

See chapter 8 of *To Err is Human*, at www.iom.edu/CMS/8089/5575.aspx, for details on these five principles.

From: Institute of Medicine. *To err is human: Building a safer health system.* Washington, DC: National Academy Press, 1999.

---

and patient complaints, day-to-day crises, morbidity and mortality conferences, regulatory body citations, and problems identified from formal quality assurance studies. Many problems can be investigated and solved in real-time by troubleshooting efforts of front line staff and administrators.

Key features of reporting systems include: (a) problem reporting, (b) logging, (c) tracking, (d) investigation, (e) prioritization, (f) corrective action, (g) dissemination and sharing of findings, and (h) cumulative learning. These elements can and should vary from organization to organization and from incident to incident. The development of knowledge and processes that are useful locally is a key element of all successful quality improvement.

Having an organized system is imperative. The data should be computerized, in a database format that facilitates ease of entry and upkeep, cross-referencing similar types of events (using some method for coding entries), and protecting confidentiality of the patient as well as (where appropriate) employees and the institution.

Building and Reinforcing a Culture of Reporting and Improvement

A nurse pages a physician, but the doctor fails to answer. She expresses her continuing frustrations with "those doctors." Another nurse, wondering why the call was not returned, double checks and finds that the wrong pager number is listed in the clinic directory. The second nurse even goes the extra mile to call the phone operator's supervisor to make sure the erroneous number is corrected. The doctor, who for weeks rarely answered his pages, starts regularly returning calls.

This common story is not about a more caring versus a more "careless" nurse. Nor is it about an irresponsible doctor who failed to ensure that the clinic had his or her correct pager number. Rather, it raises larger issues about the characteristics of the system, posed as questions rather than answers:

1. What organizational factors can nurture (or discourage) the troubleshooting behaviors displayed by the nurse who tracked down the problem?
2. Why did two nurses on the same unit react so differently to the doctor's failure to return the page?
3. What methods might the organization deploy to learn from the cumulative experience of hundreds of similar problems and responses percolating throughout its hospital or clinic?
4. What do *you* do when you uncover problems in your own organization? Do you follow-up with troubleshooting and reporting? Why or why not?

QUALITY ACTIVITY #3: IMPROVING CHRONIC DISEASE MANAGEMENT

Chronic diseases account for 70% of all deaths, 75% of health care costs, and more than one-third of all years of potential life lost before the age of 65. Yet, according to a recent RAND survey of quality-of-care process measures for more than 13,000 people, barely half received recommended care, with failing quality scores for a variety of chronic diseases.[13]

Effectively caring for chronic diseases requires a shift in emphasis from acute episodic care by physicians, to more long-term self-management by patients and their families. A redesigned superstructure to support this new type of care delivery has been advocated by practitioners such as Ed Wagner at Group Health in Seattle, and is discussed in detail in Chapter 36.[14,15]

QUALITY ACTIVITY #4: PATIENT AND STAFF EMPOWERMENT EFFORTS

A prejudicial marketplace mentality says that people get what they pay for, and that indigent patients need to make do with less. Quality suffers to the extent that such lowered expectations become internalized by both patients and staff of community clinics. In order to provide high-quality, respectful, and efficient care, both the material and mental expressions of this inequitable model must be overcome.[16,17]

Users and staff must feel and build a sense of pride and ownership in their clinic. Quality is a key factor in motivating community support; in turn, community support is critical for mobilizing resources needed for high-quality care. This mutually reinforcing dynamic operates at multiple levels, including the broader political level (advocacy for adequate funding), and accountability for individual patient-care encounters.

Only a respected clinic staff can provide respectful patient treatment. Each employee should be empowered to function as a leader. This requires: (a) employees to have a voice in decision making, (b) transparency of decision-making processes, (c) processes that genuinely encourage staff involvement, (d) employees seeing real change based on their input, and (e) a nonpunitive culture where mistakes provide opportunities for learning, not blame.

Health services for vulnerable populations also need to account for the myriad barriers to access that this population faces. Transportation difficulties, financial hurdles, complexities in the registration and scheduling process, fear of crime, substance abuse, unemployment, childcare issues, and lack of telephones all require services to be thoughtfully designed to facilitate rather than inhibit access to care. Once at the clinic, other issues arise, including communication issues related to language, cultural diversity, and varying educational and literacy levels.

Every effort possible should be made to eliminate waste. The fact that demand far outstrips supply for public health services obliges efforts to optimize human resource deployment. Quality experts estimate that 40% or more of the activities of even the best-run health care institutions currently represent waste, including overly complex processes, wasted human talents, and duplicated efforts. Staff and patients should be mobilized in this campaign, with job security as a prerequisite, so that employees do not risk being fired when they root out wasteful activities in their own work.

Tap into the creativity and experience of community members; they have already shown resilience in the face of adversity.[18] Involving community members in improving clinic operations can help the clinic work well and strengthen the community.

QUALITY ACTIVITY #5: PROCESS IMPROVEMENT FOCUS/TEAMS

Kaizen is the word Japanese industrial quality experts use to describe a work environment infused with a spirit of continuous improvement. By seeking ways to improve each step in the production process, Japanese auto manufacturers in the 1980s were able to produce cars that were 10,000 times less likely than US-made cars to have defects, yet were produced at a lower cost.[13] This paradigm can help point to ways to eliminate waste and improve quality.

The old model of assuming that things go wrong because of staff inadequacies or incompetence should be replaced by a new philosophy, based on the assumption that people are generally working quite hard but are handicapped by barriers that impede more optimal clinic functioning. Leaders of successful organizations understand that the aim of sustaining and improving the clinic is achieved only through ongoing efforts, little by little, day by day, that continuously refine work processes.

Efforts to improve work processes have revealed that quality most often falters in the hand-offs. There are many opportunities for fumbled hand-offs in health care: for example, information passing from inpatient to outpatient providers, pharmacists misreading a handwritten prescription, or patients stacked up at clinic registration while their providers wait inside for their first patient. Rather than trying to improve quality in isolation, different areas need to work across departmental boundaries to reengineer or better coordinate the way they work together.

QUALITY ACTIVITY #6: LEVERAGING EXTERNAL INFORMATION AND AGENCIES

Quality practitioners inside institutions can take advantage of two effective outside forces to leverage change and growth. The first, *environmental awareness* refers to keeping abreast of the myriad ongoing quality activities, published studies, reports, and new ideas presented at conferences in the quality field. One must reject the natural aversion to borrowing others' ideas. Staying up-to-date with relevant new research findings can help an organization translate research into practice more quickly than the current average delay of 7 to 10 years.[20]

The second external quality stimulus, which we have deliberately left for last, is *leveraging accrediting and regulatory demands*. In many practitioners' minds, quality assurance is synonymous with perfunctory compliance with mindless requirements whose sole purpose is to pass annual inspections. Nothing could be further from the truth, but the widespread belief helps create a self-fulfilling prophecy. Quality policy experts are adept at using accreditation inspections to their advantage, as many of these regulatory demands are congruent with desired internal improvement goals.[21] These regulatory functions can help infuse new resources, provide a wake-up call to complacent leadership, give more visibility to the day-to-day quality work already in place, and interject a better understanding of many important prerequisites for organizing and improving care.

SPINNING WHEELS OR ENGAGED MECHANISMS

If there were activity in each of the six quality areas, but with each working in isolation, there would be a lot of wheel-spinning (Fig. 14-1), but little real progress. A series of support tools are needed to serve as "connecting links" to get the overall program "in gear" (Fig. 14-4).

1. *Information technology.* Computerized ordering of drugs and laboratory results, clinical decision support (i.e., electronic care guidance and alerts), and electronic health records to streamline clinical documentation can record information and guide care in powerful ways.
2. *Communication and coordination.* Frequent and ongoing organization-wide communication on quality issues and initiatives, including solicitation of staff feedback, is essential for effective improvement action plans.
3. *Just-in-time processes.* "We'll get to this when we can." "We need to prioritize what is most urgent." "Poor people just have to wait—they have plenty of time anyway." These oft-heard adages are not only disrespectful of people's time, but they are also counterproductive. There are huge efficiencies to doing today's work today, rather than batching and postponing work.
4. *Quality improvement design tools.* Using four simple tools, quality practitioners can illustrate data and processes in powerful and helpful ways. These tools include: (a) control charts (discussed earlier) to help plot whether a problem is improving and differentiate special causes from random variation; (b) Pareto diagrams, which are bar graphs (histograms) drawn to display the most important problems in descending order; (c) process flow diagrams to illustrate the steps in a work process, useful for identifying overly complex or weak spots that could be simplified or improved; and (d) cause and effect ("fishbone") diagrams, which categorize causes of quality problems and display them as branching spines resembling the backbone of a fish.[22]
5. *Leadership and support.* The organization's leaders must provide sufficient resources and support, and must set the tone for a nonpunitive and committed culture through personal example.

Common Pitfalls in Quality Improvement

- *Blaming individual practitioners* rather than trying to understand deeper causes of quality problems that arise.
- Focusing on *short-term fixes* for quality problems, instead of creating long-term sustainable changes.
- Relying on *anecdotes* and *subjective impressions* rather than objective measures of quality to indicate extent, causes, and progress. Conversely, spending *excessive time on data collection,* rather than implementing real changes.
- Working on *problems in isolation* from each other, rather than connecting common threads that tie together multiple problems.

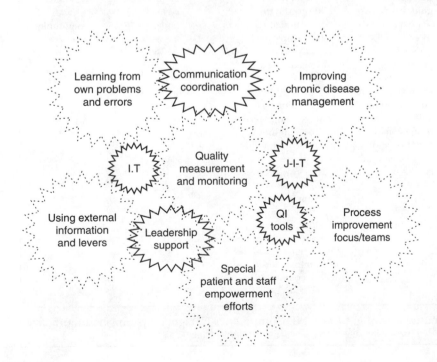

Figure 14-4. Shown are the six quality improvement activity areas and the tools that can get them "in gear" by connecting and driving them.

- *Failing to fully involve* all members of the health care team, thereby overlooking the potential of harnessing the imagination and participation of the entire community of staff and patients.

CONCLUSION

In the tension between the status quo and a changed future, quality improvement is not neutral.[23] Further, improvement is on the side of the patient, with little tolerance for complacency for poor and inefficient care. Endeavors in each of the six quality activity areas have great potential to make a difference in community clinics because such clinics are well-endowed with caring, committed staff, and an unambiguous mission to care for the neediest. Thus, in contrast to the despair of student's initial impressions, progressive change is not only possible, but is likely to have enormous impacts on patients, staff, and the community.

KEY CONCEPTS

- Many problems are very amenable to simple but systematic approaches for improvement using modern quality theory, practices, and tools.
- A profound and useful approach to quality improvement is the *structure–process–outcome* triad, which classifies aspects and measures of quality.
- Improvement comes from measuring and testing changes. This is best done by testing small-scale interventions, taking the opportunity to learn from things that go wrong, and paying special attention to day-to-day front-line experiences.
- To ensure a sustainable improvement program, efforts need to be linked across departments with leadership support and high leverage tools.

CORE COMPETENCY
Improving Quality Through Process Improvement

Measurement and Accountability*	Reduce Errors: Learn from Local Experience*	Develop Chronic Disease Management*,†	Create Systems for Change: Empower Patients and Staff†	Collaborate†	Assure Accountability: Leverage Information and Agencies†
Know your "customers": patients, staff, community, regulatory agencies	Use local examples/solve local problems	System redesign to support chronic rather than acute care	Understand your health care system	Focus on teamwork and collaborate	Keep abreast of quality field, research
Identify need based on knowledge	Create nonpunitive environment that encourages reporting errors	Provider support through guidelines etc	Build sense of ownership of clinic in patients and staff at all levels	Invest team members in cycle of improvement	Leverage regulatory demands
Be accountable: Honestly evaluate practice through measurement	Have process including problem:	Disease registries to manage populations of patients	Respectful treatment of all staff members	Work within and across systems	Work with community resources
Measurement to describe problems	• Reporting	Support patient self-management	Give employees a voice	Work across disciplines	
Use measures to show improvement	• Logging	Care teams using allied health professionals	Transparent decision-making process		
Make small steps and build on them	• Tracking	Integration and use of community resources	Encourage staff involvement in decisions		
Make measurement easy and integrated	• Investigation		Make changes based on staff input		
Involve everyone in process	• Make priorities for change		Create nonpunitive culture		
Measure for improvement not punitive judgment	• Make corrective changes		Recognize barriers for patients— transportation, registration, fear, lack of housing, money, telephones, language abilities		
Commit to continuous cycle of measure–change– measure	• Disseminate knowledge		Eliminate waste		
	• Reinforce culture change of problem solving rather than punishment		Tap community resources		

*=ACGME Competency Catagory: Practice-based learning; †= ACGME Competency Catagory: Systems-based practice.
Link above through information technology, communication and coordination, timeliness, QI tools, leadership and support.

DISCUSSION QUESTIONS

1. Where and how do you start? How do you decide what to measure, what the priority areas should be?
2. How do you involve people when institutional culture is one of workers feeling alienated from their jobs? How do you get staff to take responsibility without blaming them for things that go wrong?
3. How can you make efforts and programs sustainable, particularly in the face of severely constrained resources?
4. Is this really medicine? Do we have time for it? Or should we leave all this to the administrators and the regulators to worry about, while we clinicians concentrate on being better doctors, nurses, social workers, or pharmacists?

RESOURCES

AHRQ. Measuring Health Care Quality; Improving Safety: http://www.ahcpr.gov/qual/measurix.htm;http://psnet.ahrq.gov/

Institute for Healthcare Improvement. http://www.ihi.org/ihi

Institute of Medicine (IOM). IOM Quality Chasm Initiative: http://www.iom.edu/report.asp?id=5432

National Academy Press. To Err Is Human: Building a Safer Health System:www.iom.edu/view.asp?id=5575

Joint Commission on Accreditation of Health care Organizations (JCAHO). JCAHO Performance Measures in Health Care: http://www.jcaho.org/pms/index.htm

National Health Service (NHS). An Organisation with a Memory http://www.dh.gov.uk/PublicationsAndStatistics/Publications/PublicationsPolicyAndGuidance/PublicationsPolicyAndGuidanceArticle/fs/en?CONTENT_ID=4065083&chk=PARoiF

REFERENCES

1. Donabedian A. *An introduction to quality assurance in health care.* New York: Oxford University Press, 2003.
2. Brook R, McGlynn E, Shekelle P. Defining and measuring quality of care: A perspective from US researchers. *Int J Quality Health Care* 2000;12:281–295.
3. Liu CF, Sales AE, Sharp ND, et al. Case-mix adjusting performance measures in a veteran population: Pharmacy- and diagnosis-based approaches. *Health Serv Res* 2003; 38(5):1319–1337.
4. Denvir MA, Lee AJ, Rysdale J, et al. Comparing performance between coronary intervention centres requires detailed case-mix adjusted analysis. *J Public Health* 2004; 26(2):177–184.
5. Fiscella K, Franks P, Gold M, et al. Inequality in quality: Addressing socioeconomic, racial, and ethnic disparities in health care. JAMA 2000;283:2579–2584.
6. Sehgal AR. Impact of quality improvement efforts on race and sex disparities in hemodialysis. *JAMA* 2003;289:996–1000.
7. Betancourt J, Green A, Carrillo JE. Cultural competence in health care: Emerging frameworks and practical approaches. *Commonwealth Fund* 2002;576.
8. Mohammed MA. Using statistical process control to improve the quality of health care. *Qual Saf Health Care* 2004;13:243–245.
9. James B. Patient safety reporting systems and applications. In: *Patient safety: Setting a new standard for care.* Washington, DC: National Academy Press, 2003: 265–268.
10. Doherty JA, Reichley RM, Noirot LA, et al. Monitoring pharmacy expert system performance using statistical process control methodology. *Annu Symp Proc AMIA Symp* 2003;205–209.
11. Institute of Medicine. *To err is human: Building a safer health system.* Washington, DC: National Academy Press, 1999.
12. Institute of Medicine. *Crossing the quality chasm: A new health system for the 21st century.* Washington, DC: National Academy Press, 2001.
13. McGlynn EA, Asch SM, Adams J, et al. The quality of health care delivered to adults in the United States. *N Engl J Med* 2003;348(26):2635–2645.
14. Wagner EH, Glasgow RE, Davis C, et al. Quality improvement in chronic illness care: A collaborative approach. *Jt Comm J Qual Improv* 2001;27:63–80.
15. Bodenheimer T, Wagner EH, Grumbach K. Improving primary care for patients with chronic illness. *JAMA* 2002;288:1775–1779.
16. Schiff G, Bindman A, Brennan T. A better-quality alternative. Single-payer national health system reform. Physicians for a National Health Program Quality of Care Working Group. *JAMA* 2004;272:803–808.
17. Schiff G, Fegan C. Community health centers and the underserved: Eliminating disparities or increasing despair (editorial). *J Public Health Pol* 2003;24:307–311.
18. Berwick DM. Lessons from developing nations on improving health care. *BMJ* 2004;328:1124–1129.
19. Berwick D, Kabcenell A, Nolan T. No Toyota yet, but a start. A cadre of providers seeks to transform an inefficient industry—before it's too late. *Modern Health Care* 2005;35(5):18–19.
20. Agency for Health Care Research and Quality (March 2001). Translating Research into Practice (TRIP)-II. Fact sheet. Rockville, MD, AHRQ Publication No. 01-P017 http://www.ahrq.gov/research/trip2fac.htm
21. Joint Commission Ambulatory Care Standards Cross Walk to PCER Module II Clinical. JCAHO page. Accessed January 27, 2005. Available at: http://jcaho.org/accredited+organizations/ambulatory+care/specialized+programs/bphc_xwalk_01.pdf
22. Warmer J. Seven basic tools of quality: Applying statistical process control to education. Accessed January 27, 2005. Available at: http://www.grand-blanc.k12.mi.us/qip/sevenhelpfulcharts.htm
23. Geiger J. A health center in Mississippi: A case study in social medicine. In: Corey L, Saltman S, Epstein M, eds. *Medicine in a changing society.* Saint Louis: CV Mosby, 1972:157–167.

Chapter 15

Case Management/ Multidisciplinary Care Models

Michelle Schneidermann, MD, and Alicia Fernandez, MD

Objectives

- Review the limitations of "one-on-one" model of care for socially complex, ill patients.
- Define case management.
- Discuss the evolution of case management.
- Identify the primary functions of case management.
- Review different approaches to case management.
- Articulate the pros and cons of interdisciplinary case management teams.
- Review specific examples of current case management programs.

Patients who are poor and suffer from chronic diseases face multiple obstacles to effective health care, beginning with limited access to health services.[1] Even when health services for the poor are readily available, poor patients face multiple barriers to effective care.[2] Homelessness,[3,4] low literacy,[5,6] social isolation,[7-9] language barriers,[10-12] addiction,[13-15] and mental illness[16,17] can thwart effective treatment. Ineffective health care results in excess morbidity and mortality and in the endemic overuse of expensive services, such as acute hospitalization[18,19] and emergency department care.[20,21] As the urban poor are disproportionately from ethnic minority backgrounds, this ineffective health care contributes to the widely noted racial and ethnic disparities in chronic disease outcomes.[22]

Innovations in health care delivery, such as case management programs, have the potential to improve outcomes by helping patients overcome social and health system barriers to effective care.[23] This chapter discusses case management, stressing the potential of these programs to complement primary care services and improve the effectiveness of medical care.

FAILING CURRENT CARE

Mr. Beltran is a 56-year-old Guatemalan man who immigrates to the United States to find work. He works as a day laborer but is unable to find a steady job. Living in homeless shelters, he becomes increasingly depressed, and begins to drink heavily. After visiting the emergency room and being diagnosed with diabetes, he is referred to the resident clinic at the county hospital. Here he intermittently sees multiple physicians who adjust medications that are rarely filled, order laboratory tests that are rarely drawn, and write "lost to follow-up" over and over in the chart. The clinic nurse refers him to a Spanish-speaking social worker; she is unable to obtain benefits for him because he lacks immigration papers.

After 10 years of intermittent outpatient care, Mr. Beltran is hospitalized many times with recurrent episodes of diabetic ketoacidosis, chronic diarrhea, pancreatitis, chronic pain, and bladder obstruction requiring an indwelling Foley catheter.

After each hospitalization, he is discharged to the streets with follow-up in the resident clinic. Living on the streets with an indwelling catheter, chronic diarrhea, uncontrolled diabetes, and little access to food, water, and sanitation, Mr. Beltran is admitted to the ICU with urosepsis.

Mr. Beltran's story raises many questions. Why is he requiring frequent hospitalizations and becoming more ill despite access to primary care? What could his primary care physician do to increase the effectiveness of the medical care Mr. Beltran is receiving? What could case management offer him that the current system does not?

Conventional medical care often consists of short appointments, spaced months apart with a primary care clinician who must address multiple problems. This model works well for many people. However, for some poor people with chronic disease—certainly for those who suffer from mental illness or drug addiction—this model is fraught with challenges for patient and clinician alike.

A study of use of acute hospital services in a public hospital in San Francisco found that a subgroup of patients accounted for a larger proportion of admissions.[24] When the clinical and demographic characteristics of "high users" (patients with three or more admissions in a year), were compared to patients admitted once or twice in a year, it became clear that "high users" constitute a distinct clinical group. The most striking finding of this study was that 13% to 15% of patients accounted for close to 40% of admissions and hospital bed-days. These "high users" had a distinctive clinical profile: 77% had at least one of four chronic diseases (HIV, diabetes, COPD/asthma, or congestive heart failure); and approximately 70% suffered from concurrent alcoholism or drug addiction. In addition, approximately 15% had a psychotic illness (usually schizophrenia) and approximately 20% to 30% were homeless at the time of their last admission. These "high users" also had a distinctive pattern of health services use. Rather than avoiding primary care or specialty services, as might be hypothesized, these patients had very high rates of contact with the health care system. Their mean number of primary care visits a year was higher than that of non–high users (8.69 versus 6.13). Yet despite their high level of contact with primary care, few of the patients were getting comprehensive services: less than 20% of addicts received treatment and about half of all patients with psychotic illness received psychiatric care. In response to the high-intensity yet ineffective care described by the study, in 1995, the San Francisco Department of Public Health created a case management program for high users of emergency department services, and in 2001 an intensive case management program for high users of acute hospital services.[24]

Common Pitfalls in Delivering Quality Care to Socially Complex, Medically Ill Patients

- Lack of integration of medical, psychiatric, and addiction services constitutes a barrier to care for patients and threatens effective treatment of any kind.
- Social services are either unavailable or operate independently from medical care, leading to gaps and redundancy in care.
- Competing patient priorities (the search for food, housing, and safety) interfere with accessing medical care.
- Mental illness and/or substance use interfere with patients' abilities to follow through on treatments and appointments.
- Lack of transportation may limit patients' ability to follow-up.
- Patients often lack the social support necessary for effective self-care.
- Overcoming language differences between patient and provider may prove too cumbersome for both patient and providers.
- Real or perceived cultural biases may impede effective alliances between patients and providers.
- Patients who lack access to sanitation and hygiene are often embarrassed to seek care.
- Providers are overwhelmed by the patient's complex social situation and doubt that effective treatment is possible.

WHAT IS CASE MANAGEMENT?

Case management evolved out of two very distinct challenges to health care. The deinstitutionalization of severely mentally ill patients in the 1960s and 1970s with the closing of mental health facilities led to the development of multidisciplinary community-based programs to provide a full range of services, from housing to psychiatric care for these patients. In an unrelated trend, during the 1980s, attempts to control health care costs led insurance plans and hospitals to develop nurse-run programs for both managing and monitoring the provision of services. Common to programs developed both for the mentally ill and by insurance programs were services that coordinated and monitored care. Today case management is defined loosely as a service that coordinates and organizes care. The goals of this coordination may range from cost containment to assuring appropriate care or a combination of the two. The monitoring and coordination of care in case management programs commonly focuses on patients with a specific diagnosis or those who require extensive or expensive services. The care of patients with chronic illness complicated by poverty, addiction, or mental illness may be improved in a multitude of ways by programs designed to assess their needs and organize services to meet them.

HOW DOES IT WORK? THEORY

The Behavioral Model for Vulnerable Populations (Fig. 15-1)[25] provides a theoretical framework for understanding how case management might improve the care of underserved patients. This model describes the determinants of access to health care and health outcomes in vulnerable populations. Health behaviors (including health care use) and health care outcomes are determined, the model argues, by an individual's "predisposing," "enabling," and "need" factors. *Predisposing factors* include demographic characteristics, social structure (employment history, education), living conditions (homelessness, mobility), and underlying psychological health (mental illness, substance abuse). The *enabling factors* include personal resources (insurance, income, presence or absence of a regular source of health care) and community resources (hospital–bed–population ratio, the availability of social services). *Need factors* include self-perception of health care needs and comorbid illnesses.

Case management can assure that issues in each of these domains are addressed. By helping patients with access to housing and coordination of services, for example, case management can influence predisposing factors. Through assistance with insurance and income entitlements and by assertive outreach and facilitation of medical care, case management can enhance enabling factors. Finally, through individualized patient education and counseling, case management can change patients' perceptions of their need for medical, psychiatric, and addiction care. Attending to all three areas may influence a patient's need and ability to access care; therefore, it may translate into improved health outcomes.

PREDISPOSING: access to housing, coordination of medical and mental health services and substance services, patient education,

ENABLING: insurance and income entitlements, transportation to medical appointment, follow-up missed appointments,

NEED: enhance patient perception of need for medical, psychiatric, addiction care through education, counseling, and advocacy.

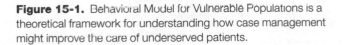

Health Behavior

↓

Outcomes

Figure 15-1. Behavioral Model for Vulnerable Populations is a theoretical framework for understanding how case management might improve the care of underserved patients.

HOW DOES IT WORK? PRACTICE

Mr. Beltran survived his hospitalization and was referred to a high-user case management program. A Spanish-speaking case manager finds him a respite bed in a shelter. The registered nurse in the program puts together a medi-set that is delivered on a weekly basis. He is reminded of his appointments and escorted to them by a team member. His primary provider adds antidepressants and nutritional supplements to his treatment. Eventually, permanent housing in a senior supportive housing facility is found for him. He is taught to use a glucometer and to straight catheterize himself. After a few months in the program, he has no further hospitalizations.

Wagner[23] has noted that interventions that improve care often share four common features: (a) they aid the patient in self-management (a critical component of chronic disease care); (b) they redesign care so as to offer the patient ready access to a health care provider (in the person of the case manager) and closer follow-up; (c) they link clinical experts to the patient's care; and (d) they collect and organize relevant data for individual patients and populations. Although different case management models generally perform the primary functions (Table 15-1), they vary in their model or approach. Especially important are the operational or process characteristics of case management programs (Box 15-1). The process characteristics of a program describe more how case management services operate, rather than what they do.

HOW DOES IT WORK? MULTIDISCIPLINARY TEAMS

The common thread among all the effective approaches to case management is the interdisciplinary team. In fact, in 2001, the Institute of Medicine's committee on the quality of health care issued a report in which a major theme was the importance of using teams to deliver quality care to patients. Unfortunately, physician education, training, and testing still stem from the outdated assumption that health care is delivered by individuals in isolation. Evidence suggests that effective teamwork does not arise spontaneously, but rather requires specific skills and development.

WHAT IS AN INTERDISCIPLINARY TEAM?

People tend to think of a team as simply being a group of people working together, but as one observer noted, "It is naïve to bring highly skilled professionals together and assume that, by calling this group a team, it will act like a team."[28] The interdisciplinary team has been defined as "a group of individuals with diverse training and backgrounds who work together as an identified unit or system. Team members consistently collaborate

Table 15-1. Primary Functions of Case Management

Function	Goal
Primary features	
Client identification and outreach	Identify and enroll clients not accessing conventional services.
Assessment	Determine a person's current and potential strengths, weaknesses, and needs.
Planning	Develop a specific, comprehensive, individualized treatment and service plan.
Linkage	Refer or transfer clients to necessary services and treatments and informal support systems.
Monitoring	Conduct ongoing evaluation of client progress and needs.
Client advocacy	Intercede on behalf of a specific client or a class of clients to ensure equity and appropriate services.
Other features	
Direct service	Some programs provide direct medical services. Others "wrap around" existing services.
Crisis intervention	Key components of case management as traditional programs often fail here.
System advocacy	Intervening with organizations or larger systems of care in order to promote more effective, equitable, and accountable services to a target client group.
Resource development	Attempt to create additional services or resources to address the needs of clients.

Adapted from: Willenbring M, Ridgely MS, Stinchfield R, et al. Application of case management in alcohol and drug dependence: Matching techniques and populations. Rockville, MD: National Institute on Alcohol Abuse and Alcoholism, 1991;
Morse G. A review of case management for people who are homeless: Implications for practice, policy, and research, in practical lessons. In: Fosburg LB, Dennis DL, eds. The 1998 National Symposium on Homelessness Research. Delmar, NY: National Resource Center on Homelessness and Mental Illness, 1999.

to solve patient problems that are too complex to be solved by one discipline or by many disciplines in sequence. Team members determine the team's mission and common goals: work interdependently to define and treat patient problems; and learn to accept and capitalize on disciplinary differences, differential power and overlapping roles."[29]

In the context of case management, interdisciplinary teams may consist of providers from multiple disciplines: a psychiatrist and a generalist, for example, along with social workers, physical and occupational therapists, nurses, outreach workers, health educators, and the like. Each member of the team addresses different aspects of patient care, working together toward a common goal for which they take joint responsibility. High-functioning teams can reach a level of synergy that enhances effectiveness and efficiency.[30]

For an interdisciplinary team to function well it must be aware of the challenges collaborative teams face in several important areas: goal and role conflict; decision making, and interpersonal communication.[29]

- *Goal conflict.* Goal conflict may arise from not clearly identifying and communication goals for all involved parties, including clients/patients, professionals on team, and the organization as a whole.
- *Role conflict.* Role conflict may stem from role ambiguity, overlapping competencies and responsibilities, preconceptions professionals have about their own role, and stereotypes of other professionals. Few professionals are aware of the scope of practice, expertise, responsibilities, and competencies of other disciplines. Professional training produces acculturation to a unique language, set of values and beliefs, and behavioral standard. Physicians, for example, do not necessarily share a common language with social workers, nurses, and medical assistants.
- *Decision making.* Decision making occurs most effectively once roles and goals are defined. Factors leading to poor decision making include an unclear statement of the problem, insufficient data about the problem, simply accepting the first option, discounting attempts at risk-taking, inattention to timeline,

Box 15-1. Case Management Process Variables[26,27]

- Duration of services
- Intensity of services (involving frequency of client contact, and client–staff ratios)
- Focus of services (from narrow and targeted to comprehensive)
- Resource responsibility (from system gatekeeper responsible for limiting use to client advocate for accessing or using multiple and frequent services)
- Availability (from scheduled office hours to 24-hour availability)
- Location of services (from all services delivered in office to all delivered in the community or home)
- Staffing pattern (from individual case loads to interdisciplinary teams with shared caseloads)

no clear commitment to action, and no agreed on responsibilities and assignments.

- *Effective communication.* Finally, avoiding conflict and successful decision making depend on effective communication. Effective communication prevents clinician burnout and allows for effective care.

CASE MANAGEMENT MODELS IN VULNERABLE POPULATIONS

Several case management models have been specifically tailored to support vulnerable populations of patients. Three models—the assertive community treatment, high-user, and chronic disease—are discussed here.

ASSERTIVE COMMUNITY TREATMENT

The oldest and most well-studied approach to case management is assertive community treatment (ACT). The ACT model was developed in the 1960s in response to the closing of psychiatric hospitals. In these models community-based, multidisciplinary teams of mental health workers provide direct treatment, rehabilitation, and support services to patients.[31] ACT teams differ from most other case management programs in that their staff is the primary provider of treatment. The goals are to minimize referrals to outside providers, provide services on a long-term care basis, deliver the vast majority of services outside of the office setting, and be available 24 hours a day.[32,33]

Evaluation of the ACT approach has found that ACT programs result in few psychiatric admissions, better independent living skills, improved symptomatology, enhanced work and social functioning, and high consumer satisfaction.[32,34] The Center for Mental Health Services within the US Dept. of Health and Human Services has published evidence-based standards for providing this type of case management. To obtain federal funding, ACT programs must demonstrate fidelity to the published standards. Although these programs are costly, cost-effectiveness studies of ACT programs have shown either cost savings or cost "neutrality." ACT programs are most cost effective when targeting the highest users of the system.[35,36]

FREQUENT USER CASE MANAGEMENT PROGRAMS

Responding to the body of evidence that emerged about ACT's success with high users of psychiatric services, physicians at San Francisco General Hospital pioneered two intensive case management programs to address the needs of patients who frequently require hospital inpatient and emergency services. "Frequent users" of the medical system tend to have multiple chronic diseases complicated by addiction, homelessness, and mental illness. The combination of severe medical and social problems leads them to fall through the cracks in the outpatient safety net system, resulting in a spiral of worse health, increased expensive health service use, and frustration for both health care providers and patients.

The frequent user programs also use multidisciplinary teams including an internist, a psychiatrist, nurses, and social workers. The goals of these community-based programs are to provide wraparound services that lead to comprehensive and effective medical, psychiatric, and addiction care while addressing the social needs of the patients. The overarching mission is to improve patients' health and avoid need for hospital and emergency room use. In this model, the social worker is at the core, assisting patients with everything from attending appointments and getting medications and treatment for mental illness or drug use to receiving entitlements and finding housing. Patients are followed closely in the hospital and out, and the team assists with communication among the many providers involved in their care: specialists, inpatient, and primary care clinicians. Evaluations of these programs have shown not only significant decreases in hospitalization, but also decreases in cost of care. Obtaining entitlements and housing are thought to be crucial aspects of care.[24]

CHRONIC DISEASE CARE MANAGEMENT

Chronic disease care management can be considered as "case management light" with important differences. In chronic disease programs, program participants are patients with a specific disease (i.e., congestive heart failure, diabetes) or particularly severe disease (patients with congestive heart failure who are hospitalized). The emphasis is on "managing the disease" rather than "managing the patient." The staffs of these programs are often nurses with high-level clinical training who help patients with self-care and identify those at need for more medical intervention.

Disease management programs have grown dramatically in number since the publication of a randomized trial of nurse case management for 281 patients discharged with congestive heart failure.[37] The program showed improved survival, decreased hospitalizations, and increase in quality of life for patients in the case management arm compared to the patients randomized to usual care. A cost analysis showed cost savings estimated at $460 per patient.[37]

Results of disease management programs have varied widely, depending on the disease and patient population targeted, as well as characteristics of the intervention. Some showed no benefit, whereas in others, the benefit was more modest. Physicians have been, on the whole, welcoming of care management programs,[38] although enthusiasm has waned recently as conflicting reports of their effectiveness have been publicized.[39–42] Nonetheless, care management programs are an important innovation in both primary and specialty care, as they facilitate greater monitoring and generally improve self-care.

CONCLUSION

Navigating the medical system is hard, particularly for patients with medical conditions complicated by mental illness and addiction. Without the benefit of resources, education, and the ability to self-advocate, these patients fail to engage in effective medical care. Paradoxically, this inadequate care, a combination of underuse and overuse, also can be quite costly and further undermine the health care system's ability to provide needed services. Recognition that we are failing to care adequately for the sickest patients has led to the development of systems such as case management to address these failures. These systems of care are one way of creating more patient-centered programs, which have built in to them an appreciation of social and medical ills that complicate patients' health the full panoply of which must be addressed. They also acknowledge that no single provider can actually provide adequate care. Although no panacea, case management programs offer patients and clinicians additional resources and multiple disciplinary perspectives that can help tackle complex situations. In moving care beyond the one-to-one model, case management programs are often successful in improving the health of patients.

KEY CONCEPTS IN CASE MANAGEMENT PROGRAMS

- Programs can target patients by disease, level of acuity, or health service use.
- Clarity of goals is essential.
- Integration with existing health care services avoids duplication of existing services and allows programs to serve a ""wrap-around"" or service extension function.
- Interdisciplinary teams contain inherent challenges, which should be addressed routinely.
- Case management programs may or may not be cost effective depending on the intensity of services, population targeted, and cost structure of parent institution.

CORE COMPETENCY
Dealing With and Avoiding Conflict When Working in Teams[29]

Avoiding goal conflict

- Clearly identify members of the team.
- Clearly identify goals (including short-term, long-term, and maintenance).
- Achieve consensus around priorities.
- Formulate action plans.
- Have all members of the team agree on action plan and follow-up steps.

Avoiding role conflict

- Clarify expectations of each team member.
- Identify professional competencies (including skills and education).
- Explore role perceptions.
- Explore overlapping responsibilities.
- Negotiate role assignments.
- Review and agree on responsibilities in carrying out action plans.

Effective decision making

- Explicitly define the problem.
- Clarify member roles and involvement in decision.
- Obtain and provide relevant data to all team members.
- Obtain input from all relevant team members.
- Generate a "differential diagnosis" for treatment; that is, multiple options and alternatives.
- Test various options.

DISCUSSION QUESTIONS

1. Think of a patient you saw recently who might benefit from case management. What makes you think so?
2. What case management programs are available in your clinical setting? How are they organized to improve care? Do you believe they are successful?
3. How should medical education be changed to create physicians effective at interdisciplinary collaboration?

RESOURCES

http://www.safetynetinstitute.org/
   The California Health Care Safety Net Institute is committed to advancing community health for California's low-income, racially and ethnically diverse populations.

http://www.nhchc.org/Network/HealingHands/1999/hh.08_99.pdf
   Healing Hands is a publication of Health Care for the Homeless Clinicians' Network, National Health Care for the Homeless Council.

http://dcahec.gwumc.edu/education/session3/

The mission of the DC Area Health Education Center is to improve the health status of the disadvantaged residents in the District of Columbia. This module is designed to assist the student in gaining an increased understanding and appreciation for interdisciplinary health care team practice.

http://www.rand.org/health/

RAND Health's goal is to advance understanding of health and health behaviors, and examine how the organization and financing of care affect costs, quality, and access.

http://www.uth.tmc.edu/sacs/bib.html

Annotated bibliography of articles on interdisciplinary or related subjects about case management.

http://www.actassociation.org/

Assertive Community Treatment Association promotes, develops, and supports high-quality Assertive Community Treatment (ACT) services that improve the lives of people with serious and persistent mental illness.

REFERENCES

1. Saha S, Bindman AB. The mirage of available health care for the uninsured. *J Gen Intern Med* 2001;16(10):714–716.
2. Weissman JS, Stern RS, Epstein AM. The impact of patient socioeconomic status and other social factors on readmission: A prospective study in four Massachusetts hospitals. *Inquiry* 1994;31(2):163–172.
3. Kushel MB, Vittinghoff E, Haas JS. Factors associated with the health care utilization of homeless persons. *JAMA* 2001;285(2):200–206.
4. O'Toole T, Gibbon J, Hanusa B, et al. Preferences for sites of care among urban homeless and housed poor adults. *J Gen Int Med* 1999;14:599–605.
5. Baker DW, Parker RM, Williams MV, et al. Health literacy and the risk of hospital admission. *J Gen Intern Med* 1998;13(12):791–798.
6. Williams DM, Counselman FL, Caggiano CD. Emergency department discharge instructions and patient literacy: A problem of disparity. *Am J Emerg Med* 1996;14(1):19–22.
7. Mistry R, Rosansky J, McGuire J, et al. Social isolation predicts re-hospitalization in a group of older American veterans enrolled in the UPBEAT Program. Unified psychogeriatric biopsychosocial evaluation and treatment. *Int J Geriatr Psychiatry* 2001;16(10):950–959.
8. Eng PM, Rimm EB, Fitzmaurice G, et al. Social ties and change in social ties in relation to subsequent total and cause-specific mortality and coronary heart disease incidence in men. *Am J Epidemiol* 2002;155(8):700–709.
9. Chesney AP, Chavira JA, Hall RP, et al. Barriers to medical care of Mexican-Americans: The role of social class, acculturation, and social isolation. *Med Care* 1982;20(9): 883–891.
10. Perez-Stable EJ, Napoles-Springer A. Interpreters and communication in the clinical encounter. *Am J Med* 2000; 108(6):509–510.
11. Derose KP, Baker DW. Limited English proficiency and Latinos' use of physician services. *Med Care Res Rev* 2000;57(1):76–91.
12. Baker DW, Hayes R, Fortier JP. Interpreter use and satisfaction with interpersonal aspects of care for Spanish-speaking patients. *Med Care* 1998;36(10):1461–1470.
13. Samet JH, Friedmann P, Saitz R. Benefits of linking primary medical care and substance abuse services: patient, provider, and societal perspectives. *Arch Int Med* 2001; 161(1):85–91.
14. O'Brien CP, McLellan AT. Myths about the treatment of addiction. *Lancet* 1996;347(8996):237–240.
15. Stein MD. Medical consequences of substance abuse. *Psychiatr Clin North Am* 1999;22(2):351–370.
16. Jeste DV, Unutzer J. Improving the delivery of care to the seriously mentally ill. *Med Care* 2001;39(9):907–909.
17. Druss BG, Rosenheck RA. Mental disorders and access to medical care in the United States. *Am J Psychiatry* 1998;155(12):1775–1777.
18. Salit SA, Kuhn EM, Hartz AJ, et al. Hospitalization costs associated with homelessness in New York City. *N Engl J Med* 1998;338(24):1734–1740.
19. Bindman AB, Grumbach K, Osmond D, et al. Preventable hospitalizations and access to health care. *JAMA* 1995; 274(4):305–311.
20. O'Brien GM, Stein MD, Zierler S, et al. Use of the ED as a regular source of care: associated factors beyond lack of health insurance. *Ann Emerg Med* 1997;30(3):286–291.
21. Stern RS, Weissman JS, Epstein AM. The emergency department as a pathway to admission for poor and high-cost patients [see comments]. *JAMA* 1991;266(16): 2238–2243.
22. Smedley BD, Stith AY, Nelson AR, eds. *Unequal treatment: Confronting racial and ethnic disparities in health care.* Washington, DC: Institute of Medicine, National Academy Press, 2002.
23. Wagner EH. More than a case manager [editorial; comment]. *Ann Int Med* 1998;129(8):654–656.
24. Okin RL, Boccellari A, Azocar F, et al. The effects of clinical case management on hospital service use among ED frequent users. *Am J Emerg Med* 2000;18(5):603–608.
25. Gelberg L, Andersen RM, Leake BD. The Behavioral Model for Vulnerable Populations: Application to medical care use and outcomes for homeless people. *Health Serv Res* 2000;34(6):1273–12302.
26. Willenbring M, Ridgely MS, Stinchfield R, et al. *Application of case management in alcohol and drug dependence: Matching techniques and populations.* Rockville, MD: National Institute on Alcohol Abuse and Alcoholism, 1991.
27. Morse G. A review of case management for people who are homeless: Implications for practice, policy, and research, in practical lessons. In: Fosburg LB, Dennis DL, eds. *The 1998 National Symposium on Homelessness Research.* Delmar, NY: National Resource Center on Homelessness and Mental Illness, 1999.
28. Baldwin DC, Tsukuda RW. Interdisciplinary teams. In: Cassell C, Walsh JR, eds. *Geriatric medicine: Fundamentals of geriatric care.* New York: Springer-Verlag, 1984.
29. Drinka TJ, Clark PG. *Health care teamwork. Interdisciplinary practice teaching.* Westport, CT: Auburn House, 2000.
30. Tsukuda RA. Interdisciplinary collaboration: Teamwork in geriatrics. In: Cassell C, Walsh JR, eds. *Geriatric medicine: Fundamentals of geriatric care.* New York: Springer-Verlag, 1990:668–675.

31. Stein LI, Test MA. Alternative to mental hospital treatment. I. Conceptual model, treatment program, and clinical evaluation. *Arch Gen Psychiatry* 1980;37(4):392–397.

32. Allness DJ. The Program of Assertive Community Treatment (PACT): The model and its replication. *New Dir Ment Health Serv* 1997;74:17–26.

33. Phillips SD, Burns BJ, Edgar ER, et al. Moving assertive community treatment into standard practice. *Psychiatr Serv* 2001;52(6):771–779.

34. Bond GR, McGrew JH, Fekete DM. Assertive outreach for frequent users of psychiatric hospitals: A meta-analysis. *J Ment Health Adm* 1995;22(1):4–16.

35. Curtis JL, Millman EJ, Struening E, et al. Effect of case management on rehospitalization and utilization of ambulatory care services. *Hosp Commun Psychiatry* 1992;43(9):895–899.

36. Rosenheck R, Neale M, Leaf P, et al. Multisite experimental cost study of intensive psychiatric community care. *Schizophr Bull* 1995;21(1):129–140.

37. Rich MW, Beckham V, Wittenberg C, et al. A multidisciplinary intervention to prevent the readmission of elderly patients with congestive heart failure. *N Engl J Med* 1995;333(18):1190–1195.

38. Fernandez A, Grumbach K, Vranizan K, et al. Primary care physicians' experience with disease management programs. *J Gen Intern Med* 2001;16(3):163–167.

39. Bodenheimer T, Fernandez A. High and rising health care costs. Part 4: Can costs be controlled while preserving quality? *Ann Intern Med* 2005;143(1):26–31.

40. Fetterolf D, Wennberg D, Devries A. Estimating the return on investment in disease management programs using a pre-post analysis. *Dis Manag* 2004;7(1):5–23.

41. Fireman B, Bartlett J, Selby J. Can disease management reduce health care costs by improving quality? *Health Aff (Millwood)* 2004;23(6):63–75.

42. Crosson FJ, Madvig P. Does population management of chronic disease lead to lower costs of care? *Health Aff (Millwood)* 2004;23(6):76–78.

Chapter 16

Health and the Community

Naomi Wortis, MD, Ellen Beck, MD, and Joanne Donsky, MSW

Objectives

- Describe the role health professionals may have in the community beyond the realm of the clinic or hospital.
- Outline how a health professional can be involved in a community, including the Community-Oriented Primary Care (COPC) model.
- Review how to define a target community.
- Describe techniques of healthy community assessment.
- Review the importance of partnering with the community.
- Discuss how health professionals can promote community empowerment.

Health depends in large part on the social context within which a person lives (see Chap. 1). This social context includes the community or communities with which the individual identifies. The term "community" is derived from the Latin *communitas*, meaning common or shared.[1] This chapter defines a community as a group of people with a shared identity.

Health professionals increasingly recognize that they have a responsibility to engage with the communities they serve, beyond the doors of their clinics or hospitals. By partnering with a community, learning about its needs and resources, and assisting a community with community-based health interventions, the health professional has the potential to improve the well-being of many more people.

This chapter reviews the common challenges faced by health professionals seeking to engage with communities and proposes some solutions to overcome them. Woven through this chapter is the story of the establishment of the San Diego–based Environmental Health Coalition and its community health worker (or *promotora*) program.

RECOGNIZING THE IMPORTANCE OF COMMUNITY

DEFINING A TARGET COMMUNITY

> Barrio Logan is a San Diego neighborhood with a mix of residences and industry, nestled between Interstate 5 and San Diego Bay's shipyards. Pollution and poverty have a negative impact on the environment and the community's health. There are strong community associations, ranging from labor unions to informal social networks of women.

The first challenge faced by a health professional wishing to address health at a community level is defining the target community. Often, a community is defined as: (a) a geographically defined neighborhood; (b) a group of people working or going to school together; or (c) a group of people with some shared sociologic characteristic such as age, language, and a shared history, cause, or identity. Commonly, health professionals define their target community as persons with a particular health problem or patients served by a particular clinical practice.

These last two definitions of target communities are problematic. People with a particular health problem or patients of a particular clinic may not feel a shared identity with others in those respective groups, and shared identity is at the heart of any definition of community. The less a community has a sense of group identity, the harder it is to engage with that community in a way that encourages community members to take responsibility for improving overall community well-being. Moreover, if a health professional limits the target community to people with a particular health problem or patients of a particular practice, the health professional may miss the opportunity to reach out to people who have not yet been diagnosed with that problem or who have not yet accessed clinical care. Many opportunities for preventing disease also are missed. This significantly decreases the potential community health impact of any intervention that is undertaken.

Involving community members in the definition of the target community is valuable. This enhances the likelihood that the target community will have a shared identity and encourages community members to take responsibility for improving overall community well-being. In addition, there are advantages to defining a target community in a way that others have before. This makes it more likely that there will be preexisting data characterizing the community. An example is a geographic community that follows census track lines, allowing census data to be used more easily.

OVERCOMING THE CULTURAL DIVIDE AND DEVELOPING TRUST

The University of California San Diego (UCSD) is located several miles north of Barrio Logan in well-to-do La Jolla. The residents of Barrio Logan are people of color, mostly Latino, and over 40% have annual household incomes of less than $10,000.

Many health professionals are not originally part of the communities they serve. This is especially likely to be true for health professionals serving vulnerable populations. Not being part of a target community often means that health professionals face a cultural divide. This divide may include race, ethnicity, language, socioeconomic status, or belief systems, to name just a few possible differences. Just as health professionals strive for cultural competence when delivering health care to individuals, they must work on learning about the realities of community life if they want to engage successfully with a target community.

Like all human beings, health professionals have their own biases, and effective community engagement, like effective patient engagement, requires self-awareness. Tervalon suggests the term "cultural humility" rather than cultural competence.[2] She describes cultural humility as incorporating "a lifelong commitment to self-evaluation and self-critique, to redressing the power imbalances in the patient-physician dynamic, and to developing mutually beneficial and nonpaternalistic clinical and advocacy partnerships with communities. . . ."

The cultural divide commonly includes the gap between the academic medical perspective and the community perspective.[3] Freeman describes the *academic perspective* as more focused on theory, analysis, and educational value; and the *community perspective* as more focused on practical solutions, service, and action. As a result of their different perspectives, academics sometimes behave in ways that are or appear to be disrespectful and generate mistrust in the community. For example, academics doing research in a community may promise to share results with that community; however, the communication of results may never happen. This missed step can represent a betrayal of trust from the community's perspective.

Another potential element of the cultural divide between health professional and community is the paternalistic role that health providers have often played with their patients. This role is sometimes extended into community work with poor results. When health professionals assume they know what would be best for the health of their target community, they may alienate and disempower community members. Conversely, taking a more collaborative approach and heeding the collective wisdom within the community is more likely to build trust and promote community empowerment.

ASSESSING A COMMUNITY

An important step in successful community engagement is assessing the target community. This means being able to describe who makes up that community, what resources already exist in the community, and what needs still exist. If this step is skipped or done superficially, the health professional may proceed with incorrect assumptions that can result in inappropriate health interventions, duplication of services, or interventions that are not sustainable. For example, there is often a temptation to start a brand-new program from scratch. It is usually better for long-term community development to work to improve the programs of an existing organization than to start a new one from scratch.

Needs-Focused Assessment

In the book, *Building Communities From the Inside Out*, Kretzmann and McKnight describe two paths to community development: needs-focused and capacity-focused.[4] They call the traditional needs-focused path "A Needs Driven Dead End." This approach to community assessment focuses solely on problems and needs, rather than including resources, and has numerous negative results at the community level, including fragmentation of services, funds being directed to service-providers rather than community members, community leaders highlighting problems rather than promoting strengths, outside experts being promoted as the only ones who can solve problems, focus on survival rather than development, and general community hopelessness.

Capacity-Focused Assessment

Kretzmann and McKnight promote a resource-centered approach that they call "Capacity-Focused Development." They highlight identifying and connecting the building blocks of "individuals, local associations, and institutions" as the keys to community development. Examples of these community assets include teens and elders; religious organizations and neighborhood groups; and local businesses, schools, and clinics. When community members identify and interconnect these assets, invest some of their own resources into the process, and take responsibility for setting priorities and finding solutions to fill gaps, the result is likely to be personal empowerment and successful community development.

Common Pitfalls

- Failing to define the target community clearly or appropriately
- Insensitivity caused by lack of awareness of the cultural divide between health professionals and community, often resulting in lack of trust
- Failing to learn about or assess the community
- Focusing only on community needs while overlooking community resources
- Failing to partner with the community, or failing to do so effectively

COMMUNITY INVOLVEMENT FOR HEALTH PROFESSIONALS

The Environmental Health Coalition (EHC), a grassroots community organization, was founded in San Diego in 1980. It initially worked with union members concerned about occupational health and safety issues and community members concerned about cancer and other environmental illnesses. Founders included industrial workers, environmentalists, health and human service providers, and university professors. Their mission statement includes: "We believe that justice is achieved when empowered communities act together to make social change."[5] Health professionals from several southern California universities, including UCSD, have been involved in many of the projects undertaken by EHC.

PARTNERING WITH THE COMMUNITY

Community health interventions by health professionals are much more likely to be effective if they are done in partnership with the community. A *community-based* project is likely to be more successful than a *community-placed* project. A community-placed project is one in which an outside "expert" assumes she or he knows what a community needs, develops an intervention without community input, and then implements it. This can lead to: (a) a project that is not valued by the community because it is not addressing one of the community's high priorities; (b) methods that are culturally inappropriate; (c) duplication of interventions that have already been tried; and (d) a project that is not sustainable beyond the expert's involvement because it does not have community support. A true community-based project is one that grows from within a community and is led by community members. Community members identify needs and resources, implement an intervention, and sustain the project. Outside experts can participate in this process through effective partnering.

Partnership with preexisting community groups or official community leaders is valuable; however, it is also essential to make sure that "grassroots" community members are consulted and involved in the project. Official community leaders are sometimes different from true community leaders. When that is the case, the health professional will find it difficult to gain the trust of the general community if she or he collaborates only with the official leaders. Also, it is important not to rely too much on one community group. The project can be undermined easily if that organization loses funding or leadership, or if internal community politics do not favor the group.

Learning how to partner with a community in order to undertake community health interventions is challenging. It takes patience and perseverance to do partnership work well, but the rewards can be tremendous. A national organization, Community-Campus Partnerships for Health, identified nine "Principles of Partnership," through an inclusive process involving members and partners.[6] These may be useful as guidelines for establishing new partnerships or as a checklist to assess existing partnerships. Highlights of these principles include: "Partners have agreed upon mission, values, goals and measurable outcomes for the partnership"; "Partners share the credit for the partnership's accomplishments"; and "Partnerships take time to develop and evolve over time."

COMMUNITY-ORIENTED PRIMARY CARE MODEL

The community-oriented primary care (COPC) model is a process through which health problems of a defined population are systematically identified and addressed. Figure 16-1A shows a diagram of the COPC process. The first step is identifying and characterizing a target community. The second step is assessing the needs and resources of that community. The third step is designing and implementing an intervention to address a prioritized need. The fourth step is evaluating the success of the intervention. Community members must be involved as partners throughout the COPC process, not merely as a source of data. Examples of this partnership include (but are not limited to) community members who define the target community, pose research questions, design survey instruments, gather and/or analyze data, design and/or staff interventions, perform evaluations, and write up results.

It should be pointed out that this COPC model is not unlike the process health professionals go through in caring for individual patients. See Figure 16-1B for a diagram of the patient care process. Obviously, patient care cannot be successful unless the health professional collaborates with the patient at each step. Patients are not only expected to provide information about their health problems. They are also expected to participate in treatment decisions, changing health behaviors, and monitoring their progress. Like patient care, the COPC process can address multiple needs simultaneously or serially. Box 16-1 reviews important tasks for health professionals embarking on COPC community collaborations.

HEALTHY COMMUNITY ASSESSMENT

In 1997, a team of community members, EHC staff, and health professionals conducted a health survey that revealed that approximately 20% of Barrio Logan's children were having severe asthma-type symptoms. Partnering with EHC, health professionals have been involved in training *promotoras* (community health workers) about a variety of health and environmental issues such as asthma and lead poisoning.

Community engagement at any level by a health professional requires some assessment of that community. Hancock and Minkler promote the idea of a "healthy community assessment" rather than the "community health assessment."[9] They build on Hancock and Duhl's definition of a healthy community, developed for the WHO: "A healthy [community] is one that is continually creating and improving those physical and social environments and expanding those community resources which enable people to mutually support each other in performing all the functions of life and in developing to their maximum potential."[10] The healthy community assessment is thus a much broader

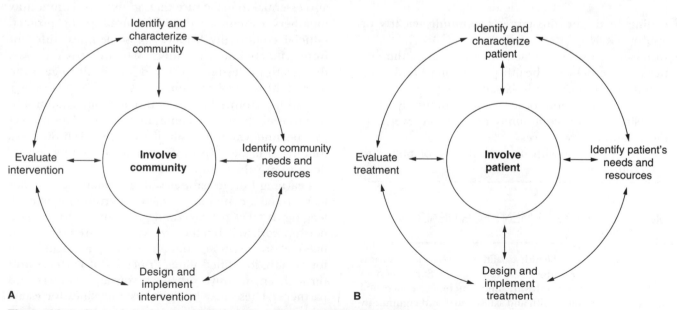

Figure 16-1. Comparison of community-oriented primary care (COPC) and patient care models. **A.** COPC process. (Adapted with permission from: Rhyne R, et al. *Community-oriented primary care: Health care for the 21st century.* Washington, DC: American Public Health Association, 1998.) **B.** Patient care process.

Box 16-1. Important Tasks when Embarking on COPC Collaborations with a Community

- **Assess** your own resources as a health professional and your interest in becoming partners with the community.
- **Engage** the community by identifying the relevant social networks and leaders.
- **Prioritize** health problems using consensus-building techniques.
- **Develop** strategies to enlist community involvement in the intervention.

- **Evaluate** outcomes, involving the community from the start.

From: Wallerstein N, Sheline B. Techniques for developing a community partnership. In: Rhyne R, Bogue R, Kukulka G, et al, eds. *Community-oriented primary care: Health care for the 21st century.* Washington, DC: American Public Health Association, 1998.[7,8]

---

assessment than a review of statistics on demographics, morbidity, mortality, and so on.

A number of methods can be used to perform a healthy community assessment, and they can be grouped in different ways: primary data versus secondary data, studies versus stories, quantitative versus qualitative, and so on. In a landmark article on community development and needs assessment, Martí-Costa and Serrano-García developed a way of grouping assessment methods based on the degree of contact with the community.[11] Hancock and Minkler[9] refined this further (see Core Competency).

No Contact Methods

"No-contact methods" consist of gathering official statistics and preexisting documents, often referred to as secondary data. These are good places to find out about demographics, health access, morbidity, and mortality. The Internet provides access to an enormous amount of data about many communities.

Minimal Contact Methods

Geographically defined communities can be assessed through a driving ("windshield") or walking tour. Health professionals might look for health clinics, hospitals, dental clinics, nursing homes, sources of mental health care, and pharmacies. It is also important to observe the people, houses, places of worship, community-based organizations, businesses, schools, parks, potential environmental hazards, police and fire services, and public transport.

Interactive Contact Methods

"Interactive contact methods" hold the potential for community empowerment through opportunities for community members to be involved and acquire new skills and knowledge. These methods of community assessment can provide valuable primary data but require significant investments of time. Conducting surveys, focus groups and interviews of key community leaders or random community members are examples

of these methods. The conducting of focus groups[12-14] and surveys[15,16] is complex, and is beyond the scope of this chapter, but there are many other sources of information on these subjects.

Participatory Methods

Examples of these methods include community members reviewing official data, conducting key informant interviews, or designing survey instruments.

Performing Community Interviews

Key informant interviews are a mainstay of interactive contact methods. The first step is determining whom to interview. Anyone who is a member of a community or who works with a community can harbor valuable information about that community and be a key informant. They may be official leaders such as a member of a community advisory board, a local politician, a religious leader, a clinic director, a teacher, the executive director of a community-based organization, a nurse, a community health worker, or a business owner.

Informal "community leaders" are not the same as the official leaders and often are not readily identifiable to an outsider. They must be sought out, because they are very valuable sources of information and may be good allies for doing work in the community. Informal community leaders are more likely than official leaders to live in the neighborhood, send their children to local schools, share the same socioeconomic status as the rest of the community, be sought out for advice by other community members, and be trusted by the community in general.

These interviews are particularly useful for learning about the history of the community, the positive aspects about the community, what resources exist, how existing services are perceived, what environmental hazards exist, and what needs are perceived. Keep in mind that key informants all come with their own biases. It is important to establish the nature and length of their association with the community. The more key informants are interviewed, the more well-rounded a view of the community is obtained.

A healthy community assessment is a necessary step for health professionals to take in the community engagement process. The depth of the assessment depends on the time and resources available. It is advisable to use multiple methods to get the fullest possible picture of the community.

COMMUNITY EMPOWERMENT

> EHC promotoras participated at San Diego Port Commission meetings and were ultimately successful in stopping methyl bromide fumigations at a fruit warehouse just a quarter mile from the Barrio Logan elementary school and local homes. Community members participated in rallies, press conferences, candlelight vigils, visits to local politicians, signed petitions, and so on to achieve their victory.

In order for a community to become healthier, community members need to lead the process. Health professionals who are partnering with a community on health projects should promote this and not inadvertently undermine it. This is analogous to the way in which health professionals must facilitate patients' taking charge of their own health. Just as the principles of patient centered care are especially important with vulnerable patients, the parallel approach to community work is especially important with vulnerable and underserved communities. It supports those communities in becoming stronger, healthier, and more empowered.

McKnight suggests the following values for health professionals working with communities:[17] (a) respect community wisdom, (b) share health expertise in the form of understandable information that enables the community to solve its own problems, (c) promote the use of system resources for the enhancement of community capacities, (d) focus on magnifying the gifts, capacities, and assets of individual community members and the community as a whole. In these ways, health professionals can promote empowered communities.

CONCLUSION

The importance of community to health is difficult to overestimate. Fostering healthy communities and partnering with communities are important roles for health professionals. Communities are dynamic places, and groups and individuals come and go. It takes time, patience, and perseverance to build trust and to do partnership work well. Through community engagement, community assessment, and community partnership, health professionals have an opportunity to promote community empowerment and reach even those who never enter the doors of the clinic. Using these approaches, health professionals have the opportunity to improve the lives of individuals and the communities in which they live and work. Doing so is enormously rewarding to all involved.

ACKNOWLEDGMENTS

The authors of this chapter would like to acknowledge the staff and members of the Environmental Health Coalition (EHC) for creating and sustaining an organization that serves as an example of successful partnering between community members and health professionals, as part of the process of improving their community's health. They would also like to acknowledge Dr. Ruth Heifetz for being an exceptional role model of a health professional partnering with EHC and other community groups and for her generous contribution of time and wisdom editing this chapter.

KEY CONCEPTS

- Engage with the community in some way.
- Use the Community-Oriented Primary Care (COPC) model, involving community members.
- Conduct broad healthy community assessment using multiple methods.
- Build partnerships with community members in all phases of work to produce a community-based project.
- Evaluate your interventions.
- Promote community empowerment whenever possible.
- Understand that partnerships take time to build and develop.

CORE COMPETENCY
Methods for Healthy Community Assessment

1. **No Contact Methods (useful preliminary step)**
   a. Review official statistics (e.g., census data, public health department data, school district data, birth/death records, crime rates)
   b. Review documents (e.g., community newspapers, newsletters, progress reports, bulletin boards)
2. **Minimal Contact Observational Methods**
   a. Driving or walking tour
   b. Visits to neighborhood businesses (e.g., a coffee shop, a store, or a nursing home)
   c. Attendance at community meetings (e.g., attend a PTA meeting or a religious service)

(Continued)

> **3. Interactive Contact Methods**
>   a. Key informant interviews
>   b. Small group methods (e.g., focus groups)
>   c. Surveys (e.g., door-to-door or other face-to-face interviews)
> **4. Participatory Methods**
>   Any of the listed methods when done in partnership with community members
>
> Adapted from: Hancock T, Minkler M. Community health assessment or healthy community assessment: Whose community? Whose health? Whose assessment? In: Minkler M, ed. *Community Organizing & Community Building for Health.* New Brunswick, NJ: Rutgers University Press, 1997;139–156.[9]

DISCUSSION QUESTIONS

Identify a community with which you would like to work.

1. How would you define that community? What are the advantages and disadvantages of defining the community in this way?
2. At what point in your work with the community would you begin to involve community partners? Why? With whom might you partner?
3. What will be some of the challenges to developing effective community partnerships? How will you overcome those challenges?
4. How will you learn more about the community? What kinds of information are you looking for? What are the best methods of getting the information you need?
5. Give some theoretical examples of community-based health interventions that you and your partners might consider implementing in this community.

RESOURCES

http://depts.washington.edu/ccph
   Community Campus Partnerships for Health (CCPH): A nonprofit organization that promotes health through partnerships between communities and higher educational institutions.

http://ctb.ku.edu/tools/en/tools_toc.htm
   Community Tool Box: This web site provides over 6,000 pages of practical skillbuilding information on over 250 different topics.

http://www.environmentalhealth.org
   Environmental Health Coalition: A grassroots organization dedicated to achieving environmental and social justice.

Minkler M, ed. *Community organizing and building for health.* New Brunswick, NJ: Rutgers University Press, 1997.

Rhyne R, et al. *Community-oriented primary care: Health care for the 21st century.* Washington, DC: American Public Health Association, 1998.

REFERENCES

1. LaBonte R. Community, community development, and forming of authentic partnerships. In Minkler M, ed. *Community organizing and community building for health.* New Brunswick, NJ: Rutgers University Press, 1997; 88.
2. Tervalon M, Murray-Garcia J. Cultural humility versus cultural competence: A critical distinction in defining physician training outcomes in multicultural education. *J Health Care Poor Underserved* 1998;9:117.
3. Freeman ER. Engaging a university: The CCHERS experience. *Metro Univ Int Forum* 2000;11:20.
4. Kretzmann J, McKnight J. *Building communities from the inside out: A path toward finding and mobilizing a community's assets.* Chicago, IL: ACTA Publications, 1993.
5. Environmental Health Coalition. Strategic plan 2002–2005. Environmental Health Coalition, 2005.
6. Community-Campus Partnerships for Health. Principles of good community-campus partnerships. Accessed December 6, 2004. Available at: http://depts.washington.edu/ccph/principles.html#principles
7. Wallerstein N, Sheline B. Techniques for developing a community partnership. In: Rhyne R, Bogue R, Kukulka G, et al, eds. *Community-oriented primary care: Health care for the 21st century.* Washington, DC: American Public Health Association, 1998.
8. Rhyne R, Bogue R, Kukulka G, et al. *Community-oriented primary care: Health care for the 21st century.* Washington, DC: American Public Health Association, 1998.
9. Hancock T, Minkler M. Community health assessment or healthy community assessment: Whose community? Whose health? Whose assessment? In: Minkler M, ed. *Community organizing and community building for health.* New Brunswick, NJ: Rutgers University Press, 1997;139.
10. Hancock T, Duhl L. Healthy cities: Promoting health in the urban context. Copenhagen: WHO Europe, 1986.
11. Martí-Costa S, Serrano-García I. Needs assessment and community development: An ideological perspective. *Prev Hum Serv* 1983;2:75.
12. Krueger RA. *Focus groups: A practical guide for applied research.* Thousand Oaks, CA: Sage, 2002.
13. Morgan DL, Krueger RA. *The focus group kit.* Thousand Oaks, CA: Sage, 1997.
14. Berkowitz B. Conducting focus groups. In: KU Work Group for Community Health and Development, University of Kansas: The Community Tool Box, 2004. Accessed December 7, 2004. Available at: http://ctb.ku.edu/tools/en/sub_section_main_1018.htm
15. Fink A. *The survey kit.* Thousand Oaks, CA: Sage, 1997.
16. Hampton C, Vilela M. Conducting surveys. In: KU Work Group for Community Health and Development, University of Kansas: The Community Tool Box, 2004. Accessed December 7, 2004. Available at: http://ctb.ku.edu/tools/en/sub_section_main_1048.htm
17. McKnight J. Two tools for well-being: health systems and communities. *J Perinatol* 1999;19:S12.

PART 3

Populations

Teresa J. Villela, MD and Margaret B. Wheeler, MD, editors

Chapter 17

Underserved Children: Preventing Chronic Illness and Promoting Health

Patricia Barreto, MD, MPH, Victor H. Perez, MD, MPH, and Neal Halfon, MD, MPH

Objectives

- Review emerging definitions of children's health.
- Describe the relationship between child health and adult health.
- Identify social and environmental factors that influence health.
- Describe the Life Course Health Development Framework and how it may guide health promotion among vulnerable populations.
- Identify groups of children with heightened vulnerability.
- Summarize strategies to tailor clinic-based assessment, education, intervention, and care coordination to vulnerable children.

Xavier is a healthy 2-year-old boy with delayed language development. His parents are immigrants and speak to him in their native language. He watches 3 hours of television a day and reads with his parents two to three times per week. His parents describe him as a normal, healthy boy.

Childhood is a critical and dynamic period of human development that that has lifelong effects on health.[1] Preventing chronic illness and promoting optimal long-term health require a special focus on optimizing functional capacity in childhood.

This chapter discusses emerging concepts of children's health and highlights the relationships among health, development, and health promotion. It proposes a framework for understanding health development over an individual's lifetime[2] and how pediatric health care providers can promote health and prevent chronic illness.

EMERGING CONCEPTS IN CHILDREN'S HEALTH

The Institute of Medicine (IOM) report, *Children's Health, the Nation's Wealth*, defines children's health as "the extent to which an individual child or groups of children are able to or enabled to: (a) develop and realize their potential; (b) satisfy their needs; and (c) develop the capacities that allow them to interact successfully with their biological, physical and social environments."[3] This definition of children's health highlights the intimate relationship between health and human development, and expands it to include not only physical, but also social and mental well-being.

CONTEXTUAL FACTORS THAT INFLUENCE HEALTH

Health development is a term that further expands the definition of health to acknowledge childhood as an unique period in which biological, behavioral, and environmental influences intertwine to influence current and future (adult) health.[2,6,7] For example, in children with asthma, environmental exposures (dust mites, smoke) cause chronic inflammation and ultimately change lung structure and function, which has implications for adult lung function and adult functional capacity. Interventions improving children's health thus potentially can prevent lifelong chronic illness.

Health development also defines health in terms of functional capacity. In so doing, it recognizes that health is a dynamic state that is influenced by multiple determinants, from genes to the environment with which they interact.[2] For example, a poorly nourished child from a low-income family who is exposed to violence and attends school in an overcrowded classroom may not reach his developmental potential, and is at greater risk for anemia, injuries, and behavioral problems. On the other hand, having parents who pay close attention to his education will mitigate some of the difficulties he faces. Positive influences on health

surrounding a more affluent child (high socioeconomic status, good schools, safe neighborhoods, and accessible healthy food) enhance health development, even if the child's parents are not attentive. These examples underscore that poverty perniciously stymies children's achievement of their maximal potentials. Termed "double jeopardy" by some, poverty presents both a multitude of risks undermining optimal health development and a dearth of resources to mitigate them.[4]

PROTECTIVE FACTORS FOR CHILD HEALTH DEVELOPMENT

Some people are able to develop mechanisms to deal successfully with the risks they face, thus enhancing their health and well-being. This quality, referred to as resilience, is critical to functional capacity.[8] Factors contributing to resilience, or protective factors, may either be intrinsic to the individual (e.g., their raw intelligence or disposition), or external (e.g., educational

Table 17-1. Individual-, Family-, and Community-Level Protective Factors

Protective Factors	Developmental Period
Individual	
Low distress/low emotionality	Infancy–adulthood
Active; alert; high vigor; drive	Infancy
Sociability	Infancy
"Easy" engaging temperament	Infancy–childhood
Advanced self-help skills	Early childhood
Average–above average intelligence	Childhood–adulthood
Ability to distance oneself; impulse control	Childhood–adulthood
Internal locus of control	Childhood–adolescence
Strong achievement motivation	Childhood–adolescence
Special talents, hobbies	Childhood–adolescence
Positive self-concept	Childhood–adolescence
Planning, foresight	Adolescence–adulthood
Strong religious orientation, faith	Childhood–adulthood
Family/community	
Small family size (<4 children)	Infancy
Mother's education	Infancy–adulthood
Maternal competence	Infancy–adolescence
Close bond with primary caregiver	Infancy–adolescence
Supportive grandparents	Infancy–adolescence
Supportive siblings	Childhood–adulthood
For girls: emphasis on autonomy with emotional support from primary caregiver	Childhood–adolescence
For boys: structure and rules in household	Childhood–adolescence
For both boys and girls: assigned chores: "required helpfulness"	Childhood–adolescence
Close, competent peer friends who are confidants	Childhood–adolescence
Supportive teachers	Preschool–adulthood
Successful school experiences	Preschool–adulthood
Mentors (elders, peers)	Childhood–adulthood

Examples of protective factors that have been identified in two or more longitudinal studies of resiliency in children and youth.
Adapted from: Werner E. Protective factors and individual resilience. In: Shonkoff J, Meisels S, eds. *Handbook of early childhood intervention*, 2nd ed. New York: Cambridge University Press, 2000:115–132.

opportunities, a supportive family). Protective qualities can be found in the individual, the family, and the community, as well as through the interactions between these groups. Like risk factors (remember the example of poverty), protective factors often occur together. Most significantly, protective factors have a greater impact on the outcomes of vulnerable children than do specific risk factors or stressful events, and some protective factors are more important than others for children at particular developmental stages[8] (Table 17-1). Supportive grandparents, siblings, teachers, and mentors all buffer children from the effects of risk factors such as poverty, substance abuse, parental mental illness, divorce, and even child abuse and neglect. Bolstering the interpersonal relationships supporting a child's health is thus one way that clinicians can promote health.[9]

Health promotion integrates broad definitions of health and development into health care to enable "individuals to increase control over and improve their health. It involves the population as a whole in the context of their everyday lives, rather than focusing on people at risk for specific diseases, and is directed toward action on the determinants or causes of health."[10]

THE LIFE COURSE HEALTH DEVELOPMENT MODEL

> Trajectory 1: Projecting forward several years, Xavier has significant language delays when he goes to school. In first grade his teachers become concerned, but it is not until third grade that he is tested and found to have language and cognitive delays. He eventually drops out of school and joins a gang.
>
> Trajectory 2: Xavier receives a comprehensive language assessment at age 2 and is placed in language and cognitive stimulation programs. He enters school with near-normal language function. He does well in school, particularly math and science.

The Life Course Health Development (LCHD) model integrates the ideas that health develops over an individual's lifetime and is influenced by environmental, physiologic, behavioral, and psychological factors into an analytic framework useful for health providers.[2] Positive or protective factors—genetic, environmental or social—act to allow an individual to attain optimal healthy functioning. Negative influences on health, on the other hand, deter a person from achieving this potential. The balance of these forces determines the health trajectory of an individual (Fig. 17-1).

Health professionals can have a significant impact on their patients' health by using the LCHD model. The LCHD model, framing health and interventions

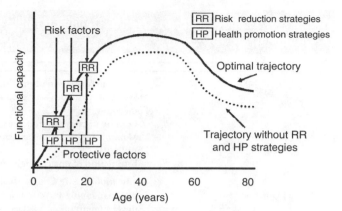

Figure 17-1. The health development trajectory: How risk reduction and health promotion strategies influence health development. This figure illustrates how risk reduction strategies can mitigate the influence of risk factors on the developmental trajectory, and how health promotion strategies can simultaneously support and optimize the developmental trajectory. In the absence of effective risk reduction and health promotion, the developmental trajectory will be suboptimal *(dotted curve).* (From: Halfon N, Hochstein M. Life course health development: An integrated framework for developing health, policy, and research. *Millbank Q* 2002;80(3):433–479.[2])

for health broadly, integrates the social factors influencing health in a way most often ignored by traditional medical models. Adoption of this framework requires a shift in clinical practice from its traditional preoccupation with a search for disease, to a perspective that searches for opportunities for prevention and the active promotion of health.

Thus, viewed from the perspectives of LCHD and health promotion, childhood represents an opportunity for health practitioners to intervene effectively to prevent disability and promote lifelong health during a developmental period in which interventions can be leveraged to improve the long-term health of the population as a whole. The integration of individual and population health promotion and disease prevention requires ongoing surveillance of the child and family in order to identify strategic opportunities to support resilience and minimize risk. Finally, LCHD and the idea of health promotion provide powerful tools for tackling the vexing health problems of underserved children (Box 17-1).

THE VULNERABILITY OF CHILDREN

Children are uniquely vulnerable because they are rapidly developing and, as nonautonomous individuals they are dependent on others for their health, safety, and well-being. Their vulnerability is dynamic because they are changing and these changes are exquisitely

Box 17-1. Linking Children's Health Definition to the Life Course Health Development Framework and Changes in Clinical Practice

Transformation of the Concept of Children's Health

Moves away from disease-based model

Focuses on:

    Optimizing development and function

    Maximizing individual and population potential

Highlights:

    Interaction of environment, contextual factors, and the individual

Application of Life Course Health Development Framework

LCDH concept: Individual, family and community level risk and protective factors interact to influence the health development of individuals over their lifetime

LCDH model: Framework for understanding how health develops over an individual's life time

    Conceptual structure to promote health among vulnerable populations

The transformed clinical practice:

Serves as a service delivery hub connected to a wide array of community resources

Utilizes community epidemiologic data to identify community-level health risk factors and guide development of targeted health service delivery pathways

Utilizes asset mapping used to identify community-level health protective factors and create external links to community-based organizations

Tailors clinic-based assessment, education, intervention and care coordination to vulnerable children

---

sensitive to external pressures. Thus, anticipating sensitive developmental periods in which children may be more vulnerable based on both their developmental capacities and their contextual environment as defined by their family, school, and community is crucial.[7]

Although all children are vulnerable, for some children this is exaggerated by poor health, social or family circumstances, or other environmental threats. For example, children who have been abused or neglected and placed into foster care often have been severely traumatized, diminishing their capacity to respond to age-specific developmental demands. Similarly, children whose parents have acute or chronic mental health or substance abuse problems can be routinely exposed to serious health and developmental threats.

Common Problems and Pitfalls

- Applying a disease-based model for health care to vulnerable populations
- Ignoring the contextual or environmental factors that influence health
- Applying individual-focused health promotion strategies to vulnerable populations
- Overlooking the inherent vulnerability of children, the dynamic nature of vulnerability, and the need to intervene at developmentally sensitive periods
- Carrying out clinical practice systems that are not organized to identify and intervene to support health protective factors and remove health risk factors

- Delivering clinic-based assessment, education, intervention, and care coordination that are not tailored to vulnerable patients

---

TRANSFORMING CLINICAL PRACTICE TO SERVE VULNERABLE CHILDREN

Evidence suggests that current clinical service delivery mechanisms fall short in key areas such as addressing children's developmental and other "nonmedical" (psychosocial, environmental) concerns.[11] These concerns are often directly linked to common morbidities (e.g., developmental delay, drug and alcohol abuse, mental and emotional disorders, family violence) that challenge families and health care providers.[12] Although these psychosocial/environmental concerns undermine health, clinicians often feel inadequate to address them.[14] Clinicians may not inquire about issues such as domestic violence, mental illness, homelessness, drug and alcohol abuse, hunger, access to high-quality child care, educational resources, or social isolation, if they cannot offer a resource or potential solution to the family.

MAKING THE CLINICAL PRACTICE THE SERVICE DELIVERY HUB

To address effectively the health risk and protective factors affecting children, a clinical practice must function

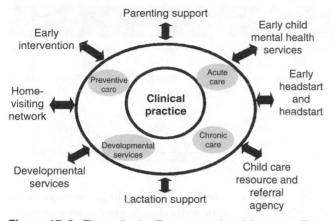

Figure 17-2. The pediatric office as a service delivery hub. The role of the clinical practice in the community. Adapted from Regalado and Halfon.[8]

as a hub or resource center that is effectively linked to community resources. Figure 17-2 illustrates the four key components of primary care of children: acute care, chronic illness care, preventive care, and developmental health services.[9] The capacity of any provider to address the needs of vulnerable children and their families is not only determined by the knowledge, skills, and resources that are available within the clinical setting, but also depends on their ability to link to other community-based resources and services such as Early Intervention Services, child care resources, developmental services and parenting support. The clinical practice is placed at the center of this service organization model because pediatric primary care providers have the unique opportunity to interact with families on a regular basis before school entry.

REVIEWING COMMUNITY EPIDEMIOLOGIC DATA

Review of community epidemiologic data is the first step in assessing the prevalence and distribution of risk in a community, as well as the identification of protective assets. Knowledge about these elements in the life of the community allows the clinician to create more individualized, context-driven assessments, education, and interventions to support individual health development (see Chap. 16).

CONDUCTING ASSET MAPPING

The asset mapping process provides a more in-depth understanding of a community's protective factors. Asset mapping focuses on the assets of a community, including "individual assets (talent, time, experience, relationships), citizen's associations (grassroots organizations, community centers), and local institutions (schools, libraries)."[15] Although a clinical practice may

not have the time or resources to complete intensive asset mapping, an asset focus is vital to identifying and supporting community-level protective factors. Practices may gather information and catalog a list of resources for their patients. Over time a practice can develop robust linkages to community-based organizations (CBOs), allowing the clinic to address health risks and support health protective factors in the community.

CREATING LINKS TO COMMUNITY-BASED ORGANIZATIONS

The community health center has been building their relationships with local CBOs, one of which focuses on developing high-quality in-home day care centers operated in the neighborhood. There is a family day care in Xavier's neighborhood whose provider speaks Xavier's family's native language. In addition, the local library has a free story-time session three times per week including weekends. The local park has a safe play area for toddlers.

Once a clinic has identified community-based resources, the next step is to create linkages to these organizations, allowing for open communication and referrals. The National Initiative for Children's Healthcare Quality (NICHQ) has developed a set of tools and procedures to help practices organize and improve health development–oriented care routines and administrative processes (see Resources).

TAILORING CLINIC-BASED ASSESSMENT, EDUCATION, INTERVENTION, AND CARE COORDINATION FOR CHILDREN WITH VARIED VULNERABILITY

The clinic reorganization strategies described in the preceding create external links allowing the clinician to identify and address community-level health risk and protective factors. The strategies and interactions that are now described address individual and family level risk and protective factors.

The health supervision guidelines outlined in *Bright Futures*[11] provides detailed, age-specific recommendations for surveillance, assessment, and intervention. These pediatric clinical services can be organized into four major categories: assessment, education, intervention, and care coordination. Each service delivery component may be tailored to patients with varying levels of vulnerability. Tailoring assessment, education, intervention, and care coordination to families with varied vulnerability requires adjusting the content (what services are delivered), the context (how services are delivered), and contacts or personnel (who delivers the services) to meet families' needs (see Core Competency).

> **Box 17-2.** Strategies for Organizing and Reengineering the Clinical Practice

- Review community epidemiological data to:
  Identify community-level health risk factors
  Guide development of targeted health service delivery pathways
- Establish external links to CBOs through an asset mapping process

- Position the practice as a service delivery hub
- Tailor practice-based assessment, education, intervention, and care coordination for the three groups of vulnerable children

CONTENT OF CARE ASSESSMENT

> Answers to questions on routine screening of Xavier reveal his language delays, a body mass index of >95%, dental caries, and mild anemia. The family interview reveals that both parents work and are unaware that there is a library and a park in the neighborhood.

Individual assessment and routine screening for diverse problems is important in caring for children. Published guidelines highlight appropriate screening topics and timing for screening.[12] A variety of assessment tools are also available to help define each child's unique resilience and vulnerability. These tools focus on the individual, family, and community context of health development of children (see Resources). For example, the *Parents' Evaluation of Developmental Status* (PEDS) and *The Ages and Stages Social and Emotional Scales*[16,17] are validated instruments that assess children's social, emotional, and behavioral development. The PEDS uses a series of questions for parents about their concerns in different domains of development. Tools such as the Family Psychosocial Screening instrument[18] are designed to identify individual psychosocial health risk and protective factors, including parental depression, parental drug and alcohol abuse, domestic violence, and available help and support.

ASSESSMENT OF VULNERABLE CHILDREN

Underserved children should receive screening that focuses on factors associated with the "double jeopardy" of childhood poverty: assessing the types and impacts of higher levels of exposure to risk factors as well as assessing available levels of resources and health services (protective and health-promoting factors). Because development is so vulnerable to external forces, all children with difficult social circumstances, particularly the poor, should be screened for developmental delay. Using clinical judgment alone only detects 30% of children with developmental disabilities[19,20] and many physicians neglect to formally screen. These facts help explain why minor developmental delays often are not detected until school entry.

In addition, a general epidemiologic assessment of the community, as described, will identify community-level risk and protective factors for all children living in the area. During the clinic visit, the provider may assess an individual child's exposure to key community-level risk and protective factors that have been identified. For example, through the epidemiologic assessment, a provider may have identified that 10% of the children in the community have asthma. With a known high prevalence of asthma and a potential high exposure to environmental pollutants, the provider may choose to carefully assess children who live in high-risk areas for asthma, thereby targeting those at risk before a major asthma exacerbation.

PARENT AND PATIENT EDUCATION

> Xavier's provider understands the multiple risks (poverty, lack of educational opportunity, poor nutritional options) and protective factors (large united family, strong sense of community and cultural identity, neighborhood with active CBOs and an active and engaged child) that contribute to Xavier's health. Xavier is a referred to Early Intervention Services; the local library; a developmentally focused child care center; local nutrition classes; and the dental van. He has his hearing and lead levels tested. His family is given guidance on Xavier's diet, exercise, and reading.

Health visits are recognized as an opportunity for informing parents about their children with a particular emphasis on prevention. When the clinician is armed with specific knowledge of the patients' experiences and potential health risk and protective factors, education and anticipatory guidance can be tailored to address the impact of those factors, allowing for more targeted and rewarding information exchange and educational intervention. For example, a child raised by a teenage parent in a community with low literacy rates and an overcrowded school system is at risk for language delay. A targeted educational intervention takes advantage of a local library with a free story time class, a clinic-based Reach Out and Read (see Resources) program, a highly involved and engaged grandparent, and access to an in-depth assessment through an Individual Education Plan (IEP) at the school.

Employing such targeted and responsive strategies when a problem has been identified also bolster parent confidence in their child-rearing skills and help parents promote the resilience of their children. Family strengths (engaged siblings, grandparents) should be captured as part of the intervention.[9] Similarly, community strengths should be incorporated into promotion of health development. Intervention not only includes clinic-based developmental education, but also demonstration (modeling book reading, and referral—local library, "mommy and me" groups, or parenting classes).

Children diagnosed with or at risk for a developmental disability may be referred to publicly funded intervention programs provided through the federal Individuals with Disabilities Education Act (IDEA). For eligible children these programs provide a comprehensive multidisciplinary evaluation to identify the needs of children and their families to assist in promoting the child's development. Services under IDEA and programs vary from state to state, based on age, risk, and level of potential disability. The National Early Childhood Technical Assistance Center web site provides details on each state's eligibility requirements and program components (see Resources).

CARE COORDINATION

Xavier's anemia improves on iron therapy. The family has not attended a nutrition class, but has stopped by the CBO and will try to attend the class soon. He is going to the library story time once a week and has started developmentally focused day care. His parents read to him daily and he has developed a few more words.

The final component of service for children is care management and coordination. There is an immediate need to have ongoing monitoring and coordination of care for children (particularly vulnerable children) to ensure that they are connected with relevant services and resources in the community. The greater the level of child and family need, and more fragmented the delivery system, the greater the need for effective care coordination. Barriers to care coordination include unclear service obligations (who is eligible and who provides services), how information is communicated to and from referral agencies, and how providers are reimbursed.[21] In addition, families often face difficulty with transportation, finances, language barriers, and confusion about services. The NICHQ Practical Guide to Implementing Office Systems for Anticipatory Guidance can guide the clinic in creating internal capacity for this activity (see Resources).

CONTEXT OF CARE

Once a child has been identified as being at risk for developmental delay, underserved, or having special health care needs, he or she often requires additional time and attention within the clinical practice. Clinical systems can be modified to create more customized clinical care pathways to allow for more effective and efficient implementation of the assessment, education, intervention, and care coordination components that outlined here (see Core Competency). For example, the front desk staff can use different scheduling algorithms to match the intensity of visit to allocated time of an appointment. Similarly, a practice may choose to schedule many of their more complex multiple-needs patients on the same day or afternoon, and alter staffing patterns to allow a nurse and clerk to be responsible for extended care coordination needs. In many regions of the United States, such extended visits can be coded and reimbursed at a higher level of intensity, thereby coupling a more responsive, effective, and efficient delivery strategy with appropriate reimbursement. The child's family may need more frequent visits to allow for medically necessary case management, and assure that they are receiving appropriate developmental services and that the services are having the expected effects. Practices and clinics that care for a number of children in specific school or child care centers also may set up direct lines of communication with designated health personnel at those institutions.

COORDINATION OF STAFF PROVIDING CARE

It is increasingly recognized that high-quality health care is a team endeavor. In this case, high-quality care for the child who is at risk for developmental delay or vulnerable by the constellation of risk factors associated with poverty includes the clinicians, nurses, front desk, and care coordination staff. In addition, there is now good evidence from a randomized control trial that for this group of children, clinical outcomes and practice-based efficiency and effectiveness can be improved by adding a developmental specialist (master's level nurse or a developmental psychologist) to the team, in order to better focus additional attention and expertise on the provision of these services.[22] For children with special circumstances or multiple vulnerabilities, the clinician often needs to coordinate a multidisciplinary team, including subspecialists and/or social work staff.

CONCLUSION

Children are an inherently vulnerable population. Individual-, family-, and community-level health risk and protective factors influence the health development of children. Traditional medical care is individual and disease focused, largely ignoring the contextual factors that impact health. Modern definitions of health call upon providers to reorganize medical practice to integrate consideration of these factors into clinical care if they care about the future well-being of children and the adults they will become.

KEY CONCEPTS IN CARING FOR CHILDREN

- Children's health is the foundation for lifelong health.
- Children's health cannot be understood apart from development and function.
- Social factors are important determinants of health; integrating them into clinical practice is of paramount importance.
- Identifying and bolstering protective factors is as important as mitigating risk factors for poor health.
- Health promotion rather than disease modification alone can have an important impact on individual and population health.
- Children are inherently vulnerable; and poor children, those with disrupted family life, abuse, and chronic illness, are particularly at risk for poor health.
- Tailoring clinical practice to care for vulnerable patients includes thorough community and individual patient assessments, education, interventions, and coordination of care.

CORE COMPETENCY
Tailoring Clinical Practice to Vulnerable Children

Population Group	Care Content	Care Context	Care Contacts
Children in the general population who are at risk for developmental problems	A: PEDS, Ages and Stages Family Psychosocial Screening E: Specific, based on assessment-use family and community-assets (e.g., book reading) I: Tailored to screening; use family and community assets (e.g., library/story time) CC: Link to community-based developmental services/development enhancing activities	Time[a] Increased time for developmental screening at selected visits Number of visits[a] Increased number of visits for children identified as at risk for developmental delay	Personnel[a] Front desk Clinician Back office
Underserved children made vulnerable by risk factors associated with poverty	A: PEDS, Ages and Stages, Family Psychosocial Screening + others as needed E: Specific, based on assessment-use family and community-assets (e.g., asthma education) I: Tailored to screening; use family and community-assets (e.g., asthma home visits) CC: Link to community-based services/health promoting activities (e.g., school-based asthma class)	Time[b] Increased time for psychosocial assessment, identification of health risk and protective factors, developmental screening at selected visits Number of visits[b] Increased number of visits for children identified as at risk	Personnel[b] Front desk Clinician Back office Developmental specialist (MA level nurse or psychologist)
Children with complex circumstances	A: PEDS, Ages and Stages, Family Psychosocial Screening E: Specific, based on assessment use family and community-assets (e.g., specific information regarding medical condition, family education regarding care of child) I: Tailored to screening; use family and community-assets (e.g., early intervention services) CC: Link to community-based services/health–function enhancing activities (e.g., physical therapy, occupational therapy)	Time[c] Maximum time for screening and education Number of visits[c] Increased number of visits to follow-up complex medical/social issues	Personnel[c] Front desk Clinician Back office Developmental specialist Subspecialist Social work

Abbreviations: A, Assessment; CC, care coordination; E, education; I, intervention; PEDS, Parents' Evaluation of Developmental Status.
Time per visit: [a]standard time intensity; [b]enhanced time intensity; [c]maximum time intensity.
Personnel: [a]standard personnel/training; [b]enhanced personnel/training; [c]maximum personnel/training.

DISCUSSION QUESTIONS

1. How does a disease-based focus influence how we think about patients and their care?
2. Why may development be used as an indicator of children's health?
3. What influence can a health care provider have on a child's health development trajectory?
4. What are the challenges to reorganizing a clinical practice to address the contextual factors that influence health?
5. Can you think of examples of health care providers who successfully address the multiple determinants/contextual factors that influence health? How have they accomplished this?

RESOURCES

This web site tracks 10 key indicators of child well-being. http://www.kidscount.org

A Practical Guide to Implementing Office Systems for Anticipatory Guidance http://www.nichq.org

This web site offers tools addressing development, mental health, vision, hearing, and oral health for use in the office setting. http://www.medicalhomeinfo.org/screening.html

The National Early Childhood Technical Assistance Center supports the national implementation of the early childhood provisions of the Individuals with Disabilities Education Act (IDEA). http://www.nectac.org

Reach Out and Read. http://www.reachoutandread.org

REFERENCES

1. Halfon N, Inkelas M, Wood DL, et al. Health care reform for children and families. In: Anderson RM, Rice TH, Kominski GF, eds. *Changing the U.S. health care system: Key issues in health services, policy, and management.* San Francisco: Jossey-Bass, 2001:261–290.
2. Halfon N, Hochstein M. Life course health development: An integrated framework for developing health, policy, and research. *Milbank Q* 2002;80(3):433–479, iii.
3. Committee on Evaluation of Children's Health. Board on Children, and Families, Division of Behavioral and Social Sciences and Education. *Children's health, the nation's wealth: Assessing and improving child health.* Washington, DC: National Academies Press, 2004.
4. Parker S, Greer S, Zuckerman B. Double jeopardy: the impact of poverty on early child development. *Pediatr Clin North Am* 1988;35(6):1227–1240.
5. Gluckman PD, Hanson MA Living with the past: evolution, development, and patterns of disease. *Science* 2004;305(5691):1733–1736.
6. Keating DP, Hertzman C, eds. *Developmental health and the wealth of nations: Social, biological, and educational dynamics.* New York: The Guilford Press, 1999.
7. Kuh D, Ben-Shlomo Y, eds. *Life course approach to chronic disease epidemiology.* New York: Oxford University Press, 2004.
8. Werner E. Protective factors and individual resilience. In: Shonkoff J, Meisels S, eds. *Handbook of early childhood intervention.* New York: Cambridge University Press, 2000: 115–132.
9. Regalado M, Halfon N. Developmental and behavioral surveillance and promotion of parenting skills. In: Osborn L, et al, eds. *Pediatrics.* Philadelphia: Elsevier Mosby, 2005:224–233.
10. Wojtczak A. Glossary of medical education terms. Institute for International Medical Education. Accessed January 1, 2005. Available at: http://www.iime.org/glossary.htm#H
11. Young KT, Davis K, Schoen C. *The Commonwealth Fund Survey of Parents with Young Children.* New York, NY: The Commonwealth Fund, 1996.
12. Green M, Palfrey JS, eds. *Bright futures: Guidelines for health supervision of infants, children, and adolescents,* 2nd ed. Arlington, VA: National Center for Education in Maternal and Child Health, 2000.
13. Mann KV, Putnam RW. Barriers to prevention: Physician perceptions versus actual practices in reducing cardiovascular risk. *Can Fam Physician* 1990;36:665–667.
14. Blumenthal D, Gokhale M, Campbell EG, et al. Preparedness for clinical practice: reports of graduating residents at academic health centers. *JAMA* 2001;286(9): 1027–1034.
15. Kretzmann JP, McKnight JL. *Building communities from the inside out: A path toward finding and mobilizing a community's assets.* Chicago: ACTA Publications, 1997.
16. Glascoe FP. Using parents' concerns to be detect and address developmental and behavioral problems. *J Soc Pediatr Nurs* 1999;4(1):24–35.
17. Squires J, et al. Revision of a parent-completed development screening tool: Ages and Stages Questionnaires. *J Pediatr Psychol* 1997;22(3):313–328.
18. Kemper KJ. Self-administered questionnaire for structured psychosocial screening in pediatrics. *Pediatrics* 1992;89(3):433–436.
19. Surveillance and Screening from the American Academy of Pediatrics' Family Voices Maternal Child Health Bureau, National Association of Children's Hospitals and Related Institutions, and The Shriners Hospitals for Children, located at: http://www.medicalhomeinfo.org/screening/Teleconference.html.
20. Palfrey JS, Singer JD, Walker DK, et al. Early identification of children's special needs: A study in five metropolitan communities. *J Pediatr* 1987;111(5):651–659.
21. Halfon N, Regalado M, McLearn KT, et al. *Building a bridge from birth to school: Improving developmental and behavioral health services for young children.* New York, NY: The Commonwealth Fund, 2003.
22. Minkovitz C, Strobino D, Hughart N, et al. Developmental specialists in pediatric practices: Perspectives of clinicians and staff. *Ambul Pediatr* 2003;3(6):295–303.

Chapter 18
Adolescence and Its Vulnerabilities

*William B. Shore, MD, FAAFP, Margaret A. Scott, RN, MSN, FNP, and
Ellen M. Scarr, RNC, MS, FNP, WHNP*

Objectives

- Describe adolescent developmental stages.
- Describe adolescent morbidity and mortality.
- Identify risk factors for adolescents.
- Describe interventions to decrease risks.
- Identify protective factors.

Jenny is a 13-year-old girl who presents for care accompanied by her mother. Jenny has vague abdominal complaints but denies nausea, vomiting, or diarrhea. Her last menstrual period was 3 or 4 months ago.

Adolescence is the process through which one experiences the transition from a dependent child to a sexually mature, independent adult. Adolescence typically begins with the physical changes of puberty and ends with the successful adoption of adult roles and responsibilities. It is a complex process involving a rapid succession of interrelated cognitive, psychosocial, and physical changes. The assumption of sexual roles and feelings can result in anxiety and concerns about the body, its functions, and disorders. Because of these rapid changes, adolescence itself can be a vulnerable developmental life stage for both adolescents and their families. Although adolescence is a time of physical wellness for most teens, the significant morbidities and mortalities of adolescence are related to high-risk behaviors. This chapter focuses on how health care providers can identify potential problems, support the maturation process and the development of a positive self-image, and address risky teen behaviors.

DEVELOPMENTAL TASKS AND STAGES IN ADOLESCENCE

The overall task for the adolescent is to become an autonomous functioning "other" adult, individuated from his or her family. Adolescent psychosocial development generally is described in three stages: early adolescence (10 to 13 years); middle adolescence (14 to 17 years); and late adolescence (17 to 21 years).[1] Developmental tasks include acceptance of sexuality (which does not necessitate being sexually active), developing future life plans, and beginning to develop life philosophies.

The principal tasks confronting the family with adolescents are to strike a changing balance between freedom and personal responsibility as adolescents mature and individuate. Although most adolescents are able to navigate these developmental tasks successfully and without lasting social and emotional consequences, for those who do not, the adverse effects can persist well into adulthood. Environmental and social factors have a significant impact on the manner in which adolescents and their families deal with these developmental tasks (Box 18-1).

ACCESS TO CARE AND CONFIDENTIALITY

Adolescents are among the most underserved populations in the US health care system.[2] Lack of confidentiality, real and perceived, can be a major barrier to

Box 18-1. Adolescent Psychosocial Development

Early adolescence (10 to 13 years)	Onset of puberty with heightened body awareness and preoccupation with rapid physical changes
	Dominance of concrete thinking with beginning abstraction
	Increasing importance of peer relationships
	Self-exploration with limited dating and intimacy
Middle adolescence (14 to 17 years)	Increased abstract thinking
	Dominance of peer relationships
	For many, sexual experimentation
Late adolescence (17 to 21 years)	Abstract thought processes predominate
	Emancipation is complete
	Individual friendships replace the peer group in importance
	Future life goals begin to be formulated
	Stable, mutually intimate relationships that have a future orientation develop

care.[3] Even with symptoms, a significant number of adolescents forego health care because of concerns over confidentiality.[4] Studies indicate that if mandatory reporting for reproductive health services were instituted, 60% of adolescents would delay or discontinue seeking reproductive health care services.[5]

Although laws vary, federal and most state regulations carry exceptions to the requirement for parental consent prior to providing care to an adolescent for reproductive health, mental health, and substance abuse and emergency situations. Adolescents may consent for their own care if they are pregnant, parenting, married, or emancipated minors.[1]

EPIDEMIOLOGY AND RISK-TAKING BEHAVIORS

After asking Jenny's mother to step out of the room, you learn that Jenny has had unprotected intercourse on several occasions with two male partners, and she is concerned she might have "something." She also tells you that she has missed many days of school and may not pass this year.

Risk-taking behaviors are defined as those potentially harmful to the initiator or others and exceed normal behavior for that developmental phase. They include delinquent behavior, gang membership, dangerous driving, truancy, risky sexual behavior, substance use and abuse, and other self-destructive behavior. The Youth Risk Behavior Surveillance System (YRBSS) 2003 reports that 70.8% of all deaths in 2001 among persons aged 10 to 24 in the United States continue to be related to behaviors that contribute to unintentional injuries and violence: motor vehicle accidents (32.3%), other unintentional injuries (11.7%), homicide (15.1%), and suicide (11.7%).[6] Vehicular accidents, the leading cause of mortality and morbidity among young people,

are increased when driving under the influence of alcohol and drugs, and when seat belts are not worn. Peer influence increases risks taken when driving.

Recent research into the neurology of risk taking suggests that changes in areas of the brain regulating romantic and sexual interests, mood lability, and emotional intensity occur relatively early in puberty, whereas those regulating cognitive development and ability to control emotional and appetitive drives develop more slowly. This "disconnect" between emotions and ability to control them helps explain the increased risk taking seen in adolescence.[7] Complicated social environments may further increase the likelihood that adolescents will engage in risky behaviors. These behaviors are tobacco use, alcohol and other drug use, unhealthy sexual and dietary behaviors, inadequate physical activity, and accidental death and injury, some of which might have been prevented by seat belt use or firearm safety.

Problems in school are problems in themselves—jeopardizing an adolescent's future employment possibilities, for example, and may be indications of other underlying troubles. Important events for health care providers to inquire about include: school phobias, truancy, academic failure, fights, poor concentration, learning disabilities, and school dropout or suspension. School problems may present with a variety of vague somatic complaints. Early identification and intervention of school problems may prevent progression to other adolescent risk behaviors.

SEXUAL ACTIVITY

Adolescents often initiate sexual activity without an understanding of reproduction, the process of conception, or the acquisition of sexually transmitted infections.[8] Approximately one half of all adolescents have had sexual intercourse, and one third of adolescents are currently sexually active, with 7.5% having initiated sexual relations (intercourse) before the age of 13.[9] Rates for African-American and Hispanic students were higher than for white students. The older the adolescent, the more likely he or she is to be sexually active.

Adolescents tend to practice "serial monogamy." They may have sexual relations with only one partner until that relationship ends, which may occur in a matter of days or weeks, and then begin another intimate relationship very soon thereafter. Consequently, 14% have had four or more partners, with older adolescents more likely to have had higher numbers of partners.[9]

SEXUALLY TRANSMITTED INFECTIONS

Annually in the United States, there are more than three million cases of sexually transmitted infections (STIs) in adolescents.[10] When compared with adolescents in other similarly developed countries, with earlier sexual initiation and more partners, adolescents in the United States have higher STI rates than other developed countries.[11]

Adolescents disproportionately carry the burden of sexually transmitted infections in the United States, and, in particular, by those who are economically disadvantaged and non-white.[12] Although public and classroom educational programs on safer sex have led to the increased use of condoms among adolescents since the early 1990s, nearly 40% of adolescents still have sexual intercourse without a condom.[9] Many adolescents feel they can judge a partner as "free from disease" by his or her good looks, reputation, a cursory examination, or the partner's reassurance that she or he is "clean." Adolescents are also more likely not to use contraception as a way of indicating the depth of their feelings for a sexual partner.

Chlamydia trachomatis is the most common bacterial sexually transmitted infection.[9] It is frequently asymptomatic in both females and males, and in women can result in pelvic inflammatory disease and increase the risk of ectopic pregnancy. In the United States, the greatest prevalence of *Chlamydia trachomatis* is in females under the age of 18, possibly because of increased susceptibility because of increased cervical ectopy.[9] Among males, the same age group is similarly affected. African-American, and to a lesser extent, Hispanic adolescents, are much more likely to be infected.[9] The incidence of gonorrhea has declined in recent years, but remains highest in adolescents 15 to 19 years of age.[9] Infection with the human immunodeficiency virus (HIV) is diagnosed in approximately eight million Americans aged 13 to 24 annually, with young women and minorities at greatest risk.[9] Some adolescents may be less concerned about sexually transmitted infections such as chlamydia

and gonorrhea, because they are curable, but remain fearful of HIV acquisition.[13]

PREGNANCY

There are approximately 900,000 adolescent pregnancies in the United States each year, affecting 10% of all adolescent girls (see Chap. 29). More than 90% of these pregnancies are unplanned; half result in live births, accounting for 13% of all births.[14] Rates for adolescents who have become pregnant or gotten someone pregnant are higher among minority youth and those from lower socioeconomic backgrounds.[10] Adolescent pregnancy rates in the United States are significantly higher than those of other developed countries, despite a similar prevalence of sexual activity.[15]

Pregnancy poses physical and social risks for adolescents. Physical risks include pregnancy-induced hypertension, anemia, and excessive overall weight gain.[16] Neonates born to adolescent mothers are more likely to be born prematurely, be of low birth weight, and have three times the mortality of neonates born to older mothers.[17] It is unclear if these untoward medical outcomes are the result of gynecologic immaturity or are related to socioeconomic factors such as poverty, low educational level, or lack of prenatal care.

Pregnancy often affects adolescents whose lives are already in turmoil. Adolescent girls who become pregnant are often poor; attend school inconsistently; live with a single parent, relative, or in foster care; and may have been physically, emotionally, or sexually abused. Many adolescents who continue their pregnancies never finish school and, subsequently, demonstrate lower literacy levels, putting their own children at educational risk.[18] The poverty rate for children born to adolescent mothers is twice that of children born to older mothers, and adolescent mothers are more likely to receive public assistance.[14]

VIOLENCE

Upon further questioning, Jenny reveals that on two occasions her boyfriend had pressured her to have intercourse, telling her that "everyone else" is having sex. She also expresses concern that he is involved with a gang, and that she does not feel safe with his friends.

Longitudinal trends show decreases in most violence-related behaviors between 1991 and 2003.[10] Nevertheless, violence remains a significant and disproportionate cause of both morbidity and mortality in adolescence, particularly for minority youth. Violence-related behaviors tracked by the YRBSS include weapon carrying, physical fighting, experiencing threats, injuries, feeling unsafe at school, and dating violence, including forced sexual behavior. Homicide, the second leading cause of adolescent mortality, disproportionately affects minority youth and is the leading cause of death for adolescent African Americans.[19] Males are significantly more likely than females to carry weapons, but rates are similar across races.[10] Identified risks for violent behaviors include substance use and abuse, aggression, delinquency, academic failure, poverty, family conflict, gang membership, and living in a neighborhood with a high prevalence of crime and drug use.[20]

Dating violence is gaining recognition as a significant problem in adolescents. Data on homicide, the most extreme form of partner violence, show that for the years 1993 to 1999, 10% of 12- to 15-year-old girls and 22% of murdered 16- to 19-year-old girls were killed by intimate partners. By contrast, only 1% of homicides in boys were perpetrated by intimate partners[21] (see Chap. 30). Nationwide, 8.9% of high school students reported being hit, slapped, or physically injured by an intimate partner, with highest rates in blacks and Hispanics. Females were significantly more likely to have been forced to have intercourse than males, 11.9% versus 6.1%, respectively.[10]

SUBSTANCE USE AND ABUSE

> When asked about substance use, Jenny denies alcohol and tobacco use, but admits to trying marijuana several times. She states that her boyfriend smokes "weed" daily, as do his friends.

Although the great majority of teens may experiment with tobacco, alcohol, and other drugs, including performance-enhancing drugs, and suffer few adverse outcomes, those who do progress to actual dependence and abuse can suffer the consequences into adulthood. Initiation of alcohol and tobacco use in adults who develop addiction most commonly occurs during adolescence, and the earlier age of use and abuse often results in greater severity and morbidity (see Chap. 33). Teens with substance use problems are at significantly increased risk for depression, academic failure, impaired family and peer relationships, and ongoing cognitive and psychological impairment.

Trends in adolescent substance use show continuing declines in drugs such as ecstasy, marijuana, methamphetamine, steroids, and LSD, but increases in use of opiate medications. Seventy-seven percent of students have consumed alcohol by the 12th grade, with 46% by eighth grade; 54% of students have tried cigarettes by 12th grade, and 24% are current smokers.[10] Prevalence

rates for use of performance-enhancing drugs are estimated at 375,000 males and 175,000 females nationally, with highest use among football players, wrestlers, bodybuilders, and weightlifters.[22]

Factors that increase the risk of progression from experimentation to abuse are multifaceted and dynamic, and include family history of alcoholism, authoritarian or permissive parenting, lack of supervision, family conflict, easy availability of drugs and alcohol, cultural or religious sanction or acceptance of use, aggressive temperament, low self-esteem, substance using peer group, poor academic performance, and lack of connectedness with school or learning.[23]

> Hank is a 15-year-old boy who comes into the homeless teen clinic complaining of a sore throat and says that he has not slept much recently. He is homeless and living in the inner city. Hank ran away from home when his parents became upset because they discovered he was having sexual relations with men. He is prostituting with men and receiving sex for drugs; he denies he is gay and has had rectal gonorrhea once. His VDRL is negative and he has refused HIV serology.

SEXUAL ORIENTATION

Some adolescents, in their search for a sexual identity, find themselves attracted to others of the same sex (see Chap. 27). For many of these youth, this is a time of great turmoil, not wanting to be "different," or fearing rejection by parents, friends, and peers. The adolescent may initiate heterosexual sexual activity to "prove" his or her heterosexuality to themselves and others. Some experiment with homosexual sex. Gay and lesbian youth have a 50% chance of being rejected by their families, and often are ejected from their homes, making up 42% of homeless youth and 28% of school dropouts.[24] These youth are frequent targets for verbal harassment and physical abuse, both in school and on the streets.[25] They are also at significant risk for substance abuse, sexually transmitted infections, depression, and suicide.[26,27]

> When asked about his mood or thoughts of harming himself, Hank admits that he has had some thoughts of suicide, but does not have a definite plan.

MENTAL HEALTH

Depression is a common symptom complex in the mood swings of adolescents. The 2003 YRBSS found that 29% of high school students reported feeling sad or hopeless for more than 2 weeks. In addition to the vegetative depressive symptoms found in adults, adolescents express depressive equivalents: increased eating and sleep disorders, aggressive behavior, delinquency, inability to concentrate, school problems, promiscuity, daredevil behavior, pregnancy, and increased alcohol and drug use. Parents often need assistance in differentiating these behaviors from normal adolescent behavior and mood swings. Adolescent depression frequently results from changes or personal loss including breakup with a partner, recent moves or a change in schools, and family dysfunctions or breakup.

In 2003, 17% of high school students seriously considered making a suicide attempt, with 8.5% actually making an attempt. Rates were highest among Hispanic females and lowest among African-American males.[10] Firearms account for 81% of teenage (ages 15 to 19) suicide deaths. There are significant increases in suicide rates in families with a history of suicide, affective disorders, alcohol and drug abuse, physical or sexual abuse, and adolescents with prior attempts. Girls make more suicide attempts, and boys complete more suicides. Depression is the most common affect that precedes teen suicide. Clues to suicide include giving away valued possessions, saying good-bye, accident proneness, poor self-image, deterioration of personal hygiene, increased isolation, and talk about attempting suicide. Adolescents frequently see a medical provider within weeks or months of a suicide attempt, often for vague somatic complaints. When the decision has been made, an unexpected elevation of mood can immediately precede a suicide attempt.[28]

HOMELESS YOUTH

There are an estimated 1.3 million youth who have run away or are homeless in the United States. The median age is 14 to 16 years, equal for males and females. They are at high risk for injuries, physical abuse, suicide, and homicide[29] (see Chap. 24).

Medical problems of homeless youth result from their lifestyle behaviors. Both males and females are involved in survival sex and prostitution with subsequent high rates of sexual transmitted infections, pregnancy, HIV disease, and substance abuse. Mental health disorders are higher than peers and many first tried alcohol or marijuana and/or cocaine under age 12, and more than 10% have attempted suicide once.[30]

Accessing health care is difficult for homeless youth. Some studies indicate that as many as 50% of street youth do not have a regular source of health care, 25% reported serious health problems, and many use emergency departments to meet their health care needs. Care is often not integrated among agencies, and homeless teens often feel isolated and have fears with regard to receiving health care.[31]

Common Pitfalls in Caring for Adolescents

- Providers treat teens as children or adults.
- Confidentiality is not respected.
- Risk behaviors are overlooked or minimized.
- School performance is not routinely assessed.
- Parental anticipatory guidance is overlooked.
- Social and environmental context is not addressed.
- Early opportunities for prevention are missed.

SOLUTIONS AND INTERVENTIONS

Parenting adolescents can be stressful for many families, and health care providers can offer anticipatory guidance to facilitate healthy outcomes. Prior to the onset of puberty, providers must clearly lay the groundwork for visits during the adolescent years. Clinicians must inform parents and children that issues will be discussed individually, with either adolescents or parents, that discussions are confidential, except in life-threatening situations, and that adolescents may be examined without the parents present. This is best done individually with parents and teens. Providing parents with written patient education materials can be helpful. Assessing for family conflict and addressing family difficulties play an important role in the prevention of high-risk behaviors. Several studies confirm that the following can be "protective" factors for adolescents, regardless of race, class, or gender: an authoritative parenting style with consistent limit setting, versus authoritarian or permissive styles; a sense of connectedness with one caring adult; involvement with parents; a positive body image; participation in extracurricular supervised activities; non–substance using peer group; and strong school affiliation.[32,33]

The Home, Education/Employment, Activities, Drugs, Sexuality, Safety and Suicide/Depression (HEADSSS) assessment is an effective screening tool to identify adolescent psychosocial risks[34,35] (see Core Competency). Asking open-ended questions at health maintenance visits pertinent to each area can identify red flags requiring further assessment, as well as referral for care, if necessary.

Because school failure can be an early indicator of adolescent risks, it is particularly important to assess school performance at every regular health maintenance visit. The evaluation for school problems includes a complete and comprehensive physical examination as well as family and social histories. Providers should be aware of resources in the schools and assistance for children with physical or mental disabilities.

SEXUAL ACTIVITY

Risks of early-onset sexual behavior should be objectively discussed, with assurances of confidentiality, during early visits and throughout adolescence. The goals of such discussions are to help adolescents make responsible decisions about their sexual behaviors, give accurate information, normalize their feelings about sexuality and attractions, and reduce risks.

PREGNANCY PREVENTION AND COUNSELING

Establishing a trusting and continuing relationship with young women promotes the comfort critical to a discussion of reproductive health needs.[40] For sexually active teens, providers should regularly offer condoms and review reliable contraceptive methods, particularly those that are long acting (see Chap. 29) Use a negative pregnancy test as an opportunity to discuss contraception, and schedule follow-up visits for teens on contraceptives frequently. Discuss and prescribe emergency contraception, the "morning after pill," and/or dispense them to those teens who are not using contraception, or who are using barrier methods exclusively. School-based clinics and organizations such as Planned Parenthood have been successful in providing confidential contraceptive counseling.

If the adolescent is pregnant, an open, frank discussion about options is essential. Outline the options of continuing or terminating the pregnancy in a nonjudgmental manner. It can be a time of great confusion and the provider must assist the adolescent to make the best individual decision, and then support her in that decision. Should the adolescent choose to continue the pregnancy, discuss the need for early prenatal care, and problem solve ways for her to tell her parents and the father of the baby of her decision, as well as means of involving either or both in prenatal and child care.

SEXUALLY TRANSMITTED INFECTIONS

Discuss the risks of various sexually transmitted infections along with prevention and common presenting symptoms and signs. The use of handouts with age- and language-appropriate information is essential. Medical treatment also should include information on how the infection is transmitted, symptoms that might suggest complications of the infection, and how to notify recent partners.

The CDC recommends annual Chlamydia screening for all active adolescents.[9] Other sexually transmitted infection screening should be performed based on geographic prevalence rates and adolescent sexual risk behaviors.

VIOLENCE

The American Academy of Pediatrics Task Force on Violence recommends violence-related assessment include the following: family and individual history of mental illness; domestic, school, or neighborhood violence; gang involvement; substance abuse; family stressors; parental disciplinary attitudes and practices; access to firearms in the home and community; history of fighting; anger threshold; dating violence; and peer involvement in violence-related activities[36] (see Chap. 30).

Anticipatory guidance for parents should include discussion of risks of weapons in the home and their removal or safe storage, use of nonviolent disciplinary action, importance of parental involvement and support, and counseling about youth access to media violence. Interventions with youth should focus on teaching strategies for weapon avoidance, conflict resolution and anger management, and encouraging involvement in productive and safe extracurricular activities.

Adolescents who have been victims of or exposed to violence may need prompt referral for additional support services; providers must be familiar with local referrals for anti-gang/violence and prevention programs. Perpetrators may also suffer depression or post-traumatic stress disorder (PTSD) and need referral for counseling and violence prevention resources.

SUBSTANCE USE AND ABUSE

To assess risks for substance abuse, providers also should routinely ask questions with the HEADSSS measures related to stressful life events, because these are strong correlates of substance use. Substance abuse by the immediate peer group and close friends strongly increases the likelihood of initiation in youth. Ask all teens about their own peers' substance use, including nicotine, alcohol, and performance-enhancing drugs. It is critical to assess family substance use and abuse history, as well as parental attitudes toward use, and availability of licit and illicit substances in the home environment. When providers identify substance abuse, the CRAFFT questionnaire (Table 18-1), can be helpful to validate the problem[38] (see Chap. 33).

Discuss the addictive potential of nicotine and offer treatment to teens who currently smoke. Given their developmental stage, many teens do not respond to warnings about the long-term adverse health outcomes of tobacco use (e.g., lung disease, cancer), but may relate to other adverse effects, such as halitosis, wrinkling, and possible effects on erectile function. In addition to discussing health-related alcohol risks, providers should routinely discuss accident prevention related to

Table 18-1. HCRAFFT Screening Tool

- Have you ever ridden in a **C**ar driven by someone (including yourself) who was high or had been using alcohol or drugs?
- Do you ever use alcohol or drugs to **R**elax, feel better about yourself, or fit in?
- Do you ever use alcohol or drugs while you are by yourself **A**lone?
- Do you ever **F**orget things you did while using alcohol or drugs?
- Do your **F**amily or Friends ever tell you that you should cut down on your drinking or drug use?
- Have you ever gotten into **T**rouble while you were using alcohol or drugs?

    Scoring 2 or more positive items indicates the need for further assessment.

Adapted from: Knight JR, et al. A new brief screen for adolescent substance abuse. *Arch Pediatr Adolesc Med* 2002;156:607.

alcohol, including zero tolerance for driving while intoxicated, designated drivers and a "no-consequences" alternative for parents when the teen may need a ride home.

Teens with identified substance abuse disorders need prompt referral for treatment to programs and resources that specifically work with teens. Research-based interventions include pharmacotherapy, cognitive-behavioral therapy, family interventions, and motivational enhancement therapy, and are most successful when they are multidisciplinary and integrated in approach[28] (see Chap. 7).

MENTAL HEALTH

Evaluation of depression must include a comprehensive and thorough history, with inquiries into any family history of depression or suicide. When diagnosing clinical depression, early referral of the adolescent and family for evaluation and therapy is critical.

Evaluate the risk of imminent suicide by determining the extent of suicidal ideation, if the teen has formulated a plan, and if there has been a recent attempt. Suicidal ideation and any attempts must be taken seriously and responded to with support and clarity. Hospitalize the patient if there are any concerns about an imminent attempt. This is a life-threatening situation in which parents must be notified regardless of the breach of confidentiality with the adolescent. Be familiar with community resources such as suicide "hotlines" and suicide prevention programs. If the youth is followed as an outpatient, there must be strong follow-up with close monitoring of any increases in suicidal ideation, plans, or attempts. Because there may be risks associated with antidepressant medications (see Chap. 28). it is important to consult with mental health specialists before prescribing them.

HOMELESS YOUTH

Youth homelessness may be prevented with early identification and referral by primary providers of families with a history of significant conflict, sexual or physical abuse, or concerns about their adolescent's sexual orientation (see Chap. 24). Providers should be aware of community resources that target this population. Outreach workers and multidisciplinary teams are best suited to work with these patients and their families.[39]

KEY CONCEPTS FOR THE CARE OF ADOLESCENTS

- Treat patients with respect.
- Do not trivialize concerns.
- Identify positive adult role model in patient's life.
- Work collaboratively with others: nurse practitioners (NPs), social workers, and teachers.
- Do not be a parent or a peer.
- Enjoy working with adolescents patients.
- Assure confidentiality of services.
- Assess school performance.
- Support parents and identify stresses of parenting adolescents.
- Express concern and compassion for healthy outcomes for adolescents.
- Become familiar with local resources for high-risk behaviors: substance abuse, violence prevention and gang task force programs, mental health services, family planning, and sexually transmitted infections.
- Be nonjudgmental.
- Normalize sexual feelings and attractions.

CONCLUSION

Reducing vulnerability in adolescence requires a multidisciplinary approach that views teens in the context of their personal characteristics, family, peer group, school environment, and community. Successful adolescent care is based on respect for the emerging autonomy of the teen, while providing for adequate assessment of family and social support, and intervening when necessary. National guidelines exist that extensively outline recommendations for routine preventive services (see Resources). The art of working with adolescents lies in identifying those who are at increased risk for preventable morbidity and mortality and working with interdisciplinary collaborative teams to intervene with appropriate resources. Providers should become familiar with community-based organizations (CBOs), such as Boys and Girls clubs, which promote prevention and adolescent development and can help teens negotiate risky environments and behaviors. Clinics that serve teens exclusively, so that they can feel comfortable, also can be a valuable resource to community physicians. Effective intervention with high-risk adolescents can prevent poor health and social outcomes when they become adults.

CORE COMPETENCY
The Psychosocial History Using **HEADSSS** Screening Questions

H	Home
	Who do you live with?
	Where do you live?
	What are relationships like at home?
	Who can you talk to at home when you are having trouble?
E	Education/Employment
	How are you doing in school (or at work)? Any recent changes?
	How are your relationships with teachers and classmates (or coworkers if employed)?
	What do you like and dislike about school or work?
	What are your future education or employment plans or goals?
A	Activities
	What do you do with your friends for fun?
	What activities (sports, clubs, groups) do you participate in?
	What are your favorite hobbies, books, music, and so on?
D	Drugs
	Have you or your friends ever tried cigarettes, alcohol, or other drugs? What have you tried?
	How often have you used them, and how much at one time?
	Do you ever drive or ride in a car when you have been using alcohol or drugs?
	Does anyone at home use tobacco, alcohol, or other drugs?
S	Sexuality
	Have you ever had a sexual relationship with anyone? With boys, girls, or both?
	How many partners have you had?
	Have you ever been pregnant or had a sexually transmitted infection?
	Have you used anything to prevent pregnancy or sexually transmitted infections?
	Have you ever been forced to have sex against your will?
S	Suicide and Depression
	What do you do when you are feeling sad, angry, or hurt?
	Have you ever felt so sad, angry, or hurt that you have wanted to hurt or kill yourself?
	Have you had any trouble with sleeping, or sleeping too much?
	Have you had any changes in appetite or concerns about eating?
S	Safety
	Do you feel safe at home and school? In your neighborhood?
	Are there guns or other weapons in your home?
	How often do you wear a seatbelt when in a car?
	Do you wear a helmet when bike riding, skateboarding, and snowboarding or skiing?

Adapted from: Goldenring JM, Cohen E. Getting into adolescent heads. *Contemp Pediatr* 1988;5:75.

DISCUSSION QUESTIONS

1. Compare the difference in approach you would use between a 13-year-old and 17-year-old pregnant patient.
2. If you had a 16-year-old pregnant patient, how would you include the father of the baby and her parents to improve her prenatal care and the outcome of the pregnancy?
3. Discuss systems that can improve access to care for adolescents and homeless youths.
4. Describe the multidisciplinary team that would best meet the needs for Hank, the homeless youth.

RESOURCES

www.ahwg.org
Toolbox for adolescent providers

http://www.youthlaw.org
The National Center for Youth Law

http://www.brightfutures.org/index.htm
Bright Futures

www.allaboutkids.umn.edu/konopka/
Community-driven partnerships with resources to develop protective factors and best practices for teens

http://www.aafp.org
American Academy of Family Physicians; Adolescent Healthcare

http://www.aap.org
American Academy of Pediatrics

http://www.adolescenthealth.org
Society for Adolescent Medicine

http://www.colorado.edu/edu/cspv
Center for the Study and Prevention of Violence

http://www.nida.nih.gov/
National Institute on Drug Abuse

http://www.ideapractices.org
Information about the Individuals with Disabilities Act, PL-101-476: with emphasis on the needs of minorities with disabilities

Neinstein LS. *Adolescent health care*, 4th ed. Philadelphia: Lippincott Williams & Wilkins, 2002.

REFERENCES

1. Slap GB Normal physiological and psychological growth in the adolescent. *J Adolesc Health* 1986;7:139.
2. Diaz A, et al. Legal and ethical issues facing adolescent health care professionals. *Mt Sinai J Med* 2004;71(3):181.
3. Bennett I, Cronholm P, Neill R, et al. Confidential reproductive care for adolescents. *Am Fam Physician* 2004; 69(5):1056.
4. Ford C, et al. Foregone health care among adolescents. *JAMA* 1999;282(23):2227.
5. Reddy D, Fleming R, Swain C. Effect of mandatory parental notification on adolescent girls' use of sexual health care services. *JAMA* 2002;288:710.
6. Centers for Disease Control. Youth risk behavior surveillance: United States, 2003. *MMWR* 2004d;53(SS-2):1 www.cdc.gov/yrbss
7. Dahl RE. Adolescent brain development: A period of vulnerabilities and opportunities. *Ann NY Acad Sci* 2004; 1021:1.
8. Kelley A, Schochet T, Landry C. Risk taking and novelty seeking in adolescence: Introduction to Part I. *Ann NY Acad Sci* 2004;1021:27.
9. Centers for Disease Control. *Sexually transmitted disease surveillance, 2003*. Atlanta, GA: U.S. Department of Health and Human Services, 2004c.
10. Centers for Disease Control. *Healthy youth: Health topics*. 2004b. http://www.cdc.gov/HealthyYouth/healthtopics/index.htm
11. Alan Guttmacher Institute. *Teenagers' sexual and reproductive health: Developed countries*. 2001. Accessed November 13, 2004. Available at: http://www.agi-usa.org/pubs/fb_teens.html
12. Chacko M, Wiemann C, Smith P. Chlamydia and gonorrhea screening in asymptomatic young women. *J Pediatr Adolesc Gynecol* 2004;17:169.
13. Connell P, McKevitt C, Low N. Investigating ethnic differences in sexual health: Focus groups with young people. *Sex Transm Infect* 2004;80:300.
14. As-Sanie S, Gantt A, Rosenthal M. Pregnancy prevention in adolescents. *Am Fam Physician* 2004;70(8):1517.
15. American Academy of Pediatrics Committee on Adolescence. Adolescent pregnancy: Current trends and issues 1998. *Pediatrics* 1999;103(2):516.
16. Treffers P, et al. Care for adolescent pregnancy and childbirth. *Int J Gynecol Obstet* 2001;75(2):111.
17. Lenders C, McElrath T, Schol T. Nutrition in adolescent pregnancy. *Curr Opin Pediatr* 2000;12(3):291.
18. Hofferth S, Reid L, Mott F. The effects of early childbearing on schooling over time. *Family Plan Perspect* 2001; 33(6):259.
19. Anderson RN, Smith BL. Deaths: Leading causes for 2001. *Natl Vital Stat Rep* 2003;52:1.
20. Soriano FI, et al. Navigating between cultures: The role of culture in youth violence. *J Adolesc Health* 2004;34:169.
21. Hickman LJ, Jaycox LH, Aronoff J. Dating violence among adolescents: Prevalence, gender distribution, and prevention program effectiveness. *Trauma Violence Abuse* 2004;5:123.
22. Yesalis CE, Bahrke MS Doping among adolescent athletes. *Baillieres Best Pract Res Clin Endocrinol Metab* 2000; 14:25.
23. Greydanus DE, Patel DR. Substance abuse in adolescents: A complex conundrum for the clinician. *Pediatr Clin North Am* 2003;50:1179.
24. Project Yes. *Statistics: Gay and lesbian youth, 2004*. http://www.yesinstitute.org/resources/statistics_and_research.php
25. Huebner D, Rebchook G, Kegeles S. Experiences of harassment, discrimination, and physical violence among young gay and bisexual men. *Am J Public Health* 2004; 94(7):1200.
26. Cochran B, et al. Challenges faced by homeless sexual minorities: Comparison of gay, lesbian, bisexual, and transgender homeless adolescents with their heterosexual counterparts. *Am J Public Health* 2002;92(5):773.
27. Noell JW, Ochs LM. Relationship of sexual orientation to substance use, suicidal ideation, suicide attempts, and other factors in a population of homeless adolescents. *J Adolesc Health* 2001;29(1):31.
28. Riggs PD. Treating adolescents for substance abuse and comorbid psychiatric disorders. *Sci Pract Perspect* 2003; August:18.
29. Klein JD, et al. Homeless and runaway youths' access to health care. *J Adolesc Health* 2000;27(5):331.
30. Rew L, Taylor-Seehafer M, Fitzgerald ML. Sexual abuse, alcohol and other drug use, and suicidal behavior in homeless adolescents. *Issues Compr Pediatr Nurs* 2001; 24(4):225.
31. Geber GM. Barriers to health care for street youth. *J Adolesc Health* 1997;21:287.
32. Blum RW, et al. The effects of race/ethnicity, income, and family structure on adolescent risk behaviors. *Am J Public Health* 2000;90:1879.
33. Tuttle J, Melnyk BM, Loveland-Cherry C. Adolescent drug and alcohol use: Strategies for assessment, intervention, and prevention. *Nurs Clin North Am* 2002;37:443.
34. Goldenring JM, Cohen E. Getting into adolescent heads. *Contemp Pediatr* 1988;July:75.
35. Reif CJ, Elster AB. Adolescent preventive services. *Prim Care* 1998;25(1):1.
36. American Academy of Pediatrics, Task Force on Violence. The role of the pediatrician in youth violence prevention in clinical practice and at the community level. *Pediatrics* 1999;103:173.
37. Denninghoff KR, et al. Emergency medicine: Competencies for youth violence prevention and control. *Acad Emerg Med* 2002;9:947.
38. Knight JR, et al. A new brief screen for adolescent substance abuse. *Arch Pediatr Adolesc Med* 2002;156:607.
39. Van Leeuwen J. Reaching the hard to reach: Innovative housing for homeless youth through strategic partnerships. *Child Welfare* 2004;83(5):453.
40. McKee MD, Karasz A, Weber CM. Health care seeking among urban minority adolescent girls: The crisis at sexual debut. *Ann Fam Med* 2004;2:549.

Chapter 19

The Family as the Context for Care

George William Saba, PhD, and Teresa J. Villela, MD

Objectives

- Describe the challenges of providing care to underserved populations in the context of family.
- Define alternative family structures.
- Define a systems model of care centered on the family.
- Outline key domains of family functioning.
- Describe the process and content of family assessment.
- Illustrate family-focused interventions.

Mrs. Escalante, a 40-year-old single parent with uncontrolled hypertension, lives with her son, Jimmy, who is 14 and has diabetes. Doctors rely on Jimmy to interpret for his mother. Medicaid covers his care, but although she works, she is undocumented, uninsured, and ineligible for Medicaid.

$\mathbf{F}$amilies play an extraordinary role in the ways people experience the world and are the principal channel for the transmission of culture. Negotiating society's demands, experiencing illness, health, and caretaking are all learned within the context of families.

However, health care in the United States is focused on the individual patient and not the family. Increasing evidence suggests that by broadening the focus to involve a patient's family, providers may be better able to understand the onset and development of disease and improve treatment outcomes.[1–6] This chapter addresses how considering the family as the context of care can improve the overall health of families in underserved populations.

DEFINING THE FAMILY

During the last century, the nuclear family—consisting of two heterosexual, legally married adults living with their biological children—was promoted as the ideal family structure. This exclusionary definition has been challenged: it sanctions only heterosexual unions and legally married partnerships, and it diminishes blended families, families with adoptive children, extended families, and kin relationships.

In fact, the traditional nuclear family has never accurately represented the "typical" family structure in the United States. Based on the 2000 census, only 36% (25.6 million) of the 71 million families who responded consisted of a married couple with children. The number of single mother families is estimated to be 9.8 million, and that of single father families 2.1 million.[7] Lesbian and gay Americans living in committed relationships in the same residence are estimated to total 3.1 million.[8] Consequently, alternative definitions of families should be recognized: a family represents a significant group of intimates with a history and a future or any group of people related biologically, emotionally, or legally.[9]

CHALLENGES TO PROVIDING CARE TO FAMILIES FROM UNDERSERVED POPULATIONS

FAMILY CAPITAL AND SOCIAL CAPITAL

All families have *capital* that helps them successfully navigate the world.[10] This capital results from economic wealth, maintaining health, and obtaining a sound education. These areas are interrelated; success in one area often determines success in the others.

A family in disarray may place its members at risk for increased financial problems, poor health, and an inability to function in society. Underserved families often store little capital (economic or educational) because of the interaction of poverty, limited access to health care, and inequality in education. However, they may be rich in *social capital;* relationships that bind individuals together, forming networks of cooperation and reciprocity. Strong family cohesion can provide sufficient critical support that might eventually lead to relative prosperity.

Significant relationships may develop between vulnerable families and those working with social institutions (e.g., social welfare offices, refugee and immigration services, county health departments, the criminal justice system). The benefits of these institutions are counterbalanced by a loss of control, privacy, and autonomy. Also, institutions can have considerable involvement in the intimate functioning of a family and, by assuming familial roles, often undermine a family's sense of competence and self-care. For example, a child with iron deficiency might be treated differently if she is from a middle-class family compared with a poor one. In the first instance, she might receive iron therapy and nutritional counseling. In the other, she and her family, appropriately or not, might face scrutiny from a social perspective (as in screening for neglect).

IMPACT OF POVERTY

In 2002, 7.2 million families (9.6%) lived below the federal poverty level (FPV). These rates differ among racial and ethnic groups: whites 8%, Latinos 22%, African Americans 24%, and Asians 10%.[11] Although the official FPV for a family of four is approx. $19,350 a year, it is estimated that this same family would need a minimum of $33,511 a year to pay for food, housing, child care, health insurance, transportation, and utilities.[12,13] (Clothing, cleaning, school supplies, etc. are notably absent from this list.)

For anyone living in poverty, going to the doctor's office incurs huge costs (e.g., transportation, taking time from work, paying for the visit, paying for prescribed medications). The additional cost of family members accompanying them may prove prohibitive. Families may make choices between paying for health care and meeting other basic needs and may postpone preventive and chronic care, feeling they can only afford services when seriously ill.

ACCESS TO CARE

The financial, physical, and emotional well-being of all members of a family is jeopardized when any individual within the family lacks health insurance coverage. In fact, 17 million of America's 85 million families are uninsured, and one in five families has at least one member who is not insured.[14] The uninsured live predominantly in working families, and two thirds are in families with incomes below 200% of the FPV. Families without full coverage are disproportionately headed by a single parent, and are more likely to be immigrants or racial/ethnic minorities.[14,16]

Lack of insurance makes it difficult for families to receive adequate health care. Compared with insured families, uninsured parents are seven times more likely to delay or not get medical care for their children and not fill their prescriptions.[15] Uninsured parents also postpone their own care to pay for their children's.[14,16]

Some families have partial insurance (e.g., a child born in the United States may have Medicaid, but his undocumented mother may not; one partner with AIDS may have health insurance, whereas the uninfected partner does not). This can lead to fragmented care: some family members can receive primary care services; others must use emergency departments to deal only with acute illnesses. Changes in a family's eligibility for health insurance may lead to disruption in care, as often happens with time-limited refugee benefits or those who work intermittently. An entire family can lose coverage overnight when an employed parent is laid off. Even a middle-class, insured family may be devastated by a critical illness or injury; half of the US families that filed for bankruptcy in 2001 cited medical causes as the chief reason for bankruptcy.[16] These shifts place many families at risk for poor access to care and poor health status; working poor families have fewer resources to supplement such abrupt and costly shifts.[14,15]

EDUCATION

Underserved families often experience poor health outcomes related to their impoverished education, low health literacy, and the inability to communicate effectively with their clinicians. The poorly educated, illiterate family may feel less empowered to take control of their care. They may fail to ask questions or admit a lack of understanding about their care for fear that their clinicians will judge them.[17] Non–English speaking patients often receive care from clinicians who do not speak their language and have minimal access to trained interpreters. Turning to English-speaking family members, often children, to interpret, they may not realize that sensitive information may be filtered, incomplete, or distorted. Clinicians might erroneously judge the family as noncompliant, unmotivated, or manipulative.[18]

CONCEPTUAL FRAMEWORKS FOR PROVIDING CARE TO FAMILIES

BIOMEDICAL MODEL

In the biomedical model, the family plays a minor role in care. This model of care greatly restricts how clinicians think about health and illness, the causes of disease, the focus of treatment, and the roles of clinicians, patients, families, and delivery systems. With some exceptions, most clinicians only consider patients' families when looking for genetic predispositions for disease or for assistance in difficult treatment decisions. Some may even prefer not to interact with family members, because it requires extra time.

The biomedical model also centers the design of health care systems on the individual patient. Examination rooms generally are large enough for only two people: the patient and the clinician. Medical charts are individually constructed and do not link the care of family members even within the same office setting. Clinicians may not realize that their patients' family members also receive care in the same health center.

CLINICIAN'S PERSONAL MODEL OF MEDICINE

In addition to the biomedical model's dominance in the culture of medicine, clinicians bring their own assumptions and values to their practice.[19] These beliefs, a complex product of one's personal family experiences, society's values, and one's professional training, influence all clinical decisions. Consciously or unconsciously, clinicians hold assumptions about what constitutes a family; the degree to which family structure and family members are responsible for the development and maintenance of illness; and what the clinician's own role and the family's role should be in the patient's care.

CROSS-CULTURAL DIFFERENCES

The culture of health care may differ considerably within families, across generations, and among family members who immigrate at different times or acculturate at different rates. Clinicians are poorly equipped to deal with such differences. Although cultural competency has

once again reached national attention, many of the offered educational interventions still rely on stereotyping the commonalities of racial and ethnic groups (e.g., "African-American families expect . . ., Latino families believe . . ., Asian families think . . ."). A more nuanced, systems-based approach acknowledges the importance of shared history within a racial, ethnic, or immigrant group while focusing on the unique experiences of an individual family, its members, and their complex relationships (see Chap. 9). Interventions that educate clinicians about skills they need for this approach are rare.[20]

Common Pitfalls in Working with Underserved Families

- Assuming an individual patient provides a meaningful view of his or her own illness and family functioning
- Assuming a stereotypic view of what constitutes a family
- Assuming the role of rescuer; that is, trying to save a family from the many challenges it faces
- Becoming inducted into a family's unproductive patterns of interaction, rather than introducing new, healthier ones
- Seeing only the challenges that families face and forgetting about their internal strengths and resources
- Forming unconscious assumptions about patients' family dynamics based on personal views of families

---

IMPROVING CARE FOR UNDERSERVED FAMILIES

Many of the challenges to optimal health for underserved families are linked to social, political, and economic forces. Understanding the resources, strengths, and limitations of a specific family can help mitigate these forces and improve the health of family members. To deliver family-oriented care, providers need to accurately define the patient's family and understand how a family functions as well as advocate for social and political change (see Chap. 41).

FAMILY SYSTEMS APPROACH

A family systems–oriented or biopsychosocial approach to care expands the biomedical model to include broader forces that influence health and significant interpersonal relationships.[12,21] This paradigm assumes that without focusing on the complex interactions among individuals, their families, and society, one cannot truly understand the individual. Providers must place people in the context of family, time, culture, and society to begin to appreciate who they are.

Clinicians should find out about their patients' intimate relationships, whether connected legally, biologically, or through shared emotional experience. Families of choice that are not legally sanctioned (e.g., same-sex partnerships, kinship foster care) face special challenges such as not sharing insurance benefits, lacking access to information, and being denied involvement in legal and health care decision making.

On the other hand, some patients may deny having any family or minimize the degree of interaction with family because of previous family strife and estrangement. However, past family interactions may still have profound effects on one's overall health. For example, sexual abuse in poor families has more devastating and longer intergenerational effects than in more affluent families, primarily because of fewer resources.[24] Even when the abuser is deceased or estranged, the relationship patterns in the family can have profound power, and a clinician can miss important information about how these patterns operate.

The biomedical model guides clinicians to examine the relationships between organ systems and physiology. The systems approach, in contrast, broadens the view to explore the relationships between these "internal" systems and an individual's "external" interpersonal and social systems. Examining these relationships allows clinicians to learn more and be more effective in their care than investigating pathophysiologic processes alone. For example, rather than considering only the level of insulin resistance complicating a patient's diabetes, clinicians can explore interconnections between insulin resistance and family and work life. Central to this analysis is discovering how a patient's view of health and illness affects the care of his or her diabetes and what role the disease plays in family interactions.

Relationships are the essence of this approach. A patient's health and illness are conceptualized in the context both of their physiologic and interpersonal functioning. The focus is on discovering how the health and illness of any one member affects the multiple relationships within each family. Even when seeing a patient alone, a clinician can inquire about family as an essential, not an optional, aspect of ongoing care.

Learning how a patient's illness affects the family and how the family affects the illness needs to be determined early and continually in clinical care. To enrich the clinician's understanding, gathering other family members' perspectives is invaluable. Asking family members their views on the patient's condition, how the illness has affected family life, and what they try to do to help reveals the similarities and discrepancies between the patient's and family's perspectives. With this knowledge, clinicians can support family patterns that aid in the patients' care and challenge

those that seem to hinder it. Too frequently, clinicians spend months or years focusing on the biomedical management of a chronic illness only to call in a family member out of frustration. Although this can be valuable, calling family members only as a last resort risks losing early opportunities to build on familial strengths and may even unwittingly provoke stressful family reactions.

CREATING A NETWORK OF CARE

The family systems paradigm attempts to move beyond the patient–clinician relationship to develop a network of care. This network creates a context for a relationship between the "patient–family" subsystem and the "clinician" subsystem. The "patient–family" subsystem can include family members, friends, community support (e.g., church, cultural groups, social clubs), institutions (e.g., social welfare, immigration and refugee health, work). The "clinician" subsystem can include the primary care clinician, nursing staff, subspecialists, interpreters, social workers, and mental health staff. This network of care operates in a particular health care context (hospital, clinic) that contributes its own influences (e.g., treatment guidelines, available resources).

Clinicians should recognize that they too have a "family context" and personal model of medical care. Reflecting on their own assumptions about underserved families, values about family structure, and beliefs about patients', families', and their own role in health care is important. A common pitfall for clinicians working with underserved families is to assume the role of rescuer. This not only can lead to clinician burnout, but also can seriously undermine the competencies of a family. Articulating one's model of medicine can shed light on points of convergence and divergence between the clinician's and patient's and family's expectations.

THE FAMILY AS THE CONTEXT OF CARE

FAMILY FUNCTIONING

Systems and Subsystems

Within a family, individuals group into various subsystems according to their identity or function (e.g., partners, parents, generations, siblings, gender). A family's rules guide interaction and function, telling *who* to do *what, how, and when it should be done.* These rules dictate patterns of behavior that become ingrained in a family's life and in turn reinforce the fabric that holds family rules in place. Family rules govern key domains of family and individual functioning that are important to how a person conceives of illness, health, and medical treatment. These key domains of family functioning include:

(a) boundaries, (b) decision making, (c) conflict, (d) roles, (e) protection, and (f) caretaking.

Boundaries

Boundaries exist between families and the external world and among members of a family. Boundaries protect the family and its members from unnecessary intrusion and allow sufficient interaction to promote its development. All major life transitions (e.g., pregnancy, adolescence, migration, disease diagnosis) require renegotiation of these boundaries.

Boundaries that are too rigid make it difficult for the family to assimilate new information, interact in new ways, and grow. This rigidity can lead to a *disengagement* of its members. Disengaged families require significant events to trigger resonance between members: a child may have to be arrested before parents recognize a problem exists; a chronically ill parent may need to be hospitalized before her family acknowledges that she is seriously ill. Some families who fear intrusion from social and public institutions develop rigid boundaries to protect themselves and, as a consequence, become isolated and unable to access available health care services.

On the other hand, boundaries that are too permeable jeopardize the ability of individual family members to operate autonomously. "Enmeshment" is the term used to describe extreme proximity and intensity in family relationships in which boundaries are not well demarcated. Permeable boundaries allow a rapid resonance of behavior from one person to another, undermining each member's autonomy. Individuals may have a difficult time distinguishing personal needs and priorities from those of other family members. For example, in an enmeshed, obese family, a child might feel it would be disloyal to attempt to lose weight.

Decision Making

Each family has rules that guide which family members are responsible for which decisions, clarifying who has power and authority. One family member may be responsible for decisions external to the family (e.g., housing, earning money), whereas a different one manages decisions within the family (e.g., how the money is spent). How families make decisions about health care (e.g., when to seek care, what treatments should be pursued) may mirror their general decision-making patterns. Challenges to decision-making patterns can cause significant family stress. Consider a woman who emigrated from Vietnam 15 years ago with her young children. When her husband escaped from a reeducation camp and joined them years later, he expected to resume his role as decision maker and she was reluctant to relinquish it, leading to an unexpected familial stress. A system-based intervention would encourage the couple to renegotiate new roles and emphasize the strengths of their bond, which survived the hardships of war and relocation.

Conflict

Families deal with conflict in various ways. Rules guide how they face conflict and whether they choose to resolve or avoid conflict. Unresolved conflict can result when families avoid acknowledging disagreements because they believe that they threaten their relationships. Unaddressed disagreements increase stress and affect overall health. Families reproduce these patterns of dealing with conflict in their relationships with health care professionals, profoundly affecting communication, decision making, and follow-through.

Consider a family (parents and young children) who emigrated from Guatemala. As the children reach adolescence, parents and children differ dramatically in expectations about independence. The adolescents, wanting to avoid conflict, choose not to tell the parents about new values and beliefs. The parents, who do not speak English and mistrust the culture their children have adopted, fear losing touch with them but are afraid to confront them and lose them altogether. This mutual avoidance of conflict leads to greater distance, which all experience as stressful. In this family system, a health problem (e.g., unplanned pregnancy in one of the teenagers) might not be addressed promptly because to do so increases conflict.

Role

Family functioning is increased when members are assigned specific roles such as nurturing, caretaking, maintaining financial security, decision making, and parenting. Roles can be guided by sociocultural values or interpreted idiosyncratically within the family. Family members may or may not agree with a role assigned to them. When someone is sick, their ability to carry out their role is compromised, and his or her tasks need to be shared, assumed by another family member, or go undone.

Consider a single parent whose work-related injury causes a long-term disability. Because she is undocumented, she cannot apply for worker's compensation and has never had health insurance. She can no longer carry out many of her roles (e.g., earning money, caring for her children). Her 16-year-old daughter leaves school to get a job, whereas her 12-year-old daughter manages the household.

Protection

Protecting its members is a key responsibility for families. Overprotection can occur in families whose internal boundaries are enmeshed and can develop in families when members face a serious chronic or life-threatening illness. A desire to prevent worsening of the illness can cause family members to protect the person from any risk, often leading to a problematic relationship. For instance, a child diagnosed with asthma at the age of 4 may warrant a high degree of protection (e.g., ensuring allergen-free environment, obtaining medication refills on time, ensuring daily dosing) that can be readily provided by his parents. However, if these patterns of protection continue into young adulthood, both parents and child will be poorly prepared for essential developmental growth.

Lack of protection can occur within and between families and the outside world. Within the family, lack of protection can lead to abuse and incest. Through neglect, members may be left vulnerable to violence and intrusion from public institutions.

Caretaking

Families develop patterns of caretaking and clear expectations for how family members are to act when sick and how responsible they are for their own care (e.g., to continue with duties without complaint, to be excused from expected tasks). For example, expectations among racial/ethnic groups receiving care in urban, public health clinics vary widely: some patients identify themselves as responsible for managing their own care, whereas others rely on their families.[22] Families bring these caretaking patterns to relationships with the health care team, often expecting clinicians to adhere to these unspoken family rules.

FAMILY ASSESSMENT

Family assessment includes formulating a *"family database,"* a detailed description of the family network; analyzing the *patterns of familial functioning* in the key domains described in the preceding section (i.e., decision making, conflict); analyzing familial *strengths* and *views* on health problems; and organizing and *charting* this information effectively. Assessment is an essential component of a family meeting (Box 19-1)

Family Database

To understand key relationships in a patient's life, clinicians need to develop and maintain a family database. They should inquire who is in the family, who lives in the household, where other key members live, and what is the frequency of contact among them. They should also clarify institutional relationships (social workers, parole officers, school counselors), including frequency of interaction and contact information.

Charting

Genograms and other methods of visually cataloging family composition and relationships can provide useful means for charting information and making it accessible for future visits. Computerized medical records could facilitate this process by allowing individual patients' charts to be linked to create a central "virtual" family record that includes important family data.

Questions may arise for clinicians about privacy and sharing of information among family members. Legal requirements should serve to guide what information should be revealed to family members or outside agencies (e.g., danger to self or others, child abuse). Beyond professional guidelines, clinicians should not share information among family members unless given permission to do so. However, clinicians can help facilitate open discussion and disclosure of important information.

FAMILY-FOCUSED INTERVENTIONS

Reframing

The family's view of how they can deal with the current health condition may be inadequate to help mobilize them toward full participation in the healing process. It may emphasize fear, weakness, and blame. Clinicians should consider whether changing the view, or reframing it, would allow the family to maintain hope and activate resources. Reframing should highlight the family's strengths to promote a sense of control.

Enactment

One intervention to help families learn new ways of interacting is called enactment. This is a structured process to help families experience new interactions around familiar issues, leading to new patterns (Box 19-2).

Tasks

Changes in behavior patterns can be reinforced between appointments through tasks (Box 19-3).

Clinicians should follow up on the outcome of assigned tasks at subsequent visits. This highlights the important message that the clinician takes the task seriously and increases the chances that a family will engage in future tasks. Any outcome of the task yields valuable information: forgot to do it; tried to do it, but failed; tried to do it, and succeeded. Why families forget or "try and fail" can reveal the complex process of achieving change. The results of a successfully completed task can reveal whether it yielded change and whether there were any unexpected negative or positive consequences (Box 19-4).

Box 19-1. Conducting a Family Meeting

- Meet and introduce all members (e.g., family, friends, other agency or health care personnel). Express appreciation for attendance.
- Clarify the purpose for the appointment and some guidelines:

    Overall treatment goal (e.g., "We wanted to get everyone together to help me best care for Eleanor. You are all very important in this process, and I would like to get your ideas on how we can all help")

    Goal for the appointment (e.g., "I want to hear from each of you, including Eleanor, how you think her illness has affected you and what you have done to try to help her.")

    How long the meeting will take and whether you will meet with everyone together for the whole time or in smaller groups

- Include everyone in your gathering of information; be attentive not to exclude children, those who may be reticent, or those who have a language or communication barrier.
- Gather each member's perspective on:

    Domains of family functioning (e.g., decision-making, conflict). ("What is your role?" "How do you handle disagreements?" "When you become symptomatic, what do you do? Do you tell anyone?")

    Family strengths (e.g., unquestionable love and trust, steadfast faith in God, ability to be creative in a crisis, strong network of friends). Families may have invoked these strengths to transcend previous difficult episodes in their lives (e.g., immigration; untimely death of a loved one; experiences of abuse, torture, or war) and are somehow unable to apply them to a current health crisis;

clinicians can ask family members to identify their own strengths and also can reflect to a family the strengths they observe.

Views of illness/problem. Individual family members may all share the same interpretation or vary in their perception, and these variations may be openly acknowledged or operate more covertly to avoid disruption or censure. Ask each member in turn: "What is *your* understanding of the problem?" "Do you think others share your perception?" "What are *you*, in particular, most worried about?"

Solutions. Include solutions that have been attempted as well as those only considered.

- Summarize and clarify the information gathered to ensure accuracy.
- Reframe the illness in the context of relationships and strengths.
- Create enactments during the appointment to experiment with and experience new interaction patterns of behavior.
- Elicit any questions or concerns.
- Develop an agreed-upon plan and clarify everyone's role, including the clinician, in the plan.
- Construct tasks for family members to engage in outside of the office that evolve from the work accomplished during the appointment; ensure understanding of the tasks and family members' agreement to do them prior to the next appointment.
- Determine the timing of the next appointment and who should attend.

Box 19-2. Central Steps in Family Enactment

1. Identify a pattern of interaction relevant to the current health issue.
2. Describe the pattern to the family, delineating the rule-governed sequences of behavior that lead to unproductive outcomes.
3. Ask the family to reengage in the pattern and suggest trying a new behavior to change the sequence.
4. When the new pattern changes how people interact, have the family repeat it either immediately or as a task at home.

Box 19-3. Tasks

- Tie in with the focus of the visit;

Prescribe tasks that:

- Are practical, measurable and doable;

- Are clear to each family member (have each person report his or her understanding of the task); and
- Include all family members, even if some members' role is simply to observe.

Box 19-4. Example of a Family Systems Approach

Jimmy's new doctor at the health center, Dr. Rodgers, speaks Spanish to include the mother. When she asks their respective views on his diabetes, Mrs. Escalante answers that he refuses eat properly and exercise.

Jimmy then answers that his mother is overprotective. He has refused to give himself his insulin injections, relying on Mrs. Escalante to do it (*Enmeshed, Caretaking, Overprotection*). They both feel hopeless that the other will change (*Family's View*).

In further family assessment, Dr. Rodgers discovers that Mrs. Escalante and Jimmy immigrated from El Salvador 12 years ago, after Jimmy's father was killed. They have relatives in El Salvador with whom they talk monthly, and she sends money to them when she can. They live in a house with another family, but are isolated. Jimmy sees a counselor at school "who at least doesn't treat me like a baby" (*Family Composition and Important People*).

The doctor notices that mother and son are emotionally close and have a strong affection for each other. They immigrated together and established themselves in the United States (*Strengths*). Doctor Rodgers suggests to Jimmy that his mother's "overprotectiveness" springs from her deep concern, and explains to both that she sees Jimmy's behavior not as "rebellious" but as "experimenting" with the normal autonomy of adolescence. She challenges them to acknowledge that they are at an important transition phase in their life, and that some of the rules that have helped them will need to change. Mrs. Escalante's intrusion and Jimmy's lack of initiative may have worked when the family was at an earlier developmental stage; but things now need to shift.

Dr. Rodgers strongly assures them that they will succeed given all that they have previously accomplished as a family (*Reframing, Strengths*). She suggests that Mrs. Escalante teach Jimmy to give himself his injections. They try this out in the visit with success (*Enactment*). They are instructed to continue this "hand over" of responsibility as a step toward a new way of being a family (*Task*).

CONCLUSION

The family remains one of the most important contexts through which the world is experienced, yet it does not hold the same place in how health care is conceptualized or delivered. Although this handicaps care for all families, underserved families experience even greater fragmentation and marginalization, given the social, cultural, economic, and political challenges they face; they may not have sufficient "family capital" of good health, solid education, or accumulated wealth to overcome barriers to care.

By introducing conceptual and practical changes into the US health care system and society, clinicians can improve the care of underserved families. Through social advocacy, they can influence the political process to facilitate equal access to services. By shifting from a biomedical approach to a systems-oriented one, they can center care within the context of each underserved family.

DISCUSSION QUESTIONS

1. Describe your personal beliefs and values about underserved families. How might these beliefs and values affect your clinical care?
2. What benefits and difficulties do you anticipate in adopting an approach to clinical care that sees patients in the context of their families?

3. How would you design a health care system based on a biopsychosocial paradigm that views the family as the context for care?

KEY CONCEPTS

Recognize the family as the context for patient care:

- Define this as the context for patients and staff.
- Seek family members' perspectives.
- Involve family members in care plans.

Identify family members and important relationships.

- Remember alternative definitions of family,
- Identify institutional subsystems.
  Assess the key domains of family functioning.
  Identify relevant patterns of interaction.
  Identify strengths.
  Chart family information.
  Reframe problems to improve working out solutions.
  Develop interventions to alter family patterns.

CORE COMPETENCY
Family FIRST: The Family Is the Context of Care

The following mnemonic is designed for assessment and documentation of family functioning in the medical record.

F—Family defined
- Identify the names and ages of family members and others living in the same household.
- Ask about relationships among family members.
- Identify institutions involved.

I—Interaction patterns (observed by clinician or reported by patient/family)
- Among family members
- Between the clinician and the family
- Between family and the health care system

R—Resources and strengths (observed by clinician or reported by patient/family)
- Identify key resources, strengths and coping skills (e.g., problem solving skills, strong support systems, community and/or faith-based resources).
- Assist patient/family in articulating their strengths.
- Provide your assessment of strengths to patient/family.

S—Stressors
Identify past and present stressors.
- Economic (employment, finances; government assistance; housing)
- Abuse history (physical, sexual, violence)
- Discrimination/racism
- Physical and mental health status of family members

Identify major life transitions.
- Migration (adjustment/acculturation; English language literacy)
- Parenting
- Separation/divorce
- Serious illness/death

T—Time
- Identify short and long-term goals and modify over time.
- Follow progress over time and identify areas of progress for family.

RESOURCES

http://www.aafp.org/
American Academy of Family Physicians (AAFP)

http://www.aamft.org/index_nm.asp
American Association for Marriage and Family Therapy (AAMFT)

http://www.cfha.net/
Collaborative Family Healthcare Coalition (CFHA). A diverse group of health care workers from primary and tertiary care settings who study, implement, and advocate for the collaborative family health care paradigm

http://www.familyprocess.org/
Family Process. A multidisciplinary international journal of research, training, and theoretical contributions in the family therapy

http://www.apa.org/journals/fsh/edboard.html
Families, Systems, & Health. A peer-reviewed journal of clinical research, training, and theoretical contributions with particular focus on collaborative family health care

REFERENCES

1. Chesla CA, Fisher L, Mullan JT, et al. Family and disease management in African-American patients with type 2 diabetes. *Diabetes Care* 2004;27:2850–2855.
2. Chesla CA, Fisher L, Skaff MM, et al. Family predictors of disease management over one year in Latino and European American patients with type 2 diabetes. *Fam Proc* 2003;42:375–390.
3. Chesla CA, Rungreangkulkij S. Nursing research on family processes in chronic illness in ethnically diverse families: A decade review. *J Fam Nursing* 2001;7:230–243.
4. Fisher L, Weihs KL. Can addressing family relationships improve outcomes in chronic disease? Report of the National Working Group on Family-Based Interventions in Chronic Disease. *J Fam Pract* 2000;49:561–566.
5. Schor EL. Family pediatrics: report of the Task Force on the Family. *Pediatrics* 2003;111:1541–1571.
6. Wen LK, Parchman ML, Shepherd MD. Family support and diet barriers among older Hispanic adults with type 2 diabetes. *Fam Med* 2004;36:423–430.
7. Fields J, Casper L. *America's families and living arrangements: March 2000. Current population reports, P20-537.* Washington, DC: U.S. Census Bureau, 2001.
8. Smith DM, Gates GJ. *Gay and lesbian families in the United States: Same-sex unmarried partner households. A preliminary analysis of 2000 United States census data.* Washington, DC: Human Campaign Report. 2001. Available at: http://www.urban.org/UploadedPDF/1000491_gl_partner_households.pdf
9. Carmichael L, Schooley S. Is where we are where we were going? A dialogue of two generations. *Fam Med* 2001;33:252–258.
10. Scholz JK, Wolf B. *How health, education, wealth, and family resources are shaping economic inequality.* Accessed on October 12, 2004. Available at: http://www.ssc.wisc.edu/irp/famcapital
11. Proctor BD, Dalaker J. U.S. *Census Bureau, current population reports, P60-222, poverty in the United States 2002.* Washington, DC: U.S. Government Printing Office, 2003.
12. Borrell-Carrio F, Suchman AL, Epstein RM. The biopsychosocial model 25 years later: principles, practice, and scientific inquiry. *Ann Fam Med* 2004;2:576–582.
13. Boushey H, Brocht C, Gundersen C, et al. *Hardships in America: The real story of working families.* Washington, DC: Economic Policy Institute, 2001.
14. Institute of Medicine. *Committee on the Consequences of Uninsurance. Health insurance is a family matter.* Washington, DC: National Academy Press, 2002.

15. Robert Wood Johnson Foundation. *Covering kids: A national health access initiative for low-income, uninsured children.* 2001. www.coveringkidsandfamilies.org/

16. Institute of Medicine. *Committee on the Consequences of Uninsurance. Coverage matters: insurance and health care.* Washington, DC: National Academy Press, 2001.

17. Himmelstein DU, Warren E, Thorne D, et al. Illness and injury as contributors to bankruptcy. *Health Aff (Millwood)* 2005 Jan-Jun;Suppl Web Exclusives:W5-63-W5-73.

18. Saba GW, Wong S, Schillinger D, et al. Shared decision-making and and the experience of partnership in primary care. *Ann Fam Med* 2006;4:54–62.

19. Fernandez A, Schillinger D, Grumbach K, et al. Physician language ability and cultural competence. An exploratory study of communication with Spanish-speaking patients. *J Gen Intern Med* 2004;19:167–174.

20. Saba GW. What do family physicians believe and value in their work? *J Am Board Fam Pract* 1999;12:206–213.

21. Rodriguez M, Saba GW. Cultural competence and intimate partner abuse: Health care interventions. In: Roberts G, Hegarty K, Feder G, eds. *Intimate partner abuse and health professionals: New approaches to domestic violence.* Oxford, UK: Elsevier, 2006.

22. Minuchin P, Colapinto J, Minuchin S. *Working with families of the poor.* New York: The Guilford Press, 1998.

23. Becker G, Beyene Y, Newsom EM, et al. Knowledge and care of chronic illness in three ethnic minority groups. *Fam Med* 1998;30:173–178.

24. Shipler DK. *The working poor: Invisible in America.* New York: Alfred A. Knopf, 2004.

Chapter 20

The Hidden Poor: Care of the Elderly

Helen Chen, MD, and C. Seth Landefeld, MD

Objectives

- Identify the vulnerabilities of the elderly.
- Review the coverage provided by Medicare, Medicaid, and the new prescription drug benefit.
- Outline strategies and resources available to assist in caring for the vulnerable elderly.

Mrs. Lee is a 75-year-old African-American woman. She has type 2 diabetes, coronary artery disease, high blood pressure, and osteoarthritis. Over the past year, she has lost 12 pounds and has fallen twice. On examination today, her blood pressure is 210/83. Mrs. Lee is typical of many vulnerable elders: She is a member of an ethnic/racial minority group and has multiple medical comorbidities and significant health care costs.

T he life expectancy of Americans continues to rise. The 2000 census identified 35 million Americans over age 65 years, a 12% increase since 1990. It is estimated that by 2030, 70 million people or 20% of the US population will be over age 65, with the largest percentage increases among the old-old, or those over 85.[1] The elderly population will also become more diverse: By 2030, 26.4% of elders are expected to be members of minority groups.[2] This growing population of older adults will present unique challenges to their physicians and caregivers because of the vulnerabilities that often accompany aging in America. This chapter describes the challenges of caring for the vulnerable elderly

and discusses strategies to effectively care for this population (Box 20-1).

THE VULNERABILITIES OF THE ELDERLY

Mrs. Lee is widowed and lives alone. She is unclear about the purpose of all her medications. "I have so many pills to take. Do I have to take them every day?" she asks. "They're so expensive." Her only insurance coverage is Medicare.

MULTIPLE CHRONIC ILLNESSES

Age is highly associated with increased burden of disease. Although 20% of all adults are affected by chronic illness, 80% of adults over age 65 report having at least one chronic condition and 52% have two or more conditions.[3] Five of the six leading causes of death in older adults are chronic illnesses: heart diseases, cerebrovascular diseases, malignant neoplasms, chronic lower respiratory diseases, and diabetes mellitus.[4] Chronic diseases also impact quality of life and functioning and can lead to institutionalization in elders. The approach to chronic disease management is well described elsewhere in this text (see Chap. 36).

Box 20-1. Factors Increasing Vulnerability of the Elderly

- Multiple chronic medical illnesses
- Economic insecurity
- Mental health issues (including occult substance use)

- Cultural and educational diversity
- Frailty and dependency (including risk of elder abuse)

IMPACT OF POVERTY ON THE MORBIDITY AND MORTALITY OF THE ELDERLY

Because of Social Security and Medicare, older adults are perceived as economically secure. However, in 2003, 10.2% of elders were living at or below the federal poverty level of $8,980 per year.[5] Although this represents a substantial improvement from the 35% poverty rate observed in 1959, when data were first officially collected, a further 28% of elders are considered "low income," defined as having incomes less than 200% of the federal poverty level. In addition, poverty in the elderly is not equally distributed across the population: Women, those who live alone, the foreign born, and members of ethnic and racial minority groups are at higher risk for living in poverty. Twenty-four percent of African-American and 21.4% of Hispanic elders live at or below the federal poverty level compared with 8.3% of whites. Twelve percent of older women versus 7.7% of older men live in poverty, likely reflecting lower salary attainment and fewer years worked, with a resultant decrease in social security or pension benefits. Therefore, the typical poor older adult is a woman from a minority group who lives alone.[6]

Poverty has a negative impact on health.[7-10] Among other factors, lower-income individuals may have less access to health insurance coverage and by extension health care. Because most of the elderly have health coverage through Medicare, it might be expected that they would be relatively protected from the negative health effects of poverty. However, this expectation is not supported by the literature.[11]

The poor have higher rates of mortality that are not fully explained. An inverse, linear relationship between income and mortality has been documented among Medicare beneficiaries, with the largest effect seen in white men.[12] In a study of socioeconomic status (SES) and mortality among the elderly in four US communities, of the SES indicators studied, low income was the most consistently associated with increased mortality.[13] Another study of elders who reported difficulty paying for food and medical bills at the time of discharge from an acute hospitalization found that those with the highest level of financial disability had a 25% higher 1-year mortality

rate.[1] Inability to meet basic needs, such as housing (independent of race or ethnicity), also has been found to be highly associated with 10-year mortality.[15]

Furthermore, older adults in the lowest income tertile (<$13,000) have been reported to have 60% higher rates of depression and twice the rate of functional limitation, and are less than half as likely to report good or very good health status.[16] The reasons for the health disparities observed in lower-income Medicare beneficiaries are likely complex and may involve the multitude of factors that comprise socioeconomic status (see Chap. 3).

CULTURAL AND EDUCATIONAL DIVERSITY

By 2030, the US Census estimates that the racial and ethnic diversity of the older population will increase substantially. The percentage of both Asian Pacific Islanders and Hispanics over age 65 will more than triple.[17] It is unknown how many of these elders will not speak English, but the challenges for health care providers will exceed the merely linguistic (see Chap. 26).

As a group, the elderly are less educated. In the 2000 census, 80% of adults older than 25 years had at least a high school diploma, and 24% had completed a bachelor's degree. However, among adults over age 75, only 61% had at least a high school education and only 13% had obtained a bachelor's degree or higher.[18]

Formal education is no guarantee that the elder will be able to adequately negotiate the health care system. In studies of older adults, 33% to 44% had marginal or inadequate health literacy.[19,20] Patients without adequate health literacy incur higher health care costs and are more likely to be hospitalized. These is not surprising as elders with low health literacy may have difficulty reading prescription bottles or appointment slips and are unlikely to understand more complex medical documents. Difficulty seeing and hearing may compound these difficulties. Seventy-six percent of Medicare beneficiaries with inadequate health literacy in one study were unable to understand the preparation instructions for a barium esophagram, and 54% were unable to understand whether to take a medication on an empty stomach (see Chap. 10).[21]

HEALTH CARE FINANCING FOR THE ELDERLY: MEDICARE AND MEDICAID

Medicare is the primary insurer for older adults. Ninety-six percent of older adults are eligible and are covered, at least by Part A. This is a higher rate of coverage than that seen in the general population: In 2003, 15% of Americans were uninsured.[22] However, Medicare does not provide comprehensive coverage, excluding such frequently needed services as eyeglasses, dentures, and long-term care. The Congressional Budget Office (CBO) estimates that Medicare covers only 45% of the health care costs for the average beneficiary. The average out-of-pocket cost for a Medicare beneficiary is $3500 per year. This amount is significantly higher than the $2230 in out-of-pocket health care costs incurred by nonelderly households.[23]

Traditionally, Medicaid has provided significant coverage for poor elders and has been the primary insurer for long-term care services. The income requirements are strict and necessitate "spending down" existing personal assets before entering the Medicaid program. There have been substantial pressures to reduce the growth of Medicaid expenditures, and in 2005 Congress voted to reduce Medicaid appropriations by $10 billion. What effect this will have on the health status of vulnerable elders remains to be seen.

Despite Medicare coverage, lower-income older adults may experience difficulties with access to care. In a survey of participants in the Cardiovascular Health Study, low-income respondents (defined as <$12,000 per year) were 2.6 times more likely to report a barrier to seeing a physician as those with incomes greater than $50,000. Those without supplemental coverage or Medicaid were 30% more likely to report a barrier to access.[24] Forty-seven percent of Medicare beneficiaries with incomes at or below 100% of the federal poverty level reported difficulty with getting care or services, or difficulty paying for medical bills.[25] Medicare beneficiaries who reside in poverty areas are also less likely to receive preventive services such as eye examinations, and more likely to have had potentially preventable hospital admissions for conditions such as congestive heart failure and diabetes.[11]

MEDICATION ISSUES AND THE MEDICARE PRESCRIPTION DRUG BENEFIT

Older adults who do not have coverage for or access to affordable medications often reduce their adherence to recommended medications because of cost concerns.

Despite Medicare coverage, a low-income beneficiary may still pay 30% or more of her income in out-of-pocket health care costs, with the bulk going toward prescription drugs.[26] Medications that are not available in generic formulations, those that treat chronic illnesses that may not present with noticeable symptoms such as hypertension, and high-cost medications such as proton pump inhibitors and statins are more likely to be reduced or stopped with predictable consequences for health. Mrs. Lee's question is not uncommon; medications may not be affordable and elders living on low fixed incomes who lack drug coverage may choose to self-ration or even forgo taking their medications.[27-31]

In 2003, as part of the Medicare Prescription Drug Improvement and Modernization Act, a voluntary prescription drug benefit was added to the standard benefit package, to begin in 2006. The prescription benefit has a built-in coverage gap. The beneficiary first pays a $250 deductible and 25% of the next $2000 in drug costs. There is no further coverage until his out-of-pocket costs reach $3600 (i.e., the total spending on drugs reaches $5100). Catastrophic coverage begins at this level and 95% of future drug costs will be covered. This gap in coverage has been referred to as the "doughnut hole." It is predicted that 10% to 15% of all beneficiaries will qualify for catastrophic coverage after reaching the higher spending threshold, but 6.9 million or approximately 25% of all beneficiaries will fall into the "doughnut hole."[23,32]

Some provisions for lower-income adults were included in the prescription drug plan. Under the new Medicare drug benefit, beneficiaries at 135% of federal poverty level (FPL) or less will have no premium or deductibles and will pay a $1 to $5 copayment per drug prescription. The low-income benefit begins to phase out between 135% and 150% FPL. At 150% of FPL, the standard benefit applies. The Congressional Budget Office estimates that 14.7 million older adults will be eligible for the low-income drug coverage provisions. The Kaiser Family Foundation estimates that the beneficiaries who qualify for the low-income subsidy will spend 83% less out of pocket on prescription drugs than they would have in the absence of a drug benefit, but that other beneficiaries will save less—approximately 28%—on drug costs.

What will the prescription drug benefit mean to patients like Mrs. Lee? Assuming that she is taking the recommended medications for her medical conditions, she is likely to be receiving at least six prescriptions, with an average monthly cost of $200 if she is not eligible for any subsidy programs. Depending on her income, Mrs. Lee may save between 50% and 94% of her out-of-pocket costs with the new Medicare drug benefit (Table 20-1). If she were eligible for only the standard

Table 20-1. Potential Cost Savings for Mrs. Lee

Benefit level	Premium/fee	Deductible	Copay	Monthly cost	Annual cost	Annual savings
No coverage[a]	None	None	None	$200	$2400	N/A
Standard Part D benefit (begins at 150% FPL)[b]	$35/month	$250/year	25% copay on next $2000 in costs after deductible: 537	101	1207	1193
135% to 150% FPL	Sliding scale	$50	15% coinsurance up to $3600 total	30	402 + premium	1998–premium
<135% FPL	None	None	$1–5 per prescription	6–30	72–360	2328–2040

[a]Assumes patient is taking six drugs: atorvastatin, benazepril, glipizide, HCTZ, ibuprofen, and metformin at the lowest doses. Costs estimated from www.cdc.gov, www.carefirst.org, and cdn.consumerreports.com/bestbuydrugs. All values on table rounded to the nearest dollar.
[b]FPL, Federal poverty level defined in 2003 dollars: $8980 per year for a single adult.

Part D benefit and had very high prescription costs (e.g., $1000/month), she would fall into the "doughnut hole" resulting in annual out-of-pocket costs of $5578.

NUTRITIONAL ISSUES

Food security is defined as "access at all times to a nutritionally adequate, culturally compatible diet that is not obtained through emergency food programs." In one 6-month period, between 8% and 16% of elders experienced food insecurity.[33] Food insecurity is highly correlated to income. The rate of food insecurity for elders below the FPL was 22.6%, compared with 1.8% of those at 185% of FPL. In addition, the rates of food insecurity were higher in minority groups, affecting 18.9% of African-American elderly and 15.4% of Hispanic elderly. In comparison, the rate of food insecurity for white elders was 3.7%. However, despite the existence of federal nutrition programs for the elderly, only 40% of eligible households participate.[34] Mrs. Lee's weight loss may be related to underlying medical problems, but she may also be limiting her intake because of financial issues.

MENTAL HEALTH ISSUES

Depression

The National Institute of Mental Health estimates that 2 million of the 35 million Americans over age 65 have major depression, and an additional 5 million have depressive symptoms.[35] In primary care settings, the prevalence of depressive symptoms in elders can be as high as 40%. In the long-term care setting, the rates of major depression can reach 30%, with an additional 30% expressing some depressive symptoms.[36] Despite its high prevalence, depression in older adults is often unrecognized and untreated because the symptoms of depression in elders can mimic medical illness or be attributed to medication effects or life events. In addition, elders themselves may be reluctant to seek mental health treatment or report symptoms.[37] The costs of untreated depression are quite high. White men over age 85 have over five times the national rate for completed suicide: 59/100,000.[35] Depressed patients have impaired functioning, worsening of their chronic medical conditions, and increased health care utilization costs.[38]

Cognitive Impairment

The prevalence of dementia in the United States is 3% to 11% in those age 65 or over and 30% to 50% in those over age 85. Dementia is costly, with annual estimates exceeding $100 billion. It is also a common reason for institutionalization and in its early stages is associated with an increased incidence of depression.[39] However, despite being common, dementia is under diagnosed. About two thirds of mild to moderate dementia is unrecognized by health care providers.[40,41]

Substance Abuse in the Elderly

The rates of substance abuse are lower in the elderly compared with the general population. Nevertheless, it is a mistake to assume that older adults are immune to drug and alcohol abuse problems. Older adults are more likely to abuse alcohol or prescription medications rather than illicit drugs. In a small study of elderly patients admitted to a drug treatment program, 72% were treated for alcohol abuse alone, 16% for prescription drug abuse, and 12% for both alcohol and prescription drugs.[42] The prevalence of alcohol abuse in hospitalized elders may be as high as 20%.[43]

It is challenging to diagnose substance abuse in the elderly as the typical DSM criteria may not apply and providers may not view substance abuse as high on the list of diagnostic possibilities. Screening instruments, such as the Michigan Alcoholism Screening Test-Geriatric version[44] and the commonly used CAGE questionnaire have been validated in geriatric

Box 20-2. Risk Assessment Questions for Elder Abuse

- Has anyone close to you tried to hurt or harm you recently?
- Do you feel uncomfortable with anyone in your family?
- Does anyone tell you that you give them too much trouble?
- Has anyone forced you to do things that you didn't want to do?
- Do you feel that nobody wants you around?

- Who makes decisions about your life, such as how or where you should live?

From: Wolf R. *Risk assessment instruments,* vol. 2005. National Center on Elder Abuse Newsletter September 2000. Accessed August 20, 2005. Available at: http://www.elderabusecenter.org/print_page.cfm?p=riskassessment.cfm

populations (see Chap. 33). The possibility of substance abuse should be evaluated in patients with sudden changes in function, unexplained injuries, late life depression, cognitive impairment, or "failure to thrive."

FRAILTY AND DEPENDENCY

There are approximately 1.5 million elderly residing in institutional care facilities, representing less than 5% of the total population over age 65.[45] Although the majority of community-dwelling elders are functionally independent, aging is associated with an increased need for assistance. Eight percent of those 65 to 69 years of age reported needing assistance because of a disability, in contrast to 35% of those 85 and older. Much of the care giving for disabled elders is provided informally in the community, often by a spouse or adult daughter. The 1997 National Alliance for Caregiving/AARP survey revealed that on average, informal caregivers provide 19 hours per week of care with 20% providing 40 hours or more per week. Using a low-to-moderate hourly wage of $8.18, the cost of this informal care giving is estimated to be $196 billion, much of it uncompensated.[46] Without informal care giving many disabled elders would require formal services or institutionalization; hence, the adage that many elderly patients are "one caregiver away" from placement in a nursing home.

As increasing age is associated with increasing dependency, frail and disabled elders are also at higher risk for victimization and abuse (see Chap. 30). Elder abuse remains under-recognized and under-reported, but in all states, health care providers are required to report observed or suspected abuse of dependent adults. Types of abuse may include: physical, sexual, psychological, mental, financial, and neglect, including self-neglect. There are no well-validated instruments for screening for elder abuse.[47] Dependent elders should be evaluated for abuse if there are unexplained injuries or delays in seeking medical care, changes in

affect, evidence of malnutrition or dehydration, or evidence of caregiver stress (Box 20-2). (see Chap. 30).

Common Pitfalls in Caring for the Elderly

- Understanding benefits is difficult for patients and providers.
- Benefits for the elderly are not comprehensive.
- Lack of appropriate nutrition is common.
- Mental illness, substance use and dementia go undetected.
- Many barriers to health care and understanding including physical and mental limitations, culture, literacy, and education are particularly significant in the elderly.
- Multiple challenges and limited reimbursement reduce the numbers of providers willing to care for the elderly.

STRATEGIES FOR CARING FOR VULNERABLE ELDERS

The vulnerable elderly present multiple challenges to health care providers. As noted, they are medically and socially complex with chronic diseases that often cannot be cured. Often, the provider is caring for the family or the caregivers in addition to the patient. It is also a truism of geriatric medicine that the mortality rate is unfailingly 100% with a significant proportion of elders relinquishing their ability to have meaningful interactions some time before death. Given these challenges, many physicians feel ill-equipped to care for these patients,[48] lacking the experience, knowledge, or practice infrastructure needed to coordinate the care required by frail elders.[49] Combined with the diminishing reimbursement from Medicare and Medicaid, short visit times, and expanding diagnostic and therapeutic options, it is little wonder that many physicians are limiting the number of older patients in their practices.[50]

REFRAMING PRACTICE

Geriatric Syndromes and Functional Assessment

If the purpose of the medical visit can be reframed as one of maximizing function as opposed to "curing" disease, the outcome can be satisfying for both the health care provider and the patient, with improved quality of life for the patient and caregivers. Many older patients present with multiple signs and symptoms that are related to several organ systems and impaired functioning in multiple domains, and defy single unifying diagnoses. These conditions have been classified as *geriatric syndromes* and include such commonly encountered problems as dizziness, falls, incontinence, and pressure ulcers. Naming a condition a "geriatric syndrome" does not imply that the provider no longer has an obligation to seek out underlying pathologic or potentially reversible disease states. It simply emphasizes the equal importance of assessing the condition's impact on the patient's level of function and mitigating existing risk factors in order to maximize function. Among others, these risks can include polypharmacy, environmental obstacles, and sensory impairments.

In assessing function it can be useful to define the nature of the functional impairment. Traditionally function has been described in terms of activities of daily living, separating out those requiring personal care assistance from those that are necessary to live totally independently. An elder's baseline functional status can be used to guide treatment, for example, or the prescription of adaptive devices. Changes in function can be followed over time and may alert a provider to the likelihood not only of decline requiring placement, but also of caregiver stress (Box 20-3).

The numerous functional domains that can be assessed—*continence, falls and immobility, hearing and vision, depression and dementia, abuse, and nutrition to name a few*—may seem daunting within the confines of the "15-minute" visit, but there are simple tools that can help the primary care provider effectively screen geriatric patients. Indeed, these tools do not have to be administered by the provider but can be delegated to other office staff. The authors offer one tool, originally developed and validated by Moore and Siu[51] and later modified by Lachs and Johnston (see Core Competency)

Focus on Goals

The typical primary care patient presents for episodic acute care, chronic disease management, and preventive services. As patients age, the variety and number of recommended interventions for both health maintenance and disease management can become quite complex and intimidating to both providers and patients. Although Americans are living longer, research to guide evidence-based practice, particularly for the "old-old" (over 85), is lacking. What then is the conscientious provider to do?

Regarding preventive services, one approach would be to recognize the effect of life expectancy on potential benefit. In general, the patient's reasonable life expectancy should be at least 5 years in order to benefit from many screening tests performed for prevention. A healthy 75-year-old woman would be expected to live another 12 years and thus, should be considered a reasonable candidate for interventions such as colon cancer screening. However, if she had other comorbidities such as moderately severe congestive heart failure or emphysema, it would be unlikely that she would live long enough to benefit from screening and should not be subjected to testing (see Table 20-2).[52]

Table 20-2. Average Life Expectancy by Age/Gender (for European Americans)

Age	Gender	50th Percentile	25th to 75th Percentile
70	Female	15.7 years	9.5–21.3
	Male	12.4 years	6.7–18
75	Female	11.9 years	6.8–17
	Male	9.3 years	4.9–14.2
85	Female	5.9 years	2.9–9.6
	Male	4.7	2.2–7.9

Walter LC, Covinsky KE Cancer screening in elderly patients: A framework for individualized decision making. *JAMA* 2001;285:2750–2756.

Box 20-3. Activities of Daily Living

Basic ADLs (BADLs)	Instrumental ADLs (IADLs)
Dressing	Shopping
Eating	Housework
Ambulating	Accounting
Transfers	Food preparation
Toileting/continence	Transportation
Hygiene	Telephone use
	Taking medications

However, even for healthy elders, a principal consideration should be the patient's values and goals for the remainder of her life.[53] It is important for the health care provider to elicit and document the elder's views regarding future goals and what constitutes an acceptable quality of life. At times, this requires the involvement of the family or the caregivers, particularly in cultures for which decision making is a shared responsibility. Knowledge of the patient's goals will inform decision making about screening and diagnostic tests and treatments. Also, near the end of life, understanding the patient's goals of care is ultimately more important than making a determination about cardiopulmonary resuscitation or intubation.

Resources to Assist in the Care of the Vulnerable Elderly

Mrs. Lee suffers a stroke and is admitted to the hospital. Her nephew is willing to help, but is concerned that he won't be able to afford the kind of care his aunt will need. The hospital social worker helps Mrs. Lee apply for Medicaid and schedules a home safety evaluation. She is also referred for care management. In conjunction with her primary care physician, the care manager arranges for Mrs. Lee to attend an adult day health care program where she is able to receive social support, meals, and physical therapy.

The patient and her family may look to the primary care provider for assistance with issues that are not traditionally medical in nature, but that may have greater impact on health and quality of life than many medical interventions. As physicians and other health care providers face caring for increasingly medically complex patients with fewer available resources, it is important to acknowledge the need for a team approach in the care of the elderly, particularly those with complex medical and psychosocial issues. As the elderly poor are at risk for worse health outcomes, existing resources that can assist health care providers in caring for their vulnerable older patients are reviewed here.

Care Management Programs

Geriatric care management is a relatively new field whose providers (often nurses or social workers) coordinate and oversee health and personal care for older adults. Private geriatric care management is unregulated, costly, and not covered by Medicare or insurance. For the low-income elderly, privately funded geriatric care management is beyond their financial reach. However, some states have opted to use Medicaid dollars to fund targeted case management for some elderly populations. In California, the *Multipurpose Senior*

Service Program (MSSP) provides care management for Medicaid eligible frail elderly who are at risk for institutionalization. In addition to care coordination, the services covered by MSSP include adult day programs, meal services, chore and personal care services, and transportation.

Elderly Nutrition Programs

Congregate and home-delivered meals are available through Title III–funded nutrition programs. There is no required means testing, although the programs target low-income and disabled seniors. There may be a small copayment or requested donation for each meal, although most elderly nutrition programs (ENPs) will not turn anyone away for inability to pay, and there is generally a waiting list for home-delivered meals. The Administration on Aging estimates that 3.1 million elders participate in ENP and receive 40% to 50% of required nutrients through the programs.

Provision of All-Inclusive Care for the Elderly (PACE) Programs

Provision of all-inclusive care for the elderly (PACE) programs target those elders covered under Medicare and Medicaid waiver programs; there is limited access for those with higher incomes. PACE provides inclusive care for enrolled patients who would otherwise qualify for nursing home level of care. Patients attend medically supervised, structured programs daily but return home at night. They also may receive in-home personal care services as well as respite care if needed.[54] Because PACE programs are capitated, the enrolled patients must agree to have all of their care assumed by the PACE program and must leave their current primary care providers. This is a barrier to PACE enrollment for some patients. To address this issue, some PACE programs have allowed limited numbers of patients to continue to be cared for by their community physicians.

Pharmaceutical Assistance Programs

Nearly 75 pharmaceutical companies offer free or reduced cost medications to patients who meet the income criteria. Fifty-three percent of the 200 most commonly prescribed medications are available through pharmaceutical assistance programs (PAPs).[55,56] The paperwork associated with each program can be cumbersome, requiring a significant degree of literacy and the willingness to disclose personal income information, often on a monthly basis. These factors may necessitate the use of health system personnel, thus increasing costs and limiting the utility of these programs. However, at one medical center, the initiation of a PAP for indigent oncology patients resulted in significant cost avoidance despite requiring the supervision of pharmacy

Table 20-3. Resources for Seniors

Resource	Services available	Cost/coverage
Senior centers	Activities, congregate meals	Free or small donation for meals ($2 to $5)
Adult day health centers	Skilled nursing, PT/OT, social activities, meals	Medicaid, self-pay, some with sliding scale
Home health aide	Personal care	$10+/hr, self-pay, Medicaid, Medicare if linked to skilled need
Respite care	Nursing home level care	Self-pay, limited Medicaid, Veterans Affairs benefits, Medicare if linked to hospice
Meals on Wheels	Delivered meals	$3 to $5/meal "donation"
Transportation	Van/taxi service	Self-pay, may be locally subsidized
Support groups	Peer support	Free
Friendly visitors	Volunteer social visits	Free

personnel.[57] Several web sites exist, some sponsored by the pharmaceutical industry that assist patients in applying for these programs. Some sites distribute the information to multiple companies after the completion of one electronic form. This may expand access to these programs for patients with access to the Internet.

Community Resources

Table 20-3 provides a partial list of community resources available to elderly patients.

CONCLUSION

Despite the financial gains achieved by older Americans in the last century, many continue to face significant health care costs that can lead to financial insecurity. As the American population continues to age, increased stress will be placed on a health care system that may not be adequately resourced or fiscally prepared to care for a substantially older, frailer, population. It remains to be seen if Medicare reforms will substantially improve the economic well-being and health of elders. In order to meet the needs of the elderly population who live in poverty, health care providers will need to be aware of the multidisciplinary resources that exist in their communities that can assist them in caring for this especially vulnerable population of older adults.

KEY CONCEPTS IN CARING FOR THE ELDERLY

- Use a patient- and family-centered approach.
- Focus on function and on goals.
- Involve caregivers.
- Ask specifically about geriatric syndromes, e.g., falls, incontinence, dementia, depression.
- Use available assessment tools.
- Use life expectancy to guide prevention efforts.
- Get help! Caring for frail elders often requires a multidisciplinary, team approach.
- Connect patients with community based resources.

CORE COMPETENCY

The Simple Geriatric Screen

History items	Action
Have you had any falls in the last year?	• Gait assessment • Osteoporosis and injury risk assess • Home evaluation • Physical therapy
Do you have trouble with stairs, lighting, bathroom, or other home hazards?	• Home evaluation • Physical therapy
Do you have a problem with urine leaks or accidents?	• Rule out reversible causes • History (stress, urge) • Physical examination • PVR
Over the past month, have you often been bothered by feeling sad, depressed, or hopeless? During the past month, have you often been bothered by little interest or pleasure in doing things?	• GDS or other depression assessment
Do you ever feel unsafe where you live?	• Explore further • Social work
Does anyone threaten you or hurt you?	• APS

Review medications that patient brought in	• Consider simplification
Key concerns:	• Medi-set or other aid
• Confusion about medications	• Consider home visit
• >5 Medications	
• Does not bring in	
• Also ask about herbs, vitamins, supplements, and nonprescription medications	
Is pain a problem for you?	• Evaluate

Do you have any problems with any of the following areas? Who assists? Do you use any devices? (for "yes" answers, consider causes, social services and/or home eval/PT/OT)

Doing strenuous activities like fast walking/bicycling?	Yes___	No___
Cooking	Yes___	No___
Shopping	Yes___	No___
Doing heavy housework like washing windows	Yes___	No___
Doing laundry	Yes___	No___
Getting to a place beyond walking distance by driving or taking a bus	Yes___	No___
Managing finances	Yes___	No___
Getting out of bed/transfer	Yes___	No___
Getting dressed	Yes___	No___
Toilet	Yes___	No___
Eating	Yes___	No___
Walking	Yes___	No___
Bathing (sponge bath, tub, or shower)	Yes___	No___

Physical Examination Items (may be performed by nursing staff in some settings)	*Abnormal*	*Action*
Weight/BMI And ask "have you lost weight? If so, how much?	BMI <21 Loss of 5% since last visit or 10% over one year	Alert provider • Nutrition evaluation • Consider medical, dental, social work evaluation
Jaeger Card or Snellen eye chart; test each eye (with glasses)	Can not read 20/40	Alert provider or refer
Whisper short sentence @ 6 to 12 inches (out of visual view) or audioscopy	Unable to hear	• Cerumen check • Retest/refer • Hearing handicap inventory
Name three objects/re-ask in 5 minutes	Misses any or unable	MMSE or other
Clock draw test		
"Rise from your chair (do not use arms to get up), walk 10 feet, turn, walk back to the chair and sit down."	Observed problem or unable to complete in <15 seconds	• Further gait and neurologic examination • Home evaluation and physical therapy
"Touch the back of your head with your hands." "Pick up the pencil."	Unable to do either	Further examination, consider OT
(Remember to ask about the three items!)		
Other areas of concern: caregiver stress, alcohol, social isolation, exercise, driving, advance directives, and health care wishes.		

Modified by C. Bree Johnston from: Lachs MS, Feinstein AR, et al. A simple procedure for general screening for functional disability in elderly patients. *Ann Intern Med* 1990;112:699–706; Moore AA, Siu AL. Screening for common problems in ambulatory elderly: clinical confirmation of a screening instrument. *Am J Med* 1996;100:438–443. Adapted and reproduced with permission from C. Bree Johnston.

DISCUSSION QUESTIONS

1. Using a patient or family member, calculate the cost of the Medicare drug benefit. Will the drug benefit result in savings?

2. Describe the resources that are available in your community for elders like Mrs. Lee.

3. If Mrs. Lee were not eligible for Medicaid, what other resources would be available?

RESOURCES

http://www.aarp.org
The web site of the American Association of Retired Persons, this site contains consumer-directed information and resources on general topics related to aging.

http://nihseniorhealth.gov
A NIH web site geared toward providing health information on topics of interest to seniors, this site has both verbal and large text options.

www.rxassist.org
RxAssist is a nonprofit site sponsored by Volunteers in Health Care, which is funded by the Robert Wood Johnson Foundation. RxAssist maintains a searchable database with information about pharmaceutical assistance programs.

www.alz.org
Alzheimer's Association: 1-800-660-1993

www.caregiver.org
Caregiver Resource Centers: 1-800-445-8106

http://www.elderabusecenter.org/default.cfm?p=statehotlines.cfm
Elder abuse: Contact local adult protective services, or for local elder abuse hotline numbers

www.AOA.gov
The US Administration on Aging maintains a comprehensive website at which provides information on resources of interest to elders, their families/caregivers, and health professionals. For specific information regarding local resources, the website provides links to state and area aging agencies as well as contact information for the nationwide Eldercare Locator service.

http://www.hrsa.gov/tpr/webcast-Sept1-2004-Case-Management-Services-by-State040825.htm
As of February 2005, a list of states with targeted case management services.

REFERENCES

1. Hetzel L, Smith A. *The 65 years and over population: Census 2000 Brief.* US Census Bureau 2001. Accessed 11/22/04. Available at: http://www.census.gov/prod/2001pubs/c2kbr01-10.pdf
2. *A profile of older Americans: 2003.* Administration on Aging. Accessed 1/15/05, 2005. Available at: http://www.aoa.gov/prof/Statistics/profile/2003/profiles2003.asp
3. Friedland RB. *Multiple chronic conditions.* Accessed May 2005. Center on an Aging Society, Georgetown University. Available at: http://ihcrp.georgetown.edu/agingsociety/pubhtml/multiple/multiple.html
4. *Older Americans 2004: Key indicators of well-being.* Federal Interagency Forum on Aging-Related Statistics. Accessed May 2005. Available at: http://www.agingstats.gov/chartbook2004/healthstatus.html
5. DeNavas-Walt C, Proctor BD, Mills RJ. *Income, poverty, and health insurance coverage in the United States: 2003.* US Census Bureau. Accessed 11/23/04, 2004. Available at: http://www.census.gov/prod/2004pubs/p60-226.pdf
6. Smith D. The older population in the United States: March 2002. Current Population Reports, US Census Bureau, 2003. Accessed August 20, 2005. Available at: http://www.census.gov/prod/2003pubs/p20-546.pdf
7. Fiscella K, Franks P. Poverty or income inequality as predictor of mortality: Longitudinal cohort study. *BMJ* 1997; 314:1724–1727.
8. Lynch JW, Kaplan GA, Shema SJ. Cumulative impact of sustained economic hardship on physical, cognitive, psychological, and social functioning. *N Engl J Med* 1997; 337: 1889–1895.
9. Stronks K, van de Mheen HD, Mackenbach JP. A higher prevalence of health problems in low income groups: Does it reflect relative deprivation? *J Epidemiol Commun Health* 1998;52:548–557.
10. Ware JE Jr, Bayliss MS, Rogers WH, et al. Differences in 4-year health outcomes for elderly and poor, chronically ill patients treated in HMO and fee-for-service systems. Results from the Medical Outcomes Study. *JAMA* 1996;276:1039–1047.
11. Asch SM, Sloss EM, Hogan C, et al. Measuring underuse of necessary care among elderly Medicare beneficiaries using inpatient and outpatient claims. *JAMA* 2000;284:2325–2333.
12. Gornick ME, Eggers PW, Reilly TW, et al. Effects of race and income on mortality and use of services among Medicare beneficiaries. *N Engl J Med* 1996;335;11:791–799.
13. Bassuk SS, Berkman LF, Amick BC, 3rd. Socioeconomic status and mortality among the elderly: findings from four US communities. *Am J Epidemiol* 2002;155:520–533.
14. Li AK, Covinsky KE, Sands LP, et al. Reports of financial disability predict functional decline and death in older patients discharged from the hospital. *J Gen Intern Med* 2005;20:168–174.
15. Blazer DG, Sachs-Ericsson N, Hybels CF. Perception of unmet basic needs as a predictor of mortality among community-dwelling older adults. *Am J Public Health* 2005;95:299–304.
16. von dem Knesebeck O, Luschen G, Cockerham WC, et al. Socioeconomic status and health among the aged in the United States and Germany: A comparative cross-sectional study. *Soc Sci Med* 2003;57:1643–1652.
17. *Addressing diversity.* Administration on Aging. Accessed 3/15/05, 2005. Available at: http://www.aoa.gov/prof/adddiv/adddiv/asp
18. Bauman KJ, Graf NL. *Educational Attainment 2000.* US Census Bureau. Accessed 6/1/05, 2005. Available at: http://www.census.gov/prod/2003pubs/c2kbr-24.pdf
19. Baker DW, Gazmararian JA, Williams MV, et al. Functional health literacy and the risk of hospital admission among Medicare managed care enrollees. *Am J Public Health* 2002; 92(8):1278–1283.
20. Howard DH, Gazmararian J, Parker RM. The impact of low health literacy on the medical costs of Medicare managed care enrollees. *Am J Med* 2005;118:371–377.
21. Gazmararian JA, Baker DW, Williams MV, et al. Health literacy among Medicare enrollees in a managed care organization. *JAMA* 1999;281:545–551.
22. *Health care and the 2004 elections: the uninsured.* Henry J. Kaiser Family Foundation. 9/14/04. Accessed 11/24/04. Available at: www.kff.org/unisured/7155.cfm

23. Mays J, M Brenner, T Neuman, et al. *Estimates of Medicare beneficiaries' out-of pocket drug spending in 2006. Modeling the impact of the MMA. Executive Summary.* 11/24/04. Accessed 11/30/04. Available at:http://www.kff.org/medicare/loader.cfm?url=/commonspot/security/getfile.cfm&PageID=48943

24. Fitzpatrick AL, Powe NR, Cooper LS, et al. Barriers to health care access among the elderly and who perceives them. *Am J Public Health* 2004;94:1788–1794.

25. Neuman P, Rowland D, Kitchman M, et al. Understanding the diverse needs of the Medicare population: Implications for Medicare reform. *J Aging Soc Policy* 1999;10:25–50.

26. Crystal S, Johnson RW, Harman J, et al. Out-of-pocket health care costs among older Americans. *J Gerontol B Psychol Sci Soc Sci* 2000;55:S51–62.

27. Federman AD, Adams AS, Ross-Degnan D, et al. Supplemental insurance and use of effective cardiovascular drugs among elderly medicare beneficiaries with coronary heart disease. *JAMA* 2001;286:1732–1739.

28. Mojtabai R, Olfson M. Medication costs, adherence, and health outcomes among Medicare beneficiaries. *Health Aff (Millwood)* 2003;22:220–229.

29. Soumerai SB, Ross-Degnan D. Inadequate prescription-drug coverage for Medicare enrollees—a call to action. *N Engl J Med* 1999;340:722–728.

30. Steinman MA, Sands LP, Covinsky KE. Self-restriction of medications due to cost in seniors without prescription coverage. *J Gen Intern Med* 2001;16:793–799.

31. Tseng CW, Brook RH, Keeler E, et al. Cost-lowering strategies used by medicare beneficiaries who exceed drug benefit caps and have a gap in drug coverage. *JAMA* 2004;292:952–960.

32. Moon M. *How beneficiaries fare under the new Medicare drug bill.* Commonwealth Fund Issue Brief, 2004June 2004. Accessed on: August 20, 2005. Available at: http://www. cmwf.org/publications/publications_show.htm?doc_id= 227453

33. Wellman NS, Weddle DO, Kranz S, et al. Elder insecurities: Poverty, hunger, and malnutrition. *J Am Diet Assoc* 1997;97;10 Suppl 2:S120–122.

34. Nord M. Food security rates are high for elderly households. *FoodReview* 2002;25:19–24.

35. *Older adults: Depression and suicide facts.* Revised May 2003. Accessed 6/1/05, 2005. Available at: http://www.nimh.nih.gov/HealthInformation/elderlydepsuicide.cfm

36. Birrer RB, Vermuri SP. Depression in later life: A diagnostic and therapeutic challenge. *AFP* 2004;69:2375.

37. Lapid MI, Rummans TA. Evaluation and management of geriatric depression in primary care. *Mayo Clin Proc* 2003; 78:1423–1429.

38. Unutzer J, Patrick DL, Simon G, et al. Depressive symptoms and the cost of health services in HMO patients aged 65 years and older. A 4-year prospective study. *JAMA* 1997; 277:1618–1623.

39. Martin LM, Fleming KC, Evans JM. Recognition and management of anxiety and depression in elderly patients. *Mayo Clin Proc* 1995 ;70:999–1006.

40. Larson EB. Recognition of dementia: discovering the silent epidemic. *J Am Geriatr Soc* 1998;46:1576–1577.

41. Siu AL. Screening for dementia and investigating its causes. *Ann Intern Med* 1991;115:122–132.

42. Finlayson RE, Davis LJ Jr. Prescription drug dependence in the elderly population: Demographic and clinical features of 100 inpatients. *Mayo Clin Proc* 1994;69: 1137 –1145.

43. Adams WL, Yuan Z, Barboriak JJ, et al. Alcohol-related hospitalizations of elderly people. Prevalence and geographic variation in the United States. *JAMA* 1993;270:1222–1225.

44. Blow FC, Brower KJ, Schulenberg JE, et al. *The Michigan Alcoholism Screening Test, Geriatric Version (MAST-G): A new elderly-specific screening instrument. Alcoholism: Clinical and Experimental Research, 1992.* 16:372. Accessed August 20, 2005. Available at: http://www.ncbi.nlm.nih.gov/ books/bv.fcgi?rid=hstat5.table.49350

45. Gabrel CS. *Characteristics of elderly nursing home current residents and discharges: Data from the 1997 National Nursing Home Survey, Advance Data no. 312.* Atlanta: Centers for Disease Control and Prevention, National Center for Health Statistics, April 25, 2000.

46. Tennsted S. *Family caregiving in an aging society.* Administration on Aging. Accessed 6/1/05, 2005. Available at: http://www.aoa.gov/prof/research/famcare.pdf

47. Wolf R. *Risk assessment instruments.* National Center on Elder Abuse Newsletter. Accessed 5/23/05, 2005. Available at http://www.elderabusecenter.org/default.cfm?p=riskassessment.cfm

48. Blumenthal D, Gokhale M, Campbell EG, et al. Prepare dness for clinical practice: Reports of graduating residents at academic health centers. *JAMA* 2001;286: 1027–1034.

49. Adams WL, McIlvain HE, Lacy NL, et al. Primary care for elderly people: Why do doctors find it so hard? *Gerontologist* 2002;42:835–842.

50. *Statement to the practicing physicians advisory council.* May 19, 2003. American College of Physicians. Accessed 10/30/04, 2004. Available at: http://cms.hhs.gov/faca/ppac/apcstmt5_03.pdf

51. Moore AA, Siu AL. Screening for common problems in ambulatory elderly: Clinical confirmation of a screening instrument. *Am J Med* 1996;100:438–443.

52. Walter LC, Covinsky KE Cancer screening in elderly patients: A framework for individualized decision making. *JAMA* 2001;285:2750–2756.

53. Sox HC. Screening for disease in older people. *J Gen Intern Med* 1998;13(6):424.

54. Bodenheimer T. Long-term care for frail elderly people—the On Lok model. *N Engl J Med* 1999;341: 1324–1328.

55. Chisholm MA, DiPiro JT. Pharmaceutical manufacturer assistance programs. *Arch Intern Med* 2002;162:780–784.

56. Montemayor K. How to help your low-income patients get prescription drugs. *Family Pract Manag* 2002;9:51–56.

57. Decane BE, Chapman J. Program for procurement of drugs for indigent patients. *Am J Hosp Pharmacol* 1994;51: 669–671.

58. Lachs MS, Feinstein AR, Cooney LM Jr, et al. A simple procedure for general screening for functional disability in elderly patients. *Ann Intern Med* 1990;112:699–706.

Chapter 21

Work, Living Environment, and Health

Janet Victoria Diaz, MD, and John R. Balmes, MD

Objectives

- Summarize occupational and environmental risks.
- Review epidemiology of occupational and environmental exposures and illness.
- Describe occupational and environmental risk assessment.
- Review preventive and therapeutic interventions to decrease environmental and occupational illness.
- Review the effect of urban and community planning on health.

Arnulfo Perez, an undocumented day laborer, receives a laceration falling off of a ladder. He works 14 hours days, primarily in construction or painting projects. He does not have a steady employer, has never received any job safety training, and has never heard about worker's compensation or unions. He shares a single room apartment with six friends. He is paid in cash. He knows that without a bank account to store his earnings, and fearful of reporting thefts to the police, he is vulnerable to being assaulted.

and at home, highlighting their disproportionate effect on vulnerable populations. This chapter presents practical approaches for preventive and therapeutic interventions.

The environmental and occupational safety of residential and work places have an enormous impact on people's health. Public health measures implemented during the 20th century have improved people's living and working environments, resulting in increased longevity. However, dangerous occupations and harmful environmental exposures continue to be major contributors to disparities in health.[1,2] Health care providers also often ignore these important risk factors for disease.[3] This chapter reviews adverse health issues attributable to environmental factors in the workplace

ENVIRONMENTAL AND OCCUPATIONAL CONTRIBUTIONS TO INJURY, ILLNESS, AND DEATH

UNEMPLOYMENT AND HEALTH

Unemployment is an important risk factor for the ill health faced by poor and minority populations. Unemployed workers have higher rates of morbidity and mortality caused by multiple diseases, most prominently cardiovascular disease and suicide.[6-9] It has been hypothesized that recessionary economic cycles, characterized by unemployment and decreased income, may have profound negative effects on population health, especially for those on the lower rungs of the socioeconomic ladder.[10] A variety of explanations has been posited. First, unskilled and semiskilled workers in cyclic industries are among the earliest to become unemployed, and remain so for the longest periods of time. Their increased morbidity and mortality may result from the stress of unemployment. Second, workers who enter long-term unemployment following a structural change in the economy (e.g., after the introduction of a new technology such as automated harvesting machinery) often have inadequate education or English language skills to obtain new jobs in different sectors when the economy recovers. Low-wage, minority, women, and older workers are particularly vulnerable to both of these economic phenomena, with substantial impact to both their mental and physical health.

RACE-BASED DISCRIMINATION IN THE WORKPLACE

Race-based discrimination at work can lead to increased stress and poor health.[11,12] Several studies suggest that stress from racial discrimination may be associated with mental health disorders, hypertension, coronary artery disease, and poorer pregnancy outcomes.[11] In a cross-sectional observational study of 356 African Americans from Atlanta, the likelihood of a physician diagnosis of hypertension increased significantly in patients who perceived high levels of stress from race-based discrimination.[12]

HOUSING AND HEALTH

More than 5 million American families live in substandard housing (i.e., deteriorating houses or apartments) that expose them to the following hazardous conditions: poor insulation, combustion appliances (gas cookers or heaters that generate nitrogen and sulfur dioxides), cockroach and rodent infestation, dust mites, hypothermia and hyperthermia, dampness, mold, dangerous levels of lead in contaminated dust, residential soil and lead-based paint.[13,14] These housing hazards have been associated with adverse health outcomes.[15] A cross-sectional analysis found that neighborhoods with a high "broken windows" index (i.e., the sum of percentages of homes with major structural damage or boarded-up vacant housing units; the percentage of streets with garbage, abandoned cars or graffiti; and number of building code violations in public high schools) also had higher rates of premature death from all causes and from several specific causes (e.g., diabetes, homicide, suicide) and higher rates of sexually transmitted diseases.[4,16]

Overcrowding and poor-quality housing also have been associated with poor mental health, developmental delay, heart disease, and even short stature.[13]

Unfortunately, the most vulnerable populations (infants, children, elderly, and chronically ill) are those who spend the most time indoors and possibly alone. Despite declines in the prevalence of lead poisoning, children aged 18 to 36 months living in poor and inner-city communities continue to be at high risk for lead poisoning. Lead poisoning can result in neurologic damage, reduced IQ, hyperactivity, increased aggression, and learning disabilities. Exposure to excessive heat during summer heat waves is another housing-quality problem that primarily affects elderly persons living in older homes with inadequate ventilation and cooling who also have limited transportation options. Distributing electric fans, providing air conditioning in specific areas of apartment buildings, and transporting the elderly to air-conditioned areas can reduce heat-related mortality.[17]

NEIGHBORHOODS AND VIOLENCE

A neglected and disorderly physical environment signals to residents that behaviors that are usually prohibited are tolerated. Homicide is the fourth leading cause of preventable deaths in the United States. Latino and African-American men aged 18 to 50 years are disproportionately represented in these deaths.[18] Economic deprivation, social disorganization, and acculturation are independent risk factors for homicide mortality among Mexicans and African Americans. Residents of public housing surrounded by green space had a stronger sense of community and reported using less violent ways of dealing with domestic conflicts.[19]

URBAN AIR POLLUTION AND HEALTH

More than 80% of the residents of poor urban centers are ethnic and racial minorities. These populations are chronically subjected to poor air quality because they live in close proximity to transportation facilities (bus depots, trucking stations, rail yards, ports), high-volume roadways, waste treatment stations, power plants, toxic waste sites, refineries, and industrial facilities.

Urban air pollutants include nitrogen dioxide (NO_2), ozone, carbon monoxide, particulate matter, sulfur dioxide, and lead (the United States Environmental Protection Agency [EPA] regulated criteria pollutants[5]), as well as toxic air contaminants.[20] These are strongly associated with excess cardiopulmonary mortality, increased health care use, asthma exacerbations, decreased lung function, increased respiratory symptoms, increased airway reactivity, and lung inflammation.[20] Other pollutants, the so-called toxic air contaminants (e.g., benzene or perchloethylene) are known to be associated with cancer and reproductive abnormalities.[20] Because lung growth continues into early adulthood, children are especially vulnerable

Box 21-1. High-Risk Occupations for Heart Disease

	Men	Women
Air traffic controllers	Paper industry workers	Bus drivers, taxi drivers
Bakers	Police, protective service workers	Cleaners
Bus drivers, taxi drivers, Truck drivers	Prison wardens	Cooks, waitresses
Butchers	Rubber and plastics workers	Rubber and plastics workers
Cannery workers	Sea pilots	Paper workers
Cooks, waiters	Warehousemen, storekeepers	Self-employed in hotel and catering
Fire fighters		Home help
Fishermen, ship's deck officers		Unskilled worker in tube, sheet, and steel construction
Foundry workers		
Hairdressers		

From: Tüchsen F, Landsbergis P. *High-risk occupations*. Forum on The Way We Work And Its Impact On Our Health. Los Angeles, April 22–23, 2004.

to respiratory tract toxicity from urban air pollution. A recent longitudinal study of children from Southern California reported that exposure to high levels of air pollutants was associated with decreased growth of lung function over an 8-year period and clinically significant decreased forced expiratory volume in 1 second (FEV_1) by age 18.[21] A number of studies also have shown adverse effects of urban air pollution on birth outcomes. For example, a prospective study of minority pregnant women in New York City reported that exposure to high levels of urban air pollutants (specifically, polycyclic aromatic hydrocarbons) was associated with decreased birth weight and head circumference among African-American newborns.[22] Finally, asthma morbidity and mortality rates are highest among African Americans, especially children, living in urban areas and are associated with high levels of ambient pollution.[23]

FATALITIES IN THE WORKPLACE

Ethnic and racial minorities are disproportionately represented in occupations with higher risks for fatal injuries.[24–26] Foreign-born workers account for 50% of the growth of the nation's labor force and their workplace fatality rate is on the rise; whereas the national workplace fatality rate has declined.[26] Latinos and younger workers suffer the highest rates of workplace fatalities and the majority worked in the following five occupations: (a) transportation and material moving; (b) handlers, equipment cleaners, helpers, and laborers; (c) farming, forestry and fishing; (d) construction trades; and (e) security. In all five industries, foreign-born workers experienced higher fatality rates than their native-born coworkers. The most common fatal events were homicide (25%), falls to a lower level (15%), and highway motor vehicle incidents (14%).

Generalizing from what is known for all US workers, workplaces associated with the highest rates of homicides are taxicab establishments, liquor stores, gas stations, detective or protective services, justice or public order establishments, and grocery and jewelry stores.[27] Other risk factors associated with homicides include: male gender, working early or late hours, working in high crime neighborhoods, and occupations engaged in the exchange of money or valuables. Finally, elderly workers and adolescents suffer from workplace homicides at a higher rate than others. Elderly workers likely are less able to defend themselves when assaulted and are at increased risk of dying from an assault. The reasons that younger workers have higher rates, is unknown.[28]

NONFATAL OCCUPATIONAL INJURIES

The construction industry carries an estimated nonfatal injury rate that is four times the average of all other industries.[25] Laborers or unskilled construction workers are more likely to suffer from serious injuries requiring hospitalizations, than are more-skilled workers.[25] Urban dwelling workers, both men and women, who are injured on the job, tend to be young and unskilled. Their injuries commonly affect the musculoskeletal system, and have an impact on their immediate ability to work and their long-term health (Box 21-1).[24]

SELECTED OCCUPATIONS AND EXPOSURES AND THEIR IMPACT ON HEALTH

MIGRANT FARM WORK AND HEALTH

The agricultural industry is another inherently dangerous industry. It employs 3% of the US workforce but is responsible for 13% of workplace fatalities.[23] The agricultural industry employs 4.2 million migrant and seasonal farm workers. A migrant farm worker establishes a temporary home in order to do seasonal agricultural work, while a seasonal worker does not migrate.[31] Migrant workers and their families are among the most underserved and understudied populations in the United States. Nearly all migrant and seasonal farm workers are ethnic and racial minorities; 90% are Latino and the remainder African American or Caribbean.[31]

Migrant workers are at risk for various work-related illnesses, including: pesticide-related illnesses, musculoskeletal strains/sprains, traumatic injuries, noninfectious respiratory diseases, dermatitis, infectious disease, cancer, eye problems, and mental health problems.[32] The burden of these problems is exacerbated by minimal access to health care.

SUBSTANDARD HOUSING FOR MIGRANTS

The migratory nature of farm workers places them at risk for social isolation and living in substandard housing. Social isolation is a result of separating nuclear families and has been associated with stress, anxiety, depression, and substance abuse.[32] Substandard housing creates crowded and unsanitary conditions and has been associated with higher rates of communicable diarrheal illnesses and tuberculosis.

PESTICIDES AND HEALTH

Pesticide exposure is estimated to annually cause 313,000 cases of illness and 1000 deaths among farm workers.[23] Exposure results from absorption through the skin, direct spraying, or accidental ingestion.[23] Although exposure to organophosphate pesticides can result in acute toxicity characterized by headache, rash, nausea, vomiting, disorientation, shock, respiratory failure or, in most severe cases, death, most exposures to pesticides are to low-moderate levels and present with dermatitis, eye irritation, or more diffuse complaints.

Although good data on the chronic health effects of low-moderate levels of pesticide exposure among migrant and seasonal farm workers are limited, some studies suggest that farm workers are at higher risk for cancer and neurological and reproductive abnormalities.[23] In all scenarios, the pesticide or its residues can be deposited on the farm workers' clothing and then be brought home to expose family members, which may include pregnant women and young children, who may be particularly vulnerable to toxic effects.[22]

To protect farm workers from pesticide exposure, the EPA implemented Worker Protection Standards (WPS) and the Occupational Safety and Health Administration (OSHA) developed regulations.[27] The WPS states that employers must centrally post information about pesticide application (name, location, date of application, re-entry period), place warning signs around fields just sprayed with a re-entry date, and provide safety training to farm workers.[32] The OSHA regulations mandate that adequate sanitation facilities be available in the field, including potable drinking water with individual cups, toilets, and hand washing facilities.[32] Similarly, farm worker housing must have adequate showering and laundry facilities.

In a survey of 514 Latino farm workers from North Carolina only 50% of respondents reported that their employer notified them where pesticides are being applied or posted warning signs around fields that were just sprayed. Just 11% knew the names of the pesticides they had ever applied.[33] Similarly, 50% of the farm workers reported a lack of field toilets, laundry facilities, or any pesticide training. Despite federal and state regulations to promote the health of migrant and seasonal farm workers, they remain at high risk for pesticide exposure and poor health, and are likely less able to access appropriate help for themselves and their families.[34]

Recognition of pesticide exposures is a challenge for prevention, treatment, and reporting, even if they are common.[35] The EPA and the National Environmental Education and Training Foundation (NEETF), in collaboration with the US Departments of Health and Human Services, Agriculture, and Labor, have created an initiative, the *National Strategies for Health Care Providers: Pesticide Initiative,* to improve the ability of health care providers to recognize pesticide exposures and manage pesticide-related health problems (see Resources section).

Pesticides are not the only toxins that might cause harm to agricultural workers. Plant toxins themselves (e.g., tobacco), animal confinement building environments, grain dusts, diesel exhaust, and solvents are examples of other types of exposures that may have serious impacts on health.[36]

APPAREL INDUSTRY AND HEALTH

Minority immigrants often find work at facilities manufacturing goods in highly competitive sectors where there is a premium on low labor costs; for example, the apparel industry, known as sweatshops. These jobs involve repetitive motion, and often are associated with a high risk of exposure to potentially harmful chemicals. Several investigations of garment workers both in the United States, and those in *maquiladoras* along the Mexican side of the US–Mexican border, have documented increased risk of musculoskeletal disorders and acute health effects consistent with excessive exposure to chemicals such as solvents.[37–39]

HOSPITALITY INDUSTRY AND HEALTH

Room cleaning jobs in the hospitality industry are characterized by increasing repetitive physical workloads, low income, low skill use, low job control, and virtually no prospects for training and career advancement. These workers are largely female, immigrants who speak a native language other than English, and over age 50.[40] The hospitality industry has experienced a wave of restructuring, consolidation, and new practices to cut costs, including lean staffing and greater performance demands on the workforce. The hospitality industry has become a major target for welfare-to-work and job training programs in cities throughout the country.[40] A recent study found an association between poor working conditions and reduced health in hotel room cleaners. Room cleaners reported increasing physical workloads in recent years, and a large proportion of room cleaners were exposed to high levels of job stress. The study also found that room cleaners have high rates of work-related pain and disability, and that self-reported general health of room cleaners is below the national average.[40]

Janitors in other work environments are also at risk of job-related illness. Many are male, immigrants who speak a native language other than English (especially Latinos), have limited literacy in native language, work multiple jobs, and usually do not have personal transportation. They tend to be unfamiliar with workplace rights, receive limited if any training and infrequently use protective equipment. Often employers use intimidation to silence workers about work place hazards, illness or injury. Many suffer deteriorating physical health, skin rashes, asthma, headaches, back injuries, repetitive motion injuries, pregnancy complications, and mental and emotional stress.

OCCUPATIONAL ASTHMA

Occupational asthma is the most common occupational lung disease. It is estimated that 15% of all adult-onset asthma is caused by occupational asthma and many more have their asthma aggravated by workplace exposure. Prognosis is directly related to the duration of time between onset of symptoms and removal of the cause. The earlier it is recognized and treated, the better the prognosis for the patients. Health care workers should ask all adult asthmatic patients about their work. Occupational asthma should be suspected in any newly diagnosed adult asthmatic; any patient with cough or wheeze that improves on weekends or holidays; any patient working in a high-risk occupation, especially if they have other symptoms of atopy; and in an otherwise unexplained exacerbation of previously well-controlled asthma.

There are more than 250 agents suspected of causing occupational asthma. At-risk occupations include spray painters, agricultural workers, bakers, health workers (allergy to latex gloves), animal handlers, and hairdressers. The key to treatment is removal from exposure. Studies have shown a direct link between length of time of exposure and persisting asthma. Reduction and removal of exposure is also important for those asthmatics whose asthma is exacerbated by workplace exposure.

Common Pitfalls in Environmental Health

- Those from poor and minority groups are at high risk for fatal and nonfatal work injuries and violence.
- Construction, migrant farm work, taxi cab driving, and retail sales work in small, all-night stores are dangerous occupations.
- Morbidity and mortality resulting from respiratory and cardiovascular disease are strongly associated with poor housing and urban air pollution.
- Health care providers often do not assess occupational and environmental risk.
- Interventions, although useful, are suggested infrequently by health care professionals.

PREVENTIVE INTERVENTIONS

Environmental justice is the belief that all people and communities have the right to live, work and play in places and communities that are safe, healthy, and free of life-threatening conditions.[14]

Each clinical encounter with a patient provides an opportunity to assess environmental and occupational health risks. Clinicians have a vital role to play by recognizing, treating, and preventing problems. Communication among health care providers, public health agencies, and researchers, employers, community organizers, and urban planners completes the process necessary to promote health and environmental justice.[14,41]

SCREENING

Failure to take an exposure history is one reason that environmental and occupational illnesses often go unrecognized. Many of these illnesses are associated with nonspecific medical complaints and without a basic exposure history may never be linked to their actual cause. All patients, but particularly poor and minority patients, should be questioned about their occupations and living environments, including job description, safety training, neighborhood, and housing. Screening

Box 21-2. Screening Questions for Occupational and Environmental Exposures

Adults

- What kind of work do you do?
- Do you think your health problems are related to work, home, neighborhood, or other location or activity?
- Are your symptoms better or worse when you are at home or at work?
- What hobbies do you have?
- Are you now or have you previously been exposed to pesticides, solvents, or other chemicals, dusts, fumes, radiation, or loud noise?
- Have you received safety training/equipment and do you follow it?
- Do you live near a major road or industrial facility?
- Does your home have water damage?

Agricultural workers

- Are pesticides being used at home or work?
- Were the fields wet when you were picking?
- Was any spraying going on while you were working in the fields?

- Do you get sick during or after working in the fields?
- Have you had problems with rashes or eye irritation after working?
- Do you have the opportunity to bathe and change clothes after work?
- Are you notified when spraying is occurring and have you received safety training/equipment?

Children

- Do you think the child's health problems are related to the home, neighborhood, day care, school, or other location or activity?
- Has there been any exposure to pesticides, solvents or other chemicals, dusts, fumes, radiation, or loud noise?
- What kind of work do the parents or other household members engage in?
- How are cleansers, pesticides, medications, and firearms stored at home?
- Was your house built before 1978? Is the paint in poor condition?

for possible occupational or environmental exposures with a few simple questions is the most practical first step (Box 21-2).

OCCUPATIONAL HISTORY

If the clinical presentation or initial medical history suggests a potential occupational or environmental exposure, a detailed exposure interview is needed. A complete job description should include specific work tasks, work hours, product(s) manufactured or service(s) provided by the employer, any exposures to dust or fumes, workplace discrimination, and stress. Linking timing of symptoms with exposures is also important. The Agency for Toxic Substances and Disease Registry (ATSDR) publishes a handy guide to taking a detailed exposure history including a useful form (see Resources).

Adequate safety training is an important intervention that can reduce risk of occupational injury or illness. If a worker has not received training (e.g., about the risks of lead intoxication from removing old house paint), then referral to an occupational medicine specialist, nurse, industrial hygienist, or safety specialist is in order. The information that needs to be provided includes the inherent risks of the job, interventions that may decrease these risks (e.g., the use of personal protective equipment such as gloves or respirators), and instruction about where to receive timely medical care and the right to workers' compensation if injured on the job. Special attention should be given to those in the most

dangerous occupations to ensure that they are receiving appropriate workplace safety training. Most local health departments have occupational and environmental health units that can provide such training.

Losing a job can have profound health consequences for a low-wage, minority worker. It is often better to try to keep such a patient working at a job that has potentially harmful occupational exposures with appropriate efforts to reduce the exposures than to advise quitting the job.

NEIGHBORHOOD AND HOUSING

Questioning about housing quality, neighborhood safety, and air pollution is also important. An adequate housing conditions history should ask about the presence of poor insulation, combustion appliances, cockroach and rodent infestation, carpets, heating availability, stove type and fuel use, moldy walls, lead paint, and unaffordable rent. If a house was built before 1978, it might well have lead paint. Peeling paint is particularly problematic. Neighborhood safety should be assessed from the patients' perception of safety and green space availability. If children are playing in areas of bare soil, concerns over lead levels are warranted.

AIR QUALITY

A complete air pollution exposure history may be difficult to elicit from the patient because many are unaware of local polluting facilities. Patients should be asked about their physical proximity to transportation facilities (bus depots, trucking stations, rail yards, and ports), high-volume roadways, waste treatment stations, power plants, refineries, and polluting industrial facilities. Given the known effects of urban air pollution on health, it is a physician's responsibility to have general knowledge of the community's pollution sources. This information should be obtained from environmental agency web sites, distributed amongst the health care providers working in the community, and then shared with patients.

Special attention should be given to patients who are elderly and those with asthma, chronic obstructive pulmonary disease (COPD), and cardiovascular disease or with young children to ensure that any housing and environmental hazards are detected. To do so, an environmental health specialist, usually from the local health department, can perform a home assessment.

PREVENTIVE ADVICE

If no clear risk is identified, health care providers should provide general preventive advice to maintain occupational and home safety. For example, firearms, cleaning products, and garden products should be stored safely and away from children's reach, and product labels should be read to assure proper use. Pregnant and breastfeeding women in particular should be advised to use chemicals cautiously (see Chap. 29). Peeling paint should be removed to minimize risk for potential lead toxicity. Carbon monoxide monitors should be installed in homes with indoor gas heaters.

THERAPEUTIC INTERVENTIONS

Once an occupational or environmental illness or injury is suspected, the clinician has two concerns: the care of the individual and the health of the community. Referral to an occupational health specialist may assist in both areas.

GENERAL GUIDELINES

If one suspects that a patient's illness or injury is related to a chemical or physical exposure, it is important to consider whether the signs, symptoms, and timing make sense for the suspected exposure. For example, a patient's exposure to asbestos from a building renovation project, even if heavy for days or weeks, should not produce any acute symptoms.

Identification of the specific agent(s) responsible for causing a health problem is often critical to effective management. If there is a concern about a chemical exposure related to a commercial product, the product label should be read carefully and, if necessary, the manufacturer contacted to obtain information about what chemicals the product contains. For products used at work, identification of chemical constituents often begins with Material Safety Data Sheets (MSDS); employers are required to keep MSDSs on file for all products that could be harmful. Once the chemicals in a product are identified, the local poison control center or web-based information systems can aid in confirming the diagnosis of chemical toxicity and managing the resultant illness.

The next step is to perform a complete history and physical examination to exclude other possible etiologies. Remember, patients with chronic diseases resulting from other factors (e.g., coronary artery disease, hypertension, or tobacco-related COPD) can have their diseases exacerbated by their occupational and living environments and control of aggravating exposures can improve outcomes.

If there is a concern about work-related respiratory illnesses, such as asthma or hypersensitivity pneumonitis, documentation of work-related variability in symptoms or lung function is important to link exposures to effects. Exposures to certain heavy metals or pesticides can be confirmed by biomarkers of exposure (e.g., blood lead or acetylcholinesterase levels).

Finally, it is important to ascertain whether other people who spend time in the home or workplace are also ill in order to identify and reduce high-risk exposures to prevent further spread of illness.

OCCUPATIONAL INJURY

When caring for a patient that has been injured at work, the goals are to minimize time out of the workforce and on long-term physical disability, and prevent future serious or even fatal injuries. If the patient is unable to return to work because of the injury, he or she should be referred to an occupational medicine specialist. There the patient can receive rehabilitation care, safety training, ergonomically improved job redesign, and assistance with workers' compensation and disability benefits, as needed.

Workers' compensation is a type of insurance system that is usually governed by state-specific rules. In general, workers who become injured or sick as a result of work-related factors are entitled to reimbursement of lost wages and for any permanent disability. The historical compromise that allowed the workers' compensation system to be developed was speedy payment of benefits to injured workers with the proviso that they gave up their right to sue employers for liability. The current system does not always live up to either side of this bargain: benefit payments often are delayed as a result of litigation. Most physicians are inadequately prepared to deal with the separate and somewhat arcane workers' compensation reporting rules and billing procedures. Perhaps the most important point for nonoccupational medicine physicians to remember is that their patients who are injured or made sick at work will likely need expert help (medical and/or legal) at navigating the workers' compensation system in their state.

ENVIRONMENTAL ILLNESS

When caring for a patient who is exposed to a hazardous living environment, therapeutic interventions tend to be more complex because the living environment is created by a complex interaction of people, organizations, and physical factors (i.e., architects, planners, landlords, bus depots, industrial sites) (see Chap. 41). The type and extent of assistance will depend on whether the concern is removing lead paint from the walls or decreasing community violence. Health care professionals can serve as a bridge to connect individuals at risk with community organizations, governmental regulatory units, and legal professionals who work with vulnerable populations to promote environmental justice.

For example, if poor housing has been identified as a health risk, national agencies such as the EPA and the US Department of Housing and Urban Development (HUD) have web-based information systems and hotlines to help patients and clinicians know how and where they can get the safety of the drinking water or soil at their homes checked or paint tested for lead. Health care providers may advocate for interventions from repair of water damage to reduce mold to improved appliances to reduce indoor air pollution, or more radically the patient may need to be relocated to a healthier unit.

If outdoor urban air pollution has been identified as the health risk, then patients should be instructed on how to access daily air pollution reports from local news sources or web-based systems. Possible interventions that can be advocated include: minimize outdoor activities during high pollution periods or traffic rush hour if living near busy roadways, attend planning meeting to voice opposition to the construction of new toxic waste sites or industrial refineries near populated communities, and in severe cases, the patient may have to relocate to a less polluted neighborhood or city. Interventions to make communities safer require that patients and health care providers direct their efforts toward local governmental and community organizations focused on these issues.

REPORTING REQUIREMENTS

Occupational injuries and illnesses generally are required to be reported by employers, but not usually by physicians. In California, physicians are required to report diagnoses of occupational injury or illness on a standard form. Elevated blood lead levels in children and often in adults must be reported in most states, but this requirement usually falls to the clinical laboratory doing the measurement rather than the physician who ordered the test. Several states (e.g., California, Washington, Texas) also require reporting of pesticide-related illness.

PUBLIC HEALTH, URBAN PLANNING, AND COMMUNITY-BASED RESEARCH

The disproportionate exposure of ethnic and racial minorities to dangerous occupations and harmful environments is caused by complex interactions of economic, social, and political factors. It is crucial that politicians, urban planners, developers, architects, and engineers recognize the link between these factors and the physical environment in which our patients live and work.[12,14,19]

In 2000, the National Center for Environmental Health issued, *Creating a Healthy Environment: The Impact of the Built Environment on Public Health*, which argued that urban planning is fundamentally linked to public health.[19] "Smart growth," which takes into account the potential health consequences of land-use decisions, was recommended. For example, enhancing community "walkability," with more sidewalks, open spaces, and safety, promotes exercise and better general health. In contrast, "sprawl" and poorly planned growth, increases use of motor vehicles, levels air pollution, and poor respiratory health.

Health care providers caring for vulnerable populations can advocate for their health by participating in community development and by providing strong public health arguments to support or oppose planning proposals (see Chap. 41).[16] Providers are also able to identify areas where research is needed to better understand the associations between exposures and health as well as assessing the potential health impacts of environmental and occupational interventions.[19]

CONCLUSION

The ultimate treatments for the heavy burden of occupational and environmental illness borne by the poor are preventive interventions occurring at a community or societal level; that is, policy changes to promote full employment, occupational health and safety, environmental justice, and smart growth. Clinicians also have a role to play in preventing, recognizing, and mitigating their effects and advocating for long-term solutions.

KEY CONCEPTS IN ENVIRONMENTAL AND OCCUPATIONAL SAFETY

Take a work and residential history.

Refer to an occupational health specialist when:

- Patients' job-related injuries keep them from working to assist with job redesign, safety training, disability evaluation, and workers' compensation
- For patients with pulmonary problems living in a polluted neighborhood or substandard housing for home environment assessment

Know your community

Environmental justice organizations

- Local polluting sources
- Waste facilities
- Crime statistics
- Availability of open spaces and recreation parks
- Neighborhood resources for healthy choices

Be alert to the connection between environment and health

Advocate for patients on the community level

CORE COMPETENCY
How to Obtain a Home Assessment

1. *Contact your local health department.* Most health departments in large cities have environmental health units that may be able to provide inspections of the housing conditions of patients for whom there is a high suspicion of illness related to home environmental exposures. If such personnel are not available, contact an occupational health clinic for assistance in arranging for an industrial hygienist to inspect the home.
2. *Document the conditions.* Either the specialists or a member of the primary health team can visit the home to document the presence poor housing conditions or the patient should take photos of the damage.
3. *Consider a therapeutic trial of changing residence.* If the inspection warrants it, try changing the environment (e.g., temporarily living with a relative) and following clinical status. If symptoms improve, then efforts to provide a more permanent change in residence are warranted.

DISCUSSION QUESTIONS

1. A 22-year-old man, who is a recent immigrant from Mexico comes to your office complaining of back pain. What are the important occupational issues that should be discussed at this visit and what interventions would you suggest?
2. A 32-year-old African-American woman who you follow for severe persistent asthma comes to your office after three emergency room visits in the past month. What are the important home environment issues that should be discussed and what interventions would you recommend?
3. The city is proposing to expand a highway to lessen traffic congestion and improve commute times. The highway expansion is to occur through one of the poorest sectors of town. Will this affect the health of the local community? What can you do to make your opinions heard?
4. Using web-based resources look up the following questions: My apartment is flea-infested. I have a 6-month-old child, can I safely have the place flea-bombed? Every time I turn on the heat in the house I get a headache. Could there be a problem with the heater?

RESOURCES

http://www.cdc.gov/niosh/topics/
This National Institute for Occupational Safety and Health web site provides information by specific hazard, occupation, or disease.

http://www.cehn.org/cehn/trainingmanual/manual-front.html
Agency for Toxic Substances and Disease Registry manual on pediatric environmental health.

http://www.epa.gov/airnow/
This US Environmental Protection Agency web site provides links to local air quality data, resources to aid in patient education and care regarding health effects of air pollutants.

http://www.hud.gov/offices/lead/hhi/index.cfm
The Healthy Homes Program web site of the US Department of Housing and Urban Development provides links to useful documents such as "Overview of Asthma and the Home Environment" and "Help Yourself to a Healthy Home."

http://www.aoec.org/
The web site of the Association of Occupational and Environmental Clinics provides contact information for clinics throughout the United States.

http://www.naccho.org/
The web site of the National Association of City and County Health Officials has a searchable web site with useful information on environmental health and justice.

http://www.cehrc.org/about/index.cfm
The Community Environmental Health Resource Center is a resource to grassroots groups working for social justice.

http://www.epa.gov/oppfead1/safety/healthcare/handbook/handbook.pdf
Recognition and management of pesticide poisons, by Roult Reigert and James Roberts.

REFERENCES

1. Health disparities experienced by Latinos: United States. *MMWR Morb Mortal Wkly Rep* 2004;53;40:935–937.
2. Health disparities experienced by black or African Americans: United States. *MMWR Morb Mortal Wkly Rep* 2005;54(1):1–3.
3. Doctors and nurses who treat kids need more training in environmental health. *Hosp Health Netw* 2004;78(12):60–61.
4. Cohen D, Spear S, Scribner R, et al. "Broken windows" and the risk of gonorrhea. *Am J Public Health* 2000;90(2):230–236.
5. Urban air pollution and health inequities: A workshop report. *Environ Health Perspect* 2001;109(Suppl 3):357–374.
6. Brenner MH. Mortality and the national economy. A review, and the experience of England and Wales, 1936–76. *Lancet* 1979;2(8142):568–573.
7. Franks PJ, Adamson C, Bulpitt PF, et al. Stroke death and unemployment in London. *J Epidemiol Community Health* 1991;45(1):16–18.
8. Bartley M. Unemployment and ill health: Understanding the relationship. *J Epidemiol Community Health* 1994;48(4):333–337.
9. Morris JK, Cook DG, Shaper AG. Loss of employment and mortality. *BMJ* 1994;308(6937):1135–1139.
10. Laporte A. Do economic cycles have a permanent effect on population health? Revisiting the Brenner hypothesis. *Health Econ* 2004;13(8):767–779.
11. Williams DR, Neighbors HW, Jackson JS. Racial/ethnic discrimination and health: Findings from community studies. *Am J Public Health* 2003;93(2):200–208.
12. Din-Dzietham R, Nembhard WN, Collins R, et al. Perceived stress following race-based discrimination at work is associated with hypertension in African-Americans. The metro Atlanta heart disease study, 1999–2001. Soc Sci Med 2004; 58(3):449–461.
13. Bashir SA. Home is where the harm is: Inadequate housing as a public health crisis. *Am J Public Health* 2002;92(5):733–738.
14. Corburn J. Confronting the challenges in reconnecting urban planning and public health. *Am J Public Health* 2004;94(4):541–546.
15. Fullilove MT, Fullilove RE 3rd. What's housing got to do with it? *Am J Public Health* 2000;90(2):183–184.
16. Cohen HW, Northridge ME. Getting political: Racism and urban health. *Am J Public Health* 2000;90(6):841–842.
17. Davis RE, Knappenberger PC, Michaels PJ, et al. Changing heat-related mortality in the United States. *Environ Health Perspect* 2003;111(14):1712–1718.
18. Krueger PM, Bond Huie SA, Rogers RG, et al. Neighbourhoods and homicide mortality: An analysis of race/ethnic differences. *J Epidemiol Community Health* 2004;58;3:223–230.
19. Jackson RJ. *Creating a healthy environment: The impact of the built environment on public health.* Washington, DC: Sprawl Watch Clearinghouse, 2000.
20. Balmes J, Tager I. Air pollution. In: Murray JF, Nadel JA, eds. *Textbook of respiratory medicine.* Philadelphia: Saunders, 2000:188–1902.
21. Gauderman WJ, Avol E, Gilliland F, et al. The effect of air pollution on lung development from 10 to 18 years of age. *N Engl J Med* 2004;351(11):1057–1067.
22. Perera FP, Rauh V, Tsai WY, et al. Effects of transplacental exposure to environmental pollutants on birth outcomes in a multiethnic population. *Environ Health Perspect* 2003;111(2):201–205.
23. Frumkin H, Walker ED, Friedman-Jimenez G. Minority workers and communities. *Occup Med* 1999;14(3):495–517.
24. Frumkin H, Williamson M, Magid D, et al. Occupational injuries in a poor inner-city population. *J Occup Environ Med* 1995;37(12):1374–1382.
25. Anderson JT, Hunting KL, Welch LS. Injury and employment patterns among Latino construction workers. *J Occup Environ Med* 2000;42(2):176–186.
26. Loh K. *Foreign-born workers: Trends in fatal occupational injuries, 1996–2001. In: Census of Fatal Occupational Injuries, 1996–2001.* Washington, DC: US Department of Labor/Bureau of Labor Statistics, 2004.
27. Alert N. *Preventing homicide in the workplace.* Washington, DC: Department of Health and Human Services, National Institute for Occupational Safety and Health, 1995.
28. Janicak CA. An analysis of occupational homicides involving workers 19 years old and younger. *J Occup Environ Med* 1999;41(12):1140–1145.
29. Tüchsen F, Landsbergis P. *High-risk occupations.* The Way We Work and Its Impact On Our Health Forum. Los Angeles, CA, April 22–23, 2004.
30. Arcury TA, Quandt SA, Dearry A. Farm worker pesticide exposure and community-based participatory research: Rationale and practical applications. *Environ Health Perspect* 2001;109(Suppl 3):429–434.
31. Arcury TA, Quandt SA, McCauley L Farm workers and pesticides: Community-based research. *Environ Health Perspect* 2000;108(8):787–792.
32. Villarejo D, Baron SL. The occupational health status of hired farm workers. *Occup Med* 1999;14(3):613–635.
33. Arcury TA, Quandt SA, Russell GB. Pesticide safety among farm workers: Perceived risk and perceived control as factors reflecting environmental justice. *Environ Health Perspect* 2002;110(Suppl 2):233–240.
34. Belson M, Kieszak S, Watson W, et al. Childhood pesticide exposures on the Texas-Mexico border: Clinical manifestations and poison center use. *Am J Public Health* 2003;93(8):1310–1315.
35. Strong LL, Thompson B, Coronado GD, et al. Health symptoms and exposure to organophosphate pesticides in farm workers. *Am J Ind Med* 2004;46(6):599–606.
36. Hoppin JA, Umbach DM, London SJ, et al. Diesel exhaust, solvents, and other occupational exposures as

risk factors for wheeze among farmers. *Am J Respir Crit Care Med* 2004;169(12):1308–1313.

37. Herbert R, Plattus B, Kellogg L, et al. The Union Health Center: A working model of clinical care linked to preventive occupational health services. *Am J Ind Med* 1997; 31(3):263–273.

38. Moure-Eraso R, Wilcox M, Punnett L, et al. Back to the future: Sweatshop conditions on the Mexico-US border. II. Occupational health impact of maquiladora industrial activity. *Am J Ind Med* 1997;31(5):587–599.

39. Burgel BJ, Lashuay N, Israel L, et al. Garment workers in California: Health outcomes of the Asian Immigrant Women Workers Clinic. *Aaohn J* 2004;52(11):465–475.

40. Lee PT, Krause N. The impact of a worker health study on working conditions. *J Public Health Policy* 2002; 23:268–285.

41. Freudenberg N. Time for a national agenda to improve the health of urban populations. *Am J Public Health* 2000;90(6):837–840.

Chapter 22
Care of the Dying Patient

LaVera M. Crawley, MD, MPH

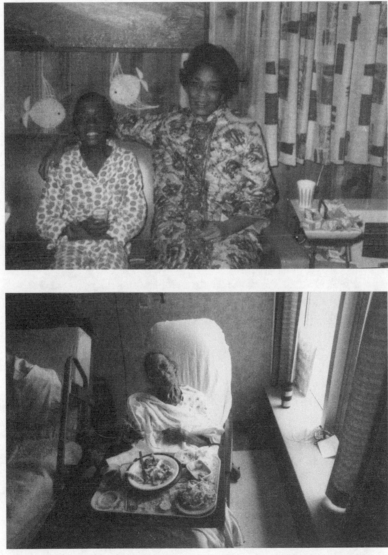

Figure 22-1. Looking back/looking ahead. (Reprinted with permission from Dr. Chip Thomas.)

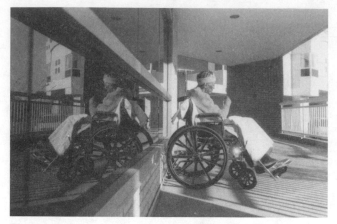

Figure 22-2. As her world contracted. (Reprinted with permission from Dr. Chip Thomas.)

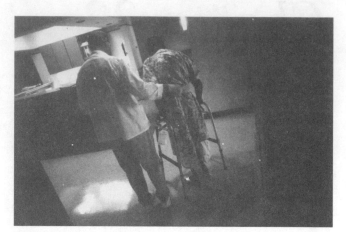

Figure 22-3. Physical therapy. (Reprinted with permission from Dr. Chip Thomas.)

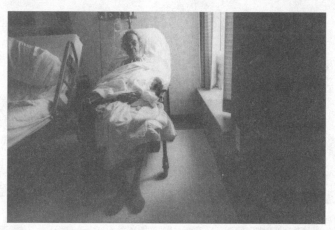

Figure 22-4. Mom's last portrait I. (Reprinted with permission from Dr. Chip Thomas.)

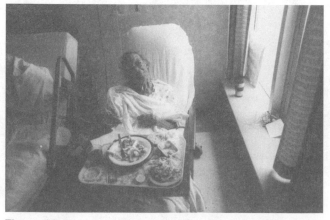

Figure 22-5. Mom's last portrait II. (Reprinted with permission from Dr. Chip Thomas.)

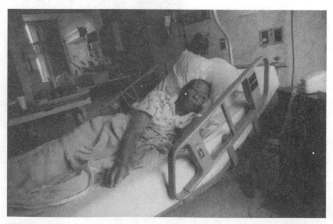

Figure 22-6. Looking homeward. (Reprinted with permission from Dr. Chip Thomas.)

Objectives

- Identify unique burdens of vulnerable persons at the end of life.
- Identify communication barriers to quality care for the dying.
- Discuss challenges to end-of-life decision making.
- Identify models of health care delivery for dying patients.
- Summarize practice guidelines and suggest other strategies to improve care of the dying patient.

Mrs. Johnson is a marginally literate 72-year-old woman who comes to your emergency room complaining of abdominal pain. You discover that she had been recently discharged from another hospital with a diagnosis of stage M2 acute myelogenous leukemia (AML M2). She tells you that she does not believe it to be true and does not want to discuss it further. Instead, she wants you to focus on her abdominal pain.

Facing one's own mortality is perhaps life's greatest challenge, one that makes all persons vulnerable to some extent. Despite the successes of the hospice movement and advances in the field of palliative medicine, many people are still at risk for physical and existential suffering at the end of life. For those marginalized by social or economic circumstances, illiteracy, or cultural or language barriers, this suffering may be compounded by additional burdens that are equally overwhelming. As a result, end-of-life care goals and priorities for marginalized patients extend beyond clinical concerns and may require providers to act as advocates on behalf of social and economic equity. This chapter identifies key issues for the dying patient focusing on difficulties encountered in medical discussions and in decision making in the face of death. Various end-of-life health care delivery models are summarized along with practice guidelines and other strategies that may improve the quality of life for dying patients.

CHALLENGES IN THE CARE OF THE DYING PATIENT

DEFINING A GOOD DEATH IN THE CONTEXT OF DISPARITIES

How does one define a "good death" for the person whose life has been constrained by disadvantage, or whose imminent death may result, in whole or in part,

from societal factors responsible for socioeconomic inequalities or racial or ethnic-based inequities?[1-4] Life expectancy among vulnerable persons is generally lower than for their more privileged counterparts.[5] Their deaths are often premature, occur at younger ages, and are associated with a markedly diminished quality of life. Many factors, including cultural and ethnic heritage, determine how one thinks about death and dying, advance directives, hospice, and the concept of a good death. Consequently, it is important for the provider to pay particular attention to these issues as they enter conversations with patients and families about a terminal illness and dying, while at the same time avoiding any temptation to engage in stereotyping by social, racial, ethnic, or cultural categories. This can be achieved by maintaining a focus on the quality of care offered to each individual or family (Table 22-1).

DIFFICULTIES IN DISCUSSING DEATH AND DYING

Using black vernacular English, Mrs. Johnson conveys that the doctor at the previous facility had told her she has cancer and that she had 3 months or less to live. Her reluctance to believe the diagnosis was caused, in part, by her misinterpretation of the hematologist's explanation of leukemia (as a disorder characterized by proliferation of abnormal cells in the bone marrow). She tells you, "My bones don't hurt and never have, so it can't be bone cancer." Furthermore, she thought it was cruel to have received a "death sentence" from a doctor whom she had only seen once.

Clear, ongoing, intelligible, and compassionate communication is essential in the care of the dying. The ability to exchange information is influenced by native language, cultural backgrounds, education, and literacy, as well as by trust, continuity, and other relational factors. The emotional and psychological nature of

Table 22-1. Common Issues to Remember When Dealing with Dying Patients and Their Families

Verbal and nonverbal signs of personal warmth are highly valued.

Illness may be denied or attributed to personal carelessness or weakness, viewed as punishment, or considered a result of external forces beyond one's control.

Patients may fear that talking about end-of-life scenarios invites disaster.

Patients may simultaneously practice traditional and Western healing methods or resort to the other when one fails.

Family members sometimes prefer to shield the patient from news about terminal illness and believe that family members should be the ones to make decisions about treatment options and the use of life support.

In the event of a terminal illness or death, certain rituals may be performed by the patient's family.

conversations about serious illness and death may interfere with patients being able to hear, understand, or remember conversations with health care providers.

Communication Barriers

Obvious communication barriers occur when patients and providers do not share the same native tongue or professional language (see Chap. 26). Highly technical medical discourse may be foreign to all but other technical experts. Less evident, but perhaps more problematic, are cases in which a patient's primary language is a dialect of a shared native tongue, such as black vernacular English or Creole. In such cases, the need for translation may not be apparent although each party may not fully perceive what is being said.

Health Literacy

Literacy is also important to effective communication, which not only entails the skill to read or write in a primary language well enough to function in society, but also may involve the ability to understand health information provided orally, including instructions for procedures or therapies (see Chap. 26). Health literacy involves the negotiation of explanatory models and some patients may not understand basic physiologic processes well enough to comprehend medical explanations, even when such explanations are presented in lay terms. Because of her limited English proficiency, coupled with health illiteracy, Mrs. Johnson misinterpreted the meaning of her diagnosis.

Terminal Illness and Discussions of Prognosis

Discussing death and delivering bad news is not an easy task, even for the seasoned provider. Doing so may require one to confront one's own mortality or unresolved grief from a personal loss. Communicating difficult news may be particularly problematic for the provider who sees death, not as an inevitable part of life, but rather as the failure of the limits of medical skill or technology. As a coping strategy, the provider may overuse technical language, defer the conversation, or worse, avoid the patient altogether.

Providers who care for large numbers of vulnerable patients may come to view death as a failure of social responsibility or worry that communicating bad news may diminish hope. The desire to maintain hope may in some way explain the general tendency for physicians to overestimate prognosis.[7-9] The consequences of these overestimates are serious and may partially account for late referrals to hospice when patients have only hours to days, rather than weeks to months, to benefit from quality palliative care.[10]

What do patients want to know about their prognosis? The question presumes that patients already know that they have a terminal or potentially fatal condition and wish to get a realistic picture of the future. Few studies have identified patient preferences regarding information sharing *before* receiving a terminal diagnosis.[11] Furthermore, the question reveals a hidden assumption about an "ideal" patient, one who shares the Western ethical precepts of truth-telling and respect for patient autonomy.[12] Not everyone embraces this normative assumption. Cultural differences may influence preferences about information sharing or the willingness to discuss prognosis. For some, discussing death may be tantamount to wishing it upon the patient.[13,14] Some families prefer that the patient never know of their condition, and that decision making be carried out by a proxy.[15,16] These values and preferences may conflict with those of the provider or others involved in care of the dying patient.

Lastly, the ability to hear, understand, and accept difficult news may be influenced by patient trust or provider or system trustworthiness. For Mrs. Johnson, the news of her diagnosis was delivered by a physician with whom she had no prior (or subsequent) relationship, and was conveyed in a manner she deemed cruel. Had she received the information in a longstanding primary care relationship, her acceptance and understanding might have been different. For some vulnerable persons, access to care is limited, making continuity of care at the level of health services or of providers an unrealistic option and uncoordinated care in resource-constrained settings more common.

Clinicians can learn to deliver bad news in a manner that can aid in patients' acceptance and facilitate participation in health care decisions. Advance preparation is a key prerequisite. Medical facts should be confirmed prior to having the discussion. A six-step protocol for delivering bad news, based on the work of oncologist Robert Buckman, has been widely adapted and endorsed.[17] By practicing the following steps in advance, the provider can increase his or her own comfort level before facing a difficult situation.

1. Prepare the environment beforehand (i.e., turning off cell phones or pagers or other sources of interruption and ensuring privacy and adequate seating).
2. Find out how much the patient already knows.
3. Find out how much the patient wants to know.
4. Deliver the information in a straightforward manner, allowing adequate time for discussion.
5. Once the news is delivered, give the patient time to take it in, and allow for emotional reactions.
6. Lastly, make plans for follow-up.

DECISION MAKING AT THE END OF LIFE

The hematologist who first diagnosed Mrs. Johnson deemed that chemotherapy or other aggressive therapies would be medically futile. You want to have a discussion with her about her wishes for resuscitation and mechanical ventilation, and other advance care plans should her condition worsen. However, because Mrs. Johnson does not believe she has leukemia, direct discussions about advance planning or desires for resuscitation are complicated.

A central tenet in medical practice is that individuals have the right to autonomous choice in receiving or refusing medical care. This presumes that such choices are intentional, informed, and free of controlling influences.[18] However, a range of circumstances that disproportionately affect the vulnerable (e.g., language, education, or literacy barriers; mental disorders; economic constraints) may challenge this assumption. Ideally, end-of-life decisions should be guided by a person's values and wishes. Various hospice and palliative care organizations promote the use of *Values History Forms* that provide a useful set of exploratory questions. However, questions such as, "What goals do you have for the future?" "How satisfied are you with what you have achieved in your life?" or "What do you fear most?" are oriented to life conditions that may not be relevant to the poor, the homeless, refugees, or other vulnerable persons.

An additional ideal is that goals of care and values be documented in a written directive, a living will, or other formal or legal document. This helps ensure that if patients are unable to speak for themselves; their autonomous wishes nonetheless will be known and carried out. Because Mrs. Johnson could not accept her cancer diagnosis, she was incapable of making informed choices about her care.[18] Persons who are deemed unable or incompetent to make informed end-of-life decisions may need to have a surrogate decide for them. When suitable family or legal guardians are available, they may be asked to provide a substituted judgment—one that is based on the wishes of the patient (and *not* on the surrogate's wishes). In some cases, there may be no one who can speak for the patient. Physicians, hospital ethics committees, or courts may then need to serve in that role. Without knowledge of the person's values and wishes, quality-of-life criteria have been applied to decisions based on what is in the best interest of the patient. These determinations can be challenging, at best. For example, consider the case of a young male victim found unconscious and badly beaten, and without any form of identification. An emergency room evaluation reveals severe nonsurgical brain injury; he is stabilized and admitted to intensive care. Two weeks later, he remains comatose. He also remains a "John Doe" with no known identifiable family members, friends, or social network. What decisions should be made about his care, particularly if his neurologic condition fails to improve and a diagnosis of persistent vegetative state is made? Who should make these decisions and whose values should guide the decision-making process on his behalf?

Values become a contestable arena for vulnerable patients at the end of life. This is particularly true for decisions involving medical futility. The American Thoracic Society defines a futile life-sustaining intervention as one that lacks medical efficacy and lacks the outcome of a *meaningful* survival.[19] The former requires the inclusion of the patient's personal values in defining what is deemed meaningful. Both the ethical principles of beneficence and nonmaleficence guide determinations of medical efficacy and meaningful survival. Ultimate decisions regarding the withdrawal or withholding of medically futile interventions may be ethically defensible but still subject to legal challenge. Furthermore, among the vulnerable, larger societal forces (e.g., poverty, war, and trauma) may have contributed to the conditions that directly or indirectly led to death in the first place. In some cases, dying patients who have lacked access to health care may view discussion of withdrawal or withholding of care as yet a further example of social injustice. In addition to principles of beneficence and nonmaleficence then, other ethical principles—most notably justice and equity—may need to be considered in such end-of-life decisions.

CLINICAL ISSUES: PAIN AND SYMPTOM MANAGEMENT

> Mrs. Johnson continued to complain of abdominal pain that went untreated.

Quality end-of-life care requires the clinician to aggressively address pain and symptom control. The landmark Study to Understand Prognoses and Preferences for Outcomes and Risks of Treatment (SUPPORT) investigation provided evidence that more than half of the 9105 seriously ill subjects enrolled in the study were in serious pain in their last days of life.[20] Even after care-related problems were identified, follow-up corrective interventions failed to show improvement in outcomes.[21]

The elderly, poor, and other vulnerable persons are at even greater risk of their pain being misdiagnosed, inadequately assessed, or poorly managed. In 2001, a physician's failure to adequately treat the pain of an elderly dying cancer patient was judged to be in violation of the California laws against elder abuse and resulted in an award of $1.5 million for the family of the deceased. In his defense, lawyers for the doctors argued that their client had not received adequate education on pain management in medical school or in subsequent training.[22] Physicians may also fear regulatory scrutiny from federal and state agencies, or they may worry about drug diversion and thus may fail to prescribe opioids for patients with serious pain (see Chap. 32). These fears, along with the lack of physician training, however, can not account for the extent of disparities in pain treatment for minority patients found in a wide range of clinical settings. In nursing hones, emergency rooms, cancer centers, and community pharmacies, racial and ethnic minority status was found to be risk factors for inadequate pain management.[23–29] In the 2002 Institute of Medicine Report titled, *Unequal Treatment: Confronting Racial and Ethnic Disparities in Health Care*, provider and health system bias directed against racial and ethnic minorities in the forms of conscious and unconscious stereotyping, prejudice, and discrimination was suggested as a potential cause of these disparities.[30]

In addition to concerns with providing adequate pain relief, providers must attend to a range of other constitutional, organ system, and psychiatric symptoms that are part of the underlying disease or that arise during the active dying process. Dyspnea, the awareness of breathlessness, is a common distressing symptom at the end of life that may worsen as death progresses. Although it is a subjective sensation, like pain, it may result from underlying pulmonary, cardiovascular, or renal disease, or caused or exacerbated by anxiety. Other common symptoms at the end of life include nausea and vomiting, constipation or diarrhea, anorexia, and dysphagia. Anxiety, delirium, and agitation also may be present as a result of drugs, metabolic disturbances, infection, or brain lesions. When the causes of any of these symptoms are not apparent or easily determined, further identification of their underlying etiology may be difficult and in some cases unwarranted. For example, patients who are imminently dying should not be subjected to a battery of invasive tests whose results may take days to weeks to return. However, appropriate management of symptoms with the goal of improving the quality of life as well as quality of dying is an absolute, inviolable priority throughout the continuum of care.

HEALTH SYSTEM ISSUES: PALLIATIVE CARE SERVICES

Quality palliative care—the total active medical, psychological, social, and spiritual care of patients who have received a diagnosis of a serious, life-threatening illness—requires a different health care system than the acute-care conventional model that is currently dominant. Multiple models of palliative care have emerged in the past decade. Palliative care provisions vary by hospital, ranging from consultative services to fully staffed wards. The funding of these services remains a challenge for most institutions.

Hospice Care

Hospice was the first comprehensive model to address the multidisciplinary needs of the dying in a coordinated fashion. Although Medicare has included hospice coverage provisions since 1983, certain requirements can create barriers to its use. For example, curative treatments are not covered and eligibility requires a prognosis of 6 months or less. Fear of indictment for Medicare fraud on the basis of patients surviving beyond the 6-month limit may make physicians and hospices reluctant to refer or enroll patients until death is imminent—often much too late to maximize the quality care services that hospice offers. This reluctance is unfortunate because provisions within Medicare do allow for coverage to be extended for 60 days and there is no limit to the number of times a patient can be recertified for this extension. Another limit, however, is that Medicare coverage is geared toward home care, which presumes that patients have adequate housing and an at-home caregiver. Vulnerable patients who are homeless, who live in substandard housing, or who live alone are disadvantaged by this requirement. Many hospitals have developed palliative care services that are available as an adjunct to, or as an alternative to curative care, thus overcoming some of the barriers of hospice eligibility.

PACE Model

The Program of All-Inclusive Care of the Elderly (PACE) model of care provides comprehensive services to disabled and nursing-home eligible elderly. Although not considered an end-of-life care provider, per se, these community-based programs have the benefit of providing continuity care and their success may result from the "all-inclusiveness" provision: patients are enrolled for the duration of their life and all medical, social, rehabilitation, psychological, and other services must be obtained through the program. As their enrollees face the end of life, coordinated comprehensive care is available to meet their needs.

Respite Care

Respite care provides a range of services to benefit both patients and their caregivers. Most programs offer daycare or short-term hospitalization that can provide temporary relief for primary caregivers. Some, such as the Boston Health Care for the Homeless Program, target the respite needs of the terminally ill homeless who are without supports or resources.

Common Pitfalls

- Health care providers avoid discussing death or do so in language that is not understood.
- Cultural and social issues are often ignored in end-of-life discussions.
- Trustworthiness of providers, an essential element to these discussions, may be a concern for underserved patients.
- Health care providers wait too long before referring patients to hospice.
- Dying patients, particularly those from minority groups, do not have their pain controlled.
- Social injustice contributes to early death and increased suffering in poor, underserved, and minority patients.

APPROACHES TO THE CARE OF THE DYING PATIENT

VALUES CLARIFICATION: PATIENT AND PROVIDER

Consumer groups have sought to empower patients to participate in decisions regarding their care. The *Five Wishes,* (available through Aging with Dignity) is one such program, developed to encourage patients to address their medical, personal, emotional, and spiritual values with their family and physicians. Recognized in most states to meet the legal requirement of an advance directive, the five wishes ascertain: the patient's proxy for health care decisions; what medical treatment, including life support, the patient wants; desired comfort measures (regarding pain and symptom control); desired care from other nonmedical personnel; and disclosure parameters (i.e., what information can be disclosed and to whom).

Perhaps the first step in caring for the dying is for providers to recognize their own mortality and to explore how their different life experiences influence interactions with patients. Indeed, personal self-awareness is a critical element in achieving cultural competence (see Chap. 9). Personnel from local hospices or other palliative care resources may be enlisted to help health care providers identify their anxieties and fears. Clinicians may benefit from asking themselves the questions comprising the *Five Wishes.* Providers should also become aware of the values they hold regarding the range of ethical issues that might arise in care for the dying. What is their own position regarding such issues as patient autonomy, truth-telling, and disclosure? They should consider how their stance might conflict with persons whose cultural values and preferences differ from their own. For example, it is important that a clinician acknowledge his or her own feelings before facing an immigrant patient's family who insists that the patient be shielded from a terminal diagnosis.

SOCIOCULTURAL COMPETENCE

Many hospice and palliative care organizations have felt the impact of changing demographic characteristics (increasing numbers of older, multicultural, and multiethnic populations) and have responded with efforts to increase the cultural competence of the palliative care workforce.[31]

Providers should become aware of the unique cultural, economic, sociopolitical, and historical backgrounds of the populations they serve. This not only may contribute to a better understanding of the clinical issues, but also may provide an opportunity for patients to tell their own story and to feel cared about. It may also enhance the perception of provider trustworthiness, an essential element in the provider–patient relationship. In turn, it is incumbent on the provider to examine negative attitudes they may hold toward certain populations and to strive to eliminate behavior that may be discriminatory.

Strategies for culturally appropriate communication are appropriate in the care of vulnerable patients, as well. In general, when language barriers arise, the use of trained medical interpreters is crucial (see Chap. 26). Even when patients and providers share the same language, it is important that the provider make explicit inquiries to check if understanding is present. Often, asking patients to offer their explanatory model of their illness can reveal gaps in health literacy that can be then addressed with appropriate information.

CLINICAL COMPETENCE

Until recently, the skills needed to manage pain and other distressing symptoms, coordinate care in interdisciplinary teams, communicate effectively with patients and families, and assess grief and loss were not part of standard medical education. Fortunately, this is changing, as demonstrated by new mandates in many states for continuing education in pain and palliative care as a requirement for physician license renewal. Several educational programs have been developed to improve the full range of end-of-life care skills and competencies. The American Medical Association's Education for Physicians on End-of-Life Care (EPEC) program combines multimedia presentations, exercises, and discussions emphasizing communication, ethical decision making, palliative care, psychosocial concerns, and symptom management with training sessions available in most major US cities or online. The APPEAL program is a useful resource that provides (as its acronym suggests) a progressive palliative care education curriculum for the care of African-Americans at life's end. Other educational programs are also available, such as the American Academy of Hospice and Palliative Medicine self-study UNIPAC curriculum. The Academy also hosts the web-based End-of-Life/Palliative Care Educational Resource Center (EPERC) that includes a comprehensive database of peer-reviewed educational materials. This includes their Fast Facts files that are continuously updated peer reviewed, one-page outlines of key information on important end-of-life clinical topics for end-of-life educators and clinicians.

CLINICAL PRACTICE GUIDELINES FOR QUALITY PALLIATIVE CARE

Care of the dying requires a multidisciplinary team approach to address the physical, psychosocial, spiritual, and practical needs of patients. The American Academy of Hospice and Palliative Medicine, the Center to Advance Palliative Care, the Hospice and Palliative Nurses Association, the former Last Acts Partnership, and the National Hospice and Palliative Care Organization worked together to establish evidence-based clinical practice guidelines for quality multi-disciplinary care.[32] These guidelines address care issues in the following domains: structures and processes; physical care; psychological and psychiatric care; social aspects; spiritual, religious, and existential issues; cultural aspects; care of the imminently dying patient; and ethical and legal aspects of care (see Core Competencies).

The goal of palliative care is to prevent and relieve suffering and to support the best possible quality of life for patients and their families, regardless of the stage of the disease or the need for other therapies.[32] Palliative care is realized through management of pain and symptoms, psychosocial distress, spiritual issues, and practical needs throughout the continuum of care.[32] However, the physical and existential suffering associated with serious and eventually fatal conditions are only one part of the overwhelming stressors with which the vulnerable patient must contend.[33–35] The guidelines also emphasize the need to share information with the patient and family about changing conditions and treatment options.

Language and literacy barriers may make information exchange particularly challenging. Although the gold standard of palliative care strives to ensure genuine coordination and continuity of care across settings, health care for the disenfranchised may be fragmented or delivered in emergency rooms or other clinical settings where time and resources are constrained. Lastly, the guidelines emphasize the value of preparing both the patient and family for the dying process, and for death, when it can be anticipated. However, a disproportionate number of vulnerable persons suffer sudden death, precluding the ability to prepare. These examples illustrate the stark contrast between the goals of palliative care and the realities of the dying vulnerable.

CONCLUSION

With the advent of the hospice movement over 30 years ago, and more recently, through grassroots, philanthropic, and special interest advocacy, care of the dying has undergone transformation in US society. Practice guidelines and continuing educational programs are available to improve clinician end-of-life care skills and competencies. The unique concerns of the vulnerable dying can be addressed by advocating for reforms in health care delivery and financing that eliminate the barriers to quality care.

KEY CONCEPTS: STRATEGIES FOR END-OF-LIFE CARE FOR VULNERABLE PERSONS

Identified Problems	Strategies
Values clarification	• Become aware of personal anxieties and fears regarding death; if necessary, seek support from local hospice or other organizations that care for the dying. • Complete a living will, *Five Wishes*, or other advance directive.
Conflicting values	• Identify personal values regarding ethical principles. • Elicit patient's expectations for care. • Identify shared values. • Be willing to modify own position to reach a mutually acceptable solution. • Seek consultation or assistance from other health care workers, institutional ethics committee, or community or religious leaders when necessary.
Communication: general concerns	• Be alert for problems, even when patient and physician share the same language or use local dialects. • Check explicitly that patient and physician have understood each other.
Language barriers	• Use trained medical interpreters. • When possible, avoid using family or friends of patient to translate.
Caring for specific populations: disparities and social justice	• Increase knowledge of the cultural, economic, sociopolitical, and historical contexts through guidebooks, community representatives, religious leaders, or professional colleagues. • Honestly examine negative attitudes they may hold toward certain populations and strive to eliminate behavior that may be discriminatory. • Respectfully inquire about past or present incidents that may have engendered mistrust. • Listen to patient's story and acknowledge the patient's experience. • Address issues that patient identifies as important.
Clinical issues	• Follow Clinical Practice guidelines developed to improve quality care.[31] • Maintain continuing education in pain and palliative care.

CORE COMPETENCY
Clinical Practice Guidelines in the Care of Dying Patients

Domain	Guideline
1. Structure and Processes of Care	1.1 The plan of care is based on a comprehensive interdisciplinary assessment of the patient and family. 1.2 The care plan is based on the identified and expressed values, goals and needs of patient and family, and is developed with professional guidance and support for decision making. 1.3 An interdisciplinary team provides services to the patient and family, consistent with the care plan. 1.4 The interdisciplinary team may include appropriately trained and supervised volunteers. 1.5 Support for education and training is available to the interdisciplinary team. 1.6 The palliative care program is committed to quality improvement in clinical and management practices. 1.7 The palliative care program recognizes the emotional impact on the palliative care team of providing care to patients with life-threatening illnesses and their families. 1.8 Palliative care programs should have a relationship with one or more hospices and other community resources in order to ensure continuity of the highest-quality palliative care across the illness trajectory. 1.9 The physical environment in which care is provided should meet the preferences, needs and circumstances of the patient and family to the extent possible.
2. Physical Aspects of Care	2.1 Pain, other symptoms and side effects are managed based upon the best available evidence, which is skillfully and systematically applied.
3. Psychological and Psychiatric Aspects of Care	3.1 Psychological and psychiatric issues are assessed and managed based upon the best available evidence, which is skillfully and systematically applied. 3.2 A grief and bereavement program is available to patients and families, based on the assessed need for services.

4. Social Aspects of Care	4.1 Comprehensive interdisciplinary assessment identifies the social needs of patients and their families, and a care plan is developed in order to respond to these needs as effectively as possible.
5. Spiritual, Religious, and Existential Aspects of Care	5.1 Spiritual and existential dimensions are assessed and responded to based upon the best available evidence, which is skillfully and systematically applied.
6. Cultural Aspects of Care	6.1 The palliative care program assesses and attempts to meet the culture-specific needs of the patient and family.
7. Care of the Imminently Dying Patient	7.1 Signs and symptoms of impending death are recognized and communicated, and care appropriate for this phase of illness is provided to patient and family.
8. Ethical and Legal Aspects of Care	8.1 The patient's goals, preferences, and choices are respected within the limits of applicable state and federal law, and form the basis for the plan of care.
	8.2 The palliative care program is aware of and addresses the complex ethical issues arising in the care of persons with life-threatening debilitating illness.
	8.3 The palliative care program is knowledgeable about legal and regulatory aspects of palliative care.

Adapted with permission from National Consensus Project for Quality Palliative Care (2004). *Clinical practice guidelines for quality palliative care.* http://www.nationalconsensusproject.org

DISCUSSION QUESTIONS

1. An elderly homeless man has a recent diagnosis of adenocarcinoma of the lung. Given the grim prognosis of this disease, what structures and processes of care are needed to insure the patient's quality of life?

2. What ethical principles should be considered in contemplating the DNR status for a patient in a persistent vegetative state if no prior advance directive is available? How might you assess the patient's values and preferences if he or she is unable to express them? In such cases, which principle, substituted judgment versus best interest, would trump the other in making that decision?

3. How can barriers to hospice referrals and utilization be overcome to make this service more widely available? What alternative delivery models for quality palliative care are available?

4. How can providers and their professional organizations advocate for changes in the health care system that meet the needs of dying patients?

RESOURCES

http://www.agingwithdignity.org/5wishes.html
Aging with Dignity: Five Wishes Program

http://www.aahpm.org/
American Academy of Hospice and Palliative Medicine

http://www.abcd-caring.org
Americans for Better Care of the Dying

http://www.appealproject.org
APPEAL: A Progressive Palliative Care Education Curriculum for the Care of African-Americans at Life's End

http://www.capc.org
Center for the Advancement of Palliative Care

http://www.epec.net/
EPEC(c): The Education in Palliative and End-of-Life Care Curriculum

http://www.aahpm.org/resources/
EPERC: EOL/Palliative Care Educational Resources

http://www.eperc.mcw.edu/ff_index.htm
Fast Facts

http://www.nationalconsensusproject.org
National Consensus Project

http://www.nhpco.org/
National Hospice and Palliative Care Organization

REFERENCES

1. Rice DP. Ethics and equity in U.S. health care: The data. *Int J Health Serv* 1991;21(4):637–651.
2. Blane D. Social determinants of health: Socioeconomic status, social class, and ethnicity. *Am J Public Health* 1995;85(7):903–905.
3. Wong MD, et al. Contribution of major diseases to disparities in mortality. *N Engl J Med* 2002;347(20): 1585–1592.
4. Winkleby MA, Cubbin C. Influence of individual and neighbourhood socioeconomic status on mortality among black, Mexican-American, and white women and men in the United States. *J Epidemiol Commun Health* 2003;57(6):444–452.
5. Anderson RN, Smith BL. Deaths: Leading causes for 2001. *Natl Vital Stat Rept* 2003;52(9):9.
6. Arias E. *United States life tables, 2002. National vital statistics reports.* Hyattsville, MD: National Center for Health Statistics, 2004.
7. Christakis NA, Lamont EB. Extent and determinants of error in doctors' prognoses in terminally ill patients: prospective cohort study. *BMJ* 2000;320(7233):469–472.
8. Lamont EB, Christakis NA. Prognostic disclosure to patients with cancer near the end of life. *Ann Intern Med* 2001;134(12):1096–1105.

9. Lamont EB, Christakis NA. Complexities in prognostication in advanced cancer: To help them live their lives the way they want to. *JAMA* 2003;290(1):98–104.

10. Weissman D. *Fast facts and concepts #30: Prognostication.* End-of-Life Physician Education Resource Center, 2005. Available online at: http://www.eperc.mcw.edu/fastFact/ff_030.htm

11. Schattner A. What do patients really want to know? *QJM* 2002;95(3):135–136.

12. Davis AJ. The bioethically constructed ideal dying patient in USA. *Med Law* 2000;19(1):161–164.

13. Carrese JA, Rhodes LA. Western bioethics on the Navajo reservation. Benefit or harm? [see comments]. *JAMA* 1995;274(10):826–829.

14. Curtis JR, Patrick DL. Barriers to communication about end-of-life care in AIDS patients. *J Gen Intern Med* 1997;12(12):736–741.

15. Blackhall LJ, Murphy ST, et al. Ethnicity and attitudes toward patient autonomy. *JAMA* 1995;274(10):820–825.

16. Lapine A, et al. When cultures clash: physician, patient, and family wishes in truth disclosure for dying patients. *J Palliat Med* 2001;4(4):475–480.

17. Buckman R. *How to break bad news: A guide for health care professionals.* Baltimore: Johns Hopkins University Press, 1992.

18. Beauchamp TL, Childress JF. *Respect for autonomy. Principles of biomedical ethics.* New York: Oxford University Press, 2001.

19. American Thoracic Society. Withholding and withdrawing life sustaining therapy. *Amer Rev Respir Dis* 1991; 144(3):726–731.

20. Desbiens NA, Wu AW. Pain and suffering in seriously ill hospitalized patients. *J Am Geriatr Soc* 2000;48(5 Suppl): S183–186.

21. Lynn J, et al. Ineffectiveness of the SUPPORT intervention: Review of explanations. *J Am Geriatr Soc* 2000;48(5 Suppl): S206–213.

22. Bureau of National Affairs. California: Jury decides undertreatment of pain was elder abuse, sets $1.5 million damages. *BNA Health Law Rpt* 2001;982(June 21):10.

23. Cleeland CS, et al. Pain and treatment of pain in minority patients with cancer. The Eastern Cooperative Oncology Group Minority Outpatient Pain Study. *Ann Intern Med* 1997;127(9): 813–816.

24. Engle V, et al. The experience of living-dying in a nursing home: Self-reports of black and white older adults. *J Am Geriatr Soc* 1998;46(9):1091–1096.

25. Anderson KO, et al. Minority cancer patients and their providers: Pain management attitudes and practice. *Cancer* 2000;88(8):1929–1938.

26. Morrison RS, et al. We don't carry that: Failure of pharmacies in predominantly nonwhite neighborhoods to stock opioid analgesics. *N Engl J Med* 2000;342(14): 1023–1026.

27. Todd KH, et al. Ethnicity and analgesic practice. *Ann Emerg Med* 2000;35(1):11–16.

28. Todd KH. Influence of ethnicity on emergency department pain management. *Emerg Med (Fremantle)* 2001;13(3): 274–278.

29. Anderson KO, et al. Cancer pain management among underserved minority outpatients: Perceived needs and barriers to optimal control. *Cancer* 2002;94(8):2295–304.

30. Smedley BD, et al, eds. *Unequal treatment: Confronting racial and ethnic disparities in healthcare.* Washington, DC: National Academies Press, 2003.

31. Crawley LM, et al. Strategies for culturally effective end-of-life care. *Ann Intern Med* 2002;136(9):673–679.

32. National Consensus Project for Quality Palliative Care. *Clinical practice guidelines for quality palliative care.* 2005. Available online at: http://www.nationalconsensusproject.org

33. Gramelspacher G. Dying poor in an urban hospital. *AMA Virtual Mentor* 2005. June 2001. Available online at: http://www.ama-assn.org/ama/pub/category/5145.html

34. Weissman DE, et al. End-of-life graduate education curriculum project: Project abstracts/progress report—year 3. *J Palliat Med* 2002;5(4):579–606.

35. Williams BR. Dying young, dying poor: A sociological examination of existential suffering among low-socioeconomic status patients. *J Palliat Med* 2004;7(1): 27–37.

Chapter 23

Clinical Care for Persons with a History of Incarceration

Emily A. Wang, MD, Jacqueline P. Tulsky, MD, and Mary C. White, RN, MPH, PhD

Objectives

- Recognize why current and former prisoners constitute a vulnerable population.
- Understand the risk factors for incarceration and ways to prevent it in patients and communities.
- Describe the health care system in prisons and jails and the barriers to providing care.
- Highlight issues unique to caring for previously incarcerated persons in the community.
- Identify ways to improve health care for currently and previously incarcerated prisoners and their families.

Mr. Xavier is a 45-year-old man who was incarcerated for 5 years. Three months after release he is referred to a primary care clinic after being hospitalized with hyperosmolar nonketotic coma.

The high prevalence of incarceration in the United States has profound implications for health both of the individual and for the community. The combination of social stigma; little access to health care before and after incarceration; inadequate health care while incarcerated; and a heavy burden of chronic and acute illnesses make this population among the most vulnerable. This chapter highlights the problems faced by prisoners and ex-offenders in obtaining health care in prison and after release. It discusses strategies for reducing the risks of incarceration, imprisonment itself, and recidivism after release.

EPIDEMIOLOGY: WHO AND WHERE ARE THE INCARCERATED?

The prisoner population in the United States has grown rapidly since the early 1980s. The United States comprises 5% of the global population, yet has 25% of the world's prisoners. About 66% of the incarcerated population is held in state or federal prison systems, with the remainder in local jails.[1] Typically, jails are run by local governments and detain individuals awaiting trial and also those sentenced to less than 1 year. In contrast, prisons detain those guilty of felony crimes and who have longer sentences. The prison systems of each state and the federal prison system are run separately.

By 2003, over 2 million persons were incarcerated in US jails and prisons, an increase of almost 400% since 1980 (Fig. 23-1). There were 482 sentenced inmates per 100,000 US residents, the highest rate among developed countries.[1] A combination of factors likely

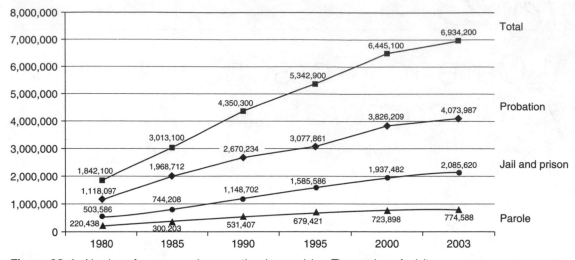

Figure 23-1. Number of persons under correctional supervision. The number of adults in the correctional population has been increasing. (From: Bureau of Justice Statistics. *Correctional surveys*. Presented in Correctional Populations in the United States, Annual, Prisoners in 2003 and Probation and Parole in the United States, 2003. Accessed July 16, 2005. Available at: http://www.ojp.usdoj.gov/bjs/)

explains why the numbers of people incarcerated have skyrocketed in the last two decades. Criminal justice policies, including the "war on drugs" and mandatory sentencing policies, gaps in care for the mentally ill, and the growing concentration of poverty in metropolitan areas all contribute.

Characteristics of the incarcerated differ considerably from the population at large. Most (93.1%) are men.[1] Likewise, the racial composition of the inmate population differs from that of the general US population. African Americans and Latinos comprised 68% of all people in prison and jail in 2003, but only 25% of the US population.[2] African-American men comprise 44% of all male inmates. An African-American man has a one in four chance of going to prison in his lifetime, a Latino man one in six, and a White man a one in 23 chance of serving time in prison.[3] Inmates have low educational attainment; 68% have no high school degree, and 31% to 40% scored in the lowest level of literacy in the National Adult Literacy Survey.[4] Thirty-one percent of state inmates and 23% of federal inmates are reported to have a learning or speech disability.[5] Over half made less than $1000 per month prior to incarceration, and 11% were homeless the year prior to incarceration.[4]

The female inmate population is rising at a faster rate than the male inmate population. Since 1995 the annual rate of growth in the number of female inmates has averaged 5.2%, higher than the 3.4% average increase of male inmates.[1] Relative to their number in the US resident population, men were about 15 times more likely than women to be incarcerated in a state or federal prison.[1]

Prisoners often are parents of dependent children. Of the nation's minor children, 2.1% had a parent in state or federal prison. African-American children were nearly nine times more likely to have a parent in prison than white children (7.0% and 0.8%, respectively), and Latino children were three times as likely as white children to have an incarcerated parent (2.6%).

HEALTH PROBLEMS OF PRISONERS AND EX-OFFENDERS

While in prison, Mr. Xavier was diagnosed with type 2 diabetes, hepatitis C, and depression. When he entered prison, his mandatory syphilis test and voluntary HIV test were both negative. When his annual skin test for tuberculosis turned positive, he received treatment for latent infection.

The likelihood of encountering patients who have been incarcerated is high; more than 11 million people have been released from the prison or jail system. Moreover, the population of prisoners and ex-offenders is increasingly ill and in need of care. The health status of the incarcerated and ex-offenders is complicated by the same risk factors that may have contributed to their being incarcerated—addiction, mental illness, poverty, low educational attainment, and racial discrimination. Despite the fact that current and former prisoners have a higher prevalence of disease, access to care when not incarcerated is limited (Box 23-1).[6]

- Nearly one third of state inmates and one fourth of federal inmates reported a physical impairment or mental condition.
- More than one in four state and federal inmates had been injured after admission to prison.
- Injuries and other medical problems increase with time in prison. Nearly half of state inmates who had served 6 or more years said they had been injured after admission.
- Medical problems and other conditions are more common among older inmates; those who had been homeless or unemployed; those who had used a needle to inject drugs; and those who were alcohol dependent.

- The most commonly reported medical problems include: HIV/AIDS, heart and other circulatory problems, cancer, kidney/liver, respiratory, neurologic, and skeletal problems, and diabetes.

These self-reported results may underestimate the prevalence rates of medical conditions.
From: Maruschak L. *HIV in prisons and jails, 2002.* Bureau of Justice Statistics Bulletin. Washington, DC: US Department of Justice 2004, NCJ 205333.[7]

COMMUNICABLE DISEASES

HIV/AIDS

In 1997, an estimated 20% to 26% of all persons living with HIV in the United States passed through a correctional facility.[8] For the incarcerated, the incidence of HIV infection was five times greater,[9,10] the incidence AIDS was four times greater, and the percent of deaths owing to AIDS was more than double[7] that of the general population. Overall, women were more likely than men (3.0% compared with 1.9%) to be HIV positive, and in some states had HIV rates over 20%.[7]

Sexually Transmitted Infections

Persons in juvenile detention facilities and jails are at higher risk than the general population for contracting sexually transmitted infections.[11] Gonorrhea and chlamydia have been found at rates as high as 20% in female adolescent detainees. Most facilities that do screen for infections treat patients with positive test results, but a large number of facilities do not screen asymptomatic prisoners despite the fact that incarceration guidelines and the Centers for Disease Control call for routine screening of detainees. Prisons tend to see less active infection, but there are documented transmissions of sexually transmitted infections in prisons among sexually active prisoners.[11,12]

Hepatitis B and C

The increased rate of incarceration for crimes related to drug use and the association of injection drug use with hepatitis C (HCV) infection have resulted in higher rates of both hepatitis B and C in the correctional settings.[13] The prevalence of chronic hepatitis B infection among inmates is two to six times that of adults in the general population.[13] HCV infection in state and federal prisons is at least 10 times higher than in the general population.[13]

Tuberculosis

The resurgence of tuberculosis in the 1980s resulted in recognition that correctional facilities were both sites for transmission and targets for case-finding and treatment.[8] An estimated 40% of all people in the nation with active tuberculosis in 1997 served time in a correctional facility that year.[8] Crowded conditions of prisons and jails, combined with high rates of HIV infection and inconsistent care both inside and outside correctional facilities, led to outbreaks of multidrug-resistant strains of tuberculosis. Latent tuberculosis infection, present in 25% to 33% of prisoners, means a risk of developing active tuberculosis disease. California jail inmates, incompletely treated for latent tuberculosis infection, were 59 times as likely to develop active disease in 5 years compared with the general population.[14]

Staphylococcus Infection

Since the late 1990s, prisons and jails have reported outbreaks of methicillin-resistant *Staphylococcus aureus* (MRSA) infections, as well as high rates of asymptomatic carriers of MRSA[21] and transmission of MRSA. Although the community is probably the initial source of MRSA, many factors in the overcrowded jail/prison setting exacerbate the problems of this potentially devastating infection. Inadequate personal hygiene (both voluntary and involuntary), barriers to medical care (specifically wound care), and failure to adequately culture and manage antibiotic treatment for wound and skin infections contribute to MRSA's pervasiveness.[11]

CHRONIC DISEASE

The US prison population is aging, reflecting the changes in society as a whole and the effects of mandatory sentencing and life without the possibility of parole. With this aging the prevalence of chronic disease is rising. The correctional health care system has had to evolve to accommodate this growing elderly population. Although some prisons in the United States have been designated for elderly inmates or for the chronically ill, many elderly and sick inmates remain in prisons that are unable to address their medical or social needs.[16] Only 26 of 41 states surveyed reported treatment protocols for prisoners with diabetes, hypertension, and asthma.[12]

Mental Illness

Mental illness is a dominant condition in prisons. Jails in New York City and Los Angeles are the largest inpatient mental health facilities in the country. Independent of substance use, 16% of state, 7% of federal, and 16% of local jail inmates, as well as 16% of probationers report either a mental condition or an overnight stay in a hospital for mental health reasons.[17] Mentally ill inmates report longer criminal histories than other inmates; about half reported three or more prior sentences and 10% to 13% reported 11 or more prior sentences. These prisoners also have high rates of homelessness—double those of persons who are not mentally ill—as well as high rates of unemployment, alcohol and drug abuse, and a history of physical and sexual abuse prior to incarceration.[17] Moreover, mental illness is not just a problem associated with crime, it is a major cause of morbidity and mortality for the incarcerated. Suicide is the third leading cause of death in state and federal prisons (behind medical illness and AIDS), and the leading cause of death in many county jails.[1]

There are unexpected racial differences in mental illness among prisoners. Nearly one fourth of white state prison and local jail inmates, and one fifth of white offenders on probation were identified as mentally ill in 1998,[17] with considerably lower rates among African-American and Latino inmates. The highest rates of identified mental illness were among white women in state prisons (29%), especially those under age 24, nearly four in 10 of whom were identified as mentally ill.[17]

Substance Abuse

The period since the 1980s was notable for its commitment to a social policy of imprisonment for drug possession or use, and lengthier or mandatory prison sentences. Although 13% of newly sentenced state prisoners in 1985 were convicted of drug offenses, by 1990 this had increased to 32%.[16] Drug- and alcohol-associated offenses also were common. One half of state and one third of federal prisoners reported committing their current offense under the influence of alcohol or drugs.[18] Although nearly 75% of prisoners report alcohol or drug abuse prior to their current offense, only 25% to 33% have ever been treated for substance abuse (see Chap. 33).[18,19]

PRISONS AND JAILS AS A RISK FACTOR: INCARCERATION MAKES PEOPLE MORE VULNERABLE

HIGH-RISK BEHAVIORS

Risky Sexual Activity or Rape

Although research is limited, prisoners' activities put them at risk for adverse health outcomes. Sexual activity between male prisoners has been reported as high as 30% in a Federal Bureau of Prisons study.[20] Little is published about women, but rates are believed to be equally high. The frequency of homosexual rape in jails and prisons is extremely difficult to estimate. A federal prison survey reported that 9% to 20% of federal inmates, especially new, homosexual, or transgender prisoners, were victims of rape.[20] With an incarcerated population of over 2 million, the US correctional system likely exposes tens of thousands of male inmates to nonconsensual, unprotected sex, and consequently to HIV/AIDS and other sexually transmitted diseases. The release of inmates from jails and prisons transforms the consequences of male rape from a correctional matter into a public health crisis.

Even for consensual sexual activity, it is difficult for a prisoner to take precautions against disease. Only five correctional institutions in the United States (three county jails and two state prison systems) make condoms available except during conjugal visits.[10] Former prisoners surveyed in New York reported using makeshift devices for safer sex, such as latex finger condoms, when condoms were not available.

Blood-Borne Infections

Use of shared needles for drug use and tattooing are a documented source of blood-borne infections in prison and jail. Intravenous drug use is common in some prisons.[20,21] Tattooing also is practiced widely in prisons and usually is done without sterilized needles, involving the reuse of sharpened and altered implements such as staples, paper clips, and plastic ink tubes. Contamination of ink has been associated with transmission of skin infections such as MRSA.[13,15]

HEALTH CARE IN PRISON: MANDATED BUT NOT OPTIMAL

> Mr. Xavier's first interaction with a primary care provider was in prison. He had been uninsured most of his adult life. Before being incarcerated he had been told during an emergency room visit that his glucose levels were high and was advised to follow up as an outpatient.

The prison riots in the New York State Penitentiary at Attica brought to national attention the inhumane

---

Box 23-2. Health Care Requirements for Inmates

- A system for intake screening
- A functioning sick call system that uses properly trained health care staff
- A means of addressing medical emergencies
- A priority system so that those most in need of care receive it first
- The development and maintenance of adequate medical records
- Liaison with outside resources for specialty and hospital care when needed

- Adequate space and supplies
- A system for staff development and training
- A quality improvement program
- Procedures for meeting the special needs of the mentally ill, disabled, and elderly
- Discharge planning

From: American Public Health Association Standards for Health Care in Correctional Institutions.[22]

---

conditions, including the state of health care, in US prison systems. By 1976, investigations and judicial intervention resulted in constitutionally guaranteed health care in the prison and jail systems. The US Supreme Court found in *Estelle v. Gamble* that "deliberate indifference" to "serious medical needs" of inmates violated the eighth amendment's protection against cruel and unusual punishment (Box 23-2).[22]

Thus, the incarcerated have a type of universal access to care on a scale not yet available to other populations in the United States. Even Medicaid and Medicare have some eligibility requirements, such as citizenship, that result in some persons being denied care. This is not true in a jail or prison. This right is the source of some tension in the public sector, in which prisoners are seen as receiving more care and services than law-abiding citizens.

Actually providing consistent health care for prisoners at a community standard has proved to be difficult for many counties and states. Reflecting overall health care costs, the costs of providing care to prisoners are mounting. It costs the state of California approximately $30,000 annually to incarcerate one prisoner and over $100,000 annually to incarcerate a prisoner with HIV. As a result, many states have turned toward private industry to lower the expense of care.[23]

SCREENING AND TREATMENT: REQUIRED BUT OFTEN INADEQUATE

In spite of the high burden of disease, screening, prevention, and treatment of these diseases are not universally promoted, vary from state to state, and are often substandard.[24] National organizations, such as the National Commission on Correctional Health Care, have been trying to implement realistic guidelines for health care in prisons and jails.[12] Unfortunately, despite successful institution in a handful of states, acceptance and implementation of the guidelines is elective. For example,

only 19 state and federal prisons have mandatory HIV screening on entry,[10] and only 45% of infected prisoners receive the recommended drug regimens.[23] Moreover, only about half of jails and 90% of prisons routinely screen for tuberculosis at intake.[8] Lack of communication between the correctional facility and the community into which prisoners are released hampers TB control efforts, despite policies requiring notification.

Women's health care often is not available in a system that typically cares for the health needs of men (see Chap. 29). Routine preventive care, including pap smears and mammograms, may not be offered even to prisoners who are incarcerated for long periods of time.[24,25] In 1996, an estimated 25% of imprisoned women were pregnant upon incarceration or had delivered in the past year.[26] A very few model programs provide pregnant, incarcerated women with appropriate prenatal care and parenting skills. Most women who deliver in prison or jail spend less than 24 hours with their baby before they are given over to foster care.[26]

INSTITUTIONAL BARRIERS TO CARE IN CORRECTIONAL FACILITIES

Even in the face of constitutional rights, there are numerous barriers to providing a community standard of health care. Many jail detainees are held for no more than 48 hours or a few days until they can post bail. Thus, inmates who are screened and/or diagnosed may be released prior to treatment being initiated or completed. This is especially problematic in the cases of tuberculosis and sexually transmitted diseases.

The emphasis on security can conflict with the provision of health care in the correctional setting.[11] Prisoners' requests to see a physician are often filtered through corrections officers, or nonmedical personnel, who determine whether their requests are legitimate. Confidentiality is extremely difficult to achieve in the corrections setting and fear of other prisoners finding out about medical conditions may prompt a prisoner to refuse screening or treatment for known infectious or chronic conditions.[11]

Correctional systems often face serious resource limitations in the provision of health care. Meeting inmate health needs can be expensive. Inmates have high rates of disease, partially because of the lack of health care they received prior to incarceration. Treating hepatitis C, for example, costs $12,000 per patient per year.[13] Administrators know that once a prisoner has been diagnosed with a disease, case law and ethics require them to provide treatment to community standards.

Finally, the systems and politics that govern health care in prisons create barriers to care for prisoners. Health policies often are dictated by the private health care vendors or pharmaceutical companies, which profit through supplying care and medications to prisons. In California and other states, prisoners who are not destitute pay a $5 copay to see the physician.[27] This system forces prisoners to choose between their health care and other basic needs. Prisons tend to be located in rural parts of the United States, and as a result correctional health care practitioners frequently are isolated from the medical community, thus making discharge planning and provider-to-provider communication difficult.

TRANSITIONAL HEALTH CARE

> Mr. Xavier is released from prison with a 1-month supply of medications. He receives no referral for primary care and does not follow up. He is unsure of where to go and how to pay for medical care and medications.

Unlike jails and prisons, there are no government guarantees for health care once inmates are released. Upon release, prisoners are lucky to be given even a limited supply of medication. Given that little or no follow-up is available in the community, patients frequently come to primary care via the emergency department.

Transitional health care programs for ex-offenders vary widely. In a survey of 33 state prison systems, transitional health care planning was reported to include at least one of the following: post-release medications, referral to community health agencies, scheduling of appointments, and instructions for the prevention of transmitting disease. The most successful transition programs have been established for prisoners with HIV. One such program in Rhode Island has even reduced the rates of recidivism by providing primary care, peer counseling, and discharge planning.[28]

Seamless care for those leaving prison or jail should include the reinstatement of entitlement benefits (Medicaid, Social Security Income) before release, providing adequate amounts of medication, transitional care for medical and mental health conditions, and access to medical records for community providers. Discharge case management is one proposed method of integrating prison and community health care.[12,28]

Common Pitfalls

- Prisoners are unlikely to be considered part of the community, despite the fact that it is extremely common to have been incarcerated or have a family member incarcerated.
- Opportunities to address health issues of prisoners are often overlooked in prison.
- Overlooking health issues of prisoners can have serious public health consequences.
- Incarceration poses health risks of its own that are overlooked if practitioners do not know about the prison or jail history.
- Jails and prisons have inconsistent and largely inadequate screening and treatment of illnesses common to inmates.
- Mental health and substance abuse issues that increase the likelihood of recidivism often are unaddressed.
- Provision of adequate health care to inmates is costly.
- Private companies that provide health care to inmates may not share wider public health goals.

MEDICAL MANAGEMENT OF FORMER PRISONERS

OBTAINING AN INCARCERATION HISTORY

Given the stigma of incarceration, it is difficult to discuss the effects of incarceration on a person's health. Former inmates differ on whether they believe that primary care physicians should ask about incarceration and if so how they should ask. Forming a therapeutic alliance between practitioner and patient that allows the ex-offender to feel safe enough to discuss these matters is crucial. In this context, obtaining the prison history can help the health care provider and patient address discrete health concerns, including prevention of future incarceration. Indeed, avoiding return to prison may be a patient's highest priority. Counseling regarding substance use, and strategies designed to prevent lapses in use of antipsychotic medications are interventions that might prevent future incarceration. Providers should be aware to avoid using medications that might trigger a parole violation (e.g., opiates). If these medications are deemed crucial, a letter to the

---

Box 23-3. Provider Advocacy for Prisoners and Ex-offenders

- Prison health care has evolved through litigation and case law. Health care providers need to take the lead in the care of this vulnerable population.
- The overall goal for prisons and jails should be to ensure the public safety and serve the cause of justice for all while encouraging rehabilitation and participation in productive educational programming.
- Facilities within prisons and jail must improve to accommodate the health care needs of prisoners.

- Health care providers should advocate for the following:
  —There should be a reduction in incarceration, especially the decriminalization of drug dependency and mental illness.
  —More drug treatment centers and mental health facilities should be established.
  —No institution or corporate entity should be permitted to profit from imprisonment.
  —Jails and prisons should be safe for all who spend time there—employees, visitors, and prisoners alike.

---

probation officer could be important in protecting a former inmate from additional problems with the system (see Core Competency). Another important component of the incarceration history is obtaining medical records from the prison or jail. State and county correctional facilities frequently have web sites with instructions for contacting the facility.

INCARCERATION SYSTEM: A MODEL OF DISEASE INTERVENTION AND PREVENTION

The prison health care system is the largest form of universal health care in this country, serving over 2 million people. As such, prisons and jails offer a unique opportunity to establish better disease control and prevention, and health education to a generally vulnerable population.[12] Prison and jail can be places where behaviors that promote healthy lifestyles are learned. The National Commission for Correctional Health Care (NCCHC) and the American Public Health Association have both created guidelines to standardize the care for chronic diseases in prisons.[12,22] Establishing systems of integrated transitional care would also improve in both correctional facilities and the community.

INDIVIDUAL PROVIDER ADVOCACY

Mr. Xavier's drug addiction and unemployment contributed to his imprisonment. Once his health care provider obtains his history, she contacts the parole officer to obtain prison medical records and learn the terms of parole. Mr. Xavier is referred to Narcotics Anonymous, a high school equivalency program, and an ex-offenders support group.

Primary care providers can help decrease the risk of incarceration and mitigate the effects of incarceration on patients, families, and communities. Advocacy for positive change in the health of patients often begins

with one individual patient (see Chap. 41). Addressing the broad-reaching influences incarceration has on employment, political participation, housing, and the custody of children is important. For example, more than 1.5 million children in the United States have parents in prison; many more have parents in jail.[29] Children of incarcerated parents are five times as likely to spend time in prison as adults as are children of non-incarcerated parents. Incarceration also can precipitate homelessness by removing a wage earner from the home and reducing family income. Additionally, current regulations of the US Department of Housing and Urban Development require public housing projects to evict families with whom a convicted felon resides, forcing some women leaving prison to abandon their children or partners or become homeless.[29] Consequently, many inmates require not only ongoing medical and mental health care, but also need referral to other community-based programs, such as substance abuse treatment, assistance with housing, child care, and other public assistance programs.[5]

Lifestyle and behavior change is a process, not an event. Individual risk for initial or repeat incarcerations is rooted in behaviors that can and should be addressed by primary providers, such as domestic violence, drug and alcohol addiction, and undertreated mental health symptoms (see Chap. 7). Finally, remembering the sacrifice of family members who have an incarcerated relative is a good way to gently bring up issues that may accompany a family who is missing the major wage earner, role model, or troubled member (Box 23-3).

CONCLUSION

Many people in the United States are incarcerated some time during their lives. Those who serve time suffer a heavy burden of illness and are exposed to further health risks because of their incarceration. Understanding the complexities of caring for patients with a history of incarceration allows primary care providers to help prevent recidivism and make a lasting impact on the health of their patients and their patients' families and communities.

KEY CONCEPTS

- Prisoners have a higher burden of mental illness, infectious diseases, and drug addiction, and present to care later in the course of chronic disease.
- Risk factors operative before and after incarceration, including poverty, homelessness, race, and illiteracy, complicate the health care of ex-offenders
- Prison health care is limited by the lack of confidentiality, informed consent, and focus on security that are inherent in the corrections setting.
- Community providers can play an important role in helping their patients transition from prison to the community and reducing rates of incarceration and recidivism.

CORE COMPETENCY

Seeing a Patient with a History of Incarceration

- Obtain an incarceration history
  —Set the Stage
    Establish a safe, non-judgmental environment
    Ask permission to inquire
    Assure the patient that your interest stems from medical concern
  —Ask about:
    When and where the person was incarcerated
    Amount of time spent in prison or jail
    Charges (relation to drugs, violence, or sex work)
    Past probation or parole
    Any current probation or parole and the specific conditions of probation or parole
    Number of previous incarcerations
- Screen for history of physical or sexual abuse, substance abuse, mental illness, gang involvement; refer to appropriate services.
- Screen for tuberculosis, hepatitis, syphilis, HIV, other sexually transmitted diseases.
- Obtain medical records from prison or jail.
- Refer to social worker for reinstatement of Medicaid, obliteration of criminal record, and federal or state aid for housing and food stamps.
- Establish goals for preventing recidivism and preventing incarceration in other family members, especially children.
- Refer to special programs (e.g., tattoo removal, vocational training)

DISCUSSION QUESTIONS

1. What makes prisoners a vulnerable population?
2. What can primary care providers do to prevent recidivism?
3. What are some ways you can ask a new patient if they have been incarcerated, to lessen the stigma of having been incarcerated?
4. How can the prison health care system be used as an opportunity to improve public health and model for universal care?

RESOURCES

http://www.allofusornone.org/
A national organizing initiative of prisoners, former prisoners and felons dedicated to prison reform and self-advocacy

http://www.aclu.org
American Civil Liberties Union

http://www.ojp.usdoj.gov/bjs
Bureau of Justice web site with federal and statewide statistics of prisons and jails

http://www.ncchc.org
National Commission on Correctional Health web site, a resource for prison health care providers

http://www.prisonlaw.com/
A nonprofit organization in California that provides free legal services and online nationwide resources for prisoners and providers
Puisis M. *Clinical practice in correctional medicine.* St. Louis: Mosby, 1998.

REFERENCES

1. Harrison PM, Karberg JC. *Prison and jail inmates at midyear 2003.* Bureau of Justice Statistics Bulletin. Washington, DC: US Department of Justice, 2004, NCJ 203947.
2. Ziedenberg J, Schiraldi V. Race and imprisonment in Texas: The disparate incarceration of Latinos and African Americans in the Lone Star State. Washington, DC: Justice Policy Institute, February 24th, 2005.
3. Bonczar TB, Beck AF. *Lifetime likelihood of going to state or federal prison.* Bureau of Justice Statistics Bulletin. Washington, DC: US Department of Justice, 1997, NCJ 1600092.
4. Harlow CW. Education and correctional populations. Bureau of Justice Statistics Bulletin. Washington, DC: US Department of Justice, 2003, NCJ 195670.
5. Maruschak L, Beck AJ. *Medical problems of inmates, 1997.* Bureau of Justice Statistics Bulletin Washington, DC: US Department of Justice 2001, NCJ 181644.
6. Conklin TJ, Lincoln T, Tuthill RW. Self-reported health and prior health behaviors of newly admitted correctional inmates. *Am J Pub Health* 2000;90:1939–1941.

7. Maruschak L. *HIV in prisons and jails, 2002.* Bureau of Justice Statistics Bulletin. Washington, DC: US Department of Justice 2004, NCJ 205333.

8. Hammett TM, Harmon MP, Rhodes W. The burden of infectious disease among inmates of and releasees from US correctional facilities, 1997. *Am J Public Health* 2002; 92:1789–1794.

9. National Commission on Correctional Health Care. *Standards for health care in prison, 2003. Standards for health care in jail, 2003.* Available at: http://www.ncchc.org

10. Spaulding A, Stephenson B, Macalino G, et al. Human immunodeficiency virus in correctional facilities: A review. *Clin Infect Dis* 2002;35:305–312.

11. Puisis M, ed. *Clinical practice in correctional medicine.* St. Louis: Mosby, 1998.

12. National Commission on Correctional Health Care. The health status of soon-to-be-released inmates: A report to congress. Chicago: March, 2002. Accessed August 1, 2005. Available at: http://www.ncchc.org/pubs/pubs_stbr.html

13. Centers for Disease Control and Prevention. Prevention and control of infections with hepatitis viruses in correctional settings. *MMWR* 2003;52(RR01):1–33.

14. White MC, Tulsky JP, Menendez E, et al. Incidence of TB in inmates with latent TB infection: 5-year follow-up. *Am J Prev Med* 2005;29(4):295–301.

15. Centers for Disease Control and Prevention. Methicillin-resistant *Staphylococcus aureus* infections in correctional facilities—Georgia, California, and Texas, 2001–2003. *MMWR* 2003;52(41):992–996.

16. Bureau of Justice Statistics Unit. *Correctional populations in the United States, 1995.* Bureau of Justice Statistics Bulletin. Washington, DC: US Department of Justice, 1997, NCJ 163916.

17. Ditton PM. *Mental health and treatment of inmates and probationers.* Bureau of Justice Statistics Bulletin. Washington, DC: US Department of Justice 1999, NCJ 174463.

18. Mumola CJ. *Substance abuse and treatment, state and federal prisoners, 1997.* Bureau of Justice Statistics Bulletin. Washington, DC: US Department of Justice, 1999, NCJ 172871.

19. Fiscella K, Pless N, Meldrum S, et al. Alcohol and opiate withdrawal in US jails. *Am J Pub Health* 2004;94: 1522–1524.

20. Nacci P, Kane T. *Sex and sexual aggression in federal prisons.* Washington, DC: Federal Bureau of Prisons, 1982.

21. Carvell AL, Hart GJ. Risk behaviors for HIV infection among drug users in prison. *BMJ* 1990;300:1383–1384.

22. APHA Task Force on Correctional Health. Standards for Health Service in Correctional Institutions, 3rd edition. Washington, DC: American Public Health Association, 2003. Available at: http://www.apha.org/media/abc2.htm#prisons

23. Kantor E. *HIV transmission and prevention in prisons.* HIV InSite Knowledge Base Chapter. February 2003. Available at http://www.hivinsite.ucsf.edu

24. Binswanger IA, White MC, Perez-Stable E, et al. Cancer screening among jail inmates: Frequency, knowledge and willingness. *Am J Pub Health* 2005;95:1781–1787.

25. Elwood Martin R, Hislop TG, Grams GD, et al. Evaluation of a cervical cancer screening intervention for prison inmates. *Can J Public Health* 2004;95:285–289.

26. Sayfer SM, Richmond L. Pregnancy behind bars. *Semin Perinatol* 1995;19:314–322.

27. Hyde R, Brumfield B. Effect of co-payment on the use of medical services by male and female prisoners. *J Correct Health Care* 2003;9:371–379.

28. Rich JD, Holmes L, Salas C, et al. Successful linkage of medical care and community services for HIV-positive detainees being released from prison. *J Urban Health* 2001;78:279–289.

29. Hirsch A, et al. Every door closed: Barriers facing parents with criminal records. Center for Law and Social Policy, May 2002. Accessed August 1, 2005. Available at: www.clasp.org/publications.php?id=10

Chapter 24

Care of the Homeless Patient

Margot Kushel, MD, and Sharad Jain, MD

Objectives

- Define homelessness and identify risks for homelessness.
- Describe the epidemiology of homelessness, including morbidity and mortality.
- Review medical conditions common among the homeless.
- Identify challenges to providing care to homeless patients.
- Identify interventions to improve care, both at the provider and system levels.

Mr. Jones rarely comes to clinic appointments and often leaves before being seen as he is afraid of not getting a shelter bed in time. He has been homeless for years. He has schizophrenia, hypertension, and has difficulty controlling his diabetes.

Being homeless has a profound effect on health. Homeless patients have higher rates of chronic illness, morbidity, and mortality than patients who have stable housing.[1-4] Lacking insurance and transportation, their access to care is limited. Obtaining food and shelter are higher priorities for the homeless person than seeking health care.[5,6] Homeless patients present for medical attention later in the course of their illness.[7,8] Comorbid conditions such as mental illness and substance abuse can complicate adherence to treatment plans. Furthermore, providers often do not incorporate the challenges faced by homeless patients into management plans. This chapter explores the relevance of homelessness to health and healthcare and presents strategies to improve the care that homeless patients receive.

EPIDEMIOLOGY

As of the mid 1990s, approximately 400,000 Americans were homeless and used homeless services on a given week, and between 2.3 and 3.5 million Americans experienced homelessness and used homeless services annually.[9] Although 1% of the US population experiences homelessness each year, approximately 10% of the poverty population is without housing. One fourth of all Americans who are homeless are children.[9]

DEFINITION AND PATTERN OF HOMELESSNESS

The most commonly accepted definition of homelessness comes from the McKinney Act, federal legislation enacted in 1987 to define who would be identified as homeless.

An individual or family who lacks a fixed, regular and adequate nighttime residence or an individual or family whose primary nighttime residence is a temporary shelter/hotel, place not ordinarily used as a regular sleeping accommodation, or who is staying temporarily with friends or family. Persons incarcerated or detained are not included.[10]

One way to conceptualize homelessness is by understanding its varied patterns. Martha Burt, a noted expert on homelessness, conceptualizes the homeless population as chronic, intermittent, or in crisis.[9]

The *chronically homeless* person usually is defined as someone who has been homeless for at least 1 year or has had four episodes in a 4-year period. Chronically homeless persons face multiple barriers to finding stable housing and employment. Although only 10% of people who experience an episode of homelessness are chronically homeless, approximately 50% of persons who are homeless at any point could be considered chronically homeless. Chronically homeless persons are more likely to be men, have mental illness and substance abuse problems, and have a history of involvement with the criminal justice system. Because of their visibility (these are the urban street and shelter sleepers), they have come to represent the face of homelessness.

The *intermittently homeless* person is someone who has had multiple, short, self-limited episodes of homelessness. Most have spent time living with friends or family prior to losing their housing. Intermittently homeless people regain housing, but tend to be precariously housed; thus, they are at high risk of becoming homeless again. Typically, intermittently homeless persons have low income, low educational attainment, and may be escaping violent situations within their own homes. The prototypical intermittently homeless person is that of a member of a female-headed household that is struggling financially to get by.

The *in-crisis homeless* person is someone who has had one episode of homelessness brought about by a major crisis: an economic, health-related, or natural disaster (fire, earthquake). In general, those with crisis homelessness regain their housing and do not lose it again.

Homeless youth, as opposed to homeless children living in families, are adolescents or young adults (12 to 25 years old), living on their own without parents. These youth have often fled abusive situations or family disapproval caused by conflicts over their sexual identity. This population is marked by high rates of substance abuse, survival sex (exchanging sex for money, drugs, or housing), suicide, and transience, with high rates of movement between different cities.

Although many of the necessary adjustments in providing health care are similar across the patterns of homelessness, each group presents unique needs and challenges.

HOMELESSNESS AS A MEDICAL PROBLEM

Many people, health care providers included, do not consider homelessness a medical problem. Reviewing the complex causes and risks of homelessness, however, helps providers to understand ways to intervene both to prevent homelessness and mitigate its risks.

CAUSES AND RISK FACTORS FOR HOMELESSNESS

The causes of homelessness are disputed. Some emphasize personal vulnerabilities (e.g., mental illness, substance abuse), and others cite systemic and structural problems (e.g., poverty, lack of affordable housing), as the root causes.[9] Homelessness can be conceptualized as resulting from a complex interaction of protective and risk factors occurring in the context of poverty and little access to housing (Table 24-1). Many of the risk factors that push people into homelessness; for example, chronic and mental illness, family violence, pregnancy, and substance use, explain why homelessness itself is an issue of concern for medical providers. Indeed, intervening to mitigate the risks and bolster the protective factors may have a profound effect on health.

Personal Vulnerabilities

Poverty is the most essential personal and social vulnerability leading to homelessness, but it is not the sole determinant. Other personal vulnerabilities in addition to those listed in the preceding include childhood and adult victimization, and "out of home" experiences as a child (e.g., involvement in the foster care system, being homeless as a child, being in the juvenile justice system, being a runaway or "throwaway" child).[10,11] Many persons leaving state or federal prisons become homeless at discharge.

Structural Factors

Important structural factors include the availability of jobs that pay enough to allow people to maintain

Table 24-1. Factors Influencing Homelessness

Protective Factors for Homelessness

- Financial resources
- Housing subsidy
- Social support
- Health
- Good housing and job availability
- Good employment history

Risk Factors for Homelessness

- Mental illness
- Chronic illness
- Partner violence
- Substance use
- Pregnancy
- Dependent children
- Poverty
- Lack of affordable housing
- Unstable employment history
- Unstable housing
- Poor social support
- History of homelessness
- History of incarceration
- Little availability of public assistance

housing (and meet other basic needs) and the presence of affordable housing for low-income individuals.

Social programs can be part of the "safety net" that prevents people from becoming homeless. Programs such as social insurance (Temporary Assistance to Needy Families, Social Security Disability Income, and county general assistance and unemployment insurance), rent subsidies (Section 8 vouchers), temporary housing, medical care, psychiatric care, and substance abuse treatment to low-income individuals can mitigate the effects of forces precipitating homelessness.

In an environment with limited low-cost housing and employment opportunities and an inadequate safety net, those lacking personal resources may become homeless; as the safety net erodes and the economy worsens, those with less vulnerability also may find themselves to be homeless.

HEALTH STATUS OF HOMELESS POPULATIONS

Homelessness is a concern for medical providers because not only may it be precipitated by medical problems, but also it puts people at risk for illness. Homeless people often are homeless because they are ill and ill because they are homeless.

Homeless persons have high rates of morbidity and mortality. More than one third of all homeless persons report their health as fair or poor. In comparison, only approximately 11% of the population at large and slightly less than one fourth of those individuals who live in poverty feel this way about their health.[8,12]

Homeless people have high rates of both acute and chronic illness. Homeless patients are more likely to contract communicable diseases such as tuberculosis,[13] and have higher rates of human immunodeficiency virus (HIV) infection and viral hepatitis because of the increased likelihood of unprotected sex and injection drug use.[14] Foot problems from walking in ill-fitting shoes, swollen legs, and poor dentition are other common problems.

Homelessness puts women and children at particular risk for poor health.[15] Many women become homeless during pregnancy. Homelessness, in turn, puts them at risk for complicated pregnancies. Homeless women are also more likely to experience difficulty obtaining and using contraception, have multiple sexual partners, and have more unintended pregnancies, and are at high risk for physical and sexual assault.[11,16] Homeless children also have poor health. They suffer from more infectious diseases such as respiratory tract infections and diarrhea and have more nutritional disorders, asthma, and developmental delay than children with homes.[15]

Rates of mental illness have varied widely among the homeless but are consistently higher than the general population. A nationally representative study of homeless individuals found that 57% of currently homeless individuals had a mental health problem in their lifetime and 39% currently suffer with a mental illness.[17] The relative prevalence of different types of psychiatric impairments mirror that in the general population, with depression, bipolar affective disorder, schizophrenia, posttraumatic stress disorder, and personality disorders being the most common.[18] Severe mental illness is more common among the chronically homeless population than other homeless populations, although rates are elevated throughout the homeless population.

In addition, homeless people have a high rate of substance abuse, which can complicate the medical care that they receive. Thirty-eight percent of currently homeless clients in a national survey were found to have a current alcohol problem, and 62% had an alcohol problem in their lifetime.[17] Approximately 25% of currently homeless persons have a problem with drug use, and 60% have a lifetime history of a drug use disorder.[17] Sixty-six percent of currently homeless persons have at least one mental health, alcohol, or drug problem; 86% have had at least one of the three problems in their lifetimes. Many have at least two of the three problems simultaneously. Thirty percent of homeless clients have a lifetime history of mental health and alcohol and drug problems.[17]

Homeless people have higher rates of inpatient hospitalizations than housed persons, likely because of delayed access to care and lower admission thresholds. Complying with both outpatient and discharge treatment plans may be more difficult, particularly if providers do not consider housing status when developing treatment plans.

Studies in the United States and Canada have shown that homeless persons have mortality rates approximately three to four times that of housed, age-matched controls, with a median age of death from 40 to 47 years old.[1,3,4,19-21]

HOMELESSNESS AND THE HEALTH CARE SYSTEM

Homeless persons are cared for both within the mainstream health care system and within a specialized system of care developed and funded to care for the homeless population (the federally financed Health Care for the Homeless system). While in the mainstream system, because of their poverty and lack of health insurance, homeless people are more likely to be cared for within the "safety net" system of community clinics, public hospitals, and Veteran Affairs hospitals, than the private health care system.[22]

Fewer than half of homeless people are insured, and almost all of these have publicly funded insurance, such as Medicaid, Medicare, and veterans' insurance. Their access to ambulatory health care is poor and they tend to receive health care through emergency department and inpatient hospitalizations.[6] In addition to insurance issues and the competing priorities of food and shelter, other barriers to health care include poverty, low health care literacy, and distrust of the medical establishment.

The health care system itself is a barrier,[23] and having a regular provider who can build a relationship with the patient, and help her or him navigate the system is of utmost importance. Despite the high prevalence of mental illness and substance abuse, for example, homeless patients often have difficulty accessing psychiatric care or substance abuse treatment. One study found that only 20% of those with mental health or substance abuse problems were receiving any treatment for these problems.[24]

STRATEGIES TO ADDRESS HOMELESSNESS AND ITS PROBLEMS

> Ms. Smith presents 1 hour late for her appointment at her community health center. Her two school-aged children are with her. She explains that since her appointment 6 months ago, she has been evicted from her apartment. She is living at her cousin's; there are now 10 people living in a 2-bedroom apartment. She has run out of her asthma medicine; in the interview she starts to cry and states that she cannot sleep at night, has no appetite, and feels hopeless. Her asthma, previously well controlled, is now flaring.

Physicians and other health care providers normally do not play an active role in the social, political, and economic issues that must be addressed to reduce or resolve homelessness. However, it is increasingly evident that the impact and outcome of homelessness is a major health care problem. Thus, finding solutions to homelessness is critical for the health of homeless patients.

The National Alliance to End Homelessness, an advocacy agency, recommends three important conceptual steps: "closing the front door," meaning identifying people at high risk for homelessness and intervening prior to their becoming homeless, "opening the back door," meaning decreasing barriers to obtaining housing for those who have lost their housing, and "building the infrastructure," meaning creating capacity for services, such as low-income housing, that will make homelessness less likely to occur.[25]

"CLOSING THE FRONT DOOR:" PREVENTION OF HOMELESSNESS

Prevention is the ideal way to address homelessness. Strategies to prevent homelessness depend on which population is being addressed. For those with "crisis" homelessness, who generally have less personal vulnerability and more resources to draw on, efforts can be made to prevent eviction and stop the cycle of homelessness early. Community services provide legal support for tenants facing eviction, emergency financial assistance to cover back rent or utility bills, or case management to assist with applying for government benefits. Helping Ms. Smith to access these resources and advocating for her could have a more profound effect on her health and that of her children than prescribing more asthma medications.

To prevent chronic homelessness, housing and case management initiatives focus on high-risk populations, such as people being released from prisons and hospitals.

"OPENING THE BACK DOOR"

"Opening the back door" aims to move people out of homelessness as quickly and permanently as possible. For "crisis" homeless persons, this means helping to smooth the way into existing low-income housing.

Outreach and Engagement

Caring for homeless patients includes reaching out to homeless persons who are not currently engaged in care. This may be direct provision of health care by nurses, midlevel providers, and physicians at alternative sites, or by using case managers or peer counselors who do outreach. The range of services provided at these sites can vary widely, ranging from full-service clinics to nursing stations in which homeless persons can receive basic health assessments, over-the-counter remedies, and referrals. Many programs do not attempt to provide primary care, instead providing urgent care services that function as a bridge between patients and the mainstream health care system. Often other services are offered to homeless persons as a way of both providing them needed services and engendering the trust that will assist in outreach efforts; for example, providing benefit counseling, mental health services, case management, food, or toiletries.

Intensive Case Management

Intensive case management is a system of care adapted from models developed for use in the severely mentally ill. Although models differ slightly, intensive case management involves a multidisciplinary team including social workers, nurses, physicians, vocational workers, and others who provide ongoing integrated care for hard-to-reach patients. Intensive case management principles include client engagement, having a low provider-to-client ratio, 24-hour availability of services, and a multidisciplinary team.

Respite Care

Much of the health care that formerly was delivered in inpatient settings (e.g., oral antibiotics for treatment of uncomplicated pneumonia and kidney infection, surgical procedures, chemotherapy) is now done in outpatient settings. Unfortunately, homeless persons cannot receive these services while staying on the street or in basic emergency shelters. Respite care is short-term housing for homeless persons who are either recovering from hospitalization or are receiving medical care for a condition that renders them too ill to be living on the street or in emergency shelters, but does not require hospitalization.

Models of respite care vary widely, but all include shelter (where homeless persons can stay all day), meals, basic nursing care, and access to medical care. Most also provide some form of case management to assist homeless persons obtain complete medical care and other necessary services, including housing, mental health care, and substance abuse treatment. The Veteran Affairs Medical Center's respite programs, known as "hoptels," have equalized lengths of stay between homeless and non-homeless veterans admitted to the hospital.[26]

Health Care for the Homeless Network

One approach to delivering comprehensive health care for the homeless has been the creation of a network of Health Care for the Homeless [HCH] sites that provide both required services and optional programs targeting the needs of the homeless. Required services include primary health care, outreach, substance abuse treatment, mental health treatment, case management, eligibility assistance, emergency services, referral for inpatient hospitalization, and housing assistance. Optional features include restorative dental services, vision and eyewear services, specialty care, complementary and alternative medicine, employment, and job training and respite care.[27]

All systems caring for homeless patients should seek to emulate the HCH network's principles of care. These include taking services to homeless people, arranging transportation for follow-up or other necessary services, provision of services without regard to ability to pay, and collaboration with other agencies to provide comprehensive services.

BUILDING THE INFRASTRUCTURE

More intensive interventions may be necessary for chronically homeless persons. A promising intervention is *supportive housing*, subsidized housing with onsite or closely linked social services, such as medical care, mental health care, substance abuse treatment, case management, and job training. This is an example of an important collaboration between health care providers and homeless service providers. Although models differ, most target the chronically homeless with both mental health impairments as well as substance abuse disorders (and many have severe chronic medical illness). Many supportive housing models are moving to a "housing-first" model, which does not require sobriety on the part of homeless persons with substance use disorders prior to housing.

GUIDELINES FOR THE CLINICAL ENCOUNTER WITH THE HOMELESS PATIENT

Mr. Jones has had an elevated blood pressure noted on many occasions and had been started on hydrochlorothiazide. When he returns to the clinic after 6 months, having missed several appointments, he tells you that he has stopped his medication because of urinary frequency. On further screening at that visit, he is found to have post-traumatic stress disorder and admits to consuming a large amount of alcohol on an almost-daily basis.

HISTORY TAKING AND PHYSICAL EXAMINATION

Health care providers can take several steps to improve the care that their homeless patients receive (Table 24-2). In general, management of illness for homeless individuals is similar to that provided to patients who are housed. These patients' competing priorities for basic needs, flexibility, and the use of community resources are critical features of an integrated management plan.

Homeless persons should be asked the standard historical questions. In addition, all patients should be asked about their current and prior housing status, specific medical conditions found more commonly in homeless persons (e.g., asthma, hypertension, HIV, mental illness), current alcohol and drug use, and any history of abuse or violence. Patients also should be asked if they have a regular source of medical care, if they have any medical insurance, and about their impressions of their prior health care. All patients should be screened for conditions with a higher prevalence among the homeless. These include substance abuse, mental illness, sexually transmitted diseases, and victimization.

In addition, providers should update contact information, including the number of a family member or friend with stable housing where mail or messages may be accessed, and who could be contacted in case of emergency.

If the patient is currently staying outside or in a homeless shelter, the patient should be asked specifically how long he or she has been without an indoor place to stay and how many different times he or she

Table 24-2. Management of Homeless Patients

Ask patients about their housing status at every visit.
Understand competing priorities and attempt to work around them.
Recommend risk reduction when possible.
Engage patients in developing treatment plans.
Keep regimens simple (e.g., once-daily medications, consider side-effects, avoid laboratory monitoring when possible).
Offer health promotion and disease prevention at each visit.
• Annual PPD testing
• Pap smears and STD testing per recommendations
• Vaccinations (influenza, Pneumovax, hepatitis A and B, and tetanus vaccine)
• Contraception
Access community resources to assist with developing and delivering a care plan.
Screen for conditions common among the homeless (including tuberculosis, psychiatric illness, and substance abuse).
• Foot care
• Dental referral
• Needle exchange referral

has been without an indoor place to stay. In addition, providers should inquire whether there is a place to stay during the day; a place to obtain, prepare, and store food; and about access to water, toileting, showering facilities, and a refrigerator. Finally, questions about personal safety should be asked, given the high rates of victimization common in the homeless population. Answers to these questions are imperative to the construction of a treatment plan based on logistic issues raised by the patient's social context and in agreement with the patient's capabilities and desires.

For homeless women, it is important to reduce obstacles to contraception: having medications and devices onsite, use the Quick Start method, and do not make prescription of methods contingent on PAP smear results (see Chap. 29).

When performing a physical examination, special emphasis should be placed on conducting a dental assessment and foot and skin examination, given the higher prevalence of these problems in homeless persons.

For Mr. Jones—the chronically homeless man with alcohol disorder, hypertension, and posttraumatic stress disorder—the clinician should focus on establishing trust, addressing underlying psychiatric and substance use issues, and finding a medication regimen that is realistic based on the patient's chaotic life: If the hypertension is to be addressed, a once-a-day drug should be used that does not cause frequent urination. In addition, the visit should focus on high-yield preventive health interventions, such as vaccinations and purified protein derivative (PPD) testing. More complicated interventions, such as colon cancer screening, may need to be deferred until the patient's social situation is stabilized.

For crisis homeless patients like Ms. Smith, there may be other issues to consider as well.

> Upon talking further with Ms. Smith, you realize that her cousins' house where she is staying has shag carpeting, two cats, and second-hand smoke, as her cousin is a smoker.

Clinicians must focus on the acute medical and mental health issues, as well as help direct patients to resources that could help them regain housing. Ms. Smith's reactive depression and worsening asthma are inseparable from her loss of housing.

Common Pitfalls in the Evaluation of the Homeless Patient

• Not considering the patient's housing status in the assessment and plan
• Not addressing the competing priorities that interfere with health care compliance
• Failing to offer preventive measures at every visit
• Developing care plans that are not realistic for patients
• Not detecting and addressing substance use and psychiatric illness
• Not coordinating care with other members of the health care team
• Not being aware of or not discussing community resources

HEALTH PROMOTION AND DISEASE PREVENTION

Because of the fragmented nature of care that homeless persons receive, providers should address health promotion and disease prevention at every visit; patients may not be able to attend follow-up appointments. Providers should follow standard health care maintenance recommendations, including screening for cancers, when feasible. In addition to these there are some homeless specific health care maintenance recommendations, including annual or semiannual screening for tuberculosis using PPD for homeless persons who stay in the street, sleep in shelters, or use food lines, or those who have been in the criminal justice system.

In addition, homeless persons should be offered pneumococcus and hepatitis A and B vaccination; they should also receive an influenza vaccine annually and a tetanus shot every 10 years.

Risk reduction practices also should be discussed routinely with patients. They should understand strategies they might use to minimize the transmission of sexually transmitted diseases as well as diseases spread through injection drug use. For example, if readily available and appropriate, information about local needle exchange programs should be distributed to patients who are injection drug users.

SELECTION OF MEDICATIONS

Providers should select medications that are administered once daily, and do not require laboratory checks or refrigeration in order to facilitate medication regimen adherence. Providers should consider the expense of the prescribed medication and its actual availability to the patient. Providers also should consider medication side-effects. For example, prescribing diuretics to homeless patients may be problematic for some given the lack of restroom facilities and the need for laboratory monitoring. Providers should assess any potential obstacles to adherence and address them (see Chap. 8).

DEVELOPING A CARE PLAN

An integrated care plan for homeless patients must ensure that both medical and nonmedical issues are addressed. Eliciting patients' priorities, with the understanding that identifying regular sources of food, shelter, and clothing may be of paramount importance, allows providers to incorporate patients' goals into the treatment plan, develops a stronger therapeutic alliance, and establishes a more successful plan. Linking patients to resources available in the community also improves care. For example, in some communities, outreach workers can visit patients who are staying in shelters or are on the street to evaluate them between clinic visits.

In addition, patients should be encouraged to seek care at sites that offer open access or that can otherwise accommodate unscheduled visits, because prescheduled clinic appointments often are difficult for homeless persons. Finally, using a multidisciplinary approach,

drawing on the expertise of social workers, mental health professionals, and substance abuse counselors, can help both patient and provider.

ESTABLISH A MONEY MANAGER FOR THE PATIENT

Identifying third parties who will take primary responsibility for managing a client's funds may be useful in cases in which an individual is too impaired by cognitive impairments, severe mental illness, or substance abuse to safely receive his or her check. These "payees" use the client's money to pay standing bills, such as rent and utility, and dispense spending money to clients in small amounts.[27]

CONCLUSIONS

Despite the challenges, it is possible for providers to deliver high-quality care to homeless patients by understanding the social context in which these patients live and their obstacles to accessing medical care. Providers must collaborate with patients to develop appropriate care plans. Given the transience of this population, providers should discuss health promotion and disease prevention at every visit and should make every effort to comply with recommended screening guidelines that have been developed for the general population. In addition, when possible, providers should attempt to develop and system-level programs, including multidisciplinary teams, outreach programs, and respite care, to facilitate the care they provide to their patients, because these approaches can improve the outcomes for their patients.

KEY CONCEPTS

- Homelessness is a medical issue.
- Homelessness can be a cause and consequence of medical problems.
- Homelessness is the consequence of the interplay between structural social problems and personal vulnerabilities.
- Health care systems often compound the difficulties that homeless patients have in accessing care.
- Prevention of homelessness should be the goal.
- Comprehensive, integrated health care decreases barriers for homeless patients.
- Accessing community resources is important to the care of the homeless.

CORE COMPETENCY

Institute of Medicine Recommendations for Addressing Health Care Disparities General Recommendations

- *Screen* for homelessness or impending homelessness.
  - —Do you feel that your housing situation is secure?
  - —In the past month, have you slept in an emergency shelter, vehicle, or place not meant for sleeping?
  - —Are you staying temporarily with family or friends because you don't have a place of your own?
  - —Have you had difficulty paying your rent, utility bills, or food expenses in the past year?
  - —Can you live in the place you are currently living for the next several months? Are you concerned about being evicted? If that happens, do you have another place to go?
- *Distinguish* between acute and chronic homelessness.
  - —Assess for how often and how long a patient has been marginally housed or homeless in the last 3 years.
  - —Ask the chronically homeless to what he or she owes homelessness.
- *Assess* for support systems: Even chronically homeless patients may have tightly knit groups of others they rely on.
- *Record* the most reliable contact information for your patient.
- *Screen* for substance use, mental illness, and domestic violence.
- *Assess* patients' current level of safety.
- *Assess* teeth and feet in routine physical examination.
- *Consider* touching your patients in a caring, professional manner; most homeless people crave personal connections.
- *Screen* for tuberculosis.
- *Offer* health care maintenance interventions at each clinical encounter.
- *Vaccinate* for influenza, pneumococcus, and hepatitis A and B.
- *Review* medications: The patient's actual ability to receive the medications—coverage, cost. Adherence. Are medications prescribed once a day? Do they require refrigeration? Are there other storage issues? Is there a need for frequent refills?
- *Refer* the patient to a social worker and benefits counselor to address whether he or she is receiving appropriate services and benefits.
- *Reduce* barriers to care. Consolidate services, onsite referral, and medications; prescribe contraception without PAP.
- *Validate* the difficulty of your patients' lives caused by homelessness.
- *Acknowledge* and *address* competing priorities that might affect access to care.
- *Advocate* for systems changes that can help accommodate homeless patients.

DISCUSSION QUESTIONS

1. Develop a care plan for a homeless woman with newly diagnosed diabetes. What self-management recommendations do you make? With what medication do you start? Are there other resources you can use to help with adherence? Is it reasonable to make dietary recommendations to her?
2. Given your experiences with the medical system, what system-level changes would you recommend to better the care that homeless patients receive? Are there ways to change your own system that would improve the health of your patients?
3. Discuss some of the barriers you have experienced in providing medical care to homeless patients. What principles do you use when developing a medical regimen for a homeless patient?

RESOURCES

http://www.bphc.hrsa.gov
Bureau of Primary Health Care

http://www.mentalhealth.org
Center for Mental Health Care Homeless Services Branch

http://www.samhsa.gov
Center for Substance Abuse Treatment

http://www.nhchc.org
National Health Care for the Homeless Council

REFERENCES

1. Hibbs JR, et al. Mortality in a cohort of homeless adults in Philadelphia. *N Engl J Med* 1994;331(5):304–309.
2. Hwang SW, et al. Causes of death in homeless adults in Boston. *Ann Intern Med* 1997;126(8):625–628.
3. Barrow SM, et al. (1999). Mortality among homeless shelter residents in New York City. *Am J Public Health* 1999;89(4):529–534.
4. Hwang SW. Mortality among men using homeless shelters in Toronto, Ontario. *JAMA* 2000;283(16):2152–2157.
5. Gelberg L, et al. Competing priorities as a barrier to medical care among homeless adults in Los Angeles. *Am J Public Health* 1997;87(2):217–220.
6. Kushel MB, et al. Factors associated with the health care utilization of homeless persons. *JAMA* 2001;285(2): 200–206.
7. Martell JV, et al. Hospitalization in an urban homeless population: The Honolulu Urban Homeless Project. *Ann Intern Med* 1992;116(4):299–303.
8. Kushel MB, et al. Emergency department use among the homeless and marginally housed: results from a community-based study. *Am J Public Health* 2002;92(5): 778–784.

9. Burt M, et al. *Helping America's homeless: Emergency shelter or affordable housing?* Washington, DC: Urban Institute Press, 2001.

10. Burt M, et al. *Homelessness: Programs and the people they serve.* Washington, DC: Urban Institute Press, 1999.

11. Kushel MB, et al. No door to lock: Victimization among homeless and marginally housed persons. *Arch Intern Med* 2003;163(20):2492–2499.

12. White MC, et al. Association between time homeless and perceived health status among the homeless in San Francisco. *J Commun Health* 1997;22(4):271–282.

13. Martens WH. A review of physical and mental health in homeless persons. *Public Health Rev* 2001;29(1):13–33.

14. Fischer PJ. *Alcohol and drug abuse and mental health problems among homeless persons: A review of the literature, 1980–1990.* Rockville, MD: National Institute on Alcohol Abuse and Alcoholism and National Institute of Mental Health, 1991.

15. Weinreb L, et al. Determinants of health and service use patterns in homeless and low-income housed children. *Pediatrics* 1998;102(3 Pt 1):554–562.

16. Gelberg L, et al. Use of contraceptive methods among homeless women for protection against unwanted pregnancies and sexually transmitted diseases: prior use and willingness to use in the future. *Contraception* 2001;63(5): 277–281.

17. Burt M, et al. *Homelessness: Programs and the people they serve.* Findings of the National Survey of Homeless Assistance Providers and Clients. The Urban Institute. Washington, DC: Urban Institute Press, 1999.

18. Robertson MJ, Winkleby MA. Mental health problems of homeless women and differences across subgroups. *Annu Rev Public Health* 1996;17:311–336.

19. Hwang SW, et al. Risk factors for death in homeless adults in Boston. *Arch Intern Med* 1998;158(13):1454–1460.

20. Kasprow WJ, Rosenheck R. Mortality among homeless and nonhomeless mentally ill veterans. *J Nerv Ment Dis* 2000;188(3):141–147.

21. Roy E, et al. Mortality in a cohort of street youth in Montreal. *JAMA* 2004;292(5):569–574.

22. Rosen MI, Rosenheck R. Substance use and assignment of representative payees. *Psychiatr Serv* 1999;50(1):95–98.

23. Plumb JD. Homelessness: Care, prevention, and public policy. *Ann Intern Med* 1997;126(12):973–935.

24. Koegel P, et al. Utilization of mental health and substance abuse services among homeless adults in Los Angeles. *Med Care* 1999;37(3):306–317.

25. National Alliance to End Homelessness. *A plan, not a dream: How to end homelessness in ten years.* Washington, DC, National Alliance to End Homelessness, 2005. Available at: http://www.endhomelessness.org/pub/tenyear/NAEH10yrplan.pdf

26. Holzwarth J. *Care for the Homeless 101: A workshop for new staff caring for people experiencing homelessness.* Nashville, TN: National Health Care for the Homeless Council, Inc. HCH Clinicians' Network. 2004. Accessed at: http://www.nhchc.org/HCH101/HCH101WebRegional21203.ppt#257,1,Health

27. Bonin E, et al. *Adapting your practice: General recommendations for the care of homeless patients.* Nashville, TN: Health Care for the Homeless Clinicians' Network, National Health Care for the Homeless Council, 2004.

Chapter 25

Immigrant Health Issues

Susana Morales, MD

Objectives

- Describe demographics and other characteristics of immigrant Americans.
- Review determinants of legal immigrant status.
- Review health issues facing immigrants.
- Review challenges to care of immigrant patients including patient, provider, and system factors.
- Discuss interventions to improve care.

Mr. Moraga fled political persecution in Guatemala. He is undocumented, speaks little English, and has been working as a janitor. Many people assume because he is undocumented, poor, and Latino that he is also uneducated. He has a Ph.D.

Multiple waves of immigration, including the prolonged importation of African slaves, account for the fact that 99% of all Americans are either immigrants or their descendents. Immigrants to the United States are a diverse group, differing in everything from their backgrounds to reasons for immigration. People have migrated to the United States searching for economic and educational opportunity and fleeing religious persecution, political and social unrest, and personal danger. Consequently, political, economic, geographic, and cultural stimuli and barriers to immigration have shaped the character and experiences of US immigrant communities.

Immigrants face increased risks of many illnesses, poor health care access, and lower-quality health. This chapter reviews these risks and the ways to help mitigate them.

IMMIGRATION: DEMOGRAPHICS

Immigration is defined as resettlement in a country to which one is not native. Immigration is as potent a force in the United States today as it was in the past. Indeed, according to the US census, in 2003 almost 12% of the population was foreign born.[1] Immigration during the 1990s reached a historic high. Approximately 1 million persons entered the United States legally per year during the 1990s. Another 200,000 to 300,000 persons a year either entered illegally, or entered legally but overstayed temporary visas.[2] All told there are about 9 million undocumented immigrants in the U.S.[2a] In contrast, the number of refugees (i.e., somebody who is seeking or taking refuge, especially from war or persecution, by going to a foreign country) has been dropping. In 2003, only 30,000 refugees entered the United States, despite burgeoning numbers of refugees globally.[2b]

FACTORS INFLUENCING THE IMMIGRATION EXPERIENCE

Mrs. Rosas left her children with her mother when she immigrated to the United States. Eventually her mother and the children are able to come to visit on a tourist visa. While in the United States, her mother suffers a debilitating stroke.

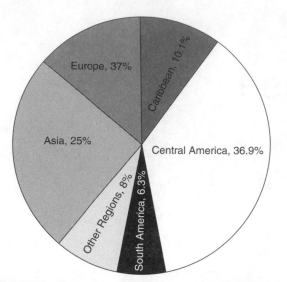
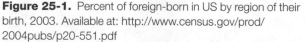

Figure 25-1. Percent of foreign-born in US by region of their birth, 2003. Available at: http://www.census.gov/prod/2004pubs/p20-551.pdf

(*Source:* Current Population Survey, Social and Economic Supplement, 2003 as cited in Larson LJ. The Foreign-Born Population in the United States, 2003. Current Population Reports P20-55.US Census Bureau, Washing DC, 2004.)

Although recent immigrants have always been a large part of the US population, in the past most came from Europe. Today's immigrants are increasingly diverse, coming mostly from Latin America and Asia. Latin Americans make up 53% of the foreign born, Asians 25%, and Europeans 12%, with the remaining from other regions (Fig. 25-1). These categories are so broad that they hide a rich diversity of nationalities, ethnicities, cultures, languages, migration histories, socioeconomic classes, and racial admixtures.[3] This diversity of factors, however, profoundly affects people's experience of immigration and the characters of the communities they form. These communities change with each wave of immigration and each generation of children.

Reviewing a patient's immigration history may help the clinician understand this experience and its possible impact on health. These experiences, as in the case of Mrs. Rosas' family, may be very different for each member. Where someone comes from, the reason for migration, whether they come alone or with family, who and what are left behind, and whether they join an immigrant community are all important. Age, culture, language, education, and legal status are also significant factors to consider.

IMPACT OF IMMIGRANTS' LEGAL STATUS

A person's documentation status has a profound effect on access to opportunities and services that affect health. Inquiring about a patient's legal status can help

clinicians understand the services their patients are entitled to and the hurdles they must face in everyday life, but must be done with sensitivity. Some patients question the clinician's motives, fearing denial of care or, even worse, that the health care provider might turn them into the immigration service. In addition, access issues are complicated when the US-born children of undocumented immigrants are granted citizenship. For example, restricted parental access to public benefits might prevent undocumented parents from seeking help for their legally entitled children.

Legal Immigrants

Legal immigrants are those who have obtained citizenship, have permanent residency status (possess a green card); temporary residency status (are part of an amnesty program); have been granted temporary protected status because of a natural disaster or civil conflict in their country; or are asylees or refugees.

Asylees Asylees are those who have been granted political asylum from fear of prosecution once they have already entered this country, and they are typically eligible for citizenship within a year.

Refugees

Refugees, on the other hand, apply to come to the United States from a country to which they have fled, fearing persecution on account of race, religion, nationality, membership in a particular social group, or political opinion in their own country. After a year of entering the United States, refugees are eligible for permanent resident status and after 5 years for citizenship. Victims of "severe trafficking," that is, those coerced into sexual or other servitude, are also eligible for refugee status.

Nonimmigrant Foreign Nationals

Nonimmigrant foreign nationals are those here on visas allowing them to work or study. They must demonstrate an ability to support themselves and claim they do not intend to stay in the United States permanently.

IMPACT OF IMMIGRATION POLICIES

Immigration issues have always been controversial: who and how people are allowed to enter legally; the causes and consequences of entering illegally; or who is eligible for refugee status are political matters. National policies determine who is legally allowed to enter the country and have a powerful influence on their experiences once here.

Before 1980, US refugee policy was heavily influenced by the Cold War. Leaving a communist state was usually sufficient justification for refugee eligibility. The Refugee Act of 1980 based refugee status less on ideology and more on evidence of persecution. Nevertheless, the president can make exceptions to the definition and allow easier access for some. The president and congress determine the total number of refugees who may be admitted to the United States each year from each of five regions, with separate quotas for each.

The 1996 Illegal Immigration Reform and Immigrant Responsibility Act significantly tightened border restrictions, changed rules on asylum, and restricted immigrant access to public benefits, including for legal immigrants.[4] This act also legislated specific vaccination and medical examination requirements for immigrants and those seeking permanent residency status. Physicians certified as Bureau of Citizenship and Immigration Services (BCIS) Designated Civil Surgeons must perform these examinations.

IMPACT OF EMPLOYMENT OPPORTUNITIES

Many of those coming to this country, legally and illegally, have come to work. Indeed, new immigrants formed about 50% of the new labor force growth in the country in the last two decades, and are thought to have provided a net economic gain for the US economy and for nonimmigrant workers.[2] Approximately 5 million immigrants are in the labor force; working predominantly in agriculture, the restaurant industry, and construction.[5] This work, particularly if the worker is undocumented, often places many immigrants at high risk for occupational injury and illness (see Chap. 21).

IMPACT OF OTHER SOCIODEMOGRAPHIC FACTORS

The diversity of immigrants is so great that it is impossible to generalize from population statistics to any one individual. Nevertheless, overall immigrants are more likely to reside in larger households, live in poverty, and lack a high school diploma than native-born Americans. Immigrants are more likely to be functionally illiterate in English and of poorer educational attainment, even in their native languages.[1] Immigrants without a high school diploma from their native lands are especially likely to have severely poor literacy in English.[6]

ISSUES AFFECTING HEALTH CARE ACCESS AND DELIVERY

HEALTH CARE ACCESS, UTILIZATION, AND QUALITY

There is a misperception that immigrants overburden the health care system.[7] Immigrants use public resources at lower rates than native-born populations and have significantly poorer access to health care. For example, immigrants comprise nearly 25% of the uninsured; and 70% of all noncitizens lacked health insurance in 1999.[8] Noncitizens receive much lower rates of medical and dental care, and go the emergency room less often. Noncitizen children in non–English speaking families were much less likely to see a doctor.[7] When they do access medical care, they are also at risk of receiving inadequate care.[7-11]

HEALTH BELIEFS AND EXPECTATIONS

The cultural diversity of immigrants may affect health care delivery. Immigrants may have culturally based health beliefs that may affect trust and adherence to provider recommendations (see Chap. 9). As with all patients, it is important for the health care providers to understand the immigrant patient's spiritual beliefs. Immigrants come from many different religious backgrounds, and religious communities are important sources of emotional and social support. Religious values influence health beliefs and values, for example about modesty, reproductive and sexual matters, and end-of-life care. For example, a Bosnian Muslim women may prefer a female provider, and in fact be unwilling to be examined by a male provider.

Immigrant patients often use alternative or complementary medications, although they may be uncomfortable about revealing this to providers. Latinos are more likely than other ethnic groups to use alternative methods because they are cheaper.[12] Use of home remedies, expectations of medical treatment, and health care delivery also are often based on patients' experiences in their home countries. For example, some immigrants may expect parenteral treatments such as injections to be administered.

In many countries, medications may be obtained without a prescription, even those considered dangerous or banned in the United States. Medications also may be outdated or adulterated. In one study of Asian patent medications available in California, 32% were found to have unlabeled medications, 14% mercury, 14% arsenic, and 10% lead.[13] Immigrants residing in the United States may use some of these medications.[14]

TRUST AND THE PROVIDER–PATIENT RELATIONSHIP

Immigrants may be wary of the health care system and its personnel. They may fear being asked about their documentation status, being misunderstood (particularly if they do not speak English), not being able to pay for care, or outright discrimination. Studies have shown that minority patients are less likely to find doctors and health systems trustworthy than white patients. Minority patients report feeling they would receive better care if they were of a different race or ethnicity, feeling they are treated with disrespect, looked down on, and that their providers do not understand their cultural origins and beliefs.[15] Not being able to speak the same language as the health care provider is also an important impediment to both trust and the receipt of high-quality medical care (see Chap. 26).[15a]

HEALTH ISSUES FACING IMMIGRANTS

The health issues facing immigrants are complicated because people are exposed to a many risks. They are at risk of the diseases and exposures that are prevalent in their country of origin, their migration itself may pose health risks, and they are at risk of the illnesses that are prevalent in the United States. The communities in which immigrants often live also have health risks of their own: more environmental risks and higher prevalence of some infectious diseases, such as tuberculosis, for example. With greater barriers to medical care, the opportunity to mitigate these risks through health care is also diminished.

"PROTECTIVE" HEALTH EFFECT OF IMMIGRATION

Despite adverse socioeconomic indicators, immigrants have been shown to have lower infant and adult mortality rates than nonimmigrant Americans. The causes of this epidemiologic paradox are unclear, but some theorize that strong social networks, traditional diets, and low rates of substance abuse, including tobacco and alcohol use, may be involved.[15b]

INFECTIOUS AND OTHER DISEASES

Infectious diseases top the list of illnesses that are prevalent in many of the developing countries from which US immigrants come. Tuberculosis, HIV, hepatitis, parasitic illnesses, rheumatic heart disease, and malaria are common problems in those coming from developing countries. Elevated lead levels have been reported in up to 50% of children from many developing countries and are common in immigrant and refugee children and pregnant women.[16] Chronic illnesses such as diabetes, hypertension, and coronary artery disease become increasingly important as people stay in the United States.

TRAVEL MEDICINE

Travel back and forth between the United States and their home countries has an impact on immigrants' health. The risk of contracting illness, particularly infectious diseases, while traveling is higher for immigrants

than for those who are merely tourists. Immigrants travel under different circumstances than tourists. Common reasons for travel include family responsibilities and emergencies, vacation, and even obtaining medical or dental services that are unaffordable in the United States. Undocumented persons may be travel or deported but return to the United States. Families may be divided by their immigration circumstances and this may be a source of severe stress. In other instances, illness may make travel impossible, creating an added layer of complexity and suffering.

Immigrants who return to visit their home countries are at increased risk of developing travel-related illnesses. Twenty percent of the population of the United States is foreign born or children of immigrants. Nearly 50% of US residents who travel abroad are foreign-born immigrants. Health care in the home country may be suboptimal, and those returning to their home country are more likely to seek care in these institutions. In addition, these travelers are more likely to engage in higher risk behavior.[17] They are more likely to visit during pregnancy or with young children, stay for longer periods of time, and eat similar to their friends and family.[18] Stress-related health problems may be exacerbated by travel or seeing ailing, impoverished family members.[18]

Health care providers often do not think of immigrant patients as traditional travelers and do not advise and appropriately manage prophylaxis. Recommendations for immigrants traveling to developing countries include treatment for diarrhea, avoiding raw fish, education on malaria prevention, and obtaining pretravel immunizations.[18] These pretravel immunizations may need to include childhood immunizations in unvaccinated adults. Prophylactic medications and immunizations for travel-related illnesses often are not covered by health insurance and the expense may be a barrier to some patients. Hence malaria prophylaxis and vaccination updating, for example, are more important in these travelers than for those who are merely tourists, but they are less likely to receive them (Box 25-1).[18,19]

MENTAL HEALTH

Many immigrants and refugees may have experienced significant trauma, including civil war, violence, and torture. Trauma may occur in the native country, during the journey to sanctuary, and in the new home country of refuge.[20] Researchers have shown that refugees may have high rates of depression, posttraumatic stress disorder, and somatization syndromes.[21]

It is estimated that between 5% and 35% of refugees and asylum seekers have been torture victims. Torture can have a severe impact on the mental and physical health of the victim as well as social well-being.[22,23] Even

Box 25-1. Advice for Travelers Visiting Friends and Relatives to Reduce Risk

For Food- and Water-Borne Illness and Diarrhea

- Advise boiling water, drinking bottled beverages, and eating peeled fruits and hot foods.
- Avoid high-risk foods such as undercooked, dairy, and raw fish.
- Frequently wash hands or use hand sanitizers.
  —Give anticipatory antibiotics such as Ciprofloxacin
  —Lower threshold for typhoid vaccine and hepatitis A vaccine

For Malaria

- Malaria prophylaxis—protective clothing, mosquito nets, DEET insect repellant, and chemoprophylaxis as recommended by the CDC.
- Traveler should be warned that malaria prophylaxis purchased abroad may be adulterated or less potent.

For Tuberculosis

- Consider PPD testing 3 to 6 months after return if PPD negative

For Sexually Transmitted Diseases

- Discuss preventive measures (avoid high-risk behavior, purchase condoms).
- Vaccinate for Hepatitis B if not immune.

For Zoonotic and Environmental Diseases: Schistosomiasis, Bites, Wood-Fire, Toxin Ingestion, Use of Medical Services, etc.

- Anticipatory advice about exposures (avoid animals, avoid sleeping at floor level, wash hands, avoid fresh water, use protective footwear)
- Anticipatory purchase of medications/supplies when necessary, such as inhalers, needles, and prescriptions. Avoid traditional medications.

For Infectious Illness and Not Having Received Complete Primary Vaccine Series

- Review vaccination history—particularly tetanus/diphtheria, polio, hepatitis A and B, measles, and varicella—and vaccinate if no serologic evidence of immunity.
- At higher risk for meningococcemia, typhoid, rabies, so consider more strongly.
- Consider rabies vaccination.

For country-by-country recommendations, see: http://www.cdc.gov/travel/
Adapted from: Bacaner N, Stauffer B, Boulware DR, et al. Travel medicine considerations for North American immigrants visiting friends and relatives. *JAMA* 2004 ;291:2856–2864.[18]

---

immigrants without official asylum status are at risk of having experienced political trauma. For example, Central American patients seeking care in California primary care clinics have reported high rates of witnessing of political violence and have psychiatric sequelae.[24]

Immigration itself is a high stress act: People may go to a new nation for a better life but the adjustments involved in such a transition may be extremely stressful. Depressive disorder is extremely prevalent worldwide but may be manifested differently by different ethnic groups, may not be understood as a disease by the patients, and may be more stigmatized in people of different cultural backgrounds. The symptoms of depression may be misinterpreted by health care providers, who may not, in fact, realize that somatization in some of their patients is related to an underlying depressive disorder. As many as half of depressed immigrants and refugees in the United States are not diagnosed or treated for depression.[25]

Immigrant and refugee children too may have posttraumatic stress disorder symptoms, including difficulty in school and unruly conduct. Cognitive behavioral therapy, art therapy, and play therapy may be useful in treating the children, and the schools have a role in detecting and supporting them.[20]

SPECIAL ISSUES THAT MAY IMPACT THE HEALTH AND HEALTH CARE OF IMMIGRANTS

Family Relationships

Most immigrant communities have close family relationships that serve as strong supports, providing an emotional and material safety net. Immigrant families often have a pioneer member or members that come to the new country first and then work to bring subsequent family members. Thus, there are also sometimes fractured relationships with families divided by visa and immigration issues, and great yearning for being reunited. Immigrants may need to return home for intervals of time and may be lonely and isolated. Medical decision making may require consulting family members not living in the United States, particularly in end-of-life decisions.

Caring for elders in the home is often a fact for immigrant families. Nearly 45% of adults in immigrant families are caring for older relatives—twice the rate as in nonimmigrant families.[26] It may be culturally unacceptable for immigrant families to place elderly relatives in nursing homes. This may place an extra strain on immigrant families who may also lack resources to have additional caregivers for disabled family members.

Acculturation

Acculturation is defined as "the process by which foreign born individuals adopt the values, customs, norms, attitudes and behaviors of the mainstream culture."[27] Immigrant families may experience conflicts because of intergenerational pressures. The first generation may especially adhere to traditional values and the second generation may be more acculturated. Differences of perspective on issues of sexuality, gender roles, intermarriage, and elder care may be particularly challenging.

Sexuality and Reproductive Health

First-generation immigrant families may adhere to more traditional values as followed in the homeland, which often include a high value placed on female sexual virtue and virginity before marriage. American-born or raised children may, on the other hand, engage in relationships, resulting in teenage pregnancy with high stress and crisis in the family. Attitudes toward homosexuality may drive gay and bisexual persons to conceal their sexuality.

Many immigrant women may have had poor access to reproductive health care in their home countries, and are less likely to have screening pap smears than other groups. Immigrant women may have had little instruction in human biology and anatomy and thus may know little about pregnancy or sexually transmitted disease prevention.

HIV and Sexually Transmitted Disease Prevention

Negotiation about issues of condom use and safer sex practices may be particularly difficult for many immigrant women where discussion of sexual practices even in the context of a sexual relationship may be culturally unacceptable. Demands for condom use may be seen as admissions of promiscuity or linked to low trust in the male partner. Immigrants also may have misconceptions about HIV transmission that interfere with safer sex practices; for example, that condoms do not work to prevent sexually transmitted diseases or HIV; that the withdrawal method is adequate to prevent HIV or sexually transmitted diseases; that a healthy physical appearance rules out infection. Sex with sex workers, especially in men who are socially isolated and far from their wives or girlfriends, may not be uncommon.

Female Circumcision

Female circumcision is practiced in many African countries, across class and religious lines. There are an estimated 100 million women who have undergone any of various forms of female circumcision (also known as *female genital mutilation*). Female circumcision is linked to cultural and sexual identity, and cultural norms may strongly favor its practice, but the World Health Organization and other international groups have condemned it.

Female circumcision is much more dangerous than male circumcision, and has both physical and psychological sequelae. It can range from partial to total clitoridectomy to infibulation (excision of the clitoris and part of or all of the labia). Infections, including sepsis and gangrene, as well as other complications have been reported. Women who have undergone this procedure may be reluctant to seek medical care because of fear of stigmatization.[28]

Border Health

Nearly 12 million people live along the Mexico–United States border. Border residents live in areas with major air quality, water quantity, and water quality problems. There are higher rates of infectious diseases such as hepatitis A, salmonella, and tuberculosis (including multi–drug resistant tuberculosis). People residing in these border regions frequently cross back and forth across the border and may obtain health care services on either side. Public health and health care delivery organizations do not routinely cooperate in planning of interventions.[29]

Violence

Immigrants may have been exposed to traumatic violence in their home countries, but because of poverty and other factors also may be exposed to violence and crime in the United States. Domestic violence also may be an important issue. In New York City, for example, immigrant women have been reported to be at increased risk for mortality in domestic violence.[30] Factors that at play may include fear of approaching the police or judicial system to seek protection from a batterer, fear of the batterer being deported, language and informational barriers about women's rights in the United States, and fear of losing custody of children if domestic violence is identified.

Common Pitfalls

- The diversity of immigrant backgrounds is not recognized.
- Immigrant experiences can vary widely, even within one family.
- Many barriers exist for immigrant patients, such as lack of insurance and low English proficiency.
- Immigrants are exposed to health risks from their home countries, migration, and the United States.

- Health care beliefs and treatments are heavily influenced by experiences in home countries.
- Immigrants who travel to their home countries do not receive appropriate prophylaxis.
- Immigrants may receive inadequate and worse treatment than native-born Americans.

STRATEGIES FOR IMPROVING IMMIGRANTS' HEALTH

MEDICAL SCREENING EXAMINATION

There are no national recommendations for the care of immigrant children and adults. However, as conditions for legal immigrant entry, the US government requires screening for infectious diseases and documentation of up-to-date immunization status. The recommendations for the medical screening examination are shown in Table 25-1.

IMPROVE PATIENT–PHYSICIAN RELATIONSHIP

Multiple issues may affect relationships between physicians and immigrant patients: language barriers, cultural

Table 25-1. Recommended Medical Screening Examination: Adult and Pediatric Immigrants and Refugees

Medical
General history
Physical examination
Children: vision and hearing screening
Developmental and nutritional assessment
Preventive health interventions
Immunization status
Tuberculosis screening
Children: safety issues
Laboratory testing
Routine
CBC with differential
HbsAg, anti-Hbs, Anti HBc
Hepatitis A serology
Urinalysis with microscopic analysis
Stool ova and parasites × 3
VDRL
HIV
Special
Hepatitis C
Malaria
Children and pregnant women: lead levels
Referrals as needed
Psychiatric
Vision and hearing
Dentistry
Psychiatric and behavioral

Adapted from: Stauffer WM, Maroushek S, Kamat D. Medical screening of immigrant children. *Clin Pediatr* 2003;42:763–773.[32]

barriers and misunderstandings, mistrust, or inability to pay for treatments. Despite all these possible impediments, immigrant patients also tend to be very grateful for attempts made to accommodate them. Inquiring about each individual's experiences of immigration, health care beliefs, and practices rather than making assumptions based on demographic probabilities is vitally important. Finding out a little about the places, political situations, and history of the countries from which patients come can enrich the experience for both patient and provider. Health care providers are often held in high esteem and are honored with intimate confidences. Hearing these confidences and bearing witness to the travails of patients who have left or fled their homes is both an exceptional privilege and an opportunity to decrease suffering.

PRACTICE LEVEL INTERVENTIONS

Reflecting the diversity of the communities served through art work, accommodating non–English speakers, and having a diverse staff are ways a practice can welcome immigrant patients. Having appointment times that are more convenient for work schedules and financial accommodations or pharmaceutical plans for those without insurance or medication coverage will help increase chances that patients will come back and take prescribed medications. Having social workers and health educators on site is also useful. Developing practice expertise in issues facing specific groups can improve care as well. For example, in Boston, one physician set up a referral clinic for women who had been circumcised. A rich network of referrals to everything from community-based organizations to immigration lawyers and low-cost dentists will help address the full panoply of issues facing immigrant patients.

Community-based primary care practices may enhance immigrant patient access to care, compared with hospital-based outpatient departments. Immigrant patients may have difficulty accessing specialty services. Instructions and consent forms for diagnostic tests and procedures often are not translated into other languages. Institutions may lack bilingual/multilingual signage and thus become labyrinths for immigrant patients. As a result, care must be taken to facilitate specialty care and diagnostic services for immigrant patients to avoid improper or inadequate informed consent or dangerous errors in preparation for procedures (e.g., not fasting; not holding anticoagulants). The use of community health promoters or advocates may enhance the ability of vulnerable immigrant patients to navigate the health care institution and system.

HEALTH CARE SYSTEM LEVEL INTERVENTIONS

Enrolling eligible patients in publicly funded health plans to expand access to care is an important step. New York City's presumptive eligibility experiment after the September 11th tragedy (computers were damaged so that presumptive Medicaid eligibility was granted pending later verification) resulted in many patients obtaining needed services. A retrospective analysis showed little if any fraudulent enrollment. Thus, streamlining enrollment procedures was extremely efficacious in expanding access to care.[31] A simple and streamlined form is essential for enrollment in the Children's Health Insurance Program (CHIP) and other expanded access programs. Outreach to immigrant populations is also important in enrollment, as has been seen in the CHIP programs nationally.

Alameda County in California instituted the "*No Wrong Door*" project, an innovative program to insure all uninsured persons in the county regardless of immigration status (www.alamedahealthconsortium.org). A variety of programs are used to obtain coverage, such as, Medi-Cal, Healthy Families, and other affordable, low-cost coverage plans for low-income families. Health promoters provided community outreach and navigation of the health care system and enrollment process.

COMMUNITY LEVEL INTERVENTIONS

Providers, practices, and health care systems might also focus on immigrant communities rather than on individual patients to improve health. These efforts might take the form of media campaigns or partnerships with community-based organizations focusing on particular issues. Media campaigns have targeted smoking cessation or HIV screening in immigrant populations. Programs training health promoters in areas as diverse as healthy eating for diabetics to screening for hepatitis, domestic violence, and cervical cancer have been shown to be successful in immigrant communities.

CONCLUSION

Immigrants are a large and diverse segment of the US population with wide-ranging health risks and needs. The stimuli and barriers to immigration; national and international politics; and personal characteristics and histories mold the immigration experience. Immigrants face increased risks of many illnesses, poor health care access, and often lower-quality health. Recognizing and attempting to understand the variety of factors that impact immigrant health will improve the health of individual patients as well as US communities.

KEY CONCEPTS

- Immigrants come from very diverse backgrounds.
- The possibility of torture should be considered in any refugee. Use a chronological method for interviewing refugees about these issues.
- Conduct culturally competent patient education.
- Develop culturally competent providers and institutions.
- Address patient concerns respectfully, and elicit concerns.
- Use trained interpreters for limited English proficiency patients.
- Screen for common infectious diseases and mental health disorders.
- Remember that immigrant travelers are high-risk travelers. Advise, provide appropriate prophylaxis, and vaccinate accordingly.
- Assess the community for resources and referral.
- Be aware of access to care problems.
  —Work with community outreach groups.
  —Help with navigation of resources.
  —Consider costs, and so on.

CORE COMPETENCY
Taking the Immigration History

Explore the patient's life history and psychosocial context.

- Does the patient use treatments or healers from the home country?
- Assess for communal decision making. Is the family a source of strength and support?
- Inquire about home remedies and alternative medical treatments.
- What is the patient's religious background, involvement in the religious community, and other community supports?
- Have there been any occupational or environmental exposures?
- When did the patient last travel abroad or to the homeland? How long was the stay?

Psychosocial assessment of immigrants and refugees

- Ask about health beliefs; do not stereotype.
- Ask how this might affect medical care, such as end-of-life issues and treatment.
- Screen for depression, anxiety, posttraumatic stress disorder (e.g., taking a complete trauma history) and examine the patient for physical findings of torture.

> **Ask about immigration status**
>
> - Ask about reasons for immigration, hardships endured, barriers, or returning plans and patterns.
> - Where is the patient from?
> - How long has the patient been in the United States?
> - Why did they come?
> - Where did the patient live before arriving here?
> - Who is still back home?
> - Who does the patient live with here?
> - How does patient support him- or herself?
> - Consider a referral to an immigration lawyer if permanent residence is desired.

DISCUSSION QUESTIONS

1. Discuss the barriers to access to care faced by immigrant patients.
2. Describe health problems faced by immigrants and refugees.
3. You are practicing in a community populated by refugees from a developing country. How would you set up a culturally competent practice to care for this community? What barriers to access would you target and how?

RESOURCES

http://www.apiahf.org/
Asian and Pacific Islander Health Forum

http://www.aapcho.org/
Association of Asian Pacific Community Health Organizations

http://www.diversityrx.org/HTML/DIVRX.htm
Diversity Rx: Promoting language and cultural competence to improve the quality of health care for minority, immigrant, and ethnically diverse communities

http://www.phrusa.org/publications/asylum_report.html
Examining asylum seekers: A physician's guide to medical and psychological evaluations of torture

http://www.migrantclinician.org/
Migrant Clinicians Network

http://www.futureofchildren.org/index.htm
Future of children. Publication devoted to issues of immigrant children put out by Woodrow Wilson School of Public Policy at Princeton and the Brookings Institute

http://www.hispanichealth.org/
National Alliance for Hispanic Health

http://www.nilc.org/
National Immigration Law Center

http://www.healthlaw.org
NHeLP: National Health Law Program

http://asianamericanhealth.nlm.nih.gov/
National Library of Medicine's Asian American Health Page

http://www.leptaskforce.org/
National Limited English Proficient (LEP) Advocacy Task Force

http://erc.msh.org/mainpage.cfm?file=1.0.htm&module=provider&language=English
The Provider's Guide to Quality and Culture

REFERENCES

1. Larson L. *The foreign born population in the U.S.: 2003 Population characteristics.* Washington, DC: U.S. Census Bureau, August, 200. Accessed September 6, 2005. Available at: http://www.census.gov/prod/2004pubs/ p20-551.pdf
2. Smith JP. The new Americans: Economic, demographic, and fiscal effects of immigration. Washington, DC: The National Academies Press, 1997.
2a. Sum A, Fogg N, Harrington P. *Immigrant workers and the great American job machine.* Washington, DC: Northeastern University, 2002.
2b. U.S. Refugee Admissions Program 2004–2005. *Interim Report. Refugee Council USA.* September. Accessed May, 2005. Available at: http://www.refugeecouncilusa.org/ 2004RCUSAinterim-w.pdf
3. Srinivasan S, Guillermo T. Toward improved health: Disaggregating Asian American and Native Hawaiian/Pacific Islander data. *Am J Public Health* 2000; 90: 1731–1734.
4. Illegal Immigration Reform and Immigrant Responsibility Act of September 30, 1996 (110 Statutes-at-Large 3009). 06/09/2003. Available at: http://uscis.gov/graphics/shared/ aboutus/ statistics/legishist/ act142.htm
5. Lowell BL, Suro R. *How many undocumented? The numbers behind the US-Mexico migration talks.* Washington, DC: Pew Hispanic Center, 2002.
6. Sum A, Kirsch I, Taggart R. *The twin challenges of mediocrity and inequality: Literacy in the U.S. from an international perspective.* Princeton, NJ: Educational Testing Service, 2002.
7. Ku L, Waidmann T. *How race/ethnicity, immigration status and language affect health insurance coverage, access to care and quality of care among the low-income population.* Kaiser Commission on Medicaid and the Uninsured. Menlo Park, CA: Kaiser Family Foundation, 2003.
8. Lillie-Blanton M, Hudman J. Untangling the Web: Race/ethnicity, immigration, and the nation's health. *Am J Public Health* 2001;91(11):1736–1738.
9. Yu SM, Huang ZJ, Singh GK. Health status and health services utilization among US Chinese, Asian Indian, Filipino, and other Asian/Pacific Islander Children. *Pediatrics* 2004,113(1 Pt 1):101–107.
10. Todd KH, Samaroo N, Hoffman JR. Ethnicity as a risk factor for inadequate emergency department analgesia. *JAMA* 1993;269:1537–1539.

11. Anderson KO, Mendoza TR, Valero V, et al. Minority cancer patients and their providers: Pain management attitudes and practice. *Cancer* 2000;88:1929–1938.

12. Graham RE, Ahn AC, Davis RB, et al. Use of complementary and alternative medical therapies among racial and ethnic minority adults: Results from the 2002 National Health Interview Survey. *J Natl Med Assoc* 2005; 97(4):535–545.

13. Ko R. Adulterants in Asian patent medications. *N Engl J Med* 1998;339:847.

14. Bonkowsky JL, Frazer JK, Buchi KF, et al. Metamizole use by Latino immigrants: A common and potentially harmful home remedy. *Pediatrics* 2002;109(6):e98.

15. Collins KS, Hughes DL, Doty MM, et al. *Diverse communities, common concerns: Assessing health care quality for minority Americans.* Findings from the Commonwealth Fund 2001 Health Care Quality Survey. New York, NY: The Commonwealth Fund, 2002.

15a. Rivadeneyra R, Elderkin-Thompson V, Silver RC, et al. Patient centeredness in medical encounters requiring an interpreter. *Am J Med* 2000;108(6):470–474.

15b. Substance Abuse and Mental Health Services Administration. *2003 National survey on drug use and health.* Available at: http://oas.samhsa.gov/nhsda/2k3nsduh/2k3Results.htm#ch2

16. Binns HJ, Kim D, Campbell C Targeted screening for elevated blood lead levels: populations at high risk. *Pediatrics* 2001;108(6):1364–1366.

17. Deren S, Kang SY, Colon HM, et al. Migration and HIV risk behaviors: Puerto Rican drug injectors in New York City and Puerto Rico. *Am J Public Health* 2003;93(5): 812–816.

18. Bacaner N, Stauffer B, Boulware DR, et al. Travel medicine considerations for North American immigrants visiting friends and relatives. *JAMA* 2004;291:2856–2864.

19. Angell SY, Behrens RH. Risk assessment and disease prevention in travelers visiting friends and relatives. *Infect Dis Clin North Am* 2005;19:49–65.

20. Fazel M, Stein A. The mental health of refugee children. *Arch Dis Child* 2002;87:366–370.

21. Hollifield M, Warner TD, Lian N, et al. Measuring trauma and health status in refugees: A critical review. *JAMA* 2002;288:611–621.

22. Keller AS. Caring and advocating for victims of torture. *Lancet* 2002.;360(Suppl):s55–56.

23. Kroll J. Posttraumatic symptoms and the complexity of responses to trauma. *JAMA* 2003;290(5):667–670.

24. Eisenman DP, Gelberg L, Liu H, et al. Mental health and health-related quality of life among adult Latino primary care patients living in the United States with previous exposure to political violence. *JAMA* 2003;290: 627–634.

25. Kleinman A. Culture and depression. *N Engl J Med* 2004;351:951–953.

26. Zahn D, Hirota S, Garcia J, et al. Valuing families and meeting them where they are. *Am J Public Health* 2003; 93:1797–1799.

27. Shelley D, Fahs M, Scheinmann R, et al. *Acculturation and tobacco use among Chinese Americans. Am J Public Health* 2004;94:300–307.

28. Toubia N. Female circumcision as a public health issue. *N Engl J Med* 1994;331:712–716.

29. Homedes N, Ugalde A .Globalization and health at the United States-Mexico border. *Am J Public Health* 2003;93: 2016–2022.

30. New York City Department of Health Bureau of Injury Epidemiology. *Femicide in New York City 1995–2002: Sortable statistics. Trends of femicide in NYC 1995–2002.* A profile of intimate partner femicide in New York City, 1995-2002. Accessed March, 2005. Available at: http://search.nyc.gov/query.html with search word "femicide."

31. Haslanger K. Radical simplification: Disaster relief Medicaid in New York City. *Health Aff (Millwood)* 2003; 22:252.

32. Stauffer WM, Maroushek S, Kamat D. Medical screening of immigrant children. *Clin Pediatr* 2003;42: 763–773.

Chapter 26

Providing Care to Patients Who Speak Limited English

Alice Hm Chen, MD, MPH, and Elizabeth A. Jacobs, MD, MPP

Objectives

- Describe the limited-English–speaking population in the United States.
- Highlight the clinical consequences of language barriers.
- Review policies pertaining to linguistic access in health care.
- Describe institutional responses to overcome language barriers.
- Summarize strategies to address language barriers in clinical practice.

We clinicians are better educated and more scientific than ever before, but we have a great failing: we sometimes do not communicate effectively with our patients or with their families.[1]

The current health care system offers some of the most technologically advanced medicine in the world. At the same time, millions of Americans have limited access to the most basic feature of good medical care: adequate communication.[2] Effective patient–provider communication is essential to providing good medical care. Taking an accurate history is fundamental to being a diagnostician; the history is the key to the final diagnosis in 56% to 82% of cases.[3] The quality of communication also affects patient and physician satisfaction, patient adherence, and clinical outcomes.[4] Unfortunately, many people in the United States are unable to reap the benefits of effective communication because they cannot speak English well.

The ability to navigate the US health care system depends in large part on the capacity to speak and understand English. Language barriers can hinder care from simple communications such as calling for an appointment, to emergent situations such as explaining symptoms to an ambulance paramedic, to more nuanced exchanges such as discussing treatment risks and benefits with a doctor. The consequences can be dire.

This chapter is designed to help readers understand the impact of language barriers on both patients and clinicians, and provide guidance to overcome them. It begins with an overview of language barriers in health care, including who faces these barriers, how language barriers affect health care, and current policies regarding linguistic access in health care settings. It concludes with practical suggestions clinicians may draw from to better care for limited-English–speaking patients.

LANGUAGE BARRIERS IN HEALTH CARE

Mikhail Tupikov immigrated to the United States 5 years ago. Despite working long days, he takes English as a second language (ESL) classes in the evenings and on weekends. He is able to say and understand basic things in English, but this becomes more difficult when he is under stress. When he presents to the emergency department with an episode of recurrent nephrolithiasis, he does not know enough English to share his past medical history, alert the nurse of his codeine allergy, or describe his symptoms in detail to his doctor.

LIMITED ENGLISH PROFICIENCY

Limited English proficiency (LEP) refers to patients such as Mr. Tupikov who cannot speak, read, write, or understand the English language at a level that permits them to interact effectively with health care providers. Since 1980, the US Census has used a set of standardized questions to ask about language ability. Anyone who reports speaking English less than "very well" (that is, "well," "not well," or "not at all") is considered to be LEP.[5]

In clinical settings, LEP status is most reliably ascertained by asking patients whether they need an interpreter, or asking what language they prefer for their health care encounter.[6] As in the case of Mikhail Tupikov, basic command of English that may suffice at the grocery store or post office may be inadequate to communicate in health care settings.[7] Given that communication is bidirectional, another important gauge of a patient's LEP status is whether or not the clinician feels confident of the quality of communication.

THE LIMITED ENGLISH–SPEAKING POPULATION IN THE UNITED STATES: LARGE, DIVERSE, AND GROWING

According to the US Census, the number of Americans aged 5 years or older who spoke a language other than English at home grew from 23.1 million in 1980 to 47 million in 2000. The percentage who were considered LEP experienced similar growth, increasing from 4.8% in 1980 to 8.1% in 2000.[5]

More than 380 different languages are spoken across the United States.[5] Although Spanish accounts for nearly 60% of people who speak a language other than English at home, because of changes in immigration patterns, other languages are increasingly likely to be encountered (Fig. 26-1). Between 1990 and 2000, Chinese jumped from the fifth most commonly spoken non-English language to second. The number of Russian speakers nearly tripled in the same decade, while the number of French/Haitian Creole speakers more than doubled.[5]

Among these various language groups, the proportion of people who are LEP varies considerably. For example, about 50% of Asian and Pacific Island language and Spanish speakers are LEP, whereas only about one third of Indo-European language speakers are LEP. The greatest concentrations of LEP residents are in the western states, particularly California, where according to the 2000 census, one in every five people is considered LEP. Other states with high percentages of LEP residents include Texas (13.9%), New York (13%), Hawaii (12.7%), New Mexico (11.9%), Arizona (11.4%), Nevada (11.2%), New Jersey (11.1%), and Florida (10.3%).[5] However, the greatest *increase* in LEP populations has been in southeastern and western states such as Georgia, North Carolina, and Nevada, all of which experienced a >200% growth between 1990 and 2000.[8] Given the relative lack of established language access services in these "emerging" LEP communities, clinicians working in these high-growth states may face particular challenges in caring for their LEP patients.

LEP individuals are more likely than English-speaking members of the same ethnic group to be older, less educated, low income, and to have been in the United States for a shorter period of time.[9] Given these demographic patterns, clinicians caring for LEP

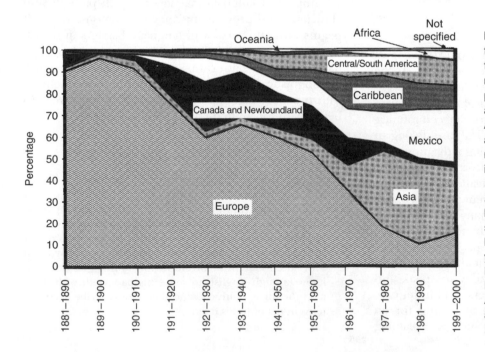

Figure 26-1. The pattern of immigration to the U.S. began to slowly shift after the turn of the 20th century, but changed rapidly after 1965, with a decline in the proportion of Europeans and Canadians associated with a rise in immigrants from Asia, Mexico, the Caribbean, and Central and South America. (From: Immigration by region, expressed as a percentage of total immigration, 1891 through 2000. *2000 Statistical Yearbook of the Immigration and Naturalization Service.* Available at: http://uscis.gov/graphics/shared/aboutus/statistics/imm00yrbk/imm2000list.htm Or http://uscis.gov/graphics/shared/statistics/yearbook/2004/table3.xls; Adapted from: Fairchild AL. Policies of inclusion: Immigrants, disease, dependency, and American immigration policy at the dawn and dusk of the 20th century. *Am J Public Health* 2004;94:528–539.)

patients often encounter concurrent challenges of poverty, uninsurance, and low functional health literacy and cross-cultural communication. However, although these issues are often intermeshed, they are also distinct, and require sensitivity to the individual patient's background. For example, a patient may speak little English, but be highly educated, literate in her or his native language, and accustomed to and accepting of western biomedical concepts.

LANGUAGE BARRIERS HAVE CLINICAL CONSEQUENCES

> Ha Lang, an elderly Cantonese-speaking woman, is hospitalized because she took too much warfarin. Late at night, she gets up to go to the bathroom. A nurse on duty stops her and tries to get her back into bed. When Mrs. Lang persists in wanting to go the bathroom, the nurse thinks she is agitated. Instead of calling for an interpreter, the nurse has Mrs. Lang put in arm restraints and gives her a sedative.

Impact on Access to Care

In studies with a wide range of LEP health consumers, language barriers are often reported as being one of the most important, if not the most important, barriers to accessing care.[13-16] When compared with English speakers, limited English–speaking patients are less likely to be insured[17,18] or know about public health insurance programs,[19] and their children are less likely to have a usual source of care.[20] Limited English–speaking patients are also less likely to receive physician visits,[21,22] dental care,[23] eye examinations,[23] mental health visits,[21] or referrals from the emergency department after discharge.[24]

Impact on Provider–Patient Relationship

Even when limited English–speaking patients are able to access care, they have been found to be less likely to understand what transpires in the clinical encounter, from basic medical terminology[7] to discharge diagnoses,[25] to prescribed medications.[10,27] They are less likely than patients who do not have language barriers to engage in active exchanges with their providers[28] or feel as if they played an active part in decision making.[29] Perhaps as a result, they are less likely to be satisfied with their medical encounters,[29-32] their individual providers,[30,33] and the institutions that provide care.[10,31]

Impact on Quality of Care

In nearly every clinical setting that has been examined, language barriers appear to result in lower-quality care. Limited-English–speaking patients are less likely to receive recommended preventive care such as mammograms,[21,34] pap smears,[34-36] colon cancer screenings,[37]

and influenza vaccinations.[21,37] In psychiatric settings, LEP status has been shown to result in inadequate evaluation and diagnosis.[38,39] In palliative care settings, LEP patients are less likely to have adequate symptom control;[40] and in obstetrical settings, they are at higher risk of experiencing a nonsterile delivery.[41] Once LEP patients present to the emergency department, they receive more diagnostic tests,[42] are more likely to be hospitalized,[18,43] and once hospitalized, tend to have a longer length of stay[44] than English-speaking patients with similar conditions.

PATIENTS HAVE A LEGAL RIGHT TO LANGUAGE ACCESS IN HEALTH CARE

There are a number of federal and state laws that give limited English–speaking patients a legal right to language assistance services in health care settings. On the federal level, Title VI of the 1964 Civil Rights Act has been interpreted by the US Department of Health and Human Services (HHS) to mean that any health care organization that receives federal money—for example, Medicare or Medicaid payments—is obligated to ensure linguistic access for its LEP patients.[45] More recently, HHS' Office for Civil Rights has issued guidelines for health care providers to follow in determining what type and extent of language assistance services to offer.[46] The Centers for Medicare and Medicaid Services (CMS) also has issued regulations that require Medicaid health plans to make interpreter services available to their enrollees free of charge.[47]

On the state level, 40 states have laws that require or encourage health care providers to address language barriers, often for a specific setting or medical condition. California alone has 63 different laws supporting linguistically appropriate care, covering settings as diverse as acute care hospitals, adult day care centers, mental health rehabilitation centers, and correctional facilities.[45] In the private sector, organizations such as the Joint Commission on Accreditation of Healthcare Organizations (JCAHO), which accredits hospitals, and the National Consortium on Quality Assurance (NCQA), which accredits health plans, have developed and are refining standards for language access.[48]

Despite legal mandates, limited-English–speaking patients continue to face barriers when they attempt to access health services. In part this results from incomplete coverage and inconsistent enforcement of federal and state laws, limited availability of trained health care interpreters, and lack of adequate financing for language access services. In the face of these challenges, it is critical that health care providers understand how they can optimize their communication with LEP patients.

Common Pitfalls in Health Care for Limited English–Speaking Patients

- Language is one of the most significant barriers to health care for immigrants in the United States.
- Limited English–speaking patients understand less of what occurs during health care visits than English speakers.
- Limited English–speaking patients receive lower quality of care than those who speak English very well.
- Using interpreters has been shown to improve understanding and quality of health care.
- Despite growing numbers of limited English–speaking patients and legal mandates requiring provision of interpreter services, these services are often lacking or inadequate.

BRIDGING THE LANGUAGE BARRIER

Michelle Nguyen was admitted from the emergency department for management of preterm labor. She was crying and distraught. Because she only spoke Vietnamese, her husband interpreted for her, reporting that she was frightened as this was her first pregnancy. A few weeks later, she was seen for follow-up care by a nurse practitioner; this time, Mrs. Nguyen's 12-year-old daughter, in tears, was able to convey that the reason her mother had come to the emergency department was that her husband had assaulted her, causing the preterm labor.

In a survey of over 4000 uninsured patients in 16 cities, more than 50% of those who needed an interpreter reported that the hospital was not able to provide one in a timely fashion.[10] A second survey of 70 hospitals from 11 regions across the country found that 56% of the time, no Spanish speaker could be found to respond to a volunteer tester's call.[49] These findings are not surprising given that another study of public and private teaching hospitals found that only 25% employed any full-time, professional interpreters. The majority used bilingual hospital staff, volunteers, and family members and friends; several reported that in emergencies, staff often called local ethnic restaurants to find someone to interpret.[50] As Mrs. Ngyuen's case demonstrates, using untrained (also referred to as "ad hoc") interpreters can be problematic.

WHO IS THE MEDICAL INTERPRETER?

The distinction between *ad hoc* untrained interpreters and trained medical interpreters is critical. *Ad hoc* interpreters have been shown to make frequent errors, including omissions, paraphrasing, use of incorrect words, substitutions, additions, and inappropriately providing their own personal views.[51–53] Family members and friends are particularly unsuitable when domestic violence or a potentially embarrassing symptom needs to be evaluated.[54] Minor children should never be used as medical interpreters, because it often places them in uncomfortable and frightening positions.

In contrast, trained medical interpreters are expected to have fluency in both English and a second language, have a command of medical terminology, understand basic medical concepts, have the necessary skills to manage a three-way conversation, be committed to interpreting accurately and completely without adding their own opinion, and abide by a code of ethics that respects patient confidentiality. Frequently they are trained in how to deal with difficult situations, such as cases of domestic violence, as well.

Each type of medical interpreter should be carefully weighed before deciding how best to proceed (Table 26-1). The following sections provide guidance on when and how to use bilingual skills, professional medical interpreters, and *ad hoc* interpreters. Clinicians also should check their organization's policy about the use of interpreters. Some organizations require the exclusive use of staff interpreters, and prohibit the use of *ad hoc* interpreters.

USING YOUR OWN BILINGUAL SKILLS

Ismelda Garcia speaks a little English, and her doctor knows a few words in Spanish. She leaves her doctor's office with a new prescription for "pression alta" (high blood pressure), which she was instructed to "take once cada dia" (each day). When she ends up in the emergency room a day later feeling lightheaded, the emergency department nurse brings in the hospital's Spanish interpreter to take a history. It turns out that the word written as "once" in English means "11" in Spanish.

Not surprisingly, when they can, LEP patients choose clinicians who can speak their language.[9] Language concordance between physicians and patients has been shown to increase patient satisfaction[55] and recall,[56] self-reported health status,[57] ratings of care,[58] and medication adherence.[59]

Given these benefits, a variety of programs have been developed to teach medical students and residents medical Spanish, ranging from 20 hours of basic language instruction to intensive, longitudinal immersion experiences.[60] Patients appreciate their clinicians' efforts to

Table 26-1. Types of Medical Interpreters

Interpreter Type	Advantages	Disadvantages
No interpreter (e.g., bilingual clinician)	• Direct communication between patient and clinician is quicker and allows for better rapport • No concerns about confidentiality, as third party is not involved in the encounter • Patients appreciate their clinicians' attempts to converse in their language	• There are a limited number of truly bilingual clinicians • Risk for miscommunication and misdiagnosis if clinicians overestimate their language skills
Bilingual staff (e.g., secretary, medical assistant, custodial staff)	• Convenient • No additional salary costs • Patients are often comfortable with health care staff	• Disrupted patient flow and inefficiencies, as staff cannot interpret and perform other duties simultaneously • Risk for inaccurate interpretation if staff do not have sufficient bilingual skills or know medical terminology
Professional interpreter (trained and tested)	• Less likely to make interpreting errors • Trained in ethics • Patients may be more likely to share sensitive information with a professional	• May require wait, particularly if there is institutional imbalance of supply and demand • Salary costs of hiring professional interpreters • Patients may not be comfortable with having a stranger involved in their communication
Ad hoc interpreter (e.g., patient's family member or friend)	• Convenient • Free for provider and institution • Patients may prefer to communicate through friends or family members	• Usually have inadequate bilingual language and interpreting skills • High rates of errors and omissions • Communication may be modified to suit the interpreter's agenda • Loss of confidentiality • Use of minor children is unethical

learn their language,[60] and respond with increased levels of trust.[61] At the same time, it is important for clinicians to have an accurate sense of their own language proficiency, and be aware of their own limitations. As in the preceding vignette, false fluency can be confusing or lead to significant miscommunication with clinical consequences.[52,54,60]

Clinicians can gauge whether they need an interpreter by considering: (a) how they learned the language and in what context, (b) how often they need to search for alternate ways to express themselves or ask patients to repeat themselves, and (c) the content and emotional tenor of the clinical exchange (See Box 26-1). An additional consideration, particularly for clinicians who grew up speaking another language at home, is familiarity with medical terminology, such as appendix, thyroid, or computed tomography scan?

The level of proficiency required may vary depending on the content and emotional tenor of the clinical exchange. A clinician with moderate language skills may be able to successfully diagnose and treat an otherwise healthy 27-year-old with a sprained ankle, but may need to call on a trained medical interpreter to evaluate an episode of syncope in a 78-year-old with multiple medical conditions. If you are uncertain, ask for an interpreter.

WORKING WITH PROFESSIONAL MEDICAL INTERPRETERS

A day in the life of an interpreter: "Before going into the room, the physician expresses to me his concern about whether the health problems claimed by this woman are real or imagined. She has been in the clinic three times before, each time with different vague and diffuse complaints, none of which makes medical sense. As we learn, the poor woman has a fistula in her rectum. In her previous visits, she could not bring herself to reveal her symptoms in the presence of . . . her son as he interprets for her. She tells me that she has been so embarrassed about her condition that she has invented other symptoms to justify her visits to the physicians. She confesses that she has been eager to have a hospital staff interpreter from the first visit, but her hope had not materialized until now.[54]

Professional medical interpreters are beneficial in a number of clinical arenas. They make fewer errors of clinical consequence,[52] improve the patient-centeredness of encounters,[63] reduce disparities in the use of preventive health services,[37] decrease the use and costs of emergency department testing,[64] and are associated with higher-quality care,[65] as well as enhanced physician and patient satisfaction with the encounter.[55,66]

Box 26-1. Assessing Your Bilingual Skills

For clinicians who use their own bilingual language skills in the patient encounter, doing a self-assessment is critical. **Is the clinician able to do the following?**

- Formulate questions easily and effectively, without frequently being stuck on vocabulary.
- Ask questions in a different way if not understood.
- Understand the response, including regional variations, nuance, and connotation.

- Explain relevant health care concepts.
- Negotiate and agree on a course of action.
- Inspire trust by communicating competence.

Adapted from: Roat C. *Addressing language access issues in your practice: A toolkit for physicians and their staff members.* San Francisco: California Academy of Family Physicians, 2005.[62]

A clinician can work with an interpreter who is either physically in the same room (a face-to-face or in-person interpreter) or is located outside the examination room (most commonly, a telephone interpreter). Although working with an in-person professional interpreter is preferred by both clinicians and patients,[66] many institutions may only have easy access to professional telephone interpreters. There are important considerations in deciding whether using a telephone interpreter will be sufficient for your needs (see Table 26-2). Similar skills are used in working with both types of trained interpreters (see Core Competency).

A caveat: the field of medical interpreting is relatively new in the United States. Although a number of medical interpreter associations have recently developed or are in the process of developing professional standards and codes of ethics[69], with the exception of Washington state there is currently no formal certification process for health care interpreters.[67] As a result, some professional interpreters may have received little or no formal training and assessment in medical interpreting, and should be treated more like *ad hoc* interpreters, as described in the following.[68]

WORKING WITH *AD HOC* INTERPRETERS

Sometimes a trained interpreter may not be available. Although the level of communication may be limited by the *ad hoc* interpreter's skills, observing certain guidelines (see Core Competency) can improve the quality of the interpretation.[62] It is important to consider the import, sensitivity, and urgency of communication when determining what kind of interpreter you use. If it is an emergency situation and there are no trained in-person interpreters immediately available, you should use a telephone or *ad hoc* interpreter rather than waiting for an in-person interpreter. With a sensitive subject, such as exposure to sexually transmitted diseases, using a trained interpreter rather than a family member or friend is more likely to elicit the critical information you need. Except in life-threatening situations, young children should never be used as interpreters.

Table 26-2. Choosing an In-person or Telephonic Interpreter

In-person	Telephonic
When delivering bad news.	When in person not available.
With patients with significant hearing loss.	With relatively straightforward encounters.
With patients from cultures unaccustomed to using telephone.	When access to an interpreter is required immediately.
For conversations with more than one person; e.g., family conference.	When privacy and confidentiality is critical, particularly in small communities.*
For psychiatric encounters psychosis is present or communication of affect critical.	When health of patient where mandates minimal exposure, e.g., immunocompromised patients.

*In small communities interpreters and patients often know each other. Using an interpreter from a telephonic interpreter service almost always guarantees patient privacy.
Adapted from: Roat C. *Addressing language access issues in your practice: A toolkit for physicians and their staff members.* San Francisco: California Academy of Family Physicians, 2005.[62]

KEY CONCEPTS

- Adequate interpretation is essential to the delivery of care to patients with limited English abilities.
- Learning to work with different types of interpreters is an essential clinical skill.
- Bilingual clinicians should learn to evaluate their language abilities and the clinical situation before forgoing the use of a trained interpreter.
- Use of professional interpreters improves quality of care.
- Except in life-threatening emergencies, young children should never be used as interpreters

CONCLUSION

The recent increase in ethnic, cultural, and linguistic diversity in the United States has been accompanied by a great need for language access services in health care settings. A growing body of research shows that language barriers result in decreased patient access, satisfaction, comprehension, and adherence, as well as an increased risk of errors, inappropriate utilization, and higher costs. Access to competent interpreter services can address these risks. Unfortunately, many health care organizations have not yet developed the internal capacity or infrastructure to provide coordinated, consistent language access for their patients. Clinicians must learn how to care for LEP patients within these limitations by recognizing the boundaries of one's personal language skills and learning how to work with both trained and untrained interpreters.

CORE COMPETENCY
Working with Trained and Ad Hoc Interpreters

Setting	Ad hoc interpreter	Trained interpreter
Before beginning the clinical encounter	1. Assess the *ad hoc* interpreter's English skills and familiarity with medical concepts. 2. Be attuned to the interpreter's limitations in the non-English language, particularly with younger people whose primary language is English. 3. Explain to the untrained interpreter that she or he will be your ears and your voice. 4. Ask him or her to interpret accurately and completely, avoid paraphrasing or answering for the patient, and let you know if she or he needs you to slow down, explain, or repeat something. 5. If the interpreter is a family member or friend, it can be helpful to let him or her know that you welcome the interpreter's opinion, but he or she needs to differentiate between his or her personal opinion and the patient's. 6. Give the untrained interpreter permission to stop and let you know if she or he is having difficulty interpreting something you or the patient is saying. Otherwise, out of fear or embarrassment, she or he may gloss over difficulties and contribute to miscommunication.	1. Briefly explain the purpose of the encounter to the interpreter. For example, "Mr. Ukomadu is here for routine follow-up of hypertension and diabetes," or "Mrs. Saleb is here to discuss her biopsy results; she has cancer." 2. Remember the interpreter is not a clinician. It is not appropriate for the clinician to hand the interpreter an informed consent form for the patient to sign, then leave the room. The patient may have questions that the interpreter cannot answer. 3. Consider the appropriateness of the interpreter. There may be historical animosities between ethnic groups that may make an interpreter unacceptable to a given patient, or regional dialects that make communication difficult. Particularly for sensitive issues, patients may feel strongly about having an interpreter of the same gender.
During the clinical encounter	1. Speak slowly and clearly, pausing between each sentence. 2. Use simply constructed sentences and plain English; avoid medical terminology and professional jargon (e.g., "workup"). 3. Speak to and look at the patient. 4. Be attuned to interpersonal dynamics between the patient and interpreter, particularly if the interpreter is a family member or friend. 5. Check in frequently with the patient using the "teach back" method. For example, after conveying a new diagnosis of diabetes, ask the patient to explain what she or he understands. 6. If the interpreter and patient get into an exchange that is not being interpreted, gently remind the interpreter that you need to know everything that is being said. Similarly, if the interpreter answers for the patient, remind the interpreter that you need her/him to interpret, even if s/he knows the answer to the question.	1. Look at and talk to your patient, not the interpreter or telephone. For example, ask Mr. Rodriguez, "How are you doing?" rather than asking the interpreter, "How is he doing?" 2. Ask one question at a time. 3. Speak at an even pace, in relatively short segments. Pause regularly to allow the interpreter time to interpret. 4. Avoid interrupting the interpretation. Many concepts have no linguistic or cultural equivalent in the patient's language, so the interpreter may need extra time to explain. 5. Pay attention to nonverbal cues that may indicate a need for further clarification or discussion.

DISCUSSION QUESTIONS

1. How does communication, or miscommunication, affect quality of care? (Try to elicit and synthesize both research evidence and personal experiences.)
2. Do you speak a language other than English? If yes, what do you think about your ability to adequately communicate with patients in that language after reading this chapter?
3. Have you ever used an *ad hoc* interpreter? What did it feel like? What could you have done to improve the patient encounter?
4. Does your institution provide professional interpreters (in-person or by telephone)? If yes, how are interactions with professional interpreters different from those with *ad hoc* interpreters?

RESOURCES

Jacobs E, Agger-Gupta N, Chen AH, et al, eds. *Language barriers in health care settings: An annotated bibliography of the research literature.* Woodland Hills, CA: The California Endowment, August 2003. Accessed January 15, 2005. Available at: http://www.calendow.org/reference/publications/pdf/cultural/LANGUAGEBARRIERSAB9-03.pdf

Grainger-Monsen M, Haslett J. *Worlds apart: A four-part series on cross cultural healthcare; Mohammad Kochi's story* (video recording). Boston, MA: Fanlight Productions, 2003.

Mutha S, Allen C, Welch M. *Toward culturally competent care: A toolbox for teaching communication strategies.* San Francisco: Center for the Health Professions, University of California, San Francisco, 2002. Available at: http://www.futurehealth.ucsf.edu/cnetwork/resources/curricula/diversity.html.

Roat C, Braganza MF. *Communicating effectively through an interpreter* (video recording). Seattle, WA: Cross Cultural Health Care Program, 1998. Available through: http://xculture.org

REFERENCES

1. Tumulty P. What is a clinician and what does he do? *NEJM* 1970;283:20–24.
2. Teutsch C. Patient-doctor communication. *Med Clin North Am* 2003;87:1115–1145.
3. Cornia PB, Lipsky BA, Dhaliwal G, et al. Clinical problem-solving. Red snapper or crab? *N Engl J Med* 2004;350:1443–1448.
4. Fortin AHT. Communication skills to improve patient satisfaction and quality of care. *Ethn Dis* 2002;12(S3):58–61.
5. Shin HB, Bruno R. *Language use and English-speaking ability Census 2000 brief.* Washington, DC: US Census Bureau, 2003. Available at: www.census.gov/prod/2003pubs/c2kbr-29.pdf
6. Giacomelli J. A review of health interpreter services in a rural community: A total quality management approach. *Aust J Rural Health* 1997;5:158–164.
7. Cooke MW, Wilson S, Cox P, et al. Public understanding of medical terminology: Non-English speakers may not receive optimal care. *J Accid Emerg Med* 2000;17:119–121.
8. Youdelman M, Kohn N, Pryor C, et al. Language services action kit: National Health Law Program & Access Project, 2003.
9. Wilson E, Chen A, Grumbach K, et al. Effects of limited English proficiency and physician language on health care comprehension. *J Gen Intern Med* 2005;20:800–806.
10. Andrulis D, Goodman N, Pryor C. *What a difference an interpreter can make. Health care experiences of uninsured with limited English proficiency.* Boston: The Access Project, 2002. Available at: www.accessproject.org/downloads/c_LEPreportENG.pdf
11. Jackson JC, Rhodes LA, Inui TS, et al. Hepatitis B among the Khmer: Issues of translation and concepts of illness. *J Gen Intern Med* 1997;12:292–298.
12. Lipton RB, Losey LM, Giachello A, et al. Attitudes and issues in treating Latino patients with type 2 diabetes: Views of healthcare providers. *Diabetes Educ* 1998;24:67–71.
13. Barrett B, Shaddick K, Schilling R, et al. Hmong/medicine interactions: Improving cross-cultural health care. *Fam Med* 1998;30:179–184.
14. Chak S, Nixon J, Dugdale A. Primary health care for Indo-Chinese children in Australia. *Aust Paediatr J* 1984;20:57–58.
15. Free C, White P, Shipman C, et al. Access to and use of out-of-hours services by members of Vietnamese community groups in South London: A focus group study. *Fam Pract* 1999;16:369–374.
16. Kelly NR, Groff JY. Exploring barriers to utilization of poison centers: A qualitative study of mothers attending an urban women, infants and children (WIC) clinic. *Pediatrics* 2000;106:199–204.
17. Doty M. *Hispanic patients' double burden: Lack of health insurance and limited English.* New York: The Commonwealth Fund, 2003.
18. Jang M, Lee E, Woo K. Income, language, and citizenship status: Factors affecting the health care access and utilization of Chinese Americans. *Health Soc Work* 1998;23:136–145.
19. Feinberg E, Swartz K, Zaslavsky A, et al. Language proficiency and the enrollment of Medicaid-eligible children in publicly funded health insurance programs. *Matern Child Health J* 2002;6:5–18.
20. Weinick R, Krauss N. Racial and ethnic differences in children's access to health care. *Am J Public Health* 2001;90:1771–1774.
21. Fiscella K, Franks P, Doescher MP, et al. Disparities in health care by race, ethnicity, and language among the insured. *Med Care* 2002;40:52–59.
22. Pitkin Derose K, Baker DW. Limited English proficiency and Latinos' use of physician services. *Med Care Res Rev* 2000;57:76–91.
23. Hu D, Covell R. Health care usage by Hispanic outpatients as a function of primary language. *West J Med* 1986;144:490–493.
24. Sarver J, Baker DW. Effect of language barriers on follow-up appointments after an emergency department visit. *J Gen Intern Med* 2000;15:256–264.
25. Baker DW, Parker RM, Williams M, et al. Use and effectiveness of interpreters in an emergency department. *JAMA* 1996;275:783–788.

26. Crane JA. Patient comprehension of doctor-patient communication on discharge from the emergency department. *J Emerg Med* 1997;15:1–7.
27. Lasater LM, Davidson AJ, Steiner JF, et al. Glycemic control in English- vs. Spanish-speaking Hispanic patients with type 2 diabetes mellitus. *Arch Intern Med* 2001;161:77–82.
28. Rivadeneyra R, Elderkin-Thompson V, Silver RC, et al. Patient centeredness in medical encounters requiring an interpreter. *Am J Med* 2000;108:470–474.
29. Small R, Rice PL, Yelland J, et al. Mothers in a new country: the role of culture and communication in Vietnamese, Turkish, and Filipino women's experiences of giving birth in Australia. *Women Health* 1999;28:77–101.
30. Baker DW, Hayes R, Fortier JP. Interpreter use and satisfaction with interpersonal aspects of care for Spanish-speaking patients. *Med Care* 1998;36:1461–1470.
31. Carrasquillo O, Orav EJ, Brennan TA, et al. Impact of language barriers on patient satisfaction in an emergency department. *J Gen Intern Med* 1999;14:82–87.
32. Weech-Maldonado R, Morales LS, Spritzer K, et al. Racial and ethnic differences in parents' assessments of pediatric care in Medicaid managed care. *Health Serv Res* 2001;36:575–594.
33. Morales LS, Cunningham WE, Brown JA, et al. Are Latinos less satisfied with communication by health care providers? *J Gen Intern Med* 1999;14:409–417.
34. Liao XH, McIlwaine G. The health status and health needs of Chinese population in Glasgow. *Scot Med J* 1995;40:77–80.
35. Harlan LC, Bernstein AB, Kessler LG. Cervical cancer screening: Who is not screened and why? *Am J Public Health* 1991;81:885–891.
36. Watt IS, Howel D, Lo L. The health care experience and health behaviour of the Chinese: A survey based in Hull. *J Public Health Med* 1993;15:129–136.
37. Jacobs EA, Lauderdale DS, Meltzer D, et al. Impact of interpreter services on delivery of health care to limited-English-proficient patients. *J Gen Intern Med* 2001;16:468–474.
38. Drennan G. Counting the costs of language services in psychiatry. *South Afr Med J* 1996;86:344–345.
39. Vasquez C, Javier R. The problem with interpreters: Communicating with Spanish-speaking patients. *Hosp Commun Psychiatry* 1991;42:163–165.
40. Chan A, Woodruff RK. Comparison of palliative care needs of English- and non-English-speaking patients. *J Palliat Care* 1999;15:26–30.
41. Devore JS, Koskela K. The language barrier in obstetric anesthesia. *Am J Obstet Gynecol* 1980;137:745–746.
42. Waxman MA, Levitt AM. Are diagnostic testing and admission rates higher in non-English-speaking versus English-speaking patients in the emergency department? *Ann Emerg Med* 2000;36:456–461.
43. Hampers LC, Cha S, Gutglass D, et al. Language barriers and resource utilization in a pediatric emergency department. *Pediatrics* 1999;103:1253–1256.
44. John-Baptiste A, Naglie G, Tomlinson G, et al. The effect of English language proficiency on length of stay and in-hospital mortality. *J Gen Intern Med* 2004;19:221–228.
45. Perkins J, Youdelman M, Wong D. *Ensuring linguistic access in health care settings: Legal rights and responsibilities,* 2nd ed. Los Angeles: National Health Law Program, 2003.
46. Office for Civil Rights. Guidance to Federal Financial Assistance Recipients Regarding Title VI Prohibition Against National Origin Discrimination Affecting Limited English Proficient Persons. *US DHHS Fed Reg* 2003;68: 47311–47323. Available at: http://www.hhs.gov/ocr/lep/revisedlep.html
47. Medicaid Program. Medicaid managed care: New provisions. *Fed Reg* 2002;67:40989–41116.
48. Cardillo J. Speaking patients' languages. As the diversity of the U.S. population grows, providers struggle to break down the barriers to communication. *Mod Healthcare* 1997;27:64–65.
49. American Institute for Social Justice. *Speaking the language of care: Language barriers to hospital access in America's cities.* Washington, DC: Association of Community Organizations for Reform Now. Accessed 2004 January 22. Available at: http://www.acorn.org/_Accomplishments/National_report.pdf
50. Ginsberg C, Martin D, Andrulis Y, et al. *Interpretation and translation services in health care: A survey of US public and private teaching hospitals.* Washington, DC: National Public Health and Hospital Institute, 1995.
51. Elderkin-Thompson V, Silver RC, Waitzkin H. When nurses double as interpreters: A study of Spanish-speaking patients in a US primary care setting. *Soc Sci Med* 2001;52:1343–1358.
52. Flores G, Laws MB, Mayo SJ, et al. Errors in medical interpretation and their potential clinical consequences in pediatric encounters. *Pediatrics* 2003;111:6–14.
53. Launer J. Taking medical histories through interpreters: Practice in a Nigerian outpatient department. *BMJ* 1978:934–935.
54. Haffner L. Cross-cultural medicine: A decade later. *West J Med* 1992;157:255–259.
55. Lee LJ, Batal HA, Maselli JH, et al. Effect of the Spanish interpretation method on patient satisfaction in an urban walk-in clinic. *J Gen Intern Med* 2002;17:641–646.
56. Seijo R, Gomez J, Freidenberg J. Language as a communication barrier in medical care for Hispanic patients. *Hispanic J Behav Sci* 1991;13:363–375.
57. Perez-Stable EJ, Napoles-Springer A, Miramontes JM. The effects of ethnicity and language on medical outcomes of patients with hypertension or diabetes. *Med Care* 1997;35:1212–1219.
58. Fernandez A, Schillinger D, Grumbach K, et al. Physician language ability and cultural competence. An exploratory study of communication with Spanish-speaking patients. *J Gen Intern Med* 2004;19:167–174.
59. Manson A. Language concordance as a determinant of patient compliance and emergency room use in patients with asthma. *Med Care* 1988;26:1119–1128.
60. Prince D, Nelson M. Teaching Spanish to emergency medicine residents. *Acad Emerg Med* 1995;2:32–37.
61. Barkin S, Balkrishnan R, Manuel J, et al. Effect of language immersion on communication with Latino patients. *NC Med J* 2003;64:258–262.
62. Roat C. *Addressing language access issues in your practice: A toolkit for physicians and their staff members.* San Francisco: California Academy of Family Physicians, 2005.
63. Henbest RJ, Fehrsen GS. Patient-centredness: Is it applicable outside the West? Its measurement and effect on outcomes. *Fam Pract* 1992;9:311–317.

64. Hampers LC, McNulty JE. Professional interpreters and bilingual physicians in a pediatric emergency department: Effect on resource utilization. *Arch Pediatr Adolesc Med* 2002;156:1108–1113.

65. Tocher M, Larosn EB. Do physicians spend more time with non-English-speaking patients? *J Gen Intern Med* 1999;14:303–309.

66. Kuo D, Fagan MJ. Satisfaction with methods of Spanish interpretation in an ambulatory care clinic. *J Gen Intern Med* 1999;14:547–550.

67. Dower C. *Health care interpreters in California*. San Francisco: UCSF Center for the Health Professions, 2003. Available at: http://www.futurehealth .ucsf.edu/pdf_files /healthinterpreters.pdf

68. Hatton DC, Webb T. Information transmission in bilingual, bicultural contexts: A field study of community health nurses and interpreters. *J Commun Health Nurs* 1993;10:137–147.

69. The National Council on Interpreting in Health Care. *A national code of ethics for interpreters in health care, 2004.* Accessed February 13, 2005. Available at: http://www.ncihc.org/NCIHC_PDF/NationalCodeofEthicsfor InterpretersinHealthCare.pdf

Chapter 27

Sexuality as Vulnerability: The Care of Lesbian and Gay Patients

Anne Rosenthal, MD, and Allison Diamant, MD, MSHS

Objectives

- Understand the social and medical context in which lesbians and gay men seek health care.
- Describe major medical and psychosocial concerns in lesbian and gay health.
- Summarize strategies to promote culturally competent care for lesbian and gay patients.

Rachel is seeing a doctor for the first time in years. She wants a doctor she can trust. She worries that the doctor will assume she is heterosexual, but also that if she makes clear that she is not, she will receive poorer care.

Sexual orientation is quite variable, and every medical provider encounters lesbian, gay, and bisexual patients. In a widely cited 1994 survey, 9.1% of men and 4.3% of women in the United States reported engaging in same-sex sexual behavior since puberty, and 2.8% of men and 1.4% of women self-identified as lesbian or gay.[1] Internationally, the prevalence appears to be similar, however, these numbers are likely underestimates, because stigmatization and fear of persecution make many people reluctant to disclose their sexuality to researchers.

Although there are no medical problems that are unique to lesbians and gay men, there is much to know about the types, prevalence, risks, and context of problems that do occur. This chapter summarizes major health concerns of lesbians and gays, and places them in a medical and psychosocial context. A major aim of this chapter is to promote cultural competence for clinicians by increasing awareness and knowledge of lesbian and gay health issues. Identifying and understanding the needs and help-seeking behaviors of lesbians and gays will improve communication, trust, and comfort for both patients and providers.

CHALLENGES TO UNDERSTANDING AND MANAGING HEALTH CONCERNS OF LESBIANS AND GAYS

RESEARCH LIMITATIONS

There are significant limitations to research findings on lesbian and gay health.[2] The generalizability of many early studies was limited by their techniques, such as nonrandom enrollment methods, a lack of heterosexual controls, low response rates, and over-representation of white and educated subjects. The term "sexual orientation" encompasses a spectrum of emotional and physical experience, including sexual desire, behavior, and identity. Classification based only on sexual behavior (i.e., men who have sex with men [MSM], women who have sex with women [WSW], and not identity (i.e., lesbian, gay male, bisexual) has resulted in homosexuality and bisexuality being combined, when in fact the health and social behaviors of these groups may be quite different. Additionally, research in the field of lesbian and gay health care is underfunded and inadequately supported. Despite the paucity of evidence and limitations in research techniques, areas of significant concern can be discussed.

ACCESS TO CARE

Lack of health insurance appears to have a larger impact on health care–seeking behaviors for lesbians than gay men, and lesbians are less likely than gay men to report a private doctor as their usual source of care.[3] For both groups, hostile attitudes from providers, manifested as verbal intolerance, or even rough gynecologic examinations for lesbians, are barriers and deterrents to care.

DISCRIMINATION AND STIGMATIZATION

Rachel's fears are not unfounded. Homophobia in medicine is widespread, mirroring society in general. Health care providers are both perpetrators and victims, and there is a great deal of prejudice against the participation of lesbian and gay people in patient care. For instance, one survey of family practice residency directors found 25% "might" or "most certainly" would rank a homosexual applicant lower than a heterosexual one.[4] A survey of practicing physicians found that 30% would oppose medical school admission for lesbians and gay men, and many felt those that were admitted should limit their practice to fields such as pathology and radiology.[5] Homophobia also has been noted commonly among nurses. A survey of female physicians found that lesbian physicians experienced four times more sexual orientation–based harassment than did heterosexual physicians.[6]

Given the degree of homophobia in the medical establishment and society at large, it is no surprise that lesbians and gay men feel vulnerable when seeking health care, and often fear disclosing or discussing their sexuality. However, disclosure rates are not only low because of patient reluctance; studies have found that even patients who wished to discuss their sexuality with their doctors did not feel comfortable or were not given an opportunity to do so. As a consequence, many opportunities are missed to test, treat, educate, and advocate about health and social problems.

SEXUAL MINORITIES AMONG RACIAL AND ETHNIC MINORITIES

Lesbian and gay racial and ethnic minorities are at risk for particularly high rates of stigmatization and discrimination. Consequently, health care providers need to be alert to the additive effects of racism, sexism, and homophobia. In addition, they should be aware that rates of disclosure of homosexual orientation to both families and health care providers, already low among gay people in general, may be even lower among minorities.

This social stigma poses threats to their own health and well-being, as well as to that of their communities. For example, the practice of being on the "down low," a term used to describe African-American men who are in relationships with women but secretly have sex with men, is directly related to the taboos against homosexuality in African-American culture, and has been responsible for numerous human immunodeficiency virus (HIV) infections among heterosexual African-American women. The social discrimination that Latino gay men experience results in poorer mental health and greater HIV risk behaviors.[7] There have been similar findings with respect to gay Asian men, for whom the degree of family and social support is associated with the likelihood of engaging in unprotected sex.[8] A study of American Indian and Alaska Native gay adolescents has suggested very high rates of abuse history and suicidality.[9] Minority lesbians also may be at higher risk for some additional health risk factors, such as obesity.[10]

OTHER ISSUES FOR LESBIANS AND GAY MEN

Adolescents

Adolescence is an especially vulnerable period, and stigmatization, confusion, and fear make it particularly so for lesbian and gay youth. Health care providers for adolescents are well positioned to provide important support, education, preventive counseling, and intervention. However, more often than not this opportunity is missed,[11] despite findings from numerous studies demonstrating lesbian and gay adolescents have a higher prevalence of mental health problems than their heterosexual peers, become sexually active at a younger age, have more sexual partners, and use more drugs and alcohol than heterosexual teenagers.[12,13] Gay youth are also at higher risk for suicidal thoughts and attempts and are more often the victims of verbal or physical assault related to their sexual orientation.[14]

Parenting

It is unknown how many lesbian and gay parents there are in the United States, or how many children have lesbian or gay parents. One researcher's broad estimate was between 1 and 9 million US children have at least one lesbian or gay parent.[15] Although many children living with gay parents were conceived during heterosexual relationships, increasingly large numbers of lesbians and gays are parenting as singles or as same-sex couples, via methods including donor insemination, surrogacy, adoption (domestic and international), foster parenting, and coparenting with other lesbians or gay men. Historically, the US legal system has been hostile to lesbian and gay parents. Recently legislation in some states has eased some restrictions, but nowhere can the nonbiological parent in a lesbian or gay couple assume the same rights as would a married heterosexual partner upon the birth of their child.

Legal discrimination against lesbian and gay parents has been based on prejudice, not data. Years of research have shown that there are no systematic differences between lesbians and gay men and heterosexual parents in emotional health or parenting skills or attitudes, and there is no evidence to support claims that children of lesbian or gay parents are in any way disadvantaged. No differences have been found in the gender identity or sexual orientation of children raised in lesbian or gay households. The psychological health and development of children of gay parents appears to be influenced by the same factors that are important to the children of heterosexual parents. Although the potential effects of stigmatization, such as teasing or abuse by peers, should be addressed with children of gay parents, health care providers, gay parents, and their children can all be assured there is no evidence for lasting psychological injury based on the homosexual orientation of a parent.[15]

Aging

The health concerns for lesbians and gay men carry into older age, and are similar to those facing the general population. Medical providers for elderly lesbians and gay men should remain alert for smoking, alcohol, and mental health–related problems, as well as an increased prevalence of cancer risk factors and lower screening rates.[16] Older gay men may experience additional stigmatization by the gay community, in which high value is placed on youth and beauty. Invisibility and isolation may be of particular concern. A number of groups are now addressing issues such as housing, health care, and long-term care, as well as support services on a local level (Gay and Lesbian Association of Retiring Persons, Lesbian and Gay Aging Issues Network, Gay and Lesbian Outreach to Elders, Old Lesbians Organizing for Change, and others). In 2002 Senior Action in a Gay Environment (SAGE) successfully advocated for the Joint Commission on the Accreditation of Healthcare Organizations (JCAHO) to add sexual orientation nondiscrimination language to accreditation requirements for US nursing homes and assisted living facilities.

Common Pitfalls in the Care of Lesbian and Gay Patients

- Heterosexuality is assumed by health care providers.
- Sexual behaviors or identity are not commonly addressed.
- Risk is assessed based on sexual orientation, not behavior.
- Substance use or mental illness is undetected.
- The importance of the relationship between sexuality and community is not appreciated.
- Same-sex partners or nontraditional family members are not included in decision making.
- It is assumed that these patients are not having or planning for children.
- Confidentiality is not addressed.

MEDICAL AND PSYCHIATRIC ISSUES

The prevalence and pattern of particular diseases and risk factors are associated with differing sexual orientations. This is true for some cancers, risk factors for cardiovascular disease, sexually transmitted infections, and some mental health and substance abuse problems.

BREAST AND OVARIAN CANCER IN LESBIANS

As in other women, there is a great deal of anxiety among lesbians about breast cancer, and many fear it is even more prevalent among homosexual than heterosexual women. Researchers have predicted an increased rate on the based on a higher prevalence of proven risk factors compared with heterosexual women in general, such as later childbearing, nulliparity, less oral contraceptive use, obesity, and possibly greater alcohol consumption. In one study, the calculated lifetime risk for lesbians was 11.1%, compared with 10.4% for their heterosexual sisters.[17] This difference was statistically significant, but the difference was smaller than might be expected based on the accumulation of known risk factors alone. The actual rate of breast cancer among lesbians is unknown because there has been no population-based study large enough make an accurate estimate.

Similarly, some of the known ovarian cancer risk factors, such as low parity, obesity, and relatively fewer years of oral contraceptive use, are more common among lesbians than heterosexual women.[18] This raises concern that ovarian cancer risk may be elevated for lesbians; but again, the incidence and prevalence have not been studied adequately.

ANAL CANCER IN GAY MEN

Gay men are increasingly aware of the risk for and development of anal cancer. Published studies cite a relative risk of 33.1 for anal cancer among men with a history of receptive anal intercourse.[19,20] This excess risk was not explained by HIV infection alone.[20] The risk factors for anal cancer are multiple sexual partners, human Papilloma virus (HPV) infection, squamous intraepithelial lesions, smoking, and immunodeficiency. HPV infection and associated intraepithelial lesions in MSM are extremely common. HPV infection rates are 93% in HIV-positive gay men, and 61% in HIV-negative gay men. Anal squamous epithelial lesions are found in 36% of HIV-positive and 7% of HIV-negative MSM.[21] Many experts now advocate for regular anal cancer screening for both HIV-positive and -negative MSM.

Additionally, it remains unknown if other types of cancer are more prevalent among lesbians and gay men. Tobacco use, alcohol consumption, and obesity rates are concerning, and may predispose lesbians and gay men to higher rates of lung and colorectal cancer.

CARDIOVASCULAR DISEASE RISKS

One consequence of higher smoking rates among lesbians and gay men may be an elevated risk for cardiovascular disease. The same is true for use of anabolic steroids, cocaine, and methamphetamines. Lesbians have been found to have a higher body mass index and higher waist to hip ratio than the general population of women.[22,23] Men in general are at higher risk for heart disease at a younger age than women. HIV-positive people may be at increased risk for cardiac events because of HIV alone, and nearly all HIV medications have been associated with metabolic effects that may result in significantly increased rates of cardiovascular disease.

SEXUALLY TRANSMITTED INFECTIONS AND SEXUAL RISK FACTORS

Rachel has not had a Pap smear in years. She is not sure that she really needs one, but, again fears she will not be able to have a frank discussion with her health care provider. She is also not sure or if there are "other things" she should discuss with or be tested for by her doctor.

Lesbians and Sexually Transmitted Infections

A broad misconception is that women who identify as lesbian are at very low risk for sexually transmitted infections because they have not been sexually active with men. Research findings indicate that most lesbians have had sex with men at some point during their lives (77% to 93%), and many during the prior 3 years (6% to 29%).[24-26]

Of note, recent sexual contact with men is more likely among younger women, and sexual contact with gay or bisexual men or injection drug users may be more common among WSW than heterosexual women.[25] Clearly, the risk of heterosexually transmitted sexually transmitted infections is significant. Additionally, there is evidence that transmission can occur between women, via mucosal contact or shared cervicovaginal secretions from orogenital or digital contact, or with sex toys. This female-to-female transmission has been demonstrated for herpes simplex virus, HPV, trichomonas, and bacterial vaginosis. Gonorrhea and Chlamydia infections occur less frequently in WSW than heterosexual women, but are detected among those who have had sexual contact with male partners. There have been at least four case reports of female-to-female orogenital transmission of HIV.[27]

Gay Men and Sexually Transmitted Infections

It is well known that gay men have a high risk for sexually transmitted infection when they practice unprotected sex. Sexually transmitted infection rates fell significantly among gay men in the United States following the identification of HIV as a sexually transmitted infection in the 1980s. However, since the late 1990s a resurgence of syphilis and gonorrhea infections among MSM has occurred, particularly in urban areas and among younger men and men of color. In 2002, MSM accounted for 93% of the primary and secondary syphilis cases in San Francisco, and 81% in Los Angeles.[28] Similar rates have been found in other US and European cities.

The increasing rates of sexually transmitted infections are attributable to an increasing frequency of unprotected sex among MSM, and there has been a less dramatic but definite accompanying increase in new HIV infections. Internet chat rooms are a common starting point for men specifically seeking unprotected anal intercourse ("barebacking").[29] Gay men who meet sex partners through the Internet are more likely to have anonymous sex, unprotected sex, sex with HIV-positive men or men of unknown HIV status, and to combine sex with drug use.[30] For one cluster of seven syphilis patients in San Francisco in 1999, an outbreak investigation found that 67% met online.[31]

Recreational drug use is also common among MSM, and has been associated with high rates of unprotected intercourse. A study of circuit parties (organized events where a large group of MSM gather to socialize and dance, often over a 2- to 3-day weekend) in San Francisco found nearly all participants used one or more drugs and 28% reported having unprotected anal sex over a 3-day period.[32] Use of methamphetamine (also called, speed, crystal meth, crystal or Tina), gamma hydroxybutyrate (GHB), "ecstasy," or other "party drugs" is associated with high numbers of sexual partners and higher rates of unprotected sex. Viagra is commonly used with other illicit drugs, and is associated with a greater number of recent sex partners and higher rates of unprotected anal intercourse.[33]

SUBSTANCE USE AND ABUSE

The literature on tobacco, alcohol, and substance use by lesbians and gay men is methodologically limited and often contradictory. However, the evidence that exists does suggest that, with the exception of alcohol use by gay men, levels of substance use, including cigarette smoking, are higher among lesbians and gay men than the general population.[13,34]

Recent population-based studies of alcohol use generally have found considerably lower rates of heavy drinking than earlier estimates. However, heavier alcohol consumption among lesbians is a consistent finding across studies, as is the finding that a greater proportion of lesbians report being in recovery or having undergone treatment for alcohol-related problems.[35] The difference between lesbian/bisexual and heterosexual women was more pronounced among younger women.

Recent studies comparing MSM and exclusively heterosexual men have found equivalent alcohol use patterns.[36,37] However, there is clearly a strong correlation between alcohol misuse and unprotected sex among MSM.

The most recent population study of drug use among lesbian and gay men, done in 1996, found higher levels of lifetime drug use among lesbians and gays across all classes of drugs. However, rates of "recent" drug use were more similar to heterosexual rates. Relative to heterosexuals, MSM were heavier users of marijuana, cocaine, and heroin in the month prior to the interview. WSW used more marijuana and analgesics, and showed a trend toward more cocaine use. Drug use patterns have changed significantly since 1996. For example, methamphetamine use has become relatively common among gay men, and is associated with high rates of risky sexual behavior.[38]

MENTAL HEALTH IN THE LESBIAN AND GAY COMMUNITY

Mental health issues for lesbians and gay men are also understudied. Higher rates of mental illness, psychological distress, and suicidal behavior have been consistently reported for lesbians gay and bisexual youth (see Adolescents), but it is unclear whether this pattern continues into adulthood. Despite methodologic limitations in the research, there appears to be a trend toward higher rates of psychological distress and mental health diagnoses among lesbians and gay men.[39] Mood (particularly depression), anxiety, and substance use disorders appear to be the most prevalent. The little data that exist on intimate partner violence in same-sex couples

(both lesbians and gay men) suggests that the prevalence and general types of violence are similar to heterosexuals,[40] although the specific expression of abusive behavior may differ.[41]

RECOMMENDATIONS FOR IMPROVING CARE

COMMUNICATION AND HISTORY TAKING

An accurate sexual history is essential, and optimizes the quality of care provided. An explanation of health risks associated with sexual activity may be helpful. Sexual history taking should focus both on self-identified sexual orientation and sexual behaviors, recognizing that there is a great deal of fluidity in sexual expression, and behavior and identity may not match. Additionally, it is important to ask your patient who in his or her family or community is aware of the patient's sexuality. Ask about, and facilitate, legal safeguards such as advanced directives and wills, that will ensure visitation rights and decision-making authority for a same-sex partner should this become necessary. Providers also should inquire about parenting plans for all patients of childbearing or child-rearing age.

PREVENTIVE HEALTH CARE

Routine Advice

Advice about regular cardiovascular physical activity is identical to that recommended for men and women in the general population, as well as age-appropriate cholesterol and diabetes screening.

Cancer Screening and Prevention

Preventive screening tests for the early diagnosis of cancer are underutilized by lesbians and gay men. Both lesbian patients and their medical providers may underestimate the need for regular gynecologic care. This combined with barriers to care results in lower rates of Pap smear testing among lesbians than heterosexual women.[42] Recommendations for preventive gynecologic care for lesbians and heterosexual women do not differ: annual Pap smears that are normal for a minimum of 3 years, followed by a longer interval (every 2 to 3 years) for those without a history of an abnormal Pap smear, an immunocompromising condition, or who are either sexually abstinent or monogamous.

Most studies reveal similar mammography rates between lesbians and heterosexual women,[43] although clinical breast examination rates may be lower among lesbians.[3] Breast cancer screening should be pursued aggressively, with annual examinations by an experienced clinician and mammography screening in keeping with the greater prevalence of risk factors.

> **Box 27-1.** Anal Pap Smear Technique
>
> Anal Pap smear collection is quite simple. A Dacron swab is moistened with water or saline and inserted 1" to 1.5" into the anal canal. It is then rotated firmly as the swab is very slowly pulled out in a tight spiral motion. The transitional zone is located approximately 1 inch (2 cm) from the anal verge. In order to get an adequate specimen it is necessary to obtain both rectal columnar cells and anal squamous cells; therefore, the swab needs to go inside further than the transitional zone. The whole sampling process should last 15 to 20 seconds.
>
> The swab is then processed identically to a cervical Pap smear, according to the requirements of your laboratory. It can be either smeared on a slide and fixed, or shaken into Thin Prep fixative. The Thin Prep method has a somewhat lower rate of air drying and artifact from debris.

Although there are currently no evidence-based recommendations for ovarian cancer screening in the general female population, lesbians may be at elevated risk. Lesbians and gay men should undergo regular screening for colorectal cancer beginning at age 50.

Anal Pap smears are an effective screening tool for precancerous and cancerous anal lesions.[44] They are easy to do (Box 27-1) and typically can be read by any cytology laboratory experienced in the reading of cervical Pap smears. Many experts are now recommending routine anal Pap screening in men who have a history of receptive anal intercourse, and particularly in HIV-infected men.[45-48] The recommended frequency for screening is currently under study, although some suggest two baseline anal Pap smears 6 months apart, to be repeated annually in HIV-positive men and every 3 years in HIV-negative men. Any patients with abnormal results should be referred to an anorectal specialist for further evaluation by high resolution anoscopy and biopsy.

Infectious Disease Prevention

Immunization of gay men deserves particular mention, as rates of hepatitis A, B, and C are all higher in MSM than in the general population.[49] The Centers for Disease Control and Prevention (CDC) recommends routine hepatitis A and B immunization for all MSM. Up to 20% of MSM have evidence of exposure to hepatitis B, but the opportunity to immunize is missed too often, and immunization rates remain low.[50] Increasing vaccination rates will require identification of MSM whenever they contact the health care system, and providing free or affordable vaccine services. Lesbians and gay men should receive tetanus boosters, flu shots, and pneumococcal vaccines and specific travel-related vaccinations according to recommendations for all adults.

CREATING A CULTURALLY COMPETENT HEALTH CARE ENVIRONMENT

A Defined Set of Values and Principles

Heterosexism is prejudice or discrimination against homosexuals based on the assumption that heterosexuality is the norm. Too frequently, often inadvertently, this assumption is made in the medical encounter. The effect is to silence patients, reinforcing their sense of invisibility and devaluation, and impairing the ability of both patient and provider to communicate effectively. A nonjudgmental attitude and willingness to ask questions and clarify relationships are important.

Health care providers can address the fear and stigma that are major barriers to accessing and receiving high-quality care by creating an environment that connotes acceptance, open-mindedness, and competence. Physical environment, medical forms, attitudes of staff and clinicians, and tone of interview all play a role in creating a comfortable and safe milieu (see Core Competency). It is helpful to ask about the nature of the relationship between a patient and a person of the same gender who accompanies him or her to an appointment. Allow partners to remain in the room, and include them in discussions if your patient desires.

Adapting forms and verbal questioning to use gender neutral words such as "partner," "significant other," or "relationship," shows that assumptions have not been made (see Core Competency). Questions for lesbian, gay, bisexual, and transgender (LGBT)–sensitive topics can be incorporated into standard intake forms about other health-related behaviors.

An assurance of confidentiality can be very important, especially to adolescents.[11] Although adolescents tend to fear unauthorized disclosure to their parents most of all, many adults fear disclosure to their community or employer. Awareness of the prevalence and power of this fear are important when addressing sexuality.

Patient Information and Education

Many medical settings have a patient information and education section connected to the waiting room, where leaflets, brochures, and referral information regarding lesbian and gay concerns can be displayed. Posters or pictures of gay couples make a strong statement. A nondiscrimination statement that includes sexual and gender identity should be prominently displayed on waiting or examination room walls. HIV/AIDS prevention or referral information is valuable in most settings, and particularly implies concern for MSM. Advertising clinic services in lesbian and gay media outlets is one way of reaching out to this patient base.

Ongoing Training of Medical Providers

An important component of promoting cultural competence and improving care for lesbian and gay patients is training medical providers. However, this is rarely done. One study that surveyed directors of family medicine departments found a mean of 2.5 hours over 4 years devoted to teaching about homosexuality or bisexuality, and 50.6% reported zero hours of such teaching.[51] Development and incorporation of curricula on lesbian and gay health into medical provider training programs is necessary to promote culturally competent care. Office staff should be trained in sensitivity to lesbian and gay patients. Openly lesbian or gay staff and providers can go a long way toward putting patients at ease.

CONCLUSION

Failure to identify lesbian and gay patients and lack of knowledge about their relevant medical and psychosocial issues seriously hinders the provision of good care. A thoughtful, informed, and nonjudgmental approach to the care of lesbian and gay patients can demonstrably improve patient care and bring both patient and provider satisfaction.

KEY CONCEPTS

- Bias against lesbians and gay men in medical settings reduces access to and quality of care. Medical providers can play a role in countering this effect.
- The risk factors for and prevalence of certain medical problems differs among lesbians and gay men than among the general population. If sexual behaviors and orientation are not identified, it is not possible to target screening and intervention.
- An understanding of the relationship between lesbian and gay patients and their families and communities is important to understand the sources of stress and support they interact with in their lives.
- Care must be taken to ensure that the environment and language of the medical encounter promote comfort and project acceptance of lesbians and gay men.

CORE COMPETENCY
Creating a Welcoming Environment for Lesbian, Gay, and Bisexual Clients

Suggestions for Creating a Welcoming Physical Environment and Conveying Acceptance of LGBT Patients

- Provide lesbian and gay informational, educational, and referral materials in waiting rooms or examination rooms.
- Display pictures or posters with lesbian or gay themes, couples, or families on the walls.
- Provide HIV/AIDS prevention and treatment information or referrals. Distribute free condoms.
- Post a nondiscrimination statement that includes gender identity and sexual orientation in a prominent place in the clinic or office.
- Train staff to be sensitive to LGB clients, and hire LGB staff members.
- Advertise in LGB media sources.
- Alter history forms and oral history taking to improve knowledge of patient sexuality and signal interest and a nonjudgmental attitude (see Sample Questions).

Sample Questions to Adapt to LGB-Sensitive History Taking or Intake Forms
Sexual Activity

- Are you sexually active?
- Are you sexually active with men, women, or both?
- Have you ever had sex with a man (woman)?
- How many sexual partners have you had in the past year?
- How many sexual partners have you had in your lifetime?

Safe Sex, Sexually Transmitted Infections, and Human Immunodeficiency Risks

- Do you use any safe sex methods?
- Do you have any questions about safe sex? With men, women, both?
- Have you ever had an STI? Which one(s)? When?
- Have you ever injected drugs, or had sex with someone you know has injected drugs?
- Have you ever had an HIV test? When? What was the result?

Sexual Identity and Relationships

- How do you identify your sexuality (circle all that apply): lesbian, gay, bisexual, transgender, heterosexual, celibate, not sure/don't know?
- Are you currently in a relationship?
- Are you: single, significantly involved, domestic partner, married, separated, divorced?
- If you are lesbian, gay, bisexual, or transgender are you "out" to: friends (all? some?), family (all? some?), work, all of the above, none of the above?

CORE COMPETENCY, CONTINUED

Living Situation, Family, and Children

- Do you live alone or with others? With whom?
- Do you have children?
- Are you interested in having children?

DISCUSSION QUESTIONS

1. What types of challenges might a lesbian or gay man face when seeking health care? What is your role in addressing these challenges?
2. Why is it often hard to discuss sexual orientation and sexual behavior in a medical visit? Discuss ways you might frame and discuss this issue with patients.
3. How might systemic barriers to accessing and receiving good care be reduced for lesbians and gay men? In your own practice, what specific measures can you take to promote comfort and open communication?

RESOURCES

http://www.amsa.org/adv/lgbtpm/
American Medical Student Association: Lesbian, Gay, Bisexual, and Transgender People in Medicine.

http://www.baphr.org
Bay Area Physicians for Human Rights. National association of gay and lesbian physicians.

http://www.glma.org/
Gay and Lesbian Medical Association home page. Information and educational materials. Links to news, publications, public policy, health care referrals, the Healthy People 2010 Companion Document for LGBT Health, and an extensive bibliography of literature on LGBT health.

http://www.lgbthealth.net/
The National Coalition for LGBT Health. Policy, education, advocacy, research.

REFERENCES

1. Laumann O, Gagnon JH, Michael RT, et al. *The social organization of sexuality: Sexual practices in the United States.* Chicago: University of Chicago Press, 1994.
2. Diamond M. Homosexuality and bisexuality in different populations. *Arch Sex Behav* 1993;22:291–310.
3. Solarz A, ed. *Lesbian health: Current assessment and directions for the future.* Washington, DC: National Academy Press, 1999.
4. Diamant AL, et al. Health behaviors, health status, and access to and use of health care: A population-based study of lesbian, bisexual, and heterosexual women. *Arch Fam Med* 2000;9(10):1043–1051.
5. Oriel KA, et al. Gay and lesbian physicians in training: Family practice program directors' attitudes and students' perceptions of bias. *Fam Med* 1996;28:720–725.
6. Mathews WC, et al. Physicians' attitudes toward homosexuality: Survey of a California County Medical Society. *West J Med* 1986;144:106–110.
7. Brogan DJ, et al. Harassment of lesbians as medical students and physicians. *JAMA* 1999;282:1290,1292.
8. Diaz RM, et al. Sexual risk as an outcome of social oppression: Data from a probability sample of Latino gay men in three U.S. cities. *Cultur Divers Ethnic Minor Psychol* 200410(3):255–267.
9. Wilson PA, Yoshikawa H. Experiences of and responses to social discrimination among Asian and Pacific Islander gay men: Their relationship to HIV risk. *AIDS Educ Prev* 2004;16:68–83.
10. Barney DD. Health risk-factors for gay American Indian and Alaska Native adolescent males. *J Homosex* 2003;46:137–157.
11. Mays VM, et al. Heterogeneity of health disparities among African American, Hispanic, and Asian American women: Unrecognized influences of sexual orientation. *Am J Public Health* 2002;92:632–639.
12. Allen LB, et al. Adolescent health care experience of gay, lesbian, and bisexual young adults. *J Adolesc Health* 1998;23:212–220.
13. Garofalo R, et al. The association between health risk behaviors and sexual orientation among a school-based sample of adolescents. *Pediatrics* 1998;101:895–902.
14. Ryan H, et al. Smoking among lesbians, gays, and bisexuals: A review of the literature. *Am J Prev Med* 2001;21:142–149.
15. Russell ST, et al. Same-sex romantic attraction and experiences of violence in adolescence. *Am J Public Health* 2001;91:903–906.
16. Perrin EC. Technical report: Coparent or second-parent adoption by same-sex parents. *Pediatrics* 2002;109:341–344.
17. Valanis BG, et al. Sexual orientation and health: comparisons in the women's health initiative sample. *Arch Fam Med* 2000;9:843–853.
18. Dibble SL, et al. Comparing breast cancer risk between lesbians and their heterosexual sisters. *Womens Health Issues* 2004;14:60–68.
19. Dibble SL, et al. Risk factors for ovarian cancer: Lesbian and heterosexual women. *Oncol Nurs Forum* 2002;29(1):E1–7.
20. Daling JR, et al. Sexual practices, sexually transmitted diseases, and the incidence of anal cancer. *N Eng J Med* 1987;317(16):973–977.
21. Koblin BA, et al. Increased incidence of cancer among homosexual men, New York City and San Francisco, 1978–1990. *Am J Epidemiol* 1996;144:916–923.
22. Palefsky JM, et al. Anal squamous intraepithelial lesions in HIV-positive and HIV–negative homosexual and bisexual men: Prevalence and risk factors. *J Acquir Immune Defic Syndr Hum Retrovirol* 1998 ;17:320–326.
23. Roberts SA, et al. Cardiovascular disease risk in lesbian women. *Womens Health Issues* 2003;13:167–174.

24. Aaron DJ, et al. Behavioral risk factors for disease and preventive health practices among lesbians. *Am J Public Health* 2001;91:972–975.

25. Diamant AL, et al. Lesbians' sexual history with men: Implications for taking a sexual history. *Arch Intern Med* 1999;159:2730–2736.

26. Fethers K, et al. Sexually transmitted infections and risk behaviours in women who have sex with women. *Sex Transm Infect* 2000;76:345–349.

27. Bailey JV, et al. Sexual behaviour of lesbians and bisexual women. *Sex Transm Infect* 2003;79:147–150.

28. Rothenberg RB, et al. Oral transmission of HIV. *AIDS* 1998;12:2095–2105.

29. Centers for Disease Control and Prevention. Trends in primary and secondary syphilis and HIV infections in men who have sex with men—San Francisco and Los Angeles, California, 1998–2002. *MMWR Morb Mortal Wkly Rep* 2004; 53:575–578.

30. Halkitis PN, Parsons JT. Intentional unsafe sex (barebacking) among HIV-positive gay men who seek sexual partners on the Internet. *AIDS Care* 2003;15:367–378.

31. Kim AA, et al. Cruising on the Internet highway. *J Acquir Immune Defic Syndr* 2001;28:89–93.

32. Klausner JD, et al. Tracing a syphilis outbreak through cyberspace. *JAMA* 2000;284:447–449.

33. Mansergh G, et al. The Circuit Party Men's Health Survey: Findings and implications for gay and bisexual men. *Am J Public Health* 2001;91:953–958.

34. Kim AA, et al. Increased risk of HIV and sexually transmitted disease transmission among gay or bisexual men who use Viagra, San Francisco 2000–2001. *AIDS* 2002;16: 1425–1428.

35. Tang H, et al. Cigarette smoking among lesbians, gays, and bisexuals: How serious a problem? (United States). *Cancer Causes Control* 2004;15:797–803.

36. Burgard SA, et al. Alcohol and tobacco use patterns among heterosexually and homosexually experienced California women. *Drug Alcohol Depend* 2005;77(1):61–70.

37. Cochran SD, Keenan C, et al. Estimates of alcohol use and clinical treatment needs among homosexually active men and women in the U.S. population. *J Consult Clin Psychol* 2000;68(6):1062–1071.

38. Stall R, et al. Alcohol use, drug use and alcohol–related problems among men who have sex with men: The Urban Men's Health Study. *Addiction* 2001;96: 1589–1601.

39. Halkitis PN, et al. Longitudinal investigation of methamphetamine use among gay and bisexual men in New York City: Findings from Project Bumps. *J Urban Health* 2005;82 (1 Suppl 1):il8–25.

40. Meyer IH. Prejudice, social stress, and mental health in lesbian, gay, and bisexual populations: Conceptual issues and research evidence. *Psychol Bull* 2003;129:674–697.

41. McClennen JC. Domestic violence between same-gender partners: Recent findings and future research. *J Interpers Violence* 2005;20:149–154.

42. National Coalition of Anti-Violence Programs. *Lesbian, gay, bisexual, and transgender domestic violence in 2001.* New York: New York City Gay and Lesbian Anti-Violence Project, 2002.

43. Matthews AK, et al. Correlates of underutilization of gynecological cancer screening among lesbian and heterosexual women. *Prev Med* 2004;38:105–113.

44. Cochran SD, et al. Cancer-related risk indicators and preventive screening behaviors among lesbians and bisexual women. *Am J Public Health* 2001;91(4):591–597.

45. Arain S, et al. The anal Pap smear: Cytomorphology of squamous intraepithelial lesions. *Cytojournal* 2005;2:4.

46. Goldie SJ, et al. Cost-effectiveness of screening for anal squamous intraepithelial lesions and anal cancer in human immunodeficiency virus-negative homosexual and bisexual men. *Am J Med* 2000;108:634–641.

47. Mathews WC. Screening for anal dysplasia associated with human Papillomavirus. *Top HIV Med* 2003;11(2):45–49.

48. Goldie S, et al. Anal cancer in HIV infection: To screen or not to screen? *AIDS Clin Care* 2004;16:53–5, 57.

49. Panther LA, et al. Spectrum of human Papillomavirus–related dysplasia and carcinoma of the anus in HIV-infected patients. AIDS Read 2005;15:79–82, 85–6, 88, 91.

50. GLMA. *Healthy People 2010 Companion Document for Lesbian, Gay, Bisexual, Transgender (LGBT) Health.* San Francisco: Gay and Lesbian Medical Association, 2001.

51. CDC (1996). Undervaccination for hepatitis B among young men who have sex with men: San Francisco and Berkeley, California, 1992–1993. *MMWR Morb Mortal Wkly Rep* 1996; 45:215–217.

52. Tesar CM, Rovi SL. Survey of curriculum on homosexuality/bisexuality in departments of family medicine. *Fam Med* 1998;30:283–287.

Chapter 28

The Medical Treatment of Patients with Psychiatric Illness

Douglas R. Price-Hanson, MD

Objectives

- Review strategies to promote screening for mental illness in general medical populations.
- Describe ways that clinicians can diagnose medical disease in patients with psychiatric disorders.
- Review principles of psychiatric risk assessment (suicidality, homicidality).
- Discuss establishing therapeutic relationships with "difficult to treat" psychiatric patients.
- Review principles for the care of psychiatric illness in the medical setting.

Delivering clinical care to patients with coexisting mental and medical illness frequently defies conventional approaches. Those with mental illness are more likely to be medically ill than the general population, have these illnesses remain undiagnosed and untreated, and die prematurely.[1] In addition, estimates suggest that approximately 25% of the adult primary care population has a psychiatric disorder, and that half of these remain undiagnosed.[2] Considering that general medical physicians provide mental health treatment to more patients than do mental health providers, clinical expertise in the recognition and treatment of both types of disease is essential.[3]

Coexisting medical and psychiatric illnesses confuse and complicate diagnosis and treatment of many patients. In schizophrenics, unmanageable emotions and paranoid thoughts may limit the ability to form strong therapeutic alliances. Patients with unexplained somatic symptoms may harbor underlying psychiatric illness yet resist inquiry into these areas. With others, especially those with various personality disorders, unproductive arguments may leave little time for medical concerns. Medical providers may not feel competent to address these and other psychiatric issues, especially those regarding suicidality and homocidality.

This chapter presents three case examples that highlight common scenarios in which psychiatric illness complicates effective medical care and for which guidance is not easily located in standard textbooks. Practical approaches are outlined for patients in whom comprehensive care is particularly difficult—schizophrenics, those with medically unexplained symptoms, and patients with borderline personality disorder—and for the problems of suicidality and risk of violence.

Common Pitfalls in Treating Those with Comorbid Illness

- Allowing psychiatric disorders to remain undiagnosed
- Proposing complicated treatment plans before establishing rapport and enlisting patient participation
- Allowing psychiatric issues to obscure the focus on medical problems

- Pursuing somatic symptoms without considering psychiatric etiologies
- Lack of experience and knowledge of psychiatric diagnosis and treatment
- Failing to monitor for medical side-effects of psychiatric medication

SCREENING FOR MENTAL ILLNESS

A number of screening tools exist to help medical providers diagnose psychiatric illness. They typically consist of a brief screening questionnaire of high sensitivity but low specificity to minimize the time of administration yet avoid missed diagnoses. The commonly used PRIME-MD[4] or streamlined version of the PRIME-MD, the Patient Health Questionnaire[2] can be administered in 8 minutes or less (Fig. 28-1). For those who screen positive, the diagnostic algorithms contained in the primary care version of the Diagnostic and Statistical Manual of Mental Disorders provide one a practical option for pursuing a specific psychiatric diagnosis.[45]

SCHIZOPHRENIA

Mr. Rutter is a 27-year-old man with schizophrenia. He has hypertension, hyperlipidemia, smokes, and is overweight. It is difficult to develop rapport with him as he is guarded and has an odd affect. He declines antipsychotic medication. He reveals he hears voices telling him to kill "aliens" who monitor him and plan him harm.

MEDICAL ILLNESS AND SCHIZOPHRENIA

People with schizophrenia are more likely to die prematurely than the general population.[5] The bulk of this mortality difference results from suicide, a potentially preventable cause of death. The remainder results from an increase in the disease-specific mortality of the same medical illnesses that cause death in the general population, headed by cardiovascular disease.[3,4] Hence, addressing modifiable risk factors for medical illness should remain a focus of ongoing care.

There is an increased prevalence of the metabolic syndrome and type 2 diabetes[9] in people with schizophrenia, as compared with the general population. In fact, schizophrenia itself is an independent risk factor for insulin resistance and diabetes.[9,11] A consensus of medical and psychiatric associations suggests that all patients with schizophrenia should be considered at high risk for diabetes and screened accordingly.[52] Other modifiable risk factors for diabetes and cardiovascular disease more common in schizophrenics include poor diet,[11] lack of exercise,[11] obesity,[12] cigarette smoking,[13] lipid abnormalities,[8,14] and hypertension.[15] All patients with schizophrenia should receive counseling on reducing these risks.[6]

Other medical conditions that are more prevalent in schizophrenics include irritable bowel syndrome, osteoporosis, polydipsia with hyponatremia, poor pregnancy outcomes, substance abuse disorders, gingival and dental disease, hepatitis B and C, and human immunodeficiency virus (HIV) and acquired immunodeficiency disease (AIDS).[5,16-19] A diagnosis of schizophrenia in itself should not preclude treatment of HIV, because adherence to antiretroviral therapy is comparable to that seen in HIV patients without schizophrenia.[20]

ASSESSING THE RISK OF VIOLENCE

Subgroups of schizophrenics are also more prone to violence than members of the general population.[21] Identifying the specific clinical variables that contribute to this risk has been elusive. Several landmark studies have found violent behavior to be driven primarily by delusions and not by isolated hallucinations.[22-24] However, these are retrospective studies and rely on self-report to identify the presence of delusions. More recent prospective data have cast doubt on the link between delusions and violent behavior, finding no such association.[25,26] Other well-designed studies have established specific personality characteristics as risk factors for violence (Box 28-1).[27]

To make clinical sense of the currently available data, violence risk may be conceptualized as a dynamic state in

---

Box 28-1. Risk Factors for Violence in Schizophrenics

- Inability to control impulses
- Difficulty controlling emotions
- Difficulty managing threats to self-esteem
- Paranoid personality style

- History of violence
- Environmental factors—substance use, lack of medication, stressful life events, lapse in therapy

Brief Patient Health Questionnaire

This questionnaire is an important part of providing you with the best health care possible. Your answers will help in understanding problems that you may have.

Name_____ Age_____ Sex: ☐ Female   ☐ Male   Today's date_____

1. Over the last 2 weeks, how often have you been bothered by any of the following problems?

	Not at all	Several days	More than half the days	Nearly every day
a. Little interest or pleasure in doing things.............................	☐	☐	☐	☐
b. Feeling down, depressed, or hopeless.................................	☐	☐	☐	☐
c. Trouble falling or staying asleep, or sleeping too much...........	☐	☐	☐	☐
d. Feeling tired or having little energy....................................	☐	☐	☐	☐
e. Poor appetite or overeating...	☐	☐	☐	☐
f. Feeling bad about yourself—or that you are a failure or have let yourself or your family down...	☐	☐	☐	☐
g. Trouble concentrating on things, such as reading the newspaper or watching television..	☐	☐	☐	☐
h. Moving or speaking so slowly that other people could have noticed? Or the opposite—being so fidgety or restless that you have been moving around a lot more than usual......................	☐	☐	☐	☐
i. Thoughts that you would be better off dead or of hurting yourself in some way..	☐	☐	☐	☐

2. Questions about anxiety.

	No	Yes
a. In the last 4 weeks, have you had an anxiety attack—suddenly feeling fear or panic?...	☐	☐

If you checked "No", go to question #3.

b. Has this ever happened before?..	☐	☐
c. Do some of these attacks come suddenly out of the blue—that is, in situations where you don't expect to be nervous or uncomfortable?...	☐	☐
d. Do these attacks bother you a lot or are you worried about having another attack?...	☐	☐
e. During your last bad anxiety attack, did you have symptoms like shortness of breath, sweating, your heart racing or pounding, dizziness or faintness, tingling or numbness, or nausea or upset stomach?...	☐	☐

3. If you checked off any problems on this questionnaire so far, how difficult have these problems made it for you to do your work, take care of things at home, or get along with other people?

Not difficult at all	Somewhat difficult	Very difficult	Extremely difficult
☐	☐	☐	☐

Figure 28-1. First page of primary care evaluation of mental disorders: brief patient health questionnaire. (From: Spitzer RL, Kroenke K, Williams JB. Related Validation and utility of a self-report version of PRIME-MD: The PHQ primary care study. Primary Care Evaluation of Mental Disorders. Patient Health Questionnaire. *JAMA* 1999;282:1737–1744.). Brief PHQ Copyright © 1999 Pfizer Inc. All rights reserved. Reproduced with permission.

which dysfunctional personality traits interact with environmental factors that can either increase (e.g., substance abuse) or decrease (e.g., medication) the likelihood of violent expression. When assessing Mr. Rutter's risk for violence, consideration is given to his personality traits, any history of violence, active substance abuse, the use of antipsychotic medication, and possibly the presence of delusions, rather than simply relying on his diagnosis or the report of auditory hallucinations.

When serious violence seems imminent, psychiatric consultation is required for complete evaluation. Consultation is advised because most medical providers have minimal experience safely managing these situations and case law does not provide clear guidance regarding the duties and responsibilities of clinicians outside of the mental health field. Involuntary psychiatric hospitalization may be required. The psychiatrist also must notify and protect any intended victims as dictated by the statutes of the state in which one practices. However, it is important for medical clinicians to have some knowledge of these issues when providing ongoing medical care to patients such as Mr. Rutter. Abstinence from drugs of abuse should be supported and vigilance maintained for any signs of relapse. Second-generation antipsychotics (listed in the following) show superior efficacy in reducing violent behavior as compared with conventional antipsychotics.[28] Adherence with antipsychotic medication and psychotherapy should be stressed and any interruption in treatment should arouse concern. Worsening emotional and behavioral control, threats to self-esteem, and increasing paranoia must be addressed. Because it is not practical to have a psychiatrist consult at every medical clinic visit, clinicians who are attentive to elevations in violence risk can more effectively consult with psychiatrists to provide the consultant with important background information, and have a positive impact on the well-being of the patient and others in the community (see Core Competency).

KEYS TO SUCCESSFUL MEDICAL MANAGEMENT

Psychotherapeutic Approaches

Of all the psychotic symptoms, paranoid delusions present some of the most challenging obstacles to successful medical management. It is difficult to provide care when one's intentions are perceived as suspect. Establishing a therapeutic alliance is of paramount importance.

Paranoid patients, such as Mr. Rutter, tend to be overwhelmed by their emotions and may project them onto others so as to make their inner worlds more manageable. For example, if his anger toward others becomes unbearable, it may be tolerable for him to believe that others harbor this anger toward him. By helping him with these uncomfortable emotions, a relationship begins to form.

A friendly but somewhat distant approach avoids emotional invasiveness that may cause discomfort. Sitting next to the patient, rather than face-to-face, avoids direct eye contact and symbolizes a relationship of two partners looking out at the world together. Questioning the specific content of delusions, such as Mr. Rutter's statement about aliens, generally is unproductive and may alienate the patient. Understanding the emotional themes underlying the delusions is important. However, directly inquiring about his emotions may be perceived as too invasive. Nonconfrontational statements such as, "Most people would be terrified by that," or "It's hard to figure out whom you can trust," or "I would be angry if someone invaded my privacy like that" may prove fruitful. Although there may be no real danger present, the threats are very real to the patient. To feign concern about the aliens, for example, would be deceptive and likely would be detected as contrived. To demonstrate empathy for his distress would be genuine. Identifying and acknowledging these emotions allows the patient to share his suffering and feel less isolated.

Focusing on the patient's emotional suffering is also the most effective way to introduce the subject of medication. Medications are offered to ameliorate symptoms that exacerbate the patient's distress. Mr. Rutter may agree to take medication if he feels it will offer some respite from the intensity of his worry about the surveillance or alleviate the hallucinations. If he feels understood, thinks of his provider as an ally, and benefits from medication, his paranoia may lessen to the point that he can entertain a more reality-based interpretation of his world.

Tip: With paranoid schizophrenics empathize with their emotional suffering instead of focusing on the content of the delusions.

Antipsychotic Medication

Medical providers must be familiar with the use of antipsychotic medications, be able to recognize medical side effects, and to assure that proper monitoring occurs. With this knowledge, the psychopharmacologic treatment of the stable patient with a clear diagnosis can be safely managed by medical clinicians, particularly when specialty care is unavailable or refused by the patient. Psychiatric consultation is advised for diagnostic uncertainty, those with unstable or severe illness, treatment resistance, and at initial presentation of psychotic illness.

Conventional antipsychotics have largely been replaced by the "second-generation antipsychotics": aripiprazole, clozapine, olanzapine, quetiapine, risperidone, and ziprasidone. Compared with conventional agents, the second-generation antipsychotics have shown equivalent efficacy in treating the symptoms of schizophrenia with olanzapine[20a] and clozaril[20b] possibly more efficacious. The second-generation antipsychotics also can improve affective symptoms and produce minimal, if any, extrapyramidal side-effects (dystonia, akathisia, parkinsonism, and tardive dyskinesia). However, it is concerning that the second-generation antipsychotics themselves have been found to be associated with cardiac risk factors such as obesity, insulin resistance, diabetes, and hyperlipidemia.[29] The degree of weight gain and lipid elevation seems to vary among agents, with clozapine and olanzapine associated with the largest increases, aripiprazole and ziprasidone the least, and quetiapine and risperidone with intermediate amounts.[12,29] For a patient such as Mr. Rutter, who is obese and has cardiac risk factors, this data may help guide medication choice.

The data showing an association of diabetes with the second-generation antipsychotics comes mostly from case reports and retrospective analyses,[30] with clozapine and olanzapine demonstrating the greatest risk.[31] Pending confirmatory studies, clinicians should monitor glycemic control according to guidelines recommended by expert consensus.[29,52] Additional monitoring should include evaluation of body mass index, lipid profiles, and extrapyramidal side effects. For patients with cardiac disease, a screening electrocardiogram should be performed prior to the use of agents associated with QTc interval prolongation, including thioridazine, mesoridazine, and ziprasidone. Patients should be asked about symptoms of prolactin elevation (sexual dysfunction, menstrual problems, galactorrhea), especially those treated with risperidone or a conventional antipsychotic. Pending more definitive evidence, those treated with quetiapine should have an annual slit-lamp examination for cataracts. Clinicians should be aware of case reports suggesting an association of clozapine with myocarditis.[29] If medication adherence is suboptimal, as has been found in 40% to 60% of schizophrenics,[32,33] psychiatric consultation may be helpful to consider transition to long-acting depot formulations.

MEDICALLY UNEXPLAINED SYMPTOMS

> Ms. Hunt is a 42-year-old woman with chronic abdominal pain. An extensive medical work-up has revealed no abnormalities. Multiple empiric trials of medications have been ineffective. She is often dejected and sad during clinic visits. She is unhappy with her medical care. She is applying for disability.

THE PATHOPHYSIOLOGY OF MEDICALLY UNEXPLAINED SYMPTOMS

In the majority of primary care visits patients present symptoms that have no identifiable pathologic cause.[34] Simple reassurance usually is sufficient to address these concerns. For some patients, however, it may seem nearly impossible to alleviate the suffering and functional limitation that accompany the physical symptom. In the absence of a medical disease, other factors must be considered that may be precipitating and sustaining the clinical presentation. Stressful life events, childhood and adult trauma, and psychiatric disorders are all associated with unexplained physical symptoms.[35–37]

Some people feel comfortable asking for help when emotionally distraught. For others, personal and sociocultural beliefs may cause them to feel that it is more acceptable to seek care for a medical symptom than an emotional need. Fear of rejection and abandonment or feeling powerless to cope with life's problems may lead a patient to complain of a physical symptom in order to elicit the desired concern and support.

It is unhelpful and too simplistic to classify unexplained symptoms as either completely organic or psychogenic. The sensations and functional limitations experienced by patients are likely caused by a complex interaction of physiologic and psychological processes. In patients seen by medical providers, there appears to be a spectrum of illness wherein most patients present with one or several medically unexplained symptoms and fewer fit criteria for DSM-IV somatoform disorders.[35]

DIFFERENTIAL DIAGNOSIS OF SOMATIC PRESENTATIONS

Many psychiatric disorders present with predominantly somatic symptoms. In fact, in primary care populations, depressive and anxiety disorders are more likely to present with somatic symptoms than psychological symptoms.[38]

Panic Disorder
People with panic disorder most commonly seek care for physical symptoms such as noncardiac chest pain, abdominal discomfort, palpitations, vertigo, and dizziness.[39] They tend to be high users of health care services, yet remain largely undiagnosed and are undertreated when they are correctly diagnosed.[39] Patients often refuse to accept that their symptoms may be caused by panic disorder. Often there is a concern that a serious illness remains undiagnosed while their symptoms are being dismissed as psychogenic and not "real"; or that having the disorder means that one is "panicky" and cannot handle stress. These concerns

often can be allayed by educating patients that panic attacks usually occur unexpectedly and that the cause, which may be biologic, remains unclear.

Posttraumatic Stress Disorder

As with panic disorder, those with posttraumatic stress disorder (PTSD) most commonly present to primary care clinics with somatic symptoms, but frequently remain undiagnosed.[40] Patients may not associate their symptoms with past trauma, as the initial event may have occurred years earlier. Endorsement of past trauma also may depend on the specific questions posed by the clinician. A diagnosis of PTSD should be considered in patients with unexplained dyspareunia, chronic pelvic pain, dyspnea, dizziness, gastrointestinal symptoms, chest pain, arthritis, and fibromyalgia.[40,41] When these symptoms are accompanied by symptoms of anxiety and depression or functional disability, as with Ms. Hunt, the likelihood of PTSD is even greater.[40] Clinicians should be aware that patients with PTSD may use self-harm (self-laceration, self-burning, urethral object insertion) as a means of coping with stress.

MANAGEMENT STRATEGIES

Eliciting the History

Exploration of symptoms of anxiety and depression, asking about previous trauma or abuse, and screening for substance abuse should occur early in the investigation of symptoms. Pursuing these issues only after the medical work-up is complete may cause patients to feel that the clinician has concluded the search for legitimate disease and has determined that the illness is imaginary. If initial attempts meet resistance, it is better to postpone these inquiries than to alienate the patient. Elicit thoughts about the cause of the symptoms. For example, a family member may have died of pancreatic cancer after developing abdominal pain and the patient fears that he or she too may have cancer.

Explore the nature of support systems and conception of illness. Do others encourage healthy functioning or relieve the patient of responsibilities, reinforcing disability? Early experiences with family members who have had chronic illnesses may influence how one copes with adversity. It may be comforting to know that many others suffer with symptoms that have no clear

explanation. Serious, life-threatening disease is unlikely and there is a large body of medical research showing that clinical improvement is possible (Box 28-2).

Physical Examination and Laboratory Testing

The physical examination should be focused and directed by the medical history. Laboratory evaluation should be kept to a minimum and limited to tests that are necessary to confirm or refute suspected medical disease. Tests obtained when there is a low pretest probability of disease are more likely to yield false-positive results that then must be pursued. Avoid establishing a pattern in which each symptom that arises is followed by exploratory testing. This conveys a message that the answer will come from ordering the correct test and it reinforces the fear of a serious illness that has yet to be diagnosed.

Establishing a Therapeutic Relationship

It cannot be overstated that the primary goal of treatment is to facilitate functioning, and not to eliminate every symptom that may occur. This requires a strong, therapeutic relationship with the patient. The clinician should show positive regard and empathy, explicitly recognizing and validating suffering. The fact that these patients are indeed suffering is often lost on clinicians. That being said, spending the rest of one's life dwelling on this agony is a dreary thought. It may be necessary to advise the patient that complete resolution of every symptom, a cure, may not be attainable. The clinician will become exasperated and resentful trying to do so, while the patient remains miserable. It is possible, however, to expect a more fulfilling and higher quality of life. Telling Ms. Hunt that she has a "more sensitive stomach than most people" may be physiologically accurate, validates her experience, and reframes the treatment. The focus turns to mobilizing her strengths so that she can forge ahead despite adversity. Working together, the clinician and patient define roles, clarify expectations, and share responsibility for setting both short-term (e.g., regular exercise) and long-term (e.g., employment) goals. Frequent unscheduled clinic visits, phone messages, and emergency care visits may indicate a need to decrease the time interval between scheduled office visits. Office visits should be time-contingent and

---

Box 28-2. Tips for Working with Patients with Medically Unexplained Symptoms

- Make appointments time not symptom contingent.
- Introduce the idea of psychiatric consultation early on in the evaluation.

- Acknowledge that the patient is truly suffering.
- Set goals of care with the patient.
- Clarify that cure may not be possible.

not symptom-contingent. Symptom-based visits begin with a focus on the symptom used to gain access to care. In a scheduled office visit, no chief complaint is needed, making it easier to proceed directly to her current functioning, sources of stress, and means of support.

If psychiatric referral is necessary, it is best to discuss this as early as possible in the treatment. When the referral is made after a negative medical work-up is complete, the patient feels that the medical provider has lost interest. It should be made explicit that the reason for referral is that a mental health specialist's input may help relieve suffering, not that the authenticity of the symptoms is questioned.

Other treatment adjuncts that may be useful include cognitive-behavioral therapy, physical therapy, relaxation training, exercise, vocational services, psychopharmacologic treatment, and the tapering of addictive medications. These modalities are discussed in detail elsewhere,[42,43] and should be considered in the comprehensive care of the patient with medically unexplained symptoms.

THE DIFFICULT PATIENT AND BORDERLINE PERSONALITY DISORDER

> Ms. Talbot, a 26-year-old woman with type 2 diabetes, has frequent angry outbursts in clinic, at times requiring the intervention of hospital security officers. She leaves phone messages and contacts the provider at inopportune times. During a stressful time she tells her doctor that she "thought of taking the whole bottle of insulin" and asks for his pager number so that she can contact him whenever she is stressed.

ESTABLISHING THE DIAGNOSIS

Every clinician has encountered the "difficult patient." Many of these patients are pejoratively and incorrectly labeled "borderlines" without a legitimate diagnosis. Conversely, primary care patients who do fit criteria for borderline personality disorder often remain undiagnosed.[44] Understanding borderline personality disorder can promote healthier relationships with patients and allow for more effective medical treatment. Medical providers also should be mindful of specific health care issues that are more common in those with borderline personality disorder, including trauma, abuse, suicidality, self-destructive behaviors, and substance abuse.[44] Although this chapter focuses on borderline personality disorder, the management principles described may be applicable to other patients as well.

Diagnosing borderline personality disorder requires familiarity with the diagnostic criteria.[45] For most medical providers, the criteria are seemingly random characteristics, difficult to memorize and without a unifying theme. Conceptualizing the core feature of the disorder as an intolerance of being alone may be more clinically useful. There is often a history of insecure early attachments to parents or other significant caregivers. Subsequent interpersonal encounters are initiated with the expectation of rejection, although the hope persists that the idealized caring person will be found. The patient's great fear is to be abandoned and unwanted. The clinician's interest and devotion to the patient is constantly being questioned and tested. The end result is that the clinician becomes "burned out," the patient feels betrayed and abandoned, interpreting this as further evidence of insignificance. As this process unfolds, she or he may become abusive and dismissive in order to preempt the forgone conclusion.

GENERAL APPROACH TO BORDERLINE PERSONALITY DISORDER

The optimal treatment of medical illness necessitates the establishment of a consistent and sustainable relationship with the patient. The nature of this relationship will depend on how central the medical provider is in the patient's life. Significant characterologic change may require years of intensive psychotherapy. General medical providers frequently do not have time to spend on this with the patient and they have not been trained as psychotherapists. Corrective personality change is probably an overly ambitious goal in primary care, but may be appropriate for mental health referral. A more attainable objective for the medical provider is to establish oneself as a reliable, predictable clinician who values the patient's health.

Limits on patient behavior and provider availability should be explicitly discussed early in the course of treatment. This negotiation should be sincere and acknowledge the patient's needs. Establishing these limits only after a significant amount of discord has developed will be perceived as punitive and indicative of the provider's loss of interest and desire to withdraw from the patient. Once limits have been agreed on, making exceptions to them is strongly discouraged. If an exception is made, even once, it will then be sought again in the future.

The degree of access considered reasonable will vary among providers. The most important guiding principle is to offer only what can be delivered on a consistent basis over time. Never make promises that can not be kept or must be reneged on in the future because they become too burdensome. If pager numbers are made available to patients, limitations need to be negotiated as to the time of day and frequency of their use. Much forethought must precede any promises of provider availability. There is no one correct approach.

Box 28-3. Tips for Working with Borderline Patients

- Negotiate availability.
- Set limits and expectations early and stick to them.
- Remain consistent and empathetic.

- All members of the treatment team should meet periodically to guarantee consistent responses to patient behavior and provide peer support.

Phone discussions or unscheduled office visits should be brief. Any such contact should then be discussed in detail during regularly scheduled office visits. Explore the reasons for the patient's call (e.g., anger, stress, testing the provider, loneliness) and what response was desired. Help to think of other coping measures; otherwise the call reinforces the feeling that the patient is incompetent, unable to solve problems without the provider's expertise and support.

The salience of expectations cannot be overstated. Patients typically assume that any lack of availability is evidence that the provider does not care about them. If the patient does not specifically articulate this, the provider must because it is such a central issue. The provider can care very much about the patient yet refuse to be called at home on the weekend. Such a thought is very difficult for some patients to conceptualize. One approach might be to simply state directly, in a nonjudgmental way, "It would help me if I knew of some of the ways that a doctor could show that he or she cares about you?" If the suggestions are reasonable, then adopt them. If not, then try to address the misconception.

Setting limits and maintaining them is difficult. Providers find themselves maligned and detested at times. The patient may "fire" a provider, possibly several times, because of accusations of delivering inadequate and incompetent care. However, if the provider remains consistent, empathetic, and can accept and acknowledge the patient's discontent, being rehired is the rule.

After repeatedly testing the provider's dedication, the patient may begin to develop a degree of trust. Trust affords an opportunity to help the patient gain insight into self-destructive behavior. For instance, the patient may realize that abusive behavior actually alienates those from whom assistance is desired. If the patient

appears able to entertain such ideas, a referral to a psychotherapist may be accepted. Consultation with a psychiatrist may be considered to explore psychopharmacologic options (Box 28-3).

SUICIDE ASSESSMENT AND MANAGEMENT

SCREENING OF MEDICAL POPULATIONS FOR SUICIDE RISK

The medical provider plays an important role in the detection and initial management of suicidality. Suicidal ideation is not uncommon in patients seen in the medical setting.[46] Up to two thirds of those who attempt or commit suicide visit a physician shortly before doing so,[46,47] and these visits are more likely to be to primary care providers than to mental health providers.[47] Vigilance for suicidality is essential in those with borderline personality: Up to 10% die by suicide.[48]

There is a paucity of data to help guide the medical provider in screening for suicide; most of the literature pertains to high-risk psychiatric populations with a previously defined risk of suicide rather than the lower-risk population of medical patients. The most recent US Preventive Services Task Force guidelines conclude that the evidence is insufficient to recommend for or against routine screening of general medical populations for suicide risk by primary care clinicians.[44] However, it may be reasonable to screen high-risk groups (see Box 28-4). The data supporting this are also meager, although one recent randomized controlled trial showed that the screening and treatment of a high-risk population, depressed elderly primary care patients, resulted in a decrease in suicidality.[50]

Box 28-4. Suicide: Identifying Those at High Risk

- Depression, hopelessness, severe anxiety, chronic medical illness
- Age >65 years (especially white men >85 years)
- Male gender
- Substance abuse
- A history of previous suicide attempts
- Being widowed or divorced, living alone

- Experiencing a recent adverse event
- A family history of suicide attempts or completions

Gaynes BN, West SL, CA Ford, et al. Screening for suicide risk in adults: A summary of the evidence for the U.S. Preventive Services Task Force. *Ann Intern Med* 2004;140(10):822–835.[33]

ASSESSMENT AND MANAGEMENT

Emergency psychiatric consultation should be obtained when encountering an acutely suicidal patient. The patient has come to the medical provider for help, so he or she should remain involved in the initial assessment and management. If the provider flees the office to call the psychiatrist at the first mention of suicide, the patient may interpret this as an indication of the provider's discomfort or disinterest in the issue. This may increase the patient's anxiety and dysphoria and decrease the likelihood of discussing such concerns with the provider in the future. The patient feels overwhelmed and is in need of support and understanding. Spending even a short amount of time with the patient prior to the arrival of an unfamiliar consultant may be very comforting.

A thorough suicide assessment consists of inquiry into specific plans, intent, methods, associated substance abuse, plans of violence to others, signs and symptoms of psychiatric disorders, previous suicide attempts, acute crises, chronic stressors, external supports, coping skills, and any future-oriented planning.[51] Although the psychiatrist will again perform this evaluation, any pertinent information obtained from the patient or collateral sources by the medical provider will be helpful to the consultant.

The provider and clinic staff are legally responsible for the patient's safety throughout the evaluation process. This may require that the patient remain in full view of monitoring staff members at all times. If the patient wishes to leave the clinic before the assessment is complete, he or she should be encouraged to stay and may need to be informed that the staff is obligated to detain suicidal patients in clinic pending a full evaluation. For patients who refuse, and proceed to leave, it is imperative to notify security personnel or police to prevent this from happening. Clinic staff should avoid directly restraining patients. If the patient does manage to abscond, local police must be notified immediately to ensure the patient's safe return. Patients who are intoxicated should be observed in a safe and secure environment until sobriety allows for a full and accurate evaluation. If there is any admission or suspicion of recent drug overdose, immediate emergency medical evaluation is warranted. At the end of the evaluation process, a detailed account of the reasons for concern and consultation obtained should be entered into the medical record.

CONCLUSION

Medical and psychiatric illnesses are often intertwined, making management of all problems more complicated. Nevertheless, being alert to the possibility of coexisting disorders and focusing on alleviating patient suffering through referral, behavioral techniques, and empathy can improve patient care and provider satisfaction.

KEY CONCEPTS

Treating Comorbid Medical and Psychiatric Illness

- Screen for mental illness.
- Consider substance use as an added comorbidity.
- Listen to the patient without distractions (i.e., reviewing the chart or writing progress notes during the visit).
- Facilitate the establishment of trust.
- Set clear limits and expectations and abide by them.
- Assess for suicidality and violence.
- See patients frequently to avoid pressure to accomplish too much in a single visit.
- Always assess for medication compliance, effectiveness, and side-effects.

CORE COMPETENCY
Managing Violent Behavior

Prevention is easier than containment.

- You, staff, and other patients can become victims.
- Recognize agitation early and deescalate.
- Consider protective measures—panic buttons, weapons searches, etc.

Train all staff and have an explicit plan for violent patients.

- Minimize provocation.
- Flag charts to alert staff and allow proactive measures.
- Minimize waits and provide patients with updated estimates.
- Arrange office space to allow easy egress for clinician and patient.

DO
- Promote self-control.
- Be polite.
- Set limits on behavior.
- Remain professional.
- Be a concerned listener.
- Allow personal space.
- Leave the office door open if necessary.
- Alert other staff before potentially violent patients are interviewed.
- Protect yourself, use security or restraints if necessary.

DON'T
- Threaten
- Physically direct
- Bargain and argue
- Ignore "gut feelings"
- Make promises you can't keep
- Turn your back on the patient

DISCUSSION QUESTIONS

1. Are patients with comorbid psychiatric illness in your clinic receiving the same quality of medical screening and treatment as those without psychiatric illness?
2. Does your health center have protocols in place to manage psychiatric emergencies (suicidality, homocidality), especially if no psychiatrist is readily available?

RESOURCES

American Psychiatric Association Treatment Guidelines. http://www.psych.org/psych_pract/treatg/

Arana GW, Hyman SE, Rosenbaum JF. *Handbook of psychiatric drug therapy,* 4th ed. Philadelphia: Lippincott Williams & Wilkins, 2000.

Stahl SM. *Essential psychopharmacolgy: The prescriber's guide.* Cambridge, UK: Cambridge University Press, 2005.

REFERENCES

1. Felker B, Yazel JJ, Short D. Mortality and medical comorbidity among psychiatric patients: A review. *Psychiatr Serv* 1996;47(12):1356–1363.
2. Spitzer RL, Kroenke K, Williams JB. Related validation and utility of a self–report version of PRIME–MD: The PHQ primary care study. Primary Care Evaluation of Mental Disorders. Patient Health Questionnaire. *JAMA* 1999;282:1737–1744.
3. Regier DA, Narrow WE, Rae DS, et al. The de facto US mental and addictive disorders service system. Epidemiologic catchment area prospective 1-year prevalence rates of disorders and services. *Arch Gen Psychiatry* 1993;50(2): 85–94.
4. Spitzer RL, Williams JB, Kroenke K, et al. Utility of a new procedure for diagnosing mental disorders in primary care. The PRIME-MD 1000 study. *JAMA* 1994;272;22:1749–1756.
5. Goldman LS. Medical illness in patients with schizophrenia. *J Clin Psychiatry* 1999;60(Suppl 21):10–5.
6. Goff DC, Cather C, Evins AE, et al., Medical morbidity and mortality in schizophrenia: Guidelines for psychiatrists. *J Clin Psychiatry* 2005;66(2):183–194; quiz 147, 273–274.
7. Enger C, Weatherby L, Reynolds RF, et al. Serious cardiovascular events and mortality among patients with schizophrenia. *J Nerv Ment Dis* 2004;192(1):19–27.
8. Toalson P, Ahmed S, Hardy T, et al. The metabolic syndrome in patients with severe mental illnesses. *Prim Care Companion J Clin Psychiatry* 2004;6(4):152–158.
9. Bushe C, Holt R. Prevalence of diabetes and impaired glucose tolerance in patients with schizophrenia. *Br J Psychiatry Suppl* 2004;47:S67–71.
10. Gough S, Peveler RC. Diabetes and its prevention: Pragmatic solutions for people with schizophrenia. *Br J Psychiatry Suppl* 2004;47:S106–111.
11. Peet M. Diet, diabetes and schizophrenia: review and hypothesis. *Br J Psychiatry* 2004;47:S102–105.
12. Allison DB, Mentore JL, Heo M, et al. Antipsychotic-induced weight gain: A comprehensive research synthesis. *Am J Psychiatry* 1999;156(11):1686–1696.
13. Lohr JB, Flynn K. Smoking and schizophrenia. *Schizophr Res* 1992;8(2):93–102.
14. McCreadie RG. Diet, smoking and cardiovascular risk in people with schizophrenia: Descriptive study. *Br J Psychiatry* 2003;183:534–539.
15. Dixon L, Postrado L, Delahanty J, et al. The association of medical comorbidity in schizophrenia with poor physical and mental health. *J Nerv Ment Dis* 1999;187(8): 496–502.
16. Friedlander AH, Marder SR. The psychopathology, medical management and dental implications of schizophrenia. *J Am Dent Assoc* 2002;133(5):603–10; quiz 624–5.
17. Rosenberg SD, Goodman LA, Osher FC, et al. Prevalence of HIV, hepatitis B, and hepatitis C in people with severe mental illness. *Am J Public Health* 2001;91(1):31–7.
18. Misra M, Papakostas GI, Klibanski A. Effects of psychiatric disorders and psychotropic medications on prolactin and bone metabolism. *J Clin Psychiatry* 2004;65(12):1607–18; quiz 1590, 1760–1.
19. Walsh E, Buchanan A, Fahy T. Violence and schizophrenia: Examining the evidence. *Br J Psychiatry* 2002;180: 490–5.
20. Walkup JT, Sambamoorthi U, Crystal S. Use of newer antiretroviral treatments among HIV-infected Medicaid beneficiaries with serious mental illness. *J Clin Psychiatry* 2004;65(9):1180–1189.
21. Link BG, Stueve A, Phelan J. Psychotic symptoms and violent behaviors: Probing the components of "threat/control-override" symptoms. *Soc Psychiatry Psychiatr Epidemiol* 1998.;33(Suppl 1):S55–60.
22. Link BG, Stueve A. Psychotic symptoms and the violent/illegal behavior of mental patients compared to community controls. In: Monahan J, Steadman HJ, eds. *Violence and mental disorder: Developments in risk assessment.* Chicago: University of Chicago Press, 1994:137–160.
23. Link BG, Andrews H, Cullen FT. The violent and illegal behavior of mental patients reconsidered. *Am Sociol Rev* 1992;57:275–292.
24. Appelbaum PS, Robbins PC, Monahan J. Violence and delusions: Data from the MacArthur Violence Risk Assessment Study. *Am J Psychiatry* 2000;157(4):566–572.
25. Stompe T, Ortwein-Swoboda G, Schanda H. Schizophrenia, delusional symptoms, and violence: The threat/control override concept reexamined. *Schizophr Bull* 2004;30(1): 31–44.
26. Nestor P. Mental disorder and violence: Personality dimensions and clinical features. *Am J Psychiatry* 2002; 159(12): 1973–1978.
27. Swanson JW, Swartz MS, Elbogen EB. Effectiveness of atypical antipsychotic medications in reducing violent behavior among persons with schizophrenia in community-based treatment. *Schizophr Bull* 2004;30(1):3–20.
28. Marder SR, Essock SM, Miller AL, et al. Physical health monitoring of patients with schizophrenia. *Am J Psychiatry* 2004;161(8):1334–1349.
28a. Lieberman JA, Stroup TS, McEnvoy JP, et al. Effectiveness of antipsychotic drugs in patients with chronic schizophrenia. *N Engl J Med* 2005;353:1205–1233.

28b. McEnvoy JP, Lieberman JA, Stroup TS, et al. Effectiveness of clozapine versus olanzapine, quetiapine, and risperidone in patients with chronic schizophrenia who did not respond to prior atypical antipsychotic treatment. *Am J Psychiatry* 2006;163:600–610.

29. Haddad, PM. Antipsychotics and diabetes: Review of non-prospective data. *Br J Psychiatry* 2004;184 (Suppl 47): S80–6.

30. Leslie DL, Rosenheck RA. Incidence of newly diagnosed diabetes attributable to atypical antipsychotic medications. *Am J Psychiatry* 2004;161:1709–11.

31. Gilmer TP, Dolder CR, Lacro JP, et al. Adherence to treatment with antipsychotic medication and health care costs among Medicaid beneficiaries with schizophrenia. *Am J Psychiatry* 2004;161(4):692–699.

32. Valenstein M, Blow FC, Copeland LA, et al. Poor antipsychotic adherence among patients with schizophrenia: Medication and patient factors. *Schizophr Bull* 2004; 30(2):255–264.

33. Kroenke K, Mangelsdorff AD. Common symptoms in ambulatory care: Incidence, evaluation, therapy, and outcome. *Am J Med* 1989;86:262–6.

34. Katon WJ, Sullivan M, Walker EA. Medical symptoms without identified pathology: Relationship to psychiatric disorders, childhood and adult trauma, and personality traits. *Ann Intern Med* 2001;134(9 Pt 2):917–925.

35. Stein MB, Lang AJ, Laffaye C, et al. Relationship of sexual assault history to somatic symptoms and health anxiety in women. *Gen Hosp Psychiatry* 2004;26(3):178–183.

36. Arnow BA. Relationships between childhood maltreatment, adult health and psychiatric outcomes, and medical utilization. *J Clin Psychiatry* 2004;65(Suppl 12):10–15.

37. Kirmayer LJ, Robbins JM, Dworkind M, et al. Somatization and the recognition of depression and anxiety in primary care. *Am J Psychiatry* 1993;150:734–41.

38. Roy-Byrne PP, Stein MB, Russo J, et al. Panic disorder in the primary care setting: Comorbidity, disability, service utilization, and treatment. *J Clin Psychiatry* 1999;60(7): 492–499; quiz 500.

39. Lecrubier Y. Posttraumatic stress disorder in primary care: A hidden diagnosis. *J Clin Psychiatry* 2004;65(Suppl 1): 49–54.

40. Dobie DJ, Kivlahan DR, Maynard C, et al. Posttraumatic stress disorder in female veterans: Association with self-reported health problems and functional impairment. *Arch Intern Med* 2004;164(4):394–400.

41. Smith RC, Lein C, Collins C, et al. Treating patients with medically unexplained symptoms in primary care. *J Gen Intern Med* 2003;18(6):478–489.

42. Walker EA, Unutzer J, Katon WJ. Understanding and caring for the distressed patient with multiple medically unexplained symptoms. *J Am Board Fam Pract* 1998; 11(5):347–356.

43. Gross R, Olfson M, Gameroff M, et al. Borderline personality disorder in primary care. *Arch Intern Med* 2002; 162(1):53–60.

44. *Diagnostic and statistical manual of mental disorders: Primary care version.* Washington, DC: American Psychiatric Association Press, 1995.

45. Gaynes BN, West SL, CA Ford, et al. Screening for suicide risk in adults: A summary of the evidence for the U.S. Preventive Services Task Force. *Ann Intern Med* 2004; 140(10): 822–835.

46. Luoma JB, Martin CE, Pearson JL. Contact with mental health and primary care providers before suicide: A review of the evidence. *Am J Psychiatry* 2002;159(6): 909–916.

47. Brodsky BS, Malone KM, Ellis SP, et al. Characteristics of borderline personality disorder associated with suicidal behavior. *Am J Psychiatry* 1997;154(12):1715–1719.

48. *Practice guideline for the assessment and treatment of patients with suicidal behaviors.* Arlington, VA: American Psychiatric Association, 2003:1–60.

49. Bruce ML, Ten Have TR, Reynolds CF 3rd, et al. Reducing suicidal ideation and depressive symptoms in depressed older primary care patients: A randomized controlled trial. *JAMA* 2004;291(9):1081–1091.

50. U.S. Preventive Services Task Force. Screening for suicide risk: Recommendation and rationale. *Ann Intern Med* 2004;140:820–821.

51. North American Association for the Study of Obesity. Consensus development conference on antipsychotic drugs and obesity and diabetes. *Diabetes Care* 2004; 27:596–601.

Chapter 29

Women's Health: Reproduction and Beyond in Poor Women

Elizabeth Harleman, MD, and Jody Steinauer, MD, MAS

Objectives

- Identify economic, social, and political causes of women's health vulnerability.
- Describe the increased burden of disease for women.
- Review barriers to effective family planning.
- Discuss innovative models for providing care to women.
- Summarize strategies to help women use contraception successfully.

Ellen Reed is a 37-year-old woman with diabetes. She has three children and works two part-time jobs. Ellen does not receive health insurance coverage from either job, and relies on Medicaid. She worries that when her children are grown she will no longer qualify for Medicaid and will have to pay for her many medicines out of pocket.

A woman's health and social position are intimately entwined. Social inequalities shape women's illnesses and their options for medical care. Women have less social and economic power than men, more limited educational and employment opportunities, and shoulder a higher burden of unpaid and hidden work (especially that related to family care and community activities). Women are more likely to work in low-wage, high-stress positions in the service industry, and lack health insurance coverage as a result. All of these inequalities place women at high risk for diseases of poverty and lack of access, but also for violence, sexually transmitted diseases and human immunodeficiency virus (HIV), body image disorders (e.g., eating disorders), mental illness, and infertility. Poor women, women of color, and elderly women are particularly affected by social disparities and their consequent impact on health. Moreover, because so much of women's lives is devoted to reproductive issues—trying to avoid pregnancy, trying to get pregnant, raising children, and being familial caretakers—women are directly affected by the politicization of reproductive health care.

This chapter discusses the factors that make women more vulnerable and the increased burden of disease they often face. In addition, it reviews the barriers to effective family planning and identifies strategies that can help women use contraception successfully. Finally, it offers models for improving the care women receive. Issues related to lesbian health are discussed in Chap. 27.

WOMEN'S HEALTH: WHY ARE WOMEN VULNERABLE?

Women in the United States have a life expectancy 5 years longer than men and lower age-adjusted death rates than men for 13 of the 15 leading causes of death.[1] However, many women's health needs are inadequately addressed.

COMPETING PRIORITIES

> Ellen is the sole breadwinner and caregiver for her family. She finds it difficult to make time for appointments with her physician. Although she knows about the importance of eating right and exercising, she often lacks the time and energy to do either.

Women's multiple roles in the family and workplace make it difficult for them to prioritize their own health care needs. Nearly one half (48%) of women ages 18 to 64 have children under age 18 at home. Mothers bear a disproportionate burden of responsibility for housework, even if they also work outside the home, as two-thirds of them do.[2] The majority of women with young children have primary responsibility for coordinating their children's health care and missing work to care for a sick child. Low-income women are particularly affected by these multiple responsibilities.[2]

In addition to caring for young children, women are often called on to care for elderly or ill parents. These women are likely to have children of their own, work outside the home, and report the presence of a chronic disease themselves. Despite their need for health care, up to 25% of women caring for elderly, disabled, or ill family members are uninsured.

POVERTY

> Last year, Ellen's combined income from her two part-time jobs was $39,500 (the poverty level for a family of four is $19,350). She barely had enough money to purchase all the resources her family required to live and she never had any discretionary income.

In 2004, the poverty rate for families was 10.2 percent, comprising almost 7.9 million families. Of all family groups, poverty is highest among those headed by single women. In 2004, 28.4 percent of all female-headed families (nearly 4 million families) were poor, compared to 5.5 percent of married-couple families (3.2 million families).[3] These figures are even more dismaying for women of color, with 51% of Latinos and 44% of African-American female-headed households falling below the poverty line, compared with 27% of whites.[2] Women also make up 70% of the elderly poor, and are 70% more likely than men to experience poverty in retirement. Poorer and less educated women have worse self-rated health status and higher rates of many chronic illnesses, including arthritis, asthma, depression, diabetes, hypertension, obesity, and osteoporosis.[4]

LACK OF HEALTH INSURANCE COVERAGE

Women are more likely than men to be uninsured (Fig. 29-1). Women perform the majority of unpaid caregiving labor in US society, which often renders them ineligible for health insurance, Social Security, and other retirement income. In addition, many women are low-wage workers in industries that do not offer benefits; consequently, they are more likely than men to be uninsured. Women who are younger and have low incomes are at greatest risk for being uninsured, especially Latinas (Fig. 29-2).[5] Furthermore, many women's access to state-supported benefits is limited to the time when they are pregnant or raising small children. Thus, once they no longer fit into these categories, it may be impossible for them to receive state-sponsored health care, no matter how poor they are.

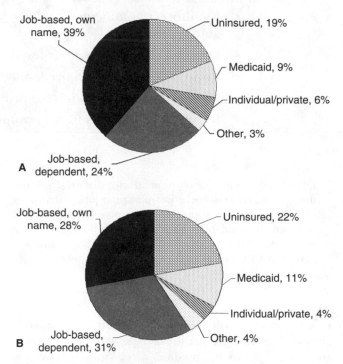

Figure 29-1. A. Health insurance coverage of women age 18 to 64 years (total = 91 million). (Other insurance includes Medicare and CHAMPUS.) Data redrawn from: *Women's health insurance coverage fact sheet #6000-0h3.* Menlo Park, CA: The Henry J. Kaiser Family Foundation. Accessed: July 8, 2005. November 2004. (Women's Health Policy Facts November 2004) Available at: http://www.kff.org/womenshealth/6000-03.cfm **B.** Health insurance coverage of women age 18 to 64 years with dependent children under age 18 in household. (Other insurance includes Medicare and CHAMPUS.) Data redrawn from: Wyn R, Ojeda V, Ranji U, et al. *Women, work, and family health: A balancing act.* The Henry J. Kaiser Family Foundation. Accessed: July 7, 2005. 2003.[2] Available at: http://www.kff.org/womenshealth/3336–index.cfm

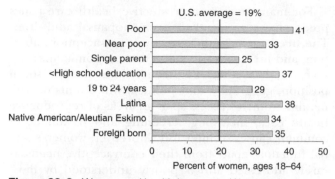

Figure 29-2. Women and health insurance. Women who are younger, poor, foreign-born, single parents, non-white, and who lack education are at risk for being uninsured. The federal poverty level was $15,260 in 2003 for a family of three. Poor indicates family income <100% of the federal poverty level. Near-poor indicates family income 101% to 200% of the federal poverty level. Data redrawn from: *Women's health insurance coverage fact sheet #6000-03.* Menlo Park, CA: The Henry J. Kaiser Family Foundation. Accessed July 8, 2005. November 2004. (Women's Health Policy Facts November 2004). Available at: http://www.kff.org/womenshealth/6000–03.cfm

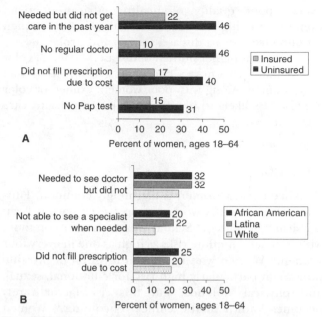

Figure 29-3. **A.** Barriers to health care based on insurance coverage. The uninsured were significantly different from the insured on all measures at $p < 0.05$. Data redrawn from: *Women's health insurance coverage fact sheet #6000-03.* Menlo Park, CA: The Henry J. Kaiser Family Foundation. Accessed: July 8, 2005. November 2004. (Women's Health Policy Facts November 2004). Available at: http://www.kff.org/womenshealth/6000–03.cfm **B.** Barriers to health care by race and ethnicity for women ages 18 to 64. The percentages are significantly different from the reference group, white women, at $p < 0.05$. Data redrawn from: Wyn R, Ojeda V, Ranji U, et al. *Racial and ethnic disparities in women's health coverage and access to care. Findings from the 2001 Kaiser Women's Health Survey.* The Henry J. Kaiser Family Foundation, March 2004. Accessed July 7, 2005. Available at: http://www.kff.org/womenshealth/7018.cfm

Uninsured women are more likely than insured women to postpone medical care, forego prescription medications, and delay or postpone important preventive care such as mammograms and Pap smears (Fig. 29-3). They have more limited contraceptive options and are less likely to receive prenatal care. Lack of adequate care leads to worse outcomes from complicated pregnancies to high infant mortality, and a higher likelihood of dying from many conditions, including breast and cervical cancer.[4]

UNCOORDINATED SERVICES

A variety of medical specialties attend to the health needs of women. Young women tend to identify generalists or obstetricians and gynecologists as their primary caregivers, whereas older women are more likely to visit family physicians or internists. The care of women's reproductive organs is often separated from other health care needs, creating an imperative to establish relationships with multiple providers or accept that some aspects of care may not be adequately covered. This fragmented care is more common in women with limited or no insurance coverage. Furthermore, providers caring for women with chronic illnesses may fail to consider their reproductive lives, resulting in lack of preconception counseling, late referrals for abortion, and inadequate contraception prescribed while taking potentially teratogenic medications. In addition, the compartmentalization of women's health

care needs among specialties may result in neglect of certain areas that do not have a clearly defined "home" such as domestic violence and eating disorders.[6]

RACIAL AND ETHNIC DISPARITIES

Racial and ethnic differences in mortality and health status are observed among women. Women of color are strikingly affected by poorer health outcomes throughout their lives. Much of this risk is attributable to the effects of poverty on health, but a differential persists after controlling for income, suggesting that race and social inequality are independent predictors of women's health status. African-American women have more complications of pregnancy and are also at higher risk for chronic illness.[4] African-American and Latina women also suffer more than white women from diabetes and overall poor quality of health.[4] African-American women have higher death rates than white women resulting from heart disease, cancer, and stroke.

Despite this higher burden of disease, women of color receive fewer preventive services and screening tests than white women. Along with poor women, women of color are also less likely to be offered important health care interventions.[7,8]

VIOLENCE

Violence against women is alarmingly common. Fifty-one percent of US women report ever having been physically assaulted.[9] Sexual assault is also common, with estimated lifetime risks as high as one in every four women.[10] Women who have been involved in prostitution are at particularly high risk for emotional, sexual, and physical violence, but this risk factor rarely becomes known in the clinical encounter.[11] Women who are the victims of violence face high rates of physical and mental illness (see Chap. 30).

ATTITUDES

Both women patients and their providers may harbor negative stereotypes that can hinder good care. Women patients may feel reluctant to report symptoms for fear of being thought of as "hypochondriacs" or reluctance to "be difficult" for the physician.

Providers also bring their own stereotypes about women patients to their interactions. Physicians may be more likely to see women patients as making excessive demands on their time, having complaints influenced by emotional factors, or having a psychosomatic component to their illness.[12] Women tend to receive more prescriptions than men for the same problems, especially obesity, and are up to four times more likely than men to be prescribed activity limitations by their physicians, even with the same complaints, personal preferences, and illness behavior.[13] Providers should be mindful of their own biases and how these may influence the therapeutic relationship.

WOMEN'S REPRODUCTIVE HEALTH CARE

Ellen asks her provider about starting Depo Provera injections on two successive visits. Her physician, concerned about Ellen's poor glycemic control and elevated blood pressure, defers the discussion until after she can review information about optimal contraceptive methods in the chronically ill. When Ellen is seen 2 months later, she is pregnant.

For many women, reproductive health care issues predominate during their premenopausal adult lives. The need for safe and effective contraception, abortion, and prenatal care cuts across economic lines, yet access to these services is strongly influenced by social position, geography, and political will. Limits on vulnerable women's access span all areas of reproductive health care, including screening and treatment of common causes of infertility. Moreover, women's sexual function, apart from their contraceptive needs, is rarely addressed and is poorly understood by most providers.[14]

UNINTENDED PREGNANCY

Unintended pregnancy has significant implications for women's health. Each year in the United States there are 6.3 million pregnancies, of which nearly half (48%) are unintended. Approximately half of these unintended pregnancies end in abortion (1.3 million). Of the women who become pregnant unintentionally, approximately 51% report using contraception at the time; either the method failed, or it was used incorrectly. In general, unintended pregnancies disproportionately affect younger and older women, women of low income, and African-American women.[15] At any given time, one fifth of homeless women are pregnant, a rate twice that of all US women of reproductive age.[16]

BARRIERS TO EFFECTIVE CONTRACEPTION

Health care providers play an important role in determining women's success with contraception. Choosing a contraceptive method requires the clinician to engage in detailed patient education, including complete information about available methods, efficacy, contraindications, and side-effects. Providing accurate information is essential to contraceptive success. Women with low literacy levels or lack of English language proficiency may find it difficult to understand much of the contraceptive information provided to them in printed form. In addition, they may not trust or feel comfortable if the provider is unfamiliar with their cultural priorities.

Providers may lack adequate time to address contraception in detail; not have a clear understanding of contraindications, efficacy, and side-effects of individual methods; and be unable to provide methods that require procedural skill, such as intrauterine device placement. These issues are particularly important for women who live in areas without dedicated family planning clinic access. If women lack the financial mobility to see a provider of choice, they may be forced to seek contraception in a setting that limits their choices (particularly of long-acting methods), is unable to provide

---

Box 29-1. Medical Barriers to Contraception Success

- Misconceptions about perceived contraindications, such as asthma or diabetes
- Concern about potential contraindications, such as stroke, blood clots, or heart attack
- Safety issues: may withhold certain contraceptive methods based on age, parity, and marital status.
- Limited provider training:
  - —Inadequate clinical experience or training
  - —Misconceptions regarding clinical practice
  - —Limited range of contraceptive options
  - —Lack of effective communications and counseling skills
- Process barriers:
  - —Protocols in place that impede a patient's access, such as a waiting period to ensure she is not pregnant

- —Unnecessary procedures prior to selecting a contraception method, such as Pap smear and other methods of cervical cancer testing
- —Unnecessary follow-up scheduling that requires frequent visits

Medical barriers to contraception are defined as ". . . practices derived at least partly from medical rationale that result in a scientifically unjustifiable impediment to or denial of contraception."[18]
Adapted from: Blumenthal P. *Contraception online. Maximizing contraceptive success.* Houston: The Center for Collaborative and Interactive Technologies (CCIT) at Baylor College of Medicine. Accessed July 7, 2005. Available at: http://www.contraceptiononline.org/slides/index.cfm[19]

---

contraceptives on site, or uniformly links contraceptive access to preventive care.

Systemic issues related to contraceptive failure include lack of public and private funding for contraceptive care and lack of access to providers. For example, funding for Title X, a federal program that provides free or low-cost family planning care to many low-income women in the United States, has decreased by 58% since 1980, limiting access for uninsured women. Even poor women with private health insurance may lack coverage, as only 24 states currently have laws that mandate contraception coverage for private insurance companies that provide prescription drugs and devices. Women with insurance for contraception often are restricted to obtaining only 1 month's supply of pills at a time, requiring regular visits to the pharmacy in order to use contraception correctly. Women may opt not to obtain contraception through their insurance because of lack of confidentiality from the primary insurance holder, who, as their partner or parent, may be unsupportive of contraception. In all of these cases, limitations on women's ability to access contraception can result in unintended pregnancy.

Barriers to contraception extend beyond funding and can directly influence the services available, even to women who have coverage. The merger of many religious and secular health care institutions, especially in communities where there are no other hospitals, has contributed to decreased access to contraception. In many such hospitals, providers are not allowed to perform tubal ligations or prescribe emergency contraception to patients in need. Faith-based clinics offering care to homeless and poor women also often do not provide contraceptive care. In some cases, pharmacists refuse to dispense contraceptives prescribed to women, citing the pharmacist's own personal code of ethics.[17]

Finally, even after choosing a method, many women do not fill prescriptions because of ambivalence, misunderstanding, lack of empowerment, or inability to pay for the method. Additional barriers to effective contraception include cultural and religious prohibitions against contraception, partner dislike of contraception, and mistrust based on medicine's historical treatment of women related to their reproductive lives (Box 29-1).

ACCESS TO ABORTION

Each year, approximately 1.31 million women undergo an abortion in the United States. Many women have limited access to abortion services, especially rural women, teens, and poor women. Ensuring the availability of safe, legal abortion care has been shown to decrease maternal mortality and morbidity.[20]

Abortion access has decreased over the last 15 years for a variety of reasons, including a shortage of practitioners who provide abortions, limited public funding for abortion services, and political restrictions. As of 2000, only 13% of US counties had an abortion provider.[21] A minority of obstetrics and gynecology (ob-gyn) and family practice residency programs provide routine abortion training,[22,23] although this number is increasing in response to ob-gyn accreditation requirements and initiatives by individual residency programs in both disciplines.

Legislative restrictions on abortion access include numerous barriers on the state level, all of which disproportionately affect poor women and young women (Table 29-1). In addition, lack of community support and violent acts directed at abortion clinics, providers, and patients all serve to limit women's access to safe abortion services.

Table 29-1. United States State Legislation Related to Abortion

Abortion-Related Legislation	Number of States	Details of Legislation
Minor access	45 states	Restrict of minors' access to privacy by requiring parental consent or notification for minors seeking abortion services
Clinic violence	16 states and the District of Columbia (DC)	Protect health care facilities from blockades, harassment, and/or other violence
Public funding	33 states and DC	Restrict low-income women's access to abortion services by restricting public funding for abortion
	17 states	Provide of public funding for abortion in all or most circumstances
Private insurance funding	17 states	Prohibit certain insurance plans from covering abortion services
Nonobjective pregnancy counseling	31 states	Require that women seeking abortion undergo biased counseling designed to dissuade them from choosing to have an abortion
Waiting periods	28 states	Require that women wait additional time after receiving counseling before they may obtain an abortion

Source: Who Decides: The Status of Womens's Reproductive Rights in the United States. NARAL Pro-Choice America. Available at http://www.prochoiceamerica.org/ choice-action-center/in_your state/who-decides/maps-and charts. Accessed May 19, 2006.

Common Pitfalls

- Poor women and women of color suffer a higher burden of disease but receive a lower quality of health care.
- Because of the competing demands of work and family, women often put their own health and well-being last.
- Women's health care needs are compartmentalized, and different providers understand each other's areas poorly.
- Effective contraception is denied because of political barriers, lack of funding, or inextricable linkage to routine health care screening.
- Women's sexual function is rarely addressed.
- Cultural preferences, language, and literacy are not incorporated when providing contraceptive information.

STRATEGIES FOR IMPROVING WOMEN'S HEALTH

ECONOMIC AND SOCIAL JUSTICE FOR WOMEN

The World Health Organization's Constitution states that "The enjoyment of the highest attainable standard of health is one of the fundamental rights of every human being without distinction of race, religion, political belief, economic or social condition."[24] However, it is increasingly well recognized that in order to achieve improved health status for women, their position in society must be improved across racial and economic lines. Access to affordable, high-quality health care is essential. The disparities that exist between women and men, and between women of color and white women, are rooted in social inequalities that must be addressed in tandem with efforts to improve health status. Because low wages are an increasingly important contributor to poverty, women and men should receive equal pay for work of equal value (Box 29-2).[24]

IMPORTANCE OF WOMEN IN FAMILY AND COMMUNITY HEALTH

Women's essential role in reproduction and the management of the family positions them to have a considerable impact on their own health and the health of children, partners, elders, and the community. Women are vastly more likely than men to take responsibility

---

Box 29-2. World Health Organization Gender Glossary

- *Gender* is used to describe those characteristics of women and men, which are socially constructed, whereas sex refers to those which are biologically determined. People are born female or male but learn to be girls and boys who grow into women and men. This learned behavior makes up gender identity and determines gender roles.
- *Gender equality* is the absence of discrimination based on a person's sex in opportunities, the allocation of resources and benefits, or access to services.

- *Gender equity* refers to fairness and justice in the distribution of benefits and responsibilities between women and men. The concept recognizes that women and men have different needs and power and that these differences should be identified and addressed in a manner that rectifies the imbalance between the sexes.

Adapted from: *WHO gender policy: Integrating gender perspectives in the work of WHO.* World Health Organization. Accessed: July 8, 2005. Available at: http://www.who.int/gender/documents/policy/en/[24]

for choosing their children's physicians and taking them to appointments, as well as making decisions regarding health insurance.[2] One means to improve women's health may be to frame a choice to care for one's own health as ensuring the health of the family as well. In addition, the ability of women (and men) to have healthy and happy families while earning income sufficient to support their needs should be ensured and defined by public policies.

FEMALE PHYSICIANS

Women patients prefer female physicians in a variety of settings, from the emergency room to obstetric care. Women physicians have higher rates of performing appropriate screening breast examinations, mammography, and pelvic examinations than do male physicians.[25] Women physicians also spend more time with patients, converse more, and appear to listen more closely, leading to greater patient satisfaction. In order for the care of women to be optimized, more women physicians need to be promoted and retained in positions of academic leadership. In addition, more emphasis should be placed on educating male physicians about how to improve their interactions with women patients and perform appropriate screening and preventive care.

COORDINATED SERVICES

> Ellen decides to continue her pregnancy. She is referred to a high-risk obstetrics clinic that accepts Medicaid. There, Ellen sees her obstetrician along with a nutritionist, social worker, and diabetes nurse. Although it is challenging to get to her appointments, she now gets more support managing her diabetes.

Given the many competing priorities in women's lives, and the resulting lack of time for self-care, offering multiple complementary services at one site is crucial. Simultaneous access to mental health services, substance abuse treatment, nutrition counseling, and social support can make it possible for a woman to address her health care needs. Simple changes such as offering evening and weekend hours, walk-in visits, and being located close to public transportation are successful innovations that enhance low-income women's ability to access health services.[26] Addressing women's care-giving responsibilities by welcoming children in the physician's office or even providing brief supervision for children and elders during visits would facilitate many women's use of care. Ensuring timely access to specialists is another important component of coordinated medical care.

COMMUNITY OUTREACH AND ADVOCACY

In addition to offering coordinated in an easily accessed location, bringing health care and information to women where they live and work is an essential part of improving outcomes. Church-based breast cancer screening programs have been shown to improve mammography rates in hard-to-reach women.[27] Providing community-based care to women is most effective when the needs and priorities of the community drive the effort.

GROUP VISITS

Social support is a critical element of effective health care for women. Group-based care is a successful model for providing services during pregnancy (see Chap. 12). Group prenatal care has been shown to improve outcomes for minority and low-income women, resulting in higher birth weights, particularly for infants born preterm.[28] The group provides a needed social support network to women who, because of the isolation imposed by poverty or immigration, might otherwise lack such a network.

ADDRESSING WOMEN'S CONTRACEPTIVE HEALTH NEEDS

In order to comfortably address women's contraceptive needs, providers should have easy access to information about contraception. There are several excellent reference guides and web sites to assist providers in understanding the variety of methods, prescribing information, contraindications, efficacy, and side-effects (see Resources).[29]

When caring for women with medical problems, providers can consult the World Health Organization guidelines (www.who.int//). These guidelines make clear recommendations about which contraceptive methods are indicated for dozens of medical diseases.

Perhaps most importantly, providers should routinely address contraception. Language- and literacy-appropriate educational materials help overcome barriers posed by a patient's beliefs, fears, or difficulties with a particular contraceptive method.

Offering triage access for refills and phone consultation about side-effects also can improve contraceptive use. Practitioners might consider "Quick Start," immediate initiation of contraception in the office, a safe management method that improves compliance with oral contraceptive pills (Box 29-3).[30,31]

Finally, emergency contraception, taken within 5 days of unprotected intercourse, decreases the risk of unintended pregnancy by up to 88% depending on method and time since intercourse (with lower efficacy associated with increased time). Emergency contraception consists of two separate doses of combined

Box 29-3. "Quick Start" of Oral Contraceptive Pill by Day of Cycle

Day 1–6
No backup necessary
Take first pill in office

Day 7–13
Give emergency contraception if unprotected sex in past 5 days
Take first pill in office
Use condoms for 7 days

Day 14–next menses
Give emergency contraception if unprotected sex in past 5 days
Take first pill in office
Use condoms for 7 days
Pregnancy test if day 25 or later
Counsel that pregnancy may be possible. The patient should repeat the pregnancy test if she does not have a period during her placebo week.

hormonal contraceptive pills totaling over 100 mcg of ethinyl estradiol per dose or progestin-only pills totaling 7.5 mg of levonorgestrel. It now appears that the entire dose of levonorgestrel emergency contraception can be taken at one time with equal efficacy.[32] Providers should offer women advanced prescriptions for emergency contraception, a simple act that has been shown to make women more likely to use emergency contraception and no less likely to use their main contraceptive method.[33]

ENSURING ABORTION ACCESS

Providers should decide whether they are trained and comfortable with offering objective pregnancy options counseling and referral within their office. If not, there are a number of referral resources, including national and local telephone hotlines. The local Planned Parenthood Federation Affiliate is able to offer counseling and referral services in almost all communities. In addition, an objective pregnancy counseling hotline administered by the National Abortion Federation is available (1-800-772-9100). Individual practitioners, including family physicians, internists, and physician assistants (in a few states), with adequate training, also can consider offering medical and/or early surgical abortion within their offices.[34-36] Even if physicians do not feel comfortable providing abortions themselves, it is important to support others in their community who do. This support can translate into patient referral, hospital backup, and inclusion in local medical societies.

Providers and/or clinic protocols may unnecessarily require women to obtain Pap smears or pelvic examinations before the initiation of hormonal birth control methods. The practice of "holding contraception hostage" to routine preventive health care may result in fewer women getting needed contraception, particularly teens or others who may have personal fears or taboos around the pelvic examination. Although linking preventive health care with contraception access may seem attractive logistically, it is not evidence-based,

and can result in more unintended pregnancies. With the exception of a blood pressure measurement prior to initiating combined hormonal contraception, no physical examination is necessary before initiating a method.[37]

ADVOCACY TO ELIMINATE BARRIERS TO EFFECTIVE FAMILY PLANNING

Advocacy on many fronts will help improve women's access to contraception. Ensuring contraceptive coverage in private and public sectors and continuing Medicaid and Title X funding for contraception are key. In nine states, women have access to emergency contraception through pharmacists, and in Washington, there is an ongoing study of direct pharmacist access for combined hormonal contraceptive methods as well.[38] Providers can make patients aware of direct emergency contraception access and support movements to replicate this work in other states. Providers also can play an important advocacy role in the protection of accessible and safe abortion services. The removal of punitive abortion restrictions and protection of the legality of this very common procedure are best accomplished by professional, legislative, and judicial efforts.

KEY CONCEPTS

- Coordinated, multidisciplinary services provide the cornerstone of outstanding care for women.
- Involving the community and welcoming the family at the site of care improves access and motivation to participate.
- Increasing patient and provider knowledge about contraceptive methods and emergency contraception can help reduce rates of unintended pregnancy.
- Advocacy to improve women's position in society and ensure access to safe and effective family planning is worth pursuing on many levels.

CORE COMPETENCY
Evidence-Based Strategies to Optimize Contraception Use

When	What to Do
Prior to the appointment	Plan to routinely discuss contraception with reproductive-aged women Have available a written or web-based reference of contraceptive contraindications, efficacy, and side-effects, to help you help women choose a method.
History	Ask your patient which contraceptive method she would like, and try to have it on hand. If she is undecided or has failed with a specific contraceptive method, consider a method that lasts longer or has greater efficacy.
Physical examination	Do not require a screening Pap smear before prescribing a method. The only required examination is a blood pressure measurement before prescribing combined hormonal methods.
Assessment and plan	Use your references to confirm contraindications. Consider starting the method in your office, "Quick Start" (see Box 29-3).
Counseling	Review expected side-effects, especially nausea and bleeding pattern. Review what to do if she forgets to use the method when scheduled. Give her literacy-appropriate handouts about her method of contraception. Give her a prescription for emergency contraception and information about how to use it.
After the appointment	Have staff readily available for questions and refills. Do not require examinations before giving refills.

CONCLUSION

The path to improving the health of women in vulnerable communities, and indeed all women, is rooted in efforts to eliminate social inequalities. Being mindful of the many personal and systemic barriers to good care and directly addressing them through personal and political advocacy, integration of services, improved access, and examining one's own perceptions about women patients are all part of providing the best possible care.

DISCUSSION QUESTIONS

1. You are involved in the planning stages of a women's clinic in a low-income community. What structural elements would you include to make your services more accessible to your target patient population?
2. Ms. Chen is a 37-year-old woman with hepatitis C who comes to you seeking contraception. How would you counsel her about her options? What resources would you consult to determine the safety of contraceptive methods in a woman with medical illness?
3. Consider the approach to providing contraception in your current practice setting. Generate a list of three specific changes you could make to improve access and compliance with contraception.

RESOURCES

http://www.arhp.org
Association of Reproductive Health Professionals (ARHP). ARHP is an organization that provides continuing medical education for health practitioners in reproductive health.

http://www.who.int
Medical Eligibility Criteria for Contraceptive Use. An online resource produced by the World Health Organization that gives clear, evidence-based guidelines about the use of contraception in women with medical illness.

http://www.healthstatus2000.com/owh/select_variables.aspx
National Women's Health Indicators Data Base is a national catalog of health indicators that highlights issues of racial, economic, and gender disparities.

Basson R. Women's sexual dysfunction: Revised and expanded definitions. *CMAJ* 2005;172(10):1327–1333.

Cantu M, Coppola M, Lindner AJ. Evaluation and management of the sexually assaulted woman. *Emerg Med Clin North Am* 2003;21(3):737–750.

Hatcher RA, Nelson AL, Zieman M, et al. *A pocket guide to managing contraception.* Tiger, GA: Bridging the Gap Foundation, 2003.

REFERENCES

1. Arias E, Anderson RN, Kung HC, et al. Deaths: Final data for 2001. In: *National Vital Statistics Report, 2003.* Hyattsville, MD: National Center for Health Statistics, 2003:1–115.
2. Wyn R, Ojeda V, Ranji U, et al. *Racial and ethnic disparities in women's health coverage and access to care. Findings from the 2001 Kaiser Women's Health Survey.* The Henry J. Kaiser Family Foundation, March 2004. Accessed July 7, 2005. Available at: http://www.kff.org/womenshealth/7018.cfm

3. *Who was poor in 2004?* University of Wisconsin-Madison, Institute for Research on Poverty. Available at: http://www.irp.wisc.edu/faqs/faq3.htm. Accessed June 2, 2006.

4. *2004 National healthcare disparities report.* U.S. Department of Health and Human Services. Accessed May, 2005. Available at: http://www.qualitytools.ahrq.gov/disparitiesreport/

5. *Women's Health Insurance Coverage* (Fact Sheet #6000-03). The Henry J. Kaiser Family Foundation. Accessed: July 8, 2005, November 2004. Available at: http://www.kff.org/womenshealth/6000-03.cfm

6. Clancy CM, Massion CT. American women's health care. A patchwork quilt with gaps. *JAMA* 1992;268:1918–1920.

7. Schneider EC, Zaslavsky AM, Epstein AM. Racial disparities in the quality of care for enrollees in medicare managed care. *JAMA* 2002;287:1288–1294.

8. Schulman KA, Berlin JA, Harless W, et al. The effect of race and sex on physicians' recommendations for cardiac catheterization. *N Engl J Med* 1999;340:618–626.

9. Tjaden P, Thoennes N. *Prevalence, incidence, and consequences of violence against women: Findings from the National Violence Against Women Survey.* Washington, DC: National Institute of Justice and Centers for Disease Control and Prevention, 1998.

10. Wilken J, Welch J. Management of people who have been raped. *BMJ* 2003;326:458–459.

11. Farley M. Prostitution is sexual violence. *Psychiatric Times* 2004;21:7–10.

12. Bernstein B, Kane R. Physicians' attitudes toward female patients. *Med Care* 1981;19:600–608.

13. Safran DG, Rogers WH, Tarlov AR, et al. Gender differences in medical treatment: The case of physician-prescribed activity restrictions. *Soc Sci Med* 1997;45:711–722.

14. Pauls RN, Kleeman SD, Segal JL, et al. Practice patterns of physician members of the American Urogynecologic Society regarding female sexual dysfunction: Results of a national survey. *Int Urogynecol J Pelvic Floor Dysfunct* 2005;16:460–467.

15. Henshaw SK. Unintended pregnancy in the United States. *Fam Plann Perspect* 1998;30:24–29, 46.

16. Gelberg L, Leake B, Lu MC, et al. Chronically homeless women's perceived deterrents to contraception. *Perspect Sex Reprod Health* 2002;34:278–285.

17. Ruetheling G. Contraceptive prescriptions at issue. *The New York Times,* April 4, 2005. Sect. 20.

18. Shelton JD, Angle MA, Jacobstein RA. Medical barriers to access to family planning. *Lancet* 1992;340:1334–1335.

19. Blumenthal P. *Contraception online. Maximizing contraceptive success.* Houston: The Center for Collaborative and Interactive Technologies (CCIT) at Baylor College of Medicine. Accessed July 7, 2005. Available at: http://www.contraceptiononline.org/slides/index.cfm

20. Cates W Jr, Grimes DA, Schulz KF. The public health impact of legal abortion: 30 years later. *Perspect Sex Reprod Health* 2003;35:25–28.

21. Finer LB, Henshaw SK. Abortion incidence and services in the United States in 2000. *Perspect Sex Reprod Health* 2003;35:6–15.

22. Almeling R, Tews L, Dudley S. Abortion training in U.S. obstetrics and gynecology residency programs, 1998. *Fam Plann Perspect* 2000;32:268–271, 320.

23. Steinauer JE, DePineres T, Robert AM, et al. Training family practice residents in abortion and other reproductive health care: A nationwide survey. *Fam Plann Perspect* 1997;29:222–227.

24. *WHO gender policy: Integrating gender perspectives in the work of WHO.* World Health Organization. Accessed: July 8, 2005. Available at: http://www.who.int/gender/documents/policy/en/

25. Lurie N, Slater J, McGovern P, et al. Preventive care for women. Does the sex of the physician matter? *N Engl J Med* 1993;329:478–482.

26. Luck J, Andersen R, Wenzel S, et al. Providers of primary care to homeless women in Los Angeles County. *J Ambul Care Manage* 2002;25:53–67.

27. Siegel JE, Clancy CM. Community-based interventions: Taking on the cost and cost-effectiveness questions. *Health Serv Res* 2000;35:905–909.

28. Ickovics JR, Kershaw TS, Westdahl C, et al. Group prenatal care and preterm birth weight: Results from a matched cohort study at public clinics. *Obstet Gynecol* 2003;102:1051–1057.

29. Hatcher RA, Nelson AL, Zieman M, et al. *A pocket guide to managing contraception.* Tiger, GA: Bridging the Gap Foundation. Accessed: July 8, 2005; 2002. Available at: http://www.managingcontraception.com/pdffiles.html

30. Bracken MB. Oral contraception and congenital malformations in offspring: A review and meta-analysis of the prospective studies. *Obstet Gynecol* 1990;76:552–557.

31. Westhoff C, Kerns J, Morroni C, et al. Quick start: Novel oral contraceptive initiation method. *Contraception* 2002;66:141–145.

32. Cheng L, Gulmezoglu AM, Oel CJ, et al. Interventions for emergency contraception. *Cochrane Database Syst Rev* 2004:CD001324.

33. Raine TR, Harper CC, Rocca CH, et al. Direct access to emergency contraception through pharmacies and effect on unintended pregnancy and STIs: A randomized controlled trial. *JAMA* 2005;293:54–62.

34. Prine L, Lesnewski R, Berley N, et al. Medical abortion in family practice: A case series. *J Am Board Fam Pract* 2003;16:290–295.

35. Schwarz EB, Luetkemeyer A, Foster DG, et al. Willing and able? Provision of medication for abortion by future internists. *Womens Health Issues* 2005;15:39–44.

36. Goldman MB, Occhiuto JS, Peterson LE, et al. Physician assistants as providers of surgically induced abortion services. *Am J Public Health* 2004;94:1352–1357.

37. Stewart FH, Harper CC, Ellertson CE, et al. Clinical breast and pelvic examination requirements for hormonal contraception: Current practice vs evidence. *JAMA* 2001;285: 2232–2239.

38. *EC Over-the-Counter Status.* Pharmacy Access Partnership. Accessed May 19, 2006. Available at: http://www.pharmacyaccess.org/ECOTCstatus.htm.

Chapter 30

Intimate Partner Violence

Leigh Kimberg, MD

Objectives

- Define intimate partner violence (IPV), childhood exposure to IPV, child abuse, and elder abuse.
- Present models that elucidate the phenomenon of IPV.
- Describe the health effects of IPV.
- Review current and recommended practices to address IPV.
- Outline challenges to addressing IPV, including patient, provider, and health system factors.
- Suggest interventions to improve the care of those affected by IPV.

Amalia and Carl have a 5-month-old daughter, Elena. When Amalia was pregnant, Carl began to criticize her and return home late, drunk, and angry. One night Carl, awakened by Elena's crying, kicked Amalia out of the bed and hit her repeatedly. Carl has hit Amalia on three other occasions, forced her to have sex, and pushed her off of the bed while she was breastfeeding Elena, knocking Elena onto the floor.

Intimate partner violence (IPV) is extremely common and has marked harmful effects on the safety, health, and well-being of those victimized. IPV extracts a high cost from women and their families physically, emotionally, and financially. Physical violence in intimate relationships is almost always accompanied by psychological and, often, sexual abuse. Many terms have been used to describe a pattern of abuse between intimate partners of all ages, including "domestic violence." The term intimate partner violence (IPV) is used to describe violence and abuse (e.g., physical, sexual, battering, or emotional abuse) between intimate partners (by a spouse, ex-spouse, or current or former boyfriend or girlfriend). Legal definitions of IPV used by the criminal and civil justice systems vary from state to state. Intimate partner violence in elderly couples is one form of elder abuse. Children are often exposed to IPV and maltreatment of children is frequently related to IPV (Table 30-1).

The health care setting presents an ideal opportunity to assist people affected by IPV by providing a confidential environment to discuss problems that patients may feel uncomfortable or unsafe addressing elsewhere. This chapter discusses the problem of IPV, including reviewing best practices and successful models for addressing IPV in the health care setting.

EPIDEMIOLOGY AND HEALTH CONSEQUENCES OF INTIMATE PARTNER VIOLENCE

Amalia sleeps poorly, suffers from daily headaches and back pain, and has fits of uncontrollable crying. Because she often complains to her doctor about her headaches and back pain, she has undergone a head computed tomography scan, lumbar puncture, spinal x-rays, and blood work. Carl injured himself when he hit Amalia. He was treated in the emergency department for the injury and chest pain diagnosed as gastroesophageal reflux disease from "stress." Elena cries often and is not nursing well.

Table 30-1. Definitions of Intimate Partner Violence, Child Abuse, and Elder Abuse

Term	Definition
Intimate partner violence	"[a] pattern of assaultive and coercive behaviors that may include inflicted physical injury, psychological abuse, sexual assault, progressive social isolation, stalking, deprivation, intimidation and threats. These behaviors are perpetrated by someone who is, was, or wishes to be involved in an intimate or dating relationship with an adult or adolescent, and are aimed at establishing control by one partner over the other".[a]
Child exposure to intimate partner violence	". . . a wide range of experiences for children whose caregivers are being abused physically, sexually, or emotionally by an intimate partner. This term includes the child who observes a parent (or guardian) being harmed, threatened, or murdered, who overhears these behaviors . . . or who is exposed to the short- or long-term physical or emotional aftermath of a caregiver's abuse without hearing or seeing a specific aggressive act. . . "[a]
Child maltreatment	"An act or failure to act by a parent, caretaker, or other person as defined under State law which results in physical abuse, neglect, medical neglect, sexual abuse, emotional abuse, or an act or failure to act which presents an imminent risk of serious harm to a child"[b]
Elder abuse	". . . a term referring to any knowing, intentional, or negligent act by a caregiver or any other person that causes harm or a serious risk of harm to a vulnerable adult."[c]

From: [a]*National Consensus guidelines on identifying and responding to domestic violence victimization in health care settings.* San Francisco: The Family Violence Prevention Fund, 2002; National Health Resource Center on Domestic Violence. *National consensus guidelines on identifying and responding to domestic violence victimization in health care settings.* Family Violence Prevention Fund, 2002. Accessed on: July 13, 2005. Available at: http://endabuse.org/health[17]
[b]National Clearinghouse on Child Abuse and Neglect Information. *What is child abuse and neglect?* Washington, DC: National Clearinghouse on Child Abuse and Neglect Information, Children's Bureau, United States Department of Health and Human Services, 2004. Accessed July 13, 2005. Available at: http://nccanch.acf.hhs.gov/pubs/factsheets/whatiscan.cfm[45]
[c]National Center on Elder Abuse. *What is elder abuse?* Washington, DC: Administration on Aging, U.S. Department of Health and Human Services, 2004. Accessed July 13, 2005. Available at: http://www.elderabusecenter.org/default.cfm[46]

IPV is exceedingly common in the United States and throughout the world. Women are far more likely than men to be IPV victims[1] and to be injured or murdered by an intimate partner[2] (see Chap. 29). Worldwide, 10% to more than 50% of women report being hit or otherwise physically harmed by an intimate male partner at some point in their lives.[3] Nearly 5.3 million intimate partner victimizations occur each year among US women ages 18 and older;[4] and 24.8% of women and 7.8% of men surveyed in the United States have been raped and/or physically assaulted by an intimate partner.[1] Rates of IPV reported in health care settings range from a lifetime prevalence of 37% to 54% in women presenting to the emergency department,[5,6] to 5.5% to 22.7% of women presenting to clinics reporting current abuse, and 28% to 66% a history of IPV.[7-9] Although lesbians and gay men experience IPV, little is known about its prevalence in these populations (see Chap. 27). As frightening as these figures appear, they are believed to *underestimate* the problem of IPV; additional efforts are needed to determine the true impact of IPV in the United States and worldwide.

In adults, IPV is correlated with poor mental health, poor physical health, low self-esteem, and numerous specific health problems[9,10] For example, poor pregnancy outcomes (low birth weight, fetal demise) are associated with IPV.[11] IPV also is associated with high-risk sexual practices, and the transmission of sexually transmitted infections, including HIV.[10,12] Although studies have found an association between substance use and IPV, further inquiry and analysis are needed to accurately define the complex relationship between them.[8-10]

In a comprehensive review on IPV, the National Center for Injury Prevention and Control reports that IPV results in nearly 2 million injuries, with more than 555,000 requiring medical attention, and more than 145,000 serious enough to warrant hospitalization. Further, it estimates that the costs of IPV against women exceed an estimated $5.8 billion each year, including $4 billion in direct costs of medical and mental health care and nearly $2 billion in indirect costs (e.g., lost productivity). In addition, IPV is the direct cause of nearly 1300 deaths each year.[4] Intimate partner homicide accounts for 40% to 50% of homicides of women and 5.9% of homicides of men.[2,13] Perpetrators of IPV also have high rates of injury, psychiatric disease, and high-risk sexual behavior.[14,15]

It is estimated that between 3 and 10 million children are exposed to IPV *each* year.[16] Children may witness physical, sexual, and emotional violence; be caught in the "crossfire" of violent acts; or be the intended victims of direct child abuse. Fifty percent of fathers who frequently beat their wives also frequently beat their children.[17] Children exposed to IPV have multiple mental health, physical health, and behavioral problems including posttraumatic stress disorder, depression, anxiety, chronic somatic complaints, learning problems, increased aggression, fearfulness, developmental problems, direct child abuse, injuries, and death.[16,18]

Adults who experienced higher levels of traumatic experiences as children (being abused as children or

Table 30-2. Risk Factors for Perpetration of Intimate Partner Violence

Individual	Relationship	Community
Young age	Marital conflict	Poverty
Low self–esteem	Marital instability	Low social capital
Low income	Male dominance in the family	Factors associated with poverty
Low academic achievement	Poor family functioning	such as overcrowding,
Involvement in aggressive or delinquent	Emotional dependence and insecurity	hopelessness, stress, frustration
behavior as a youth	Belief in strict gender roles	Weak sanctions against domestic
Alcohol use	Desire for power and control in relationships	violence
Drug use	Exhibiting anger and hostility toward a partner	
Witnessing or experiencing violence as a child		
Lack of social networks and social isolation		
Unemployment		

From: National Center for Injury Prevention and Control. *Costs of intimate partner violence against women in the United States.* Centers for Disease Control and Prevention, 2003. Accessed on July 17, 2005. Available at: http://www.cdc.gov/ncipc/pub-res/ipv_cost/IPVBook-Final-Feb18.pdf

witnessing parental violence) engage in more high-risk health behaviors (e.g., smoking cigarettes, using drugs, having a higher number of sexual partners). They also suffer more from adverse health outcomes (e.g., chronic obstructive pulmonary disease, diabetes, myocardial infarctions).[19]

FRAMEWORK FOR UNDERSTANDING INTIMATE PARTNER VIOLENCE

> Carl's father was an alcoholic who severely beat his mother, Carl, and Carl's siblings.

Multiple models of IPV have been developed.[20–22] An "ecological model" is useful to conceptualize the fact that both individual factors and larger environmental factors support the development and persistence of IPV.[3] IPV is thought of as being "passed on" from one generation to the next.[23] Although there are many risk factors for the development of IPV, witnessing parental IPV or being abused by parents are most consistently associated with perpetration of IPV as an adult (Table 30-2).

The Centers for Disease Control and Prevention have summarized "vulnerability" factors that can increase the likelihood of being victimized by an intimate partner (Box 30-1). However, it should be recognized that many IPV victims lack any of these factors, and that men and women with these factors do not necessarily experience IPV.

CHALLENGES TO ADDRESSING INTIMATE PARTNER VIOLENCE IN THE HEALTH CARE SETTING

LACK OF SCREENING

Because risk factors and vulnerability factors are such poor predictors of IPV, its identification requires adoption of routine universal screening. However, the medical community has largely failed to adopt routine screening for IPV despite multiple recommendations by professional medical associations.[18]

Box 30-1. Factors Increasing Vulnerability to Intimate Partner Violence

Individual	Relationship
History of physical abuse	Marital conflict
Prior injury from the same partner	Marital instability
Having a verbally abusive partner	Male dominance in the family
Economic stress	Poor family functioning
Partner history of alcohol or drug abuse	
Childhood abuse	
Being under the age of 24	

From: National Center for *Injury Prevention and Control. Intimate partner violence:* Fact sheet. Accessed July 12, 2005. Available at: http://www.cdc.gov/ncipc/factsheets/ipvfacts.htm[4]

Although it has been argued that there is insufficient evidence that screening for IPV improves health, it is clear that unawareness of IPV can have devastating consequences, leading to inappropriate or even life-threatening medical care. Providers may order invasive tests for physical symptoms related to IPV; patients may be given contraceptives that are not within their control to use and may endanger them if discovered by a perpetrator; couples may be referred for counseling that a perpetrator can use to exert further control over a victim.

Additionally, the vast majority of patients state that they would like their health care providers to ask them about IPV,[23] and that merely disclosing IPV privately to a trusted provider who responds compassionately is highly therapeutic.[24] Further, perpetrators of IPV are regularly seen in the health care setting, yet routine screening for perpetration is done only in rare model centers.[25]

PATIENT BARRIERS

Carl has threatened to have Amalia deported if she reveals the abuse. Amalia's provider has never asked her about IPV. The emergency department providers did not question Carl about the cause of his injury.

The Victim

The main challenge to addressing IPV is the perpetrator's persistent use of assault, coercion, psychological attacks, and other behaviors intended to maintain absolute control. The perpetrator might use physical, sexual, and emotional abuse, social isolation, economic deprivation and control, abuse of children, pets, and property to erode a victim's will and sense of worth. This abusive cycle makes disclosure of IPV and the ability to improve safety through health care interventions extraordinarily challenging. Victims report that their partners directly restrict them from obtaining medical care and threaten violence if they reveal IPV[25,26] and describe multiple barriers to disclosure, including fear of retaliation, low self-esteem and shame, sense of family responsibilities and fear of loss of custody, socioeconomic barriers, the health care provider being too busy or treating the patient negatively, and fear of consequences of mandatory reporting or police involvement.[21,22,24]

The Perpetrator

Although there are excellent guidelines for working with perpetrators of IPV in the health care setting,[25] there are no published trials of face-to-face screening for IPV perpetration. Perpetrators of IPV often minimize and deny their abusive behavior, feel that they themselves are the victims, and lack empathy for those they hurt. If perpetrators are aware of the illegal nature of their acts, they may fear disclosure to a health care provider for legal reasons.

HEALTH CARE PROVIDER BARRIERS

There is growing evidence that clinicians *do not* follow recommended guidelines for addressing IPV in the health care setting. Clinicians have described multiple barriers to addressing IPV, including concern for offending the patient, their discomfort with cultural issues (both differences and similarities), having a personal history of exposure to abuse, and frustration with screening and interventions that are seen as futile.[27-30] Providers also express practical concerns: They may not have time to screen for and respond to IPV; they fear the repercussions of mandatory reporting on patient safety; and they feel they lack adequate education and training about IPV.[28-31]

HEALTH SYSTEM BARRIERS

Among the challenges to implementing IPV screening and treatment programs is a lack of systemwide commitment to their development and implementation, partly because of the remarkable lack of health, health care utilization, and cost outcomes data for health care–related interventions for victims and/or perpetrators of IPV. Further, institutions that do not incorporate extensive system changes at every level of administration and care find it difficult to increase routine IPV screening and IPV identification rates. An ideal systemwide response would require collaboration with community services, the police, and the justice system; be culturally competent; fully coordinate family services; and include mental health, substance use, social services, and advocacy. Many practice settings lack access to trained staff and the resources required to institute an ideal, comprehensive program.

Common Pitfalls

- Failing to inquire directly about IPV
- Blaming the victim for IPV
- Advising the victim to "leave" rather than addressing safety
- Failing to give adequate attention to the needs of children affected by IPV
- Failing to respond to perpetrators of IPV by health care providers
- Failing to develop a coordinated response to IPV
- Lacking a health care response to perpetrators of IPV
- Failing to implement IPV programs in health care organizations
- Lacking culturally appropriate models for addressing IPV

APPROACH TO MANAGING VICTIMS OF INTIMATE PARTNER ABUSE

When the pediatrician sees Elena's poor growth curve and Amalia's exhausted appearance, he touches Amalia's arm and says, "You look so tired and upset. I'm worried about you. Has Carl ever hit you or hurt you in any way?" Amalia bursts into tears and says, "I'm afraid that he will hurt me if he finds out I'm talking to you."

PATIENTS: VICTIMS AND PERPETRATORS

Victims of IPV exhibit remarkable resourcefulness in staying alive and coping, despite experiencing what may be termed "domestic terrorism." Even in the face of threats, survivors of IPV do seek help. Indeed, many who survive IPV develop into skilled advocates who help others affected by IPV informally, in structured support groups, or as health care providers themselves.

On the other hand, most perpetrators seem exceedingly reluctant to acknowledge their role in IPV, much less work to change their behavior. "Batterer's treatment" reaches very few perpetrators of IPV and the dropout rates are very high even when court mandated. However, in a program in Australia, when media messages were broadcast about the damaging effects of IPV on children, many men called a Men's Domestic Violence Hotline and, after speaking with an advocate, accepted referral to a treatment center.[33] Programs are being developed to help young men learn constructive and healthy ways of relating.[31]

SCREENING FOR INTIMATE PARTNER VIOLENCE

Women

Routine screening for IPV victimization increases its identification.[5,9,35] Reporting requirements for IPV and child abuse vary widely; therefore, clinicians need to learn about them for their specific locality and state. The goal of screening is not to force disclosure of IPV; rather, it is to express genuine concern for a patient's safety and well-being, demonstrate respect for the patient's autonomy, and communicate that the health care setting is a confidential and safe place to access help. Over time, through development of a trusting, confidential relationship, this approach can reduce the patient's isolation and enhance the patient's sense of empowerment. It is important to use trained medical interpreters when necessary and ensure they are trained specifically about IPV and principles of confidentiality; often, they can provide invaluable insights into cultural beliefs about IPV.

Detailed guidelines for screening can be accessed online;[36] and multiple mnemonics and tools have been developed to facilitate screening for and assisting with IPV (Box 30-2).[37–42] In general, direct questions increase

---

Box 30-2. Tools to Screen and Assist with Intimate Partner Violence

Mnemonics	**RADAR[a]** **R**outine screening **A**lways ask **D**ocument response **A**ssess safety and lethality **R**espond **SAID[b]** **S**creen **A**ssess **I**ntervene **D**ocument **HITS[c]** tool: How often does your partner **H**urt you physically **I**nsult you **T**alk down to you **T**hreaten you with harm **S**cream or curse at you?
Direct questions	"Has your partner ever hit you or hurt you?" "Has your partner ever threatened you or frightened you?" "Has your partner ever forced you to have sex when you didn't want to?"
Questions about emotional abuse	"How does your partner treat you?" "Does your partner yell at you or frequently criticize you?"

From: [a]Committee on Violence. *Partner violence: How to recognize and treat victims of abuse. A guide for physicians and other health care professionals.* Waltham, MA. Massachusetts Medical Society, 2004. Available at: www.massmed.org
[b]Ruby J, Kimberg L, at www.leapsf.org
[c]Sherin KM, Sinacore JM, Li XQ, et al. HITS: A short domestic violence screening tool for use in a family practice setting. *Fam Med* 1998;30:508–512.

identification of IPV, whereas vague questions about safety rarely elicit disclosures of IPV. Because psychological abuse has been shown to result in poor health outcomes in both women and men,[10] questions about emotional abuse should be included. Introductory phrases can facilitate clinician and patient comfort with screening: "Because violence in relationships is so common, I ask all my patients about it. Has your partner ever hit you or hurt you?"

Men

Newer guidelines advise screening men for victimization as well.[18] These guidelines address current understanding that gay men seem to have rates of victimization equivalent to that of women, some heterosexual men are also victimized, and male victims of IPV also suffer its health consequences. Experts recommend that clinicians screening men should have the skills necessary to distinguish between perpetration and victimization or have access to staff who have this capability. Detailed guidelines for screening and intervention in men are available online.[18,36]

ASSESSMENT OF INTIMATE PARTNER VIOLENCE

Elena's pediatrician supports Amalia: "No one deserves to be treated this way. Hitting another person is never OK." He explains the confidentiality of their interaction as well as his obligation to report child abuse. He asks her about Carl's whereabouts, her immediate safety and that of Elena, and he assesses her emotional state and suicidality. He asks her what she wants to do.

Immediate

Most patients who disclose IPV will disclose *past* IPV. Assessment of past IPV includes inquiry about how the experience of IPV affected a patient's health and life, whether the patient has ongoing contact and/or threats from her or his partner, whether children were involved in the relationship, and how children are coping with the aftermath of the relationship.

In the case of *current* IPV, immediate assessment in the medical setting should include inquiry about the perpetrator (e.g., location, access to weapons) to establish whether the patient and staff are in any potential danger. The clinician can then determine the imminent risk to the victim and children, history of abuse of the children, the emotional state of the victim, and the degree of readiness or desire for change on the part of the victim. In assessing for imminent risk, it is important to inquire about threats with weapons, past use of weapons, and whether the victim thinks she or he is in danger of being killed.[13]

Over Time

The breadth of an assessment done in a primary care setting depends on the preference of the patient, the acuity and severity of the IPV, the expertise of the clinician and health care team, scheduling constraints, and the availability of community services. In some health care settings, the entire assessment and response to IPV may occur within the health care setting. In most cases, both assessment and response to IPV are shared by health care and community IPV services. Over time, it is important for the multidisciplinary team to identify the history and pattern of abuse; the physical, psychological, economic, and social effects of the abuse; and the history of injuries or hospitalizations.

Assessment can be a strong empowerment tool. Emphasizing the patient's strengths during each step of the assessment and suggesting the connection between her health problems and the abuse may help her decide to make changes that increase her safety. It is especially motivating to help a patient understand the effects of abuse on children.

INTERVENTION IN INTIMATE PARTNER VIOLENCE

Elena's pediatrician repeats supportive statements: "The abuse is not your fault. No one deserves to be treated this way." He suggests that the stress of the IPV is causing Elena's irritability and difficulty nursing, emphasizing that Carl's abusive behavior causes the stress and that both Amalia and Elena deserve to be safe. Given Elena's fall and poor growth, they will need to call Child Protective Services (CPS) together; he assures her that he will advocate for their safety. He also schedules an intake in a pioneering program that treats victimized parents and their children together.

He helps Amalia call a hotline, asks the hotline staff to do safety planning with her, provides her with the phone number of a local shelter for Latina women, and asks her whether she would like to file a police report. She is too frightened to file a police report right away but learns how to call the police and what to say to them. Amalia learns through the hotline counselor that she has legal rights to apply for citizenship independent of Carl.

The importance of providing emotional support and pointing out the patient's strengths is a critical component of intervention, and can not be emphasized enough (Box 30-3). Because a patient who is experiencing trauma may have trouble absorbing what is happening during the health care visit, repetition of messages of support is critical. Widening the circle of support for the victim by connecting her or him with supportive members of a multidisciplinary team is also vital: Each person will connect with the victim in an important, different way. In the event of life-threatening emergencies,

Box 30-3. Intervention: Guiding Principles

Regard safety of victims and their children as a priority
Respect the integrity and authority of each woman over her life choices.
Hold perpetrators responsible for the abuse and for stopping it.
Advocate on behalf of victims of domestic violence and their children.

Intervention strategies should include:

- Telephone numbers for local and national 24-hour crisis lines
- Referral to culturally appropriate community services
- An opportunity to develop a personal, specific safety plan in conjunction with the health care team, community advocates, or both

- An opportunity to file a police report; if the patient wishes, a member of the health care team or a community advocate can stay with her during the interview
- Referral to legal services; the federal "Violence Against Women Act" (VAWA) provides funding for family violence programs. It also mandates that women who are victimized may proceed with their immigration process independently; however, the burden of proof is high and requires specialized legal assistance.

From: Warshaw C, Ganley A. *Improving the health care response to domestic violence: A resource manual for health care providers.* San Francisco: Family Violence Prevention Fund, 1998. Available at: http://endabuse.org/programs/display.php3?DocID=238

police need to be summoned immediately. Leaving an abusive relationship can be *extremely* dangerous. Although it is difficult for clinicians to accept, improving safety may or may not involve separation from a partner in the near future, especially in a society in which survivors of IPV are not well protected.

There is little empirical study of the effects of interventions to assist victims of IPV. A study of telephone safety counseling by nurses increased safety behaviors adopted by victims of IPV.[40] Women who received advocacy services structured to teach and support patient self-assessment and problem-solving experienced less violence, increased social support, and higher perceived quality of life.[41] The effects of treating the sequelae of IPV are also not adequately studied, yet clinicians find that every improvement in self-care and health further empowers a victim of IPV. Referring patients to experienced mental health providers enhances safety and addresses mental health problems that may have resulted from the IPV.

Pioneering programs such as the Child Trauma Research Project at San Francisco General Hospital and the Child Witness to Violence Project in Boston are models of child–parent therapy that can help heal children and their nonabusive parents together. Each of these centers begins by focusing on safety planning, restraining orders, and other practical interventions. As safety improves, the therapist works on healing the parent and child individually, and also healing the parent–child relationship. Although there are not yet any randomized controlled trials of this dyadic therapy, initial experience appears promising.[44]

Suspected or confirmed child abuse and neglect must be reported to Child Protective Services (CPS). In some states, merely witnessing IPV is considered reportable. It is essential that the health care team advocate for the safety of both the victimized parent and the children. Some experts recommend that active CPS investigations be reserved for the most severe cases of child abuse and that childhood exposure to IPV is best treated with voluntary, community services specializing in this area.[34]

FOLLOW-UP WITH PERPETRATORS

During treatment in the parent–child program, Amalia leaves Carl. Carl drinks more heavily and is brought to the emergency department with a seizure. An astute emergency department provider suspects a history of violence and refers him to a program for perpetrators.

Clinicians with experience in identifying and intervening in IPV victimization often feel a pressing need to address perpetration as well. There is general agreement that perpetrators should at least be provided with messages that their behaviors are harmful, they are responsible for stopping these harmful behaviors, their children are at heightened risk of learning to participate in violent relationships, and they can change. Because many perpetrators of IPV continue to be involved in their children's lives, some experts have begun to explore the challenging field of "fatherhood and domestic violence."[34]

DOCUMENTATION OF INTIMATE PARTNER VIOLENCE

Elena's provider documents "IPV+" and "poor growth due to IPV" in Elena's chart. This will be useful to Amalia in court proceedings.

Guidelines have been developed that discuss the proper documentation of IPV in medical records.[43] It is essential to write legibly, document as many specifics as possible, use the victim's own words in quotes, and describe injuries with detailed descriptions, diagrams, and photographs.

INSTITUTIONAL SOLUTIONS

A "systems change" approach seems the most promising for institutionalizing IPV programs. A Kaiser-care facility implemented a multifaceted approach to IPV services to increase provider referrals of patients, patient and staff awareness, and patient satisfaction. IPV information was provided directly to patients through posters in examination rooms, pamphlets and safety cards in bathrooms, and education about IPV and self-referral to IPV services in member newsletters. Providers were given brief training on addressing IPV and how to refer patients to the services offered by mental health providers. Chart prompts, IPV guidelines, IPV "tool kits," pocket reference cards, patient information materials, and feedback on referrals made to IPV services were all introduced as part of this approach. Mental health clinicians who could perform danger assessments and safety planning, invite patients to an on-site support group, and refer patients to community-based services were made available. A community-based IPV advocacy agency agreed to provide a crisis team to the health care facility whenever needed. This multifaceted approach resulted in a 260% increase in referrals to the IPV specialist. A telephone survey to members demonstrated that on all measures of awareness of IPV services at the facility or recollection of having been asked about IPV, patient awareness increased significantly. Member satisfaction with IPV services also increased.[44] The Family Violence Prevention Fund has a checklist for scoring institutional change and a tool to assess potential cost savings associated with addressing IPV in the health care setting.[47]

VICARIOUS TRAUMATIZATION AND STAFF INTIMATE PARTNER VIOLENCE

Working with patients affected by IPV can take an emotional toll on already overworked and stressed health care providers. Medical providers and health care staff are not immune to IPV,[28] and almost invariably, during the process of implementing IPV programs, staff privately or publicly self-identify as being affected by IPV. Resources that describe workplace safety responses for staff IPV are available online at: http://endabuse.org/workplace/

CONCLUSION

IPV is a common and devastating problem that has long-term health consequences for all members in a family. Although the challenges are many, clinicians, given their access to the intimate lives of their patients, are uniquely situated to address IPV and ameliorate the suffering not only of their patients, but perhaps of generations to come as well.

KEY CONCEPTS

- **Address IPV with each patient.**
  —Ask all women about IPV (and, once experienced, ask men about IPV also).
  —Provide supportive messages to victims of IPV.
  —Provide culturally appropriate resources and referrals to victims and perpetrators of IPV.
  —Document IPV and its effects legibly and with detail (through direct quotes, diagrams, and photos).
- **Address the effects of IPV on children.**
  —Ask how children are exposed to IPV.
  —Advocate for the victimized parent's safety when Child Protective Services or other authorities are involved.
  —Advise treatment of children in a program that specializes in trauma treatment for children.
- **Use institutional supports to encourage providers to address IPV.**
  —Establish a screening, treatment, and safety protocol.
  —Provide ongoing, interactive training for all staff.
  —Incorporate written or electronic chart prompts.
  —Address patient–provider confidentiality issues.
  —Assess adherence to protocol through routine quality improvement studies.
- **Make resources available to all patients regardless of whether IPV is disclosed.**
  —Place posters prominently in health care settings.
  —Place small safety cards in private places (bathrooms, examination rooms).
  —Directly advertise and educate all patients about culturally specific and appropriate IPV services.
  —Post crisis phone numbers and the national hotline 1-800-799-SAFE.
- **Establish a mechanism for supporting health care staff.**
  —Support health care staff directly affected by IPV.
  —Support all health care staff exposed to patient trauma by routinely addressing vicarious traumatization.

CORE COMPETENCY

Intimate Partner Violence (IPV) Screening and Treatment Guidelines for Medical Providers

Screening	Assessment	Intervention	Documentation	Reporting
1. Establish privacy (screen patient alone) 2. Use staff or trained medical interpreters if needed (not family or friends) 3. Ask direct questions: • Has your partner ever hit you, hurt you, or threatened you? • Does your partner make you feel afraid? • Has your partner ever forced you to have sex when you didn't want to? 4. Ask indirect questions: • How does your partner treat you? • Do you feel safe at home? 5. Ask about past history of IPV: • Have you *ever* had a partner who hit you, hurt you, or threatened you? • Have you *ever* had a partner who treated you badly? • Have you *ever* had a partner who forced you to have sex when you didn't want to?	Assessment of current IPV Assess immediately 1. Safety in clinic • Is perpetrator with patient? 2. Current safety • Threats of homicide • Weapons involved • History of strangulation or stalking 3. Suicidality and homicidality 4. Safety of children Assess over time 1. Pattern of abuse 2. History of effects of abuse • Injuries/hospitalization • Physical and psychological health effects • Economic, social, or other effects 3. Support and coping strategies 4. Readiness for change Assessment of past IPV 1. Current safety ("Are you (and your children) safe from this person now?") 2. History of effects of abuse • Injuries/hospitalization • Physical and psychological health effects • Economic, social, or other effects	1. Give repeated messages of support 2. Offer crisis phone numbers 3. Assist in preparing a safety plan (or connect patient with a person who can) 4. Offer advocacy and counseling 5. Offer police and legal assistance 6. Arrange for follow-up visits and a safe way to contact patient 7. Expand the patient's support to multiple members of a multidisciplinary team if patient agrees (provider, community and clinic based advocates, social worker, nurse, counselor, etc.)	1. History • Write legibly • Use patient's own words in quotes • Document as much info as patient will provide regarding specific events (who, what, where, when) 2. Physical findings • Describe injuries in detail • Draw diagrams of injuries • If patient consents, take photographs of injuries • Take serial photographs of injuries over time 3. Physical evidence • If patient consents, preserve physical evidence in *paper* bag • Describe physical evidence in detail	1. If patient is injured, file a mandatory health care report to police (in CA) 2. If you suspect children are being neglected or harmed, file a CPS report. (Advocate on behalf of adult victim/survivor's safety with CPS) 3. If patient is ≥65 or a dependent adult, file an Adult Protective Services (APS) report

From: Kimberg L. Maxine Hall Health Center. Phone: 415-292-1300 (updated 2/2/05) Available at: www.leapsf.org

DISCUSSION QUESTIONS

1. Discuss how speaking limited English (or one's culture, race, ethnicity, sexual orientation) might affect one's experience with IPV and one's interaction with the health care system.
2. Discuss ways you have introduced (or could introduce) the topic of IPV with patients and then role play, asking about IPV and being supportive to a patient affected by IPV. How would you change your approach in a pediatric setting?
3. Imagine you have a patient who was severely abused as a child and presents to the health care setting in repeated abusive relationships. How would you approach this patient? How might you sustain your morale while working with this patient over time?

RESOURCES

http://endabuse.org

http://www.mincava.umn.edu

http://www.leapsf.org

http://www.cdc.gov/ncipc/factsheets/ipvfacts.htm

http://www.acestudy.org/

http://www.elderabusecenter.org/

http://nccanch.acf.hhs.gov/

Gelles RJ. *Intimate violence in families,* 3rd ed. Thousand Oaks, CA: Sage Publications, 1997.

Saakvitne KW, Pearlman LA. *Transforming the pain: A workbook on vicarious traumatization.* New York, NY: WW Norton & Company, 1996.

National Center for Injury Prevention and Control. *Intimate partner violence: Fact sheet.* Bethesda, MD: Centers for Disease Control and Prevention, 2004. Accessed July 12, 2005. Available at: http://www.cdc.gov/ncipc/factsheets/ipvfacts.htm

Nicolaides C. *Voices of survivors.* video (at endabuse.org)

Screen to end abuse. Family Violence Prevention Fund videotape (at endabuse.org).

REFERENCES

1. Tjaden P, Thoennes N. *Prevalence, incidence, and consequences of violence against women: Findings from the National Violence Against Women Survey.* National Institute of Justice and Center for Disease Control and Prevention, November 1998. Available at: www.ojp.usdoj.gov/nij/pubs-sum/172837.htm

2. Paulozzi LJ, Saltzman LE, Thompson MP, et al. Surveillance for homicide among intimate partners: United States, 1981–1998. *MMWR CDC Surveill Summ* 2001;50:1–15.

3. Heise L, Ellsberg M, Gottemoeller M. *Ending violence against women.* Center for Gender Equity and Change and Johns Hopkins University School of Public Health, Population Information Program. December 1999, Series L, No. 11. Available at: www.jhuccp.org

4. National Center for Injury Prevention and Control. *Costs of intimate partner violence against women in the United States.* Centers for Disease Control and Prevention, 2003. Accessed on July 17, 2005. Available at: http://www.cdc.gov/ncipc/pub-res/ipv_cost/IPVBook-Final-Feb18.pdf

5. Abbott J, Johnson R, Koziol-McLain J, et al. Domestic violence against women. Incidence and prevalence in an emergency department population. *JAMA* 1995;273:1763–1767.

6. Dearwater SR, Coben JH, Campbell JC, et al. Prevalence of intimate partner abuse in women treated at community hospital emergency departments. *JAMA* 1998;280: 433–438.

7. Coker AL, Smith PH, Bethea L, et al. Physical health consequences of physical and psychological intimate partner violence. *Arch Fam Med* 2000;9:451–457.

8. Gin NE, Rucker L, Frayne S, et al. Prevalence of domestic violence among patients in three ambulatory care internal medicine clinics. *J Gen Intern Med* 1991;6: 317–322.

9. McCauley J, Kern DE, Kolodner K, et al. The "battering syndrome": Prevalence and clinical characteristics of domestic violence in primary care internal medicine practices. *Ann Intern Med* 1995;123:737–746.

10. Coker AL, Davis KE, Arias I, et al. Physical and mental health effects of intimate partner violence for men and women. *Am J Prev Med* 2002;23:260–268.

11. Coker AL, Sanderson M, Dong B. Partner violence during pregnancy and risk of adverse pregnancy outcomes. *Paediatr Perinat Epidemiol* 2004;18:260–269.

12. Hillis SD, Anda RF, Felitti VJ, et al. Adverse childhood experiences and sexual risk behaviors in women: A retrospective cohort study. *Fam Plann Perspect* 2001;33: 206–211.

13. Campbell JC, Webster D, Koziol-McLain J, et al. Risk factors for femicide in abusive relationships: Results from a multisite case control study. *Am J Public Health* 2003; 93:1089–1097.

14. el-Bassel N, Fontdevila J, Gilbert L, et al. HIV risks of men in methadone maintenance treatment programs who abuse their intimate partners: A forgotten issue. *J Subst Abuse* 2001;13:29–43.

15. Gerlock AA. Health impact of domestic violence. *Issues Ment Health Nurs* 1999;20:373–385.

16. Edleson JL. Children's witnessing of adult domestic violence. *J Interpers Violence* 1999;14:839–870.

17. Straus M, Gelles R. *Physical violence in American families: Risk factors and adaptations to violence in 8,145 families.* Family Violence Prevention Fund. Piscataway, NJ: Transaction Publishers, 1990. Available at: http://endabuse.org/resources/facts/

18. National Health Resource Center on Domestic Violence. *National consensus guidelines on identifying and responding to domestic violence victimization in health care settings.* Family Violence Prevention Fund, 2002. Accessed on July 13, 2005. Available at: http://endabuse.org/health

19. Felitti VJ, Anda RF, Nordenberg D, et al. Relationship of childhood abuse and household dysfunction to the many leading causes of death in adults. The Adverse Childhood Experiences (ACE) Study. *Am J Prev Med* 1998;14: 245–248.

20. Asian Pacific Islander American Health Forum, 2005. *Domestic violence: A tightly coiled spring.* Accessed on July 13, 2005. Available at: http://www.apiahf.org/apidvinstitute/ResearchAndPolicy/analyze_b.htm

21. Duluth Model. Minnesota Program Development, Inc. Available at: http://www.duluth-model.org/documents/wheelshandout.pdf

22. Walker L. *The battered woman.* New York: Harper & Row, 1979.

23. Widom C. Does Violence Beget Violence? A Critical Examination of the Literature. *Psychological Bulletin* 1989; 106:3–28.

24. Rodriguez MA, Quiroga SS, Bauer HM. Breaking the silence. Battered women's perspectives on medical care. *Arch Fam Med* 1996;5:153–158.

25. Gerbert B, Johnston K, Caspers N, et al. Experiences of battered women in health care settings: A qualitative study. *Women Health* 1996;24:1–7.

26. Ganley A. Health care responses to perpetrators of domestic violence. In: Ganley A, Warshaw C, eds. *Improving the health care response to violence: A resource manual for health care providers.* San Francisco: Family Violence Prevention Fund, 1998.

27. McCauley J, Yurk RA, Jenckes MW, et al. Inside "Pandora's box": Abused women's experiences with clinicians and health services. *J Gen Intern Med* 1998;13:549–555.

28. deLahunta EA, Tulsky AA. Personal exposure of faculty and medical students to family violence. *JAMA* 1996;275: 1903–1906.

29. Rodriguez MA, Bauer HM, McLoughlin E, et al. Screening and intervention for intimate partner abuse: Practices and attitudes of primary care physicians. *JAMA* 1999a;282:468–474.

30. Sugg NK, Inui T. Primary care physicians' response to domestic violence. Opening Pandora's box. *JAMA* 1992;267:3157–3160.

31. Sugg NK, Thompson RS, Thompson DC, et al. Domestic violence and primary care. Attitudes, practices, and beliefs. *Arch Fam Med* 1999;8:301–306.

32. Rodriguez MA, McLoughlin E, Bauer HM, et al. Mandatory reporting of intimate partner violence to police: Views of physicians in California. *Am J Public Health* 1999b;89:575–578.

33. Gibbons L, Paterson D. *Freedom from fear campaign against domestic violence: An innovative approach to reducing crime.* August 2000. Available at: http://www.aic.gov.au/conferences/ criminality/gibbons.pdf

34. Jaffe P, Baker L, Cunningham A. *Protecting children from domestic violence: Strategies for community intervention.* New York: The Guilford Press, 2004.

35. McFarlane J, Christoffel K, Bateman L, et al. Assessing for abuse: Self-report versus nurse interview. *Public Health Nurs* 1991;8:245–250.

36. Groves BM, Augustyn M, Lee D, et al. Identifying and responding to domestic violence: Consensus recommendations for child and adolescent health. The Family Violence Prevention Fund, 2002. Available at: http://endabuse.org/programs/healthcare/files/Pediatric.pdf

37. Committee on Violence. *Partner violence: How to recognize and treat victims of abuse. A guide for physicians and other health care professionals.* Waltham, MA. Massachusetts Medical Society, 2004. Available at: www.massmed.org

38. McFarlane J, Parker B, Soeken K, et al. Assessing for abuse during pregnancy. Severity and frequency of injuries and associated entry into prenatal care. *JAMA* 1992;267:3176–3178.

39. Sherin KM, Sinacore JM, Li XQ, et al. HITS: A short domestic violence screening tool for use in a family practice setting. *Fam Med* 1998;30:508–512.

40. McFarlane J, Malecha A, Gist J, et al. Increasing the safety-promoting behaviors of abused women. *Am J Nurs* 2004;104:40–50.

41. Sullivan C. Using the ESID Model to Reduce Intimate Male Violence Against Women. *Am J Community Psychol* 2003;32:295–303.

42. Groves BM. *Children who see too much: Lessons from the Child Witness to Violence Project.* Boston: Beacon Press, 2002.

43. Warshaw C, Ganley A. *Improving the health care response to domestic violence: A resource manual for health care providers.* Family Violence Prevention Fund, 1998. Accessed July 17, 2005. Available at: http://endabuse.org/programs/display.php3?DocID=238

44. McCaw B, Berman WH, Syme SL, et al. Beyond screening for domestic violence: A systems model approach in a managed care setting. *Am J Prev Med* 2001;21:170–176.

45. National Clearinghouse on Child Abuse and Neglect Information. *What is child abuse and neglect?* Washington, DC: National Clearinghouse on Child Abuse and Neglect Information, Children's Bureau, United States Department of Health and Human Services, 2004. Accessed July 13, 2005. Available at: http://nccanch.acf.hhs.gov/pubs/factsheets/whatiscan.cfm

46. National Center on Elder Abuse. *What is elder abuse?* Washington, DC: Administration on Aging, U.S. Department of Health and Human Services, 2004. Accessed July 13, 2005. Available at: http://www.elderabusecenter.org/default.cfm

47. Family Violence Prevention Fund and Physicians for a Violence Free Society. *New tools to make the business case for domestic violence programs.* Family Violence Prevention Fund. Accessed on July 18, 2005. Available at: http://endabuse.org/programs/display.php3?DocID=9932

Chapter 31

Obesity as a Clinical and Social Problem

Ann Smith Barnes, MD, Marisa Rogers, MD, MPH, and Cam-Tu Tran, MD, MS

Objectives

- Define obesity.
- Describe the populations most affected by obesity.
- Describe the health consequences of obesity.
- Discuss the difficulties with losing weight, including patient and health care provider challenges.
- Suggest ways for health care providers to discuss weight loss with patients.
- Describe strategies for weight loss.

Esmeralda, a 15-year-old girl, requests a written excuse to skip school physical education classes. Her body mass index (BMI) of 32 reveals that she is in the highest weight category for girls her age. She often skips breakfast and eats most meals in front of the television. Her family members are also all obese and have type II diabetes.

Americans young and old are being affected by obesity and its complications. Indeed, the obesity "epidemic" may be one of the most significant challenges to the health of the nation. Lacking resources to eat healthily and exercise adequately, poor families are particularly affected.

Tackling the obesity epidemic will be no easy feat: Its causes are complex, bridging societal issues (such as governmental subsidies of high caloric food), and personal ones (how active people are). Although health care providers need to be engaged in the wider public health and community efforts addressing obesity, helping patients as they strive to lose weight or suffer from its consequences remains equally important. This chapter discusses both the challenges and strategies of addressing obesity.

DEFINITIONS OF OBESITY

The most widely used classification system for obesity—an abnormal accumulation of body fat—in adults is the body mass index (BMI). The BMI estimates the amount of body fat through a calculation that adjusts weight for height (see Resources for online BMI calculator). A normal adult BMI is between 18.5 and 24.9. BMIs between 25 and 29.9 indicate overweight, a BMI greater than 30 indicates obesity, and a BMI greater than 40 indicates morbid obesity. Increasing BMI is associated with an increased risk of death from cancers and cardiovascular disease, particularly in nonsmokers with no history of disease.[1]

BMI for children, unlike adults, is both age and gender specific because children's bodies change dramatically as they grow, and these changes differ between boys and girls. Assessments of BMI for children, also

Classification	BMI-for-Age
Underweight	<5th percentile
Normal	5th percentile to <85th percentile
At risk of overweight	85th percentile to <95th percentile
Overweight	>95th percentile

From: *Body mass index*. Bethesda, MD: Centers for Disease Control and Prevention, 2005. Available at: http://www.cdc.gov/nccdphp/dnpa/bmi/bmi-for-age.htm[2]

called BMI-for-age, avoid using the term obese and categorize children as underweight, normal, at risk for becoming overweight, or overweight (Box 31-1).[2]

In adults the *waist circumference*—the body circumference measured at the level of the superior iliac crest—is another measurement that some argue better explains obesity-related health risk. Increased waist circumference, a measure of central adiposity, has been shown to be a marker for increased risk even in persons of normal weight. A waist circumference greater than 40 inches in men, and 35 inches in women is considered abnormal and increases the risk of developing hypertension, dyslipidemia, and metabolic syndrome.[3]

EPIDEMIOLOGY OF OBESITY

The number of overweight and obese people in the United States has significantly increased in recent decades (Fig. 31-1). In 2001 to 2002, 65.7% of adults were either overweight or obese. Of these, 30.6% of adults were obese and 5.1% morbidly obese. Close to 50% of children between the ages of 6 and 19 are considered to be abnormally heavy. In general, the highest rates of obesity are found in some Native American groups, Latinos, and African Americans as well as populations with less education and lower income levels.[4] This is true for children as well, with

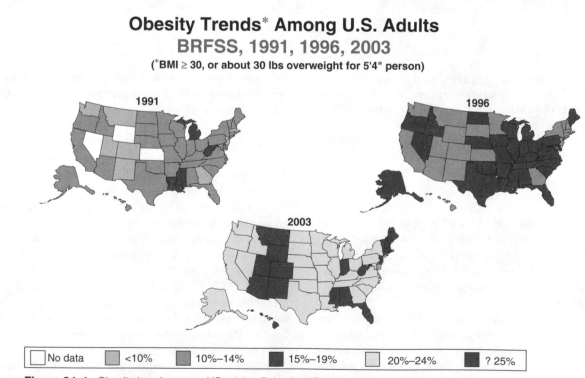

Obesity Trends* Among U.S. Adults
BRFSS, 1991, 1996, 2003
(*BMI ≥ 30, or about 30 lbs overweight for 5'4" person)

| No data | <10% | 10%–14% | 15%–19% | 20%–24% | ? 25% |

Figure 31-1. Obesity trends among US adults. Behavioral Risk Factor Surveillance System, 1991, 1996, 2003. (*BMI ≥ 30, or about 30 lbs overweight for 5'4" person) (*Source:* Behavioral Risk Factor Surveillance System, CDC. Accessed July 12, 2005. Available at: http://www.cdc.gov/nccdphp/dnpa/obesity/trend/maps/index.htm)

Table 31-1. Common Health Consequences of Obesity

Illness	Pediatric	Adult
Hypertension[a]	*	*
Hyperlipidemia[a]	*	*
Type 2 diabetes[a]	*	*
Obstructive sleep apnea	*	*
Gallbladder disease	*	*
Osteoarthritis		*
Cancer (endometrial, colon, breast, prostate)		*

[a]Cardiovascular risk factor.

more African-American and Latino boys and girls in the higher weight categories.

HEALTH CONSEQUENCES OF OBESITY

The health consequences of obesity for both adults and children are significant (Table 31-1). Complications such as hypertension, diabetes, elevated cholesterol levels, and sleep apnea increase the risk of cardiovascular disease, which remains the leading cause of death in both men and women. Not surprisingly, those with the highest rates of obesity suffer from the highest rates of these cardiovascular diseases as well.[5] The same trend even extends to children. For example, nearly half of the newly diagnosed diabetes cases in pediatric populations are type 2 diabetes. This increase is attributable to increasing rates of obesity in children and is highest in African Americans, Mexican Americans, and Native Americans.[6] Other complications of obesity, such as osteoarthritis or depression, may not be as life threatening, but may be crippling. Remember that arthritis is the most common cause of disability in the United States.

Some of the health consequences of obesity can be mitigated by physical fitness. Those who are obese but physically fit have better mortality rates than their sedentary counterparts. However, both groups have mortality rates greater than individuals who are physically fit and not obese.[7,8] Therefore, patients and health care providers should note that although physical activity is beneficial, it is not a substitute for weight loss.

LOSING WEIGHT IS HARD TO DO

Esmeralda's mother works two sedentary jobs. She has failed at multiple attempts to lose weight. The family eats cheap, fatty, high-calorie food. No one in the family feels they have the money, time, or energy to exercise.

PATIENT CHALLENGES

The battle to lose weight is often thwarted by lack of time to prepare food at home and the resources to make healthy choices.

Diet

Eating out at restaurants and eating prepared food have become common and perhaps necessary occurrences as women have exchanged household work for paid labor. The National Restaurant Association reports the typical American household spent an average 34% to 49% of their total food dollars on food away from home in 2002.

Both the larger portion sizes and poorer nutritional quality of the food prepared or consumed outside the home encourage higher energy and fat intake than home-cooked foods. Portion sizes have been increasing both in prepackaged, ready-to-eat products and at restaurants. Consumption is fueled by these larger sizes, which, marketed as giving you more for your money, may appeal especially to low-income families.[9]

Food Prices

Food prices influence food consumption. In the United States, income is associated with the type of food consumed, not the quantity. Calorie-dense foods like sodas, fruit drinks, and snack foods are cheap. Healthier foods, such as fruits and vegetables, are sold more frequently in grocery stores in wealthier neighborhoods and, not surprisingly, are more expensive. Ironically, government subsidies favoring corn syrup production underlie some of these price differences.

Physical Activity

Lack of physical activity hampers efforts at weight control and health maintenance. Longer work hours and increasing time devoted to television viewing and other related media (videos and computers) have been cited as important factors the decline in physical activity. A 2003 study found that 54% of US parents say they have little or no time, or wish they had more time to spend in physical activities with their children. Approximately 3.5 million households caring for more than 7 million US children spend an hour or less per week doing physical activities with their children.[10]

If spending time with children is hard to do, finding time for physical activity is almost impossible for many working parents. The 2000 National Health Interview Survey showed that those at the greatest risk for obesity, women and people with lower education and income levels, have both little control and little activity in their daily routines.[11]

Environmental Barriers

Watching television is problematic not only because it is a sedentary activity, but television and radio advertisements highlight quick and easy access to food that is already prepared and of low nutritional value. Children in particular are targeted for advertising, even in schools. Some school districts, in search of extra revenue, have contracted with soft drink companies who have vending machines throughout the school district. Some schools also have eliminated recess and physical education, decreasing children's daily physical activity. Adults do not fare much better, as long workdays and increasing family demands serve as barriers to regular exercise.

Low-income urban neighborhoods impose other impediments to healthy lifestyles as well. The dearth of grocery stores offering fresh produce and lean meat and plethora of fast food restaurants and convenience stores encourage high-fat, low-fiber diets. Ability to exercise may be compromised by insufficient playgrounds, and parks and trails for walking or biking. Existing areas may not be perceived to be safe. Major fitness centers rarely open exercise facilities in low-income areas, and their membership costs are expensive in any case.

Cultural Norms

Patients' motivation to lose weight is also influenced by cultural norms and expectations. Many studies have demonstrated that African Americans and some Latinos are more accepting of a larger body size than whites and Asian Americans.[12-16] Consequently, some obese women may not recognize themselves as having a weight problem. An example of a body size rating scale is shown in Fig. 31-2.

The degree of acculturation can influence desired body size preference. A study of Latina women showed that those who immigrated to the United States after the age of 17 were more accepting of larger sizes than those born in the United States or who immigrated at an earlier age.[17] These perceptions also may influence children's weight. For example, a recent study demonstrated that Latina women were less likely to recognize obesity in their children and perceived their children to be too thin if they were in the 50th and 75th percentiles of BMI-for-age and only slightly overweight if they were in the >97th percentile.[18]

The role of food in many cultures also can have an enormous impact on diet, and subsequently, weight control. In focus groups with mothers from low socioeconomic strata, they admitted to using sweets to bribe their children or reward good behavior and to encouraging them to eat more even when they were full.[19] The use of food as reward, bribe, or pacifier and the notion of "cleaning the plate" are issues that need to be addressed in discussions of diet because they relate to healthful eating within families.

Discrimination Based on Weight

Although little studied, obese people's experiences suggest that their weight has contributed to negative treatment by strangers and friends, at job interviews, in the work place, in social settings, at exercise facilities, and by health care providers.[20,21] Many of the same groups that suffer discrimination based on race, socioeconomic status, and education are more likely to be obese, and consequently suffer an inordinate amount of prejudice.

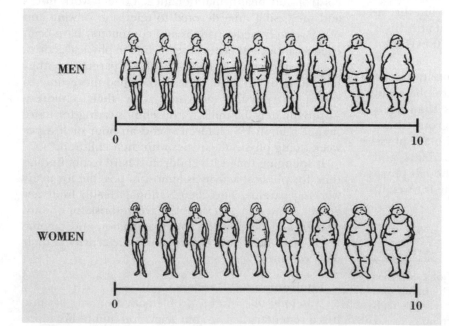

Figure 31-2. Figure rating scale. Reprinted from: Stunkard T, Schulsinger F. Use of the Danish Adoption Register for the study of obesity and thinness. In: Kety SS, Rowland LP, Sidman RL, et al, eds. *The genetics of neurological and psychiatric disorders.* New York: Raven Press, 1983:115–120.

It is important to acknowledge that subtle forms of discrimination exist in the health care setting (scales that do not weigh individuals over 300 pounds, chairs with arm rests that are too narrow for obese patients, blood pressure cuffs that are too small for proper measurements). In addition, health care providers often are guilty of blaming the obese patient for their weight problems and rarely consider the environmental, economic, and social influences on the weight of their patients.[22] Obese patients may feel that health care providers are not genuinely concerned about them or their health when simple courtesies are neglected. The feeling of second-class treatment or being blamed for a medical problem can negatively affect a person's interest in discussing weight loss with a provider. Recognizing and discussing an obese patient's discomfort in the medical setting can open lines of communication and foster trust relating to all health issues, including weight.

HEALTH CARE PROVIDER CHALLENGES

Obesity is a preventable disease and often is described as the second leading cause of preventable death (tobacco use is the first) in the United States. However, in addition to the difficulties faced by patients, providers have their own struggles in assisting patients with weight loss.

Identifying Obesity as a Health Issue

Although overweight and obesity can be identified through the BMI calculation, practitioners identify, document, and counsel only a fraction of patients whose BMI classifies them as obese.[23,24] Without identification of obesity, management strategies cannot be planned.

Conflicting Priorities

Providers must choose among many patient problems to address. Although obesity often underlies many health problems faced by patients, these acute medical problems generally become the focus of care. When faced with high blood glucose, clinicians usually choose to treat the diabetes and save discussions of weight loss for later.

Barriers to Weight Loss Counseling

Health providers have themselves identified barriers to weight loss counseling: insufficient time, disbelief that counseling will help, and lack of skills to provide counseling.[25,26] In addition to obesity, low-income and minority patients often have multiple medical and nonmedical issues limiting time for weight reduction counseling. Furthermore, many patients from these groups have not been as successful with weight loss as white participants

in large (nonculturally tailored) weight loss trials.[27] Therefore, health care provider expectations of success may be low, which further hinders clinician initiation of counseling. Despite brief intervention methods that have demonstrated success with weight loss,[25] providers have not learned how to implement counseling in their practices.

Common Pitfalls

- Neglecting patient time and cost concerns in counseling efforts
- Not addressing need for family involvement in weight loss efforts
- Not recognizing environmental barriers to healthy lifestyles
- Not incorporating cultural expectations of ideal weight into weight loss goals
- Not regularly providing identification of obesity as a health problem
- Allowing the health consequences of obesity to overwhelm clinical encounters, leaving little time for weight reduction counseling
- Lacking the skills to counsel patients on weight loss

TIPPING THE SCALE IN FAVOR OF HEALTH

APPROACH TO WEIGHT CONTROL

Identify the Problem with Patients

Each patient encounter is an opportunity to address weight management. Height, weight, and BMI should be recorded at every visit. For children, BMI should be plotted onto an age-specific-BMI growth chart (Box 31-1).[2] Cardiac risk factors and comorbidities related to obesity should be assessed.

Obese and overweight adults with obesity-related comorbidities or cardiac risk factors, and children who are overweight or at risk of overweight should be targeted. Elderly patients also should be advised to lose weight: Weight reduction has similar effects in improving cardiovascular disease risk factors in older and younger adults.

The provider should communicate to the patient the specific BMI and the related diagnosis, actually using the term *obesity* if applicable. Also inform patients that obesity puts them at risk for related comorbidities and how it impacts their current health conditions (Table 31-2).

Personalizing the message can be a useful tool. For example, patients may respond more to the message that weight puts them at risk for diabetes if they have family members who have suffered complications from

Table 31-2. Classification of Overweight and Obesity by Body Mass Index (BMI), Waist Circumference, and Associated Disease Risks

| Classification | BMI (kg/m²) | Obesity Class | Disease Risk for Type 2 Diabetes, Hypertension, and Cardiovascular Disease Relative to Normal Weight and Waist Circumference[a] | |
			Men 102 cm (40 in) or less Women 88 cm (35 in) or less	Men >102 cm (40 in) Women >88 cm (35 in)
Underweight	<18.5		—	—
Normal	18.5–24.9		—	—
Overweight	25.0–29.9		Increased	High
Obesity	30.0–34.9	I	High	Very high
	35.0–39.9	II	Very high	Very high
Extreme obesity	>40.0	III	Extremely high	Extremely high

[a]Increased waist circumference can also be a marker for increased risk even in persons of normal weight.
Adapted from: *Aim for a healthy weight.* Bethesda, MD: National Heart, Lung, and Blood Institute. Available at: http://www.nhlbi.nih.gov/health/public/heart/obesity/lose_wt/bmi_dis.htm[40]

diabetes. Patients' concerns about being overweight should be elicited as well. In all interactions, a non-judgmental and supportive attitude is essential in effectively communicating about weight control.

Motivate the Patient (and Family) to Make Changes

Behavioral changes are difficult to achieve. If patients are not ready to make the necessary adjustments that losing weight requires, providers' counseling efforts can fall on deaf ears. The Prochaska and DiClemente stages—precontemplation, contemplation, action, and maintenance—can be used to assess patients' motivation for weight loss (see Chap. 7). A precontemplative patient is not ready to lose weight and may not recognize how his or her behavior contributes to the problem. The contemplative patient is considering but not committed to change. In the precontemplative and contemplation phases, providers should focus on increasing readiness to lose weight. In the action phase, a patient is either losing weight or is ready to: This is the time to target weight loss. The maintenance patient has lost weight and is trying to keep it off. With children, the entire family must be ready for change. Because children can gain weight quickly, frequent visits can be helpful in reassessing family motivation.

Set Realistic Goals with Patients

Patients often have unrealistic weight loss goals. In most weight loss interventions, participants rarely lose and maintain more than 10% of their body weight, although many patients want to lose much more of their current body weight.[28] To minimize disappointment, providers should help patients set realistic and attainable goals. Decreasing body weight by 5% to 10%

over 6 months generally can be obtained by a weight loss of 1 to 2 pounds per week depending on a patient's BMI. A change in BMI that moves patients from the obese to overweight category is a success. In growing children, stabilizing weight gain is a desirable and attainable goal. Weight loss should only be attempted in adolescents who have completed their sexual maturity and bone growth.

Goals should not be limited to weight loss. For some patients preventing further weight gain or maintaining a lower weight for the long term are appropriate goals. Goals not involving weight also can serve as motivating influences. Some examples of realistic and attainable non–weight loss goals include fitting into a certain clothing size, taking a regular walk with family after dinner, adding daily fresh fruits or vegetables, or simply feeling better about oneself.

Counsel on Improving Diet

Any successful weight loss effort incorporates changes in diet. Despite lack of formal training and time constraints, providers can and should play an active role in this area.

Elicit Useful, Accurate Information A food diary—a detailed record of everything eaten during the day—provides the most accurate information about what the patient is eating, although they are difficult to complete. Alternatively, the patient can be asked to name everything eaten in the past 24 hours, including beverages and snacks. Other useful information includes: how often the patient eats out, at what types of restaurants (making sure to specifically ask about fast food), what beverages are typically consumed, and how meals are prepared (e.g., fried, baked, broiled). The information gleaned can be used to provide personalized messages about healthier eating. For example, a teenager eating fast food several times a week can be counseled to reduce intake and replace high-calorie food such as french fries and milk shakes with a side salad and water.

Portion Size Most people eat too much as an individual serving. Unfortunately this is fueled by US restaurants, which often serve two to three times as much as the appropriate serving. A simple teaching plate diagram can help educate patients about portions, instructing patients that for lunch and dinner half of the plate should be comprised of fruits and vegetables, a quarter meat or other source of protein, and a quarter carbohydrate (Fig. 31-3). This results in larger servings of fruits and vegetables and decreases in meat and starches. Appropriate serving sizes also can be equated with everyday objects. For example, a serving of meat should be roughly the size of a deck of cards, a serving of rice, pasta, or potato the size of a half a baseball, and a baked potato the size of a fist.[29]

Fad Diets It is important to counsel patients appropriately about fad diets. The data suggest that low-carbohydrate diets cause people to lose more weight in the short term, but that at 1 year the amount of weight lost is similar to more conventional low-fat diets.[30] These diets are difficult to maintain. For patients who are very interested in trying a fad diet, the initial weight loss can serve as a kick-start, but patients must realize that better long-term eating habits will be necessary to keep weight off.

A Balanced, Healthful Diet When counseling patients about diet options, healthier approaches that recommend a well-balanced eating plan of fresh fruits and vegetables, whole grains, low-fat dairy, and lean protein are best.

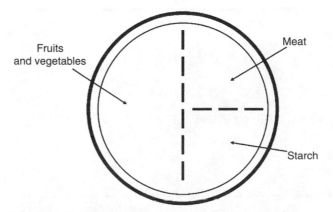

Figure 31-3. Plate diagram. Food portions: What your plate should look like.

Counting Calories To lose weight, calories expended must exceed calories taken in. To lose 1 pound per week, one must have a deficit of 500 kcal/day. Often, this can be achieved by a diet of 1200 to 1500 kcal/day for women and 1500 to 1800 kcal/day for men. Selecting whole grain products for carbohydrates, reducing soda and juice, moderating alcohol, and increasing water consumption are other steps that can help.

Patient's Long-Term Commitment Commitment to change is essential, but need not occur overnight. In fact, gradual change is more likely to be sustainable. Keeping track of dietary intake increases awareness of what a person is eating and problem eating patterns. Support is indispensable. Congratulate and reward patients' successes, comfort them when they have setbacks, and encourage them to keep trying.

Additional Resources Providers can use many resources to aid in diet counseling efforts. Dietitians educate patients in healthy eating behaviors and can provide detailed patient-specific advice. Unfortunately, depending on regional variations and insurance coverage, patients may have difficulty accessing these services. Books and web sites are more widely accessible (see Resources). A review of commercial weight loss programs found little data to support their use based on efficacy and cost effectiveness.[31] The sole exception was Weight Watchers, which resulted in a modest weight reduction, but more weight loss at 2 years than a self-help group that received minimal structured education.[32]

Counsel on Physical Activity

Although exercise alone is not enough to cause substantial weight loss, in some studies it has resulted in greater weight loss than diet alone and regular physical activity is essential in prevention of weight regain. The benefits of exercise include increased cardiovascular fitness, lower blood pressure, increased lean body mass, boosting energy, stress relief, and improved sleep. Joining a gym or jumping right into a rigorous exercise program is unappealing and unwise for most seasoned couch potatoes. It is important to start slowly. Using everyday activities to increase exercise is an easy first step: taking the stairs instead of the elevator, getting off the bus a stop early and walking the extra blocks, or exercising while watching television. Without costly memberships or a significant time commitment, these steps can significantly increase physical activity when done consistently.

Exercise can be incorporated into family life; both increasing health and fostering bonding. Families can take walks after dinner or take classes together.

Children should be encouraged to participate in after-school programs or extracurricular activities in which they can be physically active. Parents can serve as role models for good health behaviors by being physically active.

Counsel on Smoking Cessation

Cigarette smoking and obesity appear to compound the risk for cardiopulmonary disease. Often, patients are reluctant to stop smoking because they fear additional weight gain. Nevertheless, smoking cessation is a major goal of risk factor management that is especially important in obese patients.

PHARMACOTHERAPY FOR WEIGHT LOSS

Both patients and health care providers eagerly seek the "miracle weight loss pill." Unfortunately, none of the commonly used prescription weight loss medications has proved to be miraculous in its effects. Nonetheless, the modest reductions in weight associated with the two most commonly prescribed FDA-approved weight loss medications are worth considering in the management of obesity because each pound lost improves health.

Who should receive weight loss medications? Guidelines have been established to aid practitioners with the appropriate use of weight loss medications.[33] Information about the two safest and most efficacious medications currently on the market is included in Table 31-3. Weight loss medications always should be given in addition to behavioral therapy (diet and exercise). Their use can be considered in patients with a BMI of 27 and comorbidities (e.g., hypertension, diabetes, hyperlipidemia, obstructive sleep apnea), or a BMI ≥30.

BARIATRIC SURGERY FOR WEIGHT LOSS

Bariatric surgery is the most extreme as well as the most effective method available to assist patients with weight loss. In general, the goal of bariatric surgery is to decrease the size of the stomach to limit the intake of food and decrease the absorption of foods eaten. There are many types of bariatric procedures. The one deemed superior by most US surgeons is the Roux-en-Y gastric bypass. The average cost of bariatric surgery is $25,000 (www.bariatric-surgery.info). Some insurance providers, including Medicaid and Medicare, cover the surgery if it is deemed a medical necessity and the NIH criteria outlined in Box 31-2 are met; however, for low-income individuals without insurance, the cost of surgery can be prohibitive.

Recently, several pediatric hospitals around the country began performing bariatric surgery in morbidly obese adolescents who have reached skeletal maturity and who have comorbid conditions that would benefit from sustained weight loss. It is generally recommended that adolescents considering bariatric surgery seek care in a well-established pediatric obesity center.[35]

Benefits of Bariatric Surgery

Patients can lose between 20 and 40 kg through bariatric surgery.[36] The health outcomes for patients who have undergone bariatric surgery have been well established and often include 5 to 10 years of follow-up data. Although there have been no randomized controlled trials of surgical weight loss, most observational studies demonstrate improvement in diabetes, hypertension, and lipid profile (hypertriglyceridemia and low HDL).[37]

Postoperative Complications and Care

There are several common post-bariatric surgery complications. The most common complications are

Table 31-3. Weight Loss Medications

	Mechanism	Side Effects	Use in Children	Dosing	Effect	Cost
Orlistat (Xenical)	Lipase inhibitor: decreased fat absorption	GI: flatus, incontinence, bloating Impaired vitamin absorption	? use in children	120 mg TID with meals	15 lb wt loss (4.5 >placebo	$120–$170/ month
Sibutramine (Meridia)	Serotonin and norepinephrine reuptake inhibitor: appetite suppression	Headache, dry mouth, insomnia, diarrhea, Increased blood pressure and heart rate	FDA approval for use in adolescents	10–15 mg QD	11.5 lbs 7.5 lbs > placebo	$100–$120/ month

From Dietz WH, Robinson TN. Clinical practice. Overweight children and adolescents. *N Engl J Med* 2005;352:2100–2109; Poston, Haddock CK, Poston WS, et al. Pharmacotherapy for obesity: a quantitative analysis of four decades of published randomized clinical trials. *Int J Obes Relat Metab Disord* 2002;26:262–273; McMahon FG, Fujioka K, et al. Efficacy and safety of sibutramine in obese white and African American patients with hypertension: a 1-year, double-blind, placebo-controlled, multicenter trial. *Arch Intern Med* 2000;160:2185–2191; Poston WS, Reeves RS, et al. (2003). Weight loss in obese Mexican Americans treated for 1-year with orlistat and lifestyle modification. *Int J Obes Relat Metab Disord* 2003;27:1486–1493.

Box 31-2. Who Is a Candidate for Bariatric Surgery?

- Have had obesity for at least 5 years
- Have a BMI >40 kg/m² or >35 kg/m² with two comorbid conditions that would benefit from weight loss (e.g., hypertension, diabetes, hyperlipidemia, steatohepatitis, coronary artery disease, obstructive sleep apnea)

- Have failed medically supervised nonsurgical methods of weight loss
- Have no significant psychopathology

From: Collazo-Clavell ML. Safe and effective management of the obese patient. *Mayo Clin Proc* 1999;74:1255–1259.

iron and B_{12} deficiencies. Consequently, providers should follow a patient's CBC and iron profile every 3 months for a year and then yearly and should provide appropriate supplementation. Osteoporosis can occur in post-bariatric surgical patients. Its cause is unclear, although it may involve the impaired absorption of calcium and vitamin D. Primary care providers should consider evaluating patients for osteoporosis and treating them with calcium and vitamin D when necessary.[38] Gallstone formation (cholelithiasis) is a common occurrence after major weight loss of any kind; therefore, it is particularly common in patients who undergo bariatric surgery. In addition to close medical monitoring, patients should be involved in a postoperative program to assist with weight loss maintenance. For many patients, the changes in diet and eating patterns (small frequent meals) can be quite different from their usual eating styles or those of their families.

MULTIDISCIPLINARY AND INTERDISCIPLINARY APPROACHES TO WEIGHT CONTROL

Esmeralda is referred for psychiatric evaluation and her family is assigned a case manager. A dietitian and physical therapist help design plans for the family. Esmeralda receives an excuse for not taking swimming at school because of her refusal to wear a bathing suit in front of other students. However, she agrees to take part in other physical activities that do not require exposing her body.

Because social, biological, and psychological factors interact in the development of obesity, a team approach may be necessary to cope with this multifactorial problem. For some patients with longstanding relationships with primary care providers, evaluating the contributing factors and giving suggestions to alter these factors may be all it takes to bring about healthy changes. However, for other patients who may not receive regular medical care or have complicated issues, multidisciplinary or interdisciplinary treatment can be an effective way to manage weight issues.

The necessary components of a weight loss treatment program should address social, biological, and psychological factors. Hence, a multifaceted treatment program should include psychological education, advice for healthy diet and exercise, and behavior management. In addition, parenting training, social skills training, and possibly psychiatric intervention may need to be added. Multidisciplinary approaches and interdisciplinary group classes and visits may be useful in this regard (see Chaps. 12 and 15). Clinicians can devote their time to individual problems, knowing that the basic information for obesity control has been acquired in group sessions.

PUBLIC HEALTH APPROACHES TO WEIGHT CONTROL

Although individual approaches to weight loss serve to improve a single person's health, larger public health approaches can effect change on a population level. Community, school-based, and health policy initiatives can inspire healthy lifestyle behaviors in large numbers of people.

Community approaches include considering fitness in the design of neighborhoods and buildings: building office and commercial space with well-lit, easily accessible stairs or designing neighborhoods with sidewalks and trails for biking and walking. In already established communities, local governments can make funding for recreational centers and safe playgrounds a priority. Employers can provide on-site exercise facilities or incentives for their employees to join fitness centers or take classes promoting healthy behaviors. The education of key community figures, such as religious leaders, can serve to disseminate health messages in an efficient and effective manner. Partnerships among academic medical centers, community organizations, and local governments can facilitate the creation, implementation, and evaluation of weight control public health efforts.

Schools are particularly important places for healthy behavior initiatives. Ridding schools of soda and unhealthy snacks in vending machines have been adopted by many US cities in attempts to lower rates of childhood obesity. Ensuring that school breakfasts and lunches adhere to the US Department of Agriculture food pyramid can further this goal as well. Educational initiatives such as age-appropriate and culturally sensitive nutrition classes should be required in schools. Teachers, support staff, and parents should be educated on the benefits of proper nutrition and physical activity. Reinstating recess and physical education classes in schools and encouraging participation in extracurricular activities that involve sustained movement can emphasize the role of physical activity. Lastly, health promotion messages can take the place of fast food and soft drink advertising near school grounds.

Policy initiatives could have a significant impact on the obesity issue. Culturally sensitive media campaigns emphasizing healthy behaviors could easily reach millions of Americans. Mandatory labeling of prepared foods with nutritional information would make healthy choices easier. Fast food and soft drink advertising could be prohibited during children's television programs. Taxes could be levied on fast food, soft drinks, and other unhealthy snacks, whereas fruits and vegetables and healthy food options could be subsidized. The food and beverage industry could be required to provide reasonable portion sizes in restaurants.[39]

CONCLUSION

Over one half of US adults and nearly one third of children are overweight or obese. Weight loss can be an extremely difficult process. Time commitments, the cost of healthy foods, limited opportunities for physical activity, and lack of awareness of the negative effects of obesity can all be barriers to weight loss. Health care providers have an important opportunity to assist patients with this health issue through care of their individual patients and support of community and public health initiatives. Together with health care providers and patients, large-scale efforts will help reverse the trend of ever-increasing rates of obesity.

KEY CONCEPTS

- Identify obesity in patients.
  - Calculate BMI.
  - Explicitly address the issue of obesity.
- Motivate patients to lose weight.
- Consider cultural norms and time constraints specific to individual patients and their families.
- Set realistic goals.
- Counsel on diet and physical activity modifications.

CORE COMPETENCY
Action Plan for Weight Loss

Pre-Action Plan:

- Provide an accurate weight assessment.
- Assess readiness for change.
  —Precontemplators:

  Counsel weight maintenance.
  Review the health consequences of obesity.
  Assess confidence in ability to change and importance of need to do so.

  —Contemplators

  Tip the balance: strengthen reasons for weight loss.
  Assess confidence and importance.

Action Phase: Make the Action Plan

- Have patient identify *his or her* reasons for weight loss.
- Brainstorm on achievable goals: *Walk 10 extra minutes a day three times a week; drink diet soda instead of regular soda.*
- Identify desirable, nonfood rewards as motivation to achieve goals.
- Outline a dietary plan: *"I will eat breakfast every day." "I will restrict eating out to once weekly."*
- Outline a physical activity plan: *"I will park at the far end of the parking lot at the grocery store," "I will play soccer with my children on Saturday mornings."*
- Review additional supportive resources (nutritionist referral, weight loss medications, family counseling, etc.).
- Brainstorm on ways for the patient to keep weight off once it has been lost.

DISCUSSION QUESTIONS

1. Discuss three of the many factors that make it difficult for you or someone you know to lose weight. How might you overcome those difficulties?
2. Describe the steps a health care provider should take to help a patient lose weight.
3. Esmeralda's mother has been your patient for 5 years. She happily reports to you that her daughters have both been losing weight over the last year. Your medical record shows that she has gained 5 pounds in the last year and her diabetes control has worsened (Hbg A1C has risen from 7.5 to 9.0). Describe how you might approach your patient's weight gain.

RESOURCES

Weight-control Information Network: A website produced by NIH and the National Heart, Lung, Blood Institute to assist patients and providers with weight loss. http://win.niddk.nih.gov

A website with information for African-American women regarding BMI, physical activity, nutrition, and weight loss goals. http://www.blackwomenshealth.com

A website by the USDA that allows individuals to determine their nutritional needs based on physical activity level and age. http://www.mypyramid.gov

An electronic guide to recent, high-quality resources and information tools for overweight in children and adolescents. http://www.mchlibrary.info/knowledgepaths

BMI calculator. http://www.cdc.gov/nccdphp/dnpa/bmi/calc-bmi.htm#English

REFERENCES

1. Calle EE, et al. Body-mass index and mortality in a prospective cohort of U.S. adults. *N Engl J Med* 1999; 341:1097–1105.
2. *Body mass index.* Bethesda, MD: Centers for Disease Control and Prevention, 2005.
3. Janssen I, et al. Waist circumference and not body mass index explains obesity-related health risk. *Am J Clin Nutr* 2004;79:379–384.
4. Hedley AA, et al. Prevalence of overweight and obesity among US children, adolescents, and adults, 1999–2002. *JAMA* 2004;291:2847–2850.
5. Ferdinand KC. Managing cardiovascular risk in minority patients. *J Natl Med Assoc* 2005;97:459–466.
6. Dietz WH, Robinson TN. Clinical practice. Overweight children and adolescents. *N Engl J Med* 2005; 352: 2100–2109.
7. Stevens J, Cai J, et al. Fitness and fatness as predictors of mortality from all causes and from candiovascular disease in men and women in the lipid research clinics study. *Am J Epidemiol* 2002;156:832–841.
8. Hu, FB, Li TY, et al. Television watching and other sedentary behaviors in relation to risk of obesity and type 2 diabetes mellitus in women. *JAMA* 2003;289;1785–1791.
9. French SA, et al. Environmental influences on eating and physical activity. *Annu Rev Public Health* 2001;22:309–335.
10. KidsPeace annual meaningful time check-up on U.S. children & families. Available at: http://www.kidsday.net.
11. Barnes PM, Schoenborn CA. *Physical activity among adults: United States, 2000.* Advance Data from Vital and Health Statistics, no. 333. Hyattsville, Maryland; National Center for Health Statistics, no. 333. Hyattsville, Maryland: National Center for Health Statistics, 2003.
12. Collins ME Body figure perceptions and preferences among preadolescent children. *Int J Eating Disord* 1991;10: 199–208.
13. Harris SM. Racial differences in predictors of college women's body image attitudes. *Women Health* 1994;21: 89–104.
14. Lawrence CM, Thelen MH. Body image, dieting, and self-concept: Their relation in African-American and Caucasian children. *J Clin Child Psychol* 1995;24:41–48.
15. Mayville S, et al. Assessing the prevalence of body dysmorphic disorder in an ethnically diverse group of adolescents. *J Child Fam Stud* 1999;8:357–362.
16. Yates A, et al. Ethnic differences in BMI and body/self-dissatisfaction among Whites, Asian subgroups, Pacific Islanders, and African-Americans. *J Adolesc Health* 2004;34:300–307.
17. Lopez E, et al. Body image of Latinas compared to body image of non-Latina White women. *Health Values* 1995;19:3–10.
18. Contento IR, et al. Body image, weight, and food choices of Latina women and their young children. *J Nutr Educ Behav* 2003;35:236–248.
19. Sherry B, et al. Attitudes, practices, and concerns about child feeding and child weight status among socioeconomically diverse white, Hispanic, and African-American mothers. *J Am Diet Assoc* 2004;104:215–221.
20. Cossrow NH, et al. Understanding weight stigmatization: A focus group study. *J Nutr Educ* 2001;33(4):208–214.
21. Rogge MM, et al. Obesity, stigma, and civilized oppression. *ANS Adv Nurs Sci* 2004;27:301–315.
22. Ogden J, et al. General practitioners' and patients' models of obesity: Whose problem is it? *Patient Educ Couns* 2001;44:227–233.
23. Heywood A, et al. Correlates of physician counseling associated with obesity and smoking. *Prev Med* 1996;25: 268–276.
24. O'Brien SH, et al. Identification, evaluation, and management of obesity in an academic primary care center. *Pediatrics* 2004;114:e154–159.
25. Bowerman S, et al. Implementation of a primary care physician network obesity management program. *Obes Res* 2001;9(Suppl 4):321S–325S.
26. Huang J, et al. Physicians' weight loss counseling in two public hospital primary care clinics. *Acad Med* 2004;79: 156–161.
27. Kumanyika SK, et al. Weight-loss experience of black and white participants in NHLBI-sponsored clinical trials. *Am J Clin Nutr* 1991;53(6 Suppl):1631S–1638S.
28. O'Neil PM, et al. The perceived relative worth of reaching and maintaining goal weight. *Int J Obes Relat Metab Disord* 2000;24:1069–1076.
29. *Portion distortion: Do you know how food portions have changed in 20 years?* Bethesda, MD: National Heart, Lung, and Blood Institute, 2005.
30. Foster GD, Wyatt HR, et al. A randomized trial of a low-carbohydrate diet for obesity. *N Engl J Med* 2003;348: 2082–2090.
31. Tsai AG, Wadden TA. Systematic review: An evaluation of major commercial weight loss programs in the United States. *Ann Intern Med* 2005;142:56–66.
32. Heshka S, et al. Weight loss with self-help compared with a structured commercial program: A randomized trial. *JAMA* 2003;289:1792–1798.
33. National Institutes of Health. Clinical guidelines on the identification, evaluation, and treatment of overweight and obesity in adults: The evidence report. *Obes Res* 1998;6(Suppl 2):51S–209S.
34. Collazo-Clavell ML. Safe and effective management of the obese patient. *Mayo Clin Proc* 1999;74:1255–1259.
35. Inge TH, et al. Bariatric surgery for severely overweight adolescents: Concerns and recommendations. *Pediatrics* 2004;114:217–223.
36. Maggard MA, et al. Meta-analysis: Surgical treatment of obesity. *Ann Intern Med* 2005;142:547–559.

37. Buchwald H, et al. Bariatric surgery: A systematic review and meta-analysis. *JAMA* 2004;292:1724–1737.

38. Presutti RJ, et al. Primary care perspective on bariatric surgery. Mayo Clin Proc 2004;79:1158–1166.

39. Nestle M, Jacobson MF. Halting the obesity epidemic: A public health policy approach. *Public Health Rept* 2000;115:12–24.

40. *Aim for a healthy weight.* Bethesda, MD: National Heart, Lung, and Blood Institute. Available at: http://www.nhlbi.nih.gov/health/public/heart/obesity/lose_wt/bmi_dis.htm

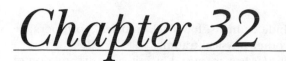

Chapter 32
Chronic Pain Management in Vulnerable Populations

Michael B. Potter, MD, Yeva Johnson, MD, and Barry D. Zevin, MD

Objectives

- Describe the disproportionate burden of chronic pain in medically vulnerable populations.

- Describe comorbidities that can present challenges in the management of chronic pain.

- Describe a general approach to the evaluation and management of chronic pain.

- Review common treatments, with a special focus on the role of opiates in the management of chronic pain.

- Suggest practical tools to improve the provision and documentation of safe and effective care for chronic pain.

Chronic pain usually serves little or no physiologic role and, in contrast to acute pain, it is perhaps best viewed as a disease state, not a symptom. Nine out of 10 US citizens aged 18 or older suffer pain at least once a month, 42% report experiencing pain every day, and nearly 1 in 10 adults lives in moderate to severe chronic pain.[1,2] Chronic pain affects both physical and mental health and leads people to rate their health as poor;[3] hence, its social and economic costs are considerable. Pain-related problems, particularly chronic pain management, are among the most challenging clinical problems confronted by clinicians.[4] This chapter reviews general principles of chronic pain management, emphasizing special circumstances confronted by clinicians caring for medically vulnerable populations.

DISPROPORTIONATE BURDEN OF PAIN IN VULNERABLE POPULATIONS

Thuy Nguyen suffers from chronic back and neck pain following an assault that occurred 6 months prior to her visit. Because of the pain, she has lost her job as a cleaning person for a small business in her neighborhood. She has no medical insurance and her landlord is trying to evict her for nonpayment of rent.

The burden of moderate to severe chronic pain is highest among the poor, the uninsured, and those belonging to ethnic minorities.[5-7] Poor individuals may be more subject than others to hazardous and more physically demanding work or living conditions that may lead to physical injury. Chronic pain itself can create economic or social disparities by causing disability or loss of health insurance.[8] Thus, costly evaluations and treatments that could reduce or manage their symptoms are often unattainable. Even living in a poor neighborhood can make it more difficult to obtain some treatments; for example, pharmacies in low-income neighborhoods might be less likely to stock expensive pain medications. Pain sufferers who are poor or uninsured may have difficulty understanding how to navigate the health care system to obtain proper treatment. Further, mental health conditions such as depression and anxiety are more prevalent among underserved medical populations and may further limit appropriate management of their pain.[6] Finally, personal interaction styles, discordant cultural beliefs, and stereotypes held by both clinicians and patients may impede communication that could lead to effective pain treatment.[9]

CLASSIFICATIONS OF CHRONIC PAIN

> Thuy does not speak English well, but she tells you that her pain is always there, and gets worse when she works. It is "sometimes tingling and sometimes aching." The only abnormality on physical examination is that her neck muscles are tender to palpation.

The International Association for the Study of Pain (IASP) takes into account that pain is a combined sensory, emotional, and cognitive phenomenon, defining it as "an unpleasant sensory and emotional experience that we primarily associate with tissue damage or describe in terms of such damage, or both." Pain becomes chronic when it persists beyond the time normally associated with healing from an acute or subacute injury (usually 4 to 12 weeks). It may be constant, intermittent, or related to physical activity. Most pain (acute or chronic) can be further classified as nociceptive, neuropathic, or mixed.[10] Chronic pain sufferers may experience many types of pain. Whatever its cause, pain can be thought of as including three distinct components: a sensory-discriminatory component (e.g., location, intensity, quality), a motivational-affective component (e.g., depression, anxiety), and a cognitive-evaluative component (e.g., thoughts concerning the cause and significance of the pain).[1]

Nociceptive pain (i.e., caused by or responding to a painful stimulus) is the most common type of chronic pain. Nociceptors can be found in skin, muscle, joints, and visceral tissue, and the pain is associated with an inflammatory response to tissue damage. The quality of the pain may be sharp, aching, or throbbing, and often worsens with movement or palpation. Common etiolo-gies include arthritis, low back injuries, postoperative pain, or other physical trauma.

Neuropathic pain is caused by injury or dysfunction of the peripheral or central nervous system, often from conditions such as diabetic or HIV-related neuropathy, post-herpetic neuralgia, or spinal cord injury. In contrast to nociceptive pain, neuropathic pain tends to cause a sensation of burning or tingling, and it often appears to be severe in proportion to physical evidence of injury. Because of the limited healing potential of nerve tissue, neuropathic pain can be more challenging to treat than nociceptive pain.

CHALLENGES IN DIAGNOSIS OF CHRONIC PAIN

> Since the assault, Thuy has been unable to sleep and has spent most of her time alone. She is diagnosed with chronic musculoskeletal pain exacerbated by depression and posttraumatic stress disorder. Treatment for both her physical and emotional symptoms is necessary for her to feel better.

Clinicians must rely primarily on patient report of the presence pain and its severity. Although at once universal and subjective, pain varies in its expression both among and within individuals.[7,11] The response to pain may be histrionic or stoic, panicked or accepting, help-seeking or highly skeptical of help.[12] Assessing and classifying it can be challenging, but is a necessary step in selecting the right treatment. Often there are multiple potential causes of physical or emotional pain. Patients may have trouble communicating their subjective symptoms or may exaggerate the extent of their symptoms. Hence, a holistic understanding of the patient is often as important as defining pain according to traditional classifications.

Having the patient keep a pain diary (i.e., written record of the pain, when it occurs, how it feels and any drugs he or she is taking) can be helpful in making a more accurate diagnosis. In addition, the treatment of chronic pain is rarely amenable to a "quick fix." Clinicians or patients must systematically test a variety of therapies to achieve successful pain control.

CHRONIC PAIN AND EMOTIONAL SUFFERING

When added to the daily hardships of living in poverty, pain may make the simple act of living one's life extremely difficult. Because many causes of pain are incurable, efforts to ameliorate these other hardships may make living with pain more bearable.

Pain can be modulated by a variety of external factors, including the effect of the pain on current life activities; learned behaviors and beliefs from family, cultural, or socioeconomic background; the meaning of the event that caused the pain; and underlying mental health disorders. Pain may lead to anxiety or depression, and primary anxiety and depression often amplify or even cause complaints of physical pain.[13]

CHRONIC PAIN AND SUBSTANCE ABUSE

Chronic pain is common among patients with substance use disorders.[14] Injuries occur more commonly in people who are impaired by alcohol and drugs. Various substances also may cause neurophysiologic changes that make chronic pain more common. Alcohol abuse and chronic stimulant abuse can cause depression and anxiety that is associated with and may exacerbate pain. Finally, chronic opioid abuse may alter pain perception at the level of opiate receptors, lending some truth to the maxim that addicts "hurt worse."

Common Pitfalls in the Care of Chronic Pain Patients

- Because pain is a subjective experience, treatment goals are rarely achieved without a trusting relationship between clinician and patient.
- A narrow focus on the patient's primary complaint may miss the big picture.
- Unrealistic expectations for symptom relief may interfere with setting and achieving realistic goals.
- Failure to understand the trial and error nature of pain treatment may cause patients and clinicians to give up on their goals prematurely.
- Failure to address associated mental health problems may impede progress in managing chronic pain.
- Social and medical taboos may limit the selective and appropriate use of opioids for intractable chronic pain.
- Limited specialty resources and/or failure to refer for specialty help early in the course of chronic pain may impede successful symptom management.

GENERAL APPROACH TO THE DIAGNOSIS OF CHRONIC PAIN

The first steps for the clinician are to obtain a complete history of events that triggered the pain, ascertain how the pain interferes with the patient's daily functioning and quality of life, determine the level of pain, and review prior diagnostic evaluations and treatments.

PAIN HISTORY

Patient history should include questions about onset, quality, duration, and ameliorating or exacerbating factors. The level of pain should be assessed to understand what the patient is experiencing and measure the effectiveness of treatment. The most common assessment tool asks the patient to rate pain intensity on a scale from 0 to 10, in which 0 represents no pain and 10 represents unbearable pain. Pictorial scales have been used and are particularly useful for children, adults with low literacy, and elderly patients.[15] In addition, these scales are helpful for clarifying the relationship between pain and activity, the effectiveness of pain treatments, and the pattern of the patient's pain (Fig. 32-1). More elaborate and comprehensive pain assessment scales have been developed, for example, the McGill Pain Questionnaire. They take longer to administer and some patients who are cognitively impaired or poorly educated may find these difficult to complete.

FUNCTIONAL ASSESSMENT

Common functional limitations caused by chronic pain include sleep disturbance, reduced mobility, sexual dysfunction, and decreased ability to perform well in social or work situations.[1] Failure to address functional limitations can lead to declining overall physical well-being, loss of important social and work relationships, and may trigger or exacerbate anxiety or depression. Evaluating work disability caused by pain and providing documentation may qualify a patient for entitlements that could improve his or her living situation. When caring for a patient with chronic pain, advocacy for disability benefits, vocational retraining, and other community services are all appropriate activities.

MENTAL HEALTH ASSESSMENT

Symptoms and their associated distress are real to the patient, and should be taken seriously. Patients with chronic pain should be screened for affective mental health disorders (anxiety, depression, or other affective or psychological disorders), because treatment of comorbid mental health problems is likely to result in better clinical outcomes.[16]

PHYSICAL EXAMINATION

A thorough physical examination is essential to the evaluation, and should include observations of the patient's appearance, behavior and responses to physical maneuvers that might elicit or relieve pain. Specific attention should be given to the musculoskeletal and neurologic evaluation, as well as potential syndromes of referred pain. However, objective findings on physical examination should not be relied on solely to confirm or disprove the patient's subjective complaint of pain.

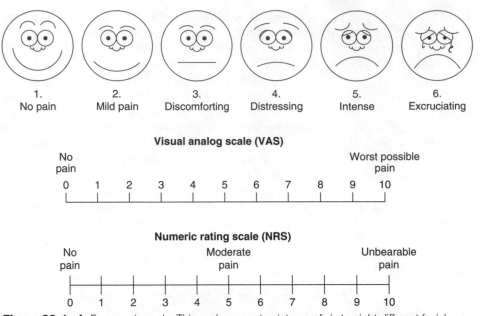

Figure 32-1. A. Faces pain scale. This scale presents pictures of six to eight different facial expressions depicting a range of emotions. From: Wong DL, Hockenberry-Eaton M, Wilson D, et al. Wong's essentials of pediatric nursing, 6th ed. St. Louis: Mosby, 2001:1301. **B.** Visual analog scale (VAS). The VAS is a validated approach to pain measurement. The most common VAS consists of a 10-cm line with one end labeled "no pain" and the other end labeled "worst pain imaginable." The patient marks the line at the point that best describes the pain intensity. The length of the line to the patient's mark is measured and recorded in millimeters. **C.** Numeric rating scale (NRS). The NRS is simple to use and is one of the most common approaches for quantifying pain. Patients indicate their pain intensity on a scale of 0 to 10, with 0 indicating no pain and 10 the worst pain imaginable. This scale is more sensitive to treatment induced changes than the VRS. The NRS can be a helpful technique for clarifying the relationship between pain and activity, the effectiveness of pain treatments, and the pattern of the patient's pain. Adapted from: American Medical Association Module 1. *Pain management: Pathophysiology of pain and pain assessment.* Accessed December 11, 2005. Available at: www.ama-cmeonline.com/pain_mgmt/module01/pdf/ama_painmgmt_m1.pdf

GENERAL APPROACH TO MANAGEMENT OF CHRONIC PAIN

Thuy's depression improves with use of an antidepressant and participation in a support group for assault victims. She continues with daily neck pain. She has difficulty taking many first-line medications and asks for something a little stronger or safer (?)

The history also should elicit the patient's broader life experiences with pain. Careful attention may provide insight into what is needed for effective treatment. Pain associated with a psychologically traumatic event may require treatment for the emotional impact of that trauma or loss. Pain that interferes with work may respond to vocational retraining. Pain caused by an underlying chronic disease may improve through education or support groups that bolster coping skills.

A mutually agreed upon treatment plan should address four important factors: the underlying cause of pain, level of pain, functional limitations, and realistic treatment goals. The treatment plan should allow both the clinician and patient to make priorities among treatment strategies and assess the success of treatments that are chosen.

FORMING A THERAPEUTIC ALLIANCE

The clinician should try to form a partnership with the patient (and his or her support people) that is marked by mutual trust and an understanding of the challenges that may lie ahead. Effective pain management—often requiring extensive evaluations and treatments that never fully eliminate pain or completely restore physical function—is one such challenge.

NONPHARMACOLOGIC THERAPIES FOR CHRONIC PAIN

Patients often seek complementary therapies either before or concurrently with conventional medical treatments.[17] Clinicians should elicit information about these therapies and incorporate them into their treatment plan when appropriate, as well as protect patients from potentially harmful side-effects.

Various components of physical therapy, chiropractic or osteopathic manipulation, acupuncture, massage, and biofeedback are promising. Pain experts often advocate cognitive behavioral approaches to chronic pain management.[18] Treatment may include individual or group psychotherapy, pharmacologic treatment, or combinations. Unfortunately, access to these therapies for vulnerable populations often is lacking because of economic and other barriers.

PHARMACOTHERAPY FOR CHRONIC PAIN

The three-step analgesic ladder, developed by the World Health Organization for the treatment of cancer pain, often guides pharmacotherapy for chronic pain (Fig. 32-2). In this model, mild pain is best treated with analgesics such as acetaminophen or a nonsteroidal antiinflammatory drug (NSAID), with or without adjuvant

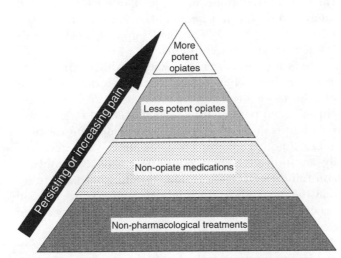

Figure 32-2. World Health Organization pain ladder. To maintain freedom from pain, drugs should be given "by the clock;" that is, every 3 to 6 hours rather than on demand. This multiple-step approach of administering the right drug in the right dose at the right time is inexpensive and 80% to 90% effective. Step 1: Nonpharmacologic treatments: massage, physical therapy, behavioral modification. Step 2: Nonopiate medications (pain persisting or increasing): Acetaminophen, acetylsalicylic acid (ASA); nonsteroidal antiinflammatory drugs (NSAIDs), tricyclic antidepressants, anticonvulsants, topical preparations. Step 3: Less potent opiates (for mild or moderate pain): codeine, oxycodone (least invasive administration—oral or transdermal—with appropriate agents to control and minimize side-effects). Step 4: More potent opiates (for moderate or severe pain): fentanyl, morphine, methadone, oxycodone (via intravenous route if necessary). Adapted from: *World Health Organization analgesic ladder: Cancer pain relief,* 2nd ed. Geneva: World Health Organization, 1996.

analgesics. Opioids are reserved for more severe pain, or when there are contraindications to less potent medications. In clinical practice, acetaminophen or NSAIDs are more likely to be effective first- or second-line agents for nociceptive pain, whereas adjuvant analgesics such as anticonvulsants and antidepressants are more likely to be effective first- or second-line treatments for neuropathic pain. Opioids are effective for both nociceptive and neuropathic pain, but because of their side-effects and potential for diversion and abuse, usually they are reserved for moderate to severe pain and/or pain that is unresponsive to other therapies. In practice, combinations of these agents typically are used together and multiple empiric trials often are required to find the best treatment.

Adjuvant Analgesics

Adjuvant analgesics include muscle relaxants, antidepressants, tricyclic antidepressants, anticonvulsants, and alternative medications such as glucosamine sulfate, topical analgesics, and intraarticular steroids. Muscle relaxants (e.g., baclofen, carisoprodol, cyclobenzaprine, and others) are used primarily as adjuvant therapy for musculoskeletal pain, especially back pain and muscle spasm of the neck and shoulders. The efficacy of these agents usually is modest, and they can be sedating or habit forming.[19] For chronic osteoarthritis pain of the knee and hip, glucosamine sulfate appears to be as effective for some patients, with potentially lower risk of side-effects than NSAIDs.[20] Systemic corticosteroids can successfully treat pain resulting from some inflammatory disorders and cancer-related syndromes, but their use for chronic pain usually is limited by the risk of serious side-effects. Intraarticular glucocorticoid injections with or without hyaluronic acid also can be offered for arthritis pain, although relief usually is only temporary.[21,22] For inflammatory arthritis, potent disease-modifying therapies are now available, and early referral for treatment may reduce pain and improve other disease-related outcomes.[23] Tricyclic antidepressants and anticonvulsants frequently are used for neuropathic pain.[24] The analgesic effect of tricyclic antidepressants is independent of their antidepressant effect, although their antidepressant effect may be helpful in patients with comorbid depression. Antidepressants acting on noradrenergic neurotransmitters are thought to have additive effects on the treatment of pain. Selective serotonin reuptake inhibitors do not possess these properties, but they can be effective in managing pain-associated depression with relatively fewer side-effects. Topical therapies such as capsaicin, lidocaine patch, and others may be useful for certain localized pain syndromes, such as postherpetic neuralgia or osteoarthritis. Long-term use of benzodiazepines usually should be avoided because of the potential risk of adverse effects. A serial trial of different adjuvant therapies is often required.

Some states have passed laws that allow for the use of marijuana for chronic pain.[25] There are plausible mechanisms by which cannabinoids might produce analgesia.[26] However, given the limited data on the efficacy and safety of marijuana and the persistent legal controversies concerning its use, it is unlikely to play a central role for most patients.

OPIOIDS

Opioids are effective treatment for nociceptive or neuropathic pain, as well as pain caused by mixed etiologies, such as cancer.[27] Short-acting opioid preparations can be useful for treating pain that is sporadic or intermittent. Typically, short-acting opioid preparations containing acetaminophen are used for this purpose. Tramadol is a short-acting low-potency opioid with the added benefit of inhibiting the reuptake of serotonin and norepinephrine, although it also has its own unique drug safety issues.[28]

For constant pain, once a stable daily opioid requirement has been established using short-acting opioids, a switch can be made to longer-acting opioids (e.g., sustained release morphine, methadone, fentanyl patch). Because of the unpredictable half-lives of their metabolites, long-acting opioids should be introduced at low doses and tapered up gradually over several days or weeks. Simultaneously, short-acting opioids should be tapered down, and reserved for occasional or episodic breakthrough pain.

Opioid Side-Effects

Constipation is probably the most common adverse effect of opioid therapy, and may lead to bowel obstruction if not treated proactively. When opioids are prescribed, a simultaneous prescription for a gentle laxative, such as senna, in combination with a stool softener, such as docusate sodium, should be part of the regimen. However, fiber-based bowel preparations should be avoided as a sole treatment for constipation in these patients, because they may increase the bulkiness of stools without promoting bowel motility.

Nausea and vomiting also are common opioid side-effects, although these usually can be managed by titrating opioid doses slowly and coadministering antiemetics such as metoclopramide or promethazine when needed.

Sedation is another common side-effect. However, this symptom usually dissipates over time and most patients on a stable dose of opioids are able to engage in their usual activities, including driving or operating machinery after adjusting to a stable dose.[29] Pruritus is a less common side-effect, but when it occurs it can be effectively managed with antihistamines.

Respiratory depression is very uncommon when opioids are begun at low doses and titrated slowly. Overdose or death most commonly occur in the setting of interaction with other sedating medications or alcohol, and patients should be educated accordingly.[30] Clinicians should be aware of equianalgesic doses of the most commonly used opioids to avoid unwanted side-effects or complications of opioids. At higher doses, opioids may have neurotoxic effects such as hyperalgesia or delirium. Therefore, clinicians should exercise caution when patients seem to require very high doses of opioids to control their pain.[31] When available, a pain specialist should be consulted.

Special Considerations When Prescribing Opioids

Many physicians refuse to prescribe potent or long-acting opioids for chronic nonmalignant pain under any circumstances.[32] An understanding of the true risks and potential benefits of opioids in selected patients with intractable pain should enable physicians to overcome ill-founded barriers to the use of opioids for legitimate pain relief.

For example, physicians often cite fear of medication tolerance or physical dependence as a reason not to prescribe opioids for chronic pain.[32,33] Both effects can certainly result when opioids are dosed around the clock. However, these effects can often be managed safely and should not be a contraindication to the use of opioids in patients who have significant pain that is refractory to other treatments.

Medication tolerance is a state in which exposure to a drug induces changes that result in a diminution of one or more of the drug's effects over time. Most chronic pain patients can be managed on stable doses for months or years without the development of tolerance. Although tolerance may occur, it is not necessarily an indication that continued use of opioids is contraindicated. In addition, diminishing pain relief may be an indication that the underlying disease process has gotten worse, rather than secondary to the development of tolerance. Tolerance also raises the doses of opiates required to achieve adequate pain control in the treatment of acute pain for those who use opiates chronically, be it for treatment of chronic pain, heroin, or methadone use.

Physical dependence occurs when a withdrawal syndrome can be produced by abrupt cessation or rapid dose reduction of a drug. Opioid withdrawal can be very unpleasant for patients, but usually it can be avoided by tapering opioids slowly when indicated, and it is not a contraindication to the use of opioids in chronic pain patients.

Addiction, Diversion, and Pseudoaddiction

Addiction is a set of behaviors distinguished by persistent craving of a drug, compulsive use, or continued use of a substance or drug despite evidence of harm. Addiction or diversion should be suspected in patients who are unable to take opioids according to an agreed-upon schedule, frequently report lost or stolen prescriptions, or seek opioid prescriptions from multiple doctors. Patients with a history of past or current substance abuse may legitimately warrant the use of opioids for chronic pain, but they also require careful evaluation of their pain syndrome, history with prescribed opioids, and current addiction status. An evaluation by an addiction specialist is very desirable.

Diversion of prescription opioids is an important law enforcement and public health problem in many communities. From a medical point of view, the greatest fear is that potent opioids will be taken by nontolerant persons, causing overdose or death.

Drug-seeking behavior also may result from an iatrogenic condition termed *pseudoaddiction*.[34] Pseudoaddictive behaviors can occur when a patient with unrelieved pain becomes focused on obtaining medications on time or even turns to the use of illicit drugs when he or she cannot receive enough pain medication from the physician. Pseudoaddiction can be distinguished from true addiction in that it resolves when the pain is effectively relieved.

Chronic pain patients who have no prior history of substance abuse generally have a much lower potential for addiction. Clinicians should make sure that patients understand the relatively low potential for abuse in this situation, because a patient's fear of addiction may prevent him or her from accepting opioids even when they could be beneficial.

Preventing Abuse or Diversion

When prescribing opioids, a relatively simple set of clinical procedures may reduce the risk of unwittingly contributing to drug abuse or diversion.[35] Begin by explaining to patients the potential risks and benefits of opioid medications, and setting out clear guidelines and consequences for the use or misuse chronic opioid prescriptions. Opioid prescriptions should be logged and documented in a central location in the clinical chart so that clinicians and staff who work together can easily monitor the amount of drug that is prescribed or dispensed. Patients should be seen frequently, especially when opioids are initiated, to monitor efficacy and side-effects. Avoid prescribing opioids to patients without complete or current clinical information (e.g., over the telephone or in on-call situations). Establish a single clinic or clinician as the sole prescriber of opioids by setting and communicating clear rules from the outset with the patient and other clinicians caring for the patient. Although pain medicine, addiction medicine, and subspecialty resources may be limited in many communities, clinicians should not hesitate to pursue consultation with a specialist as a precondition to the continued prescription of opioids, especially for patients with aberrant behaviors or suspected drug abuse. Some states now offer clinical databases on patients prescribed controlled substances that can be consulted if a clinician suspects unauthorized use of multiple prescribers or "doctor shopping."

Mandatory random urine drug testing also can be a useful tool for monitoring both the presence of unexpected drugs of abuse and the absence of prescribed opioids.[36]

Discussing the consequences of unexpected positve results before they occur is useful. For example, continued prescription of opiates might be made contingent on the patient entering drug use treatment. When performing urine drug testing, it is important to remember that rapid immunoassays do not reliably detect synthetic or semisynthetic opioids. Therefore, in addition to sending urine for a rapid urine immunoassay to screen for unexpected substances of abuse, clinicians should simultaneously order specific urine testing for the drug in question using gas chromatography, mass spectroscopy, or high-performance liquid chromatography.

It is important to understand that unexpected results cannot always be interpreted as abuse or diversion. For example, certain over-the-counter medications may lead to false-positive results for amphetamines on immunoassays, and unexpectedly negative results on specific drug testing may result from an improperly high threshold for detection in the laboratory assay. Therefore, to avoid improper interpretation of results, unexpected results should always be discussed both with the laboratory that performs the test and the patient.

Finally, many clinics incorporate their protocols for controlled substances into a written agreement that is signed by both the clinician and patient. Excellent examples of written agreements are available on the Internet (Table 32-1).[37]

Medicolegal Issues and Documentation Requirements

Many physicians are reluctant to prescribe opioids because of rare but well-publicized cases of inappropriate investigations by the US Drug Enforcement Agency. At the same time, there also has been a public outcry about the undertreatment of pain triggered by patients who have successfully sought damages for inadequate pain treatment through the courts. In 1997, California became the first state to legally enact a "Pain Patient's Bill of Rights." These opposing forces have heightened the anxiety that physicians may feel about the use of opioids for chronic pain.

In 1998, in order to encourage the appropriate use of opioids when indicated, the Federation of State Medical Boards published guidelines for the use of controlled substances that recently have been updated and are now endorsed by most state medical boards.[38] The guidelines recommend chart documentation of a thorough patient evaluation and treatment plan; informed consent and agreement for treatment; all

Table 32-1. Sample Provider/Patient Agreement for Controlled Substances for Pain[a]

I, . . . (*patient name*) . . . and . . . (*provider name*) . . . have decided to use a controlled substance for management of chronic pain or other medical condition caused by _____.

Good faith efforts to diagnose and treat the condition have been done and will continue. Appropriate consultations will occur when indicated. This treatment will not be a substitute for other modalities, including nonpharmacologic therapy.

The current medications are:

Medication	Instructions	Number/week/month	Start date	Discontinued

- I agree to other pain management strategies as necessary.
- I agree that I will reliably attend my appointments with the health care provider.
- I agree that this medication will be used only by me.
- I agree to take this medication as prescribed.
- I agree that I will notify the prescriber if I have side-effects from the medication (e.g., sedation) and will not drive or operate machinery while taking this medication if feeling impaired.
- I understand that if I run out of medication because I increased the dose without speaking to the prescriber, the prescription will not be filled early.
- I understand that spilled, lost, or stolen medications will not be replaced.
- I will not seek controlled substances from other sources.
- Pharmacy records may be reviewed to confirm prescriptions.
- Medications will be refilled only during usual office hours.
- Urine or blood screening may be performed randomly for drug testing.
- This contract will be reviewed every __ weeks/months.
- Other terms:

Consequences: If any of the preceding rules are broken, medications will no longer be prescribed.

Signatures of provider and patient, with dates

[a]Adapted from the Community Health Network and San Francisco General Hospital Medical Center Controlled Substance Contract.

treatments offered or provided (including date, type, dosage, and quantity prescribed); consultation with specialists when needed; and periodic review of progress toward treatment goals.

CONCLUSION

Four months later, Thuy continues to have some bad days, but these are helped by hydrocodone prescribed to use when she needs it. Acupuncture, support group meetings, and fluoxetine also have helped and she is working again.

Few primary care clinicians seem to enjoy working with patients in chronic pain.[32] Yet, clinicians have an ethical responsibility to provide compassionate and appropriate care to their patients with chronic pain, even and especially when access to specialty resources or expensive treatments is limited. Well-informed clinicians can contribute greatly to the amelioration of chronic pain among their patients. On a broader level,

clinicians can be important advocates for appropriate pain management resources within health care organizations that provide services to medically underserved communities.

KEY CONCEPTS

- Ask your patients about pain or you may never know about it.
- Understand the context and meaning of pain for the patient, and diagnose comorbid conditions such as depression or substance abuse.
- Create a goal-oriented treatment plan to address the underlying cause of pain, the level of pain, and the functional limitations caused by the pain.
- Periodically review the treatment plan to make sure it remains realistic and relevant to patient goals.

- Treatment of chronic pain is often a trial-and-error process.
- An understanding of the potential risks and benefits of opioid therapy can help primary care clinicians rationally select and safely monitor patients who may benefit from them.
- Opioids can be prescribed to patients with intractable pain and a history of substance abuse, provided that close monitoring and specialty evaluation are included in the treatment plan.
- Explicit office policies, written agreements, prescription drug logs, and random urine drug testing can support clinicians and patients in adhering to treatment guidelines.
- At every visit in which opioids are prescribed, document the five As: analgesia, activities of daily living, adverse effects, aberrant behaviors, and affective disorders.

Nausea can be treated with antiemetics or by changing to a different opioid.
Watch for tolerance and dependence when prescribing opioids—but recognize that these are not contraindications to use!

—Consider written agreements and random urine drug testing.
—Monitor pain.
—Use equianalgesic dosing when converting medications.
- Address and document the five As at each clinical visit:
—Analgesia
—Activities of daily living
—Adverse effects
—Aberrant behaviors
—Affective disorders

CORE COMPETENCY
Management of Chronic Pain

- Ask about pain. Use a scale, monitor treatment effectiveness
- Successful pain management requires several issues to be addressed simultaneously:
—The underlying cause of pain
—The pain itself
—Functional limitations caused by the pain
—Comorbidities such as depression or substance abuse that make treatment more complex
—Contextual issues such as employment, insurance, cultural beliefs, and social supports that may influence the ability to obtain appropriate care
- A therapeutic alliance is especially important.
—Trust, realistic expectations and mutual goals are important
- Treatment of chronic pain often involves trial and error.
—Distinguish between nociceptive, neuropathic, or mixed etiologies of pain.

Base treatment on etiology of pain.
Use adjuvant treatments.
Consider specialty consultation.

- Opioids can be effective medication for chronic pain, but must be prescribed with care.
—Manage side-effects.

Constipation may be prevented with docusate and senna.
Itching may be prevented or treated with antihistamines.

DISCUSSION QUESTIONS

1. Discuss the reasons why chronic pain is more prevalent in medically underserved populations.
2. What can you do in your own practice to make it easier for your patients to talk to you about pain?
3. What practice tools can help you manage pain once it is recognized?
4. If Thuy's pain were more severe or persistent, would you have prescribed long-acting opioids? Why or why not? If so, how would you have monitored her care?

RESOURCES

http://www.painmed.org
The American Academy of Pain Medicine

http://www.ampainsoc.org
American Pain Society

http://www.asam.org
American Society of Addiction Medicine

http://www.medsch.wisc.edu/painpolicy/
Pain and Policy Studies Group

REFERENCES

1. American Medical Association Module 1. *Pain management: Pathophysiology of pain and pain assessment.* Accessed December 11, 2005. Available at: www.ama-cmeonline.com/pain_mgmt/module01/pdf/ama_pain mgmt_m1.pdf
2. Gureje O, Von Korff M, Simon GE, et al. Persistent pain and well-being: A World Health Organization Study in Primary Care. *JAMA* 1998;280(13):1142.
3. Mantyselka PT, Turunen JH, Ahonen RS, et al. Chronic pain and poor self-rated health. *JAMA* 2003;290:2435–2442.

4. Meldrum ML. A capsule history of pain management. *JAMA* 2003;290(18):2470–2475.

5. Sturm R, Gresenz CR. Relations of income inequality and family income to chronic medical conditions and mental health disorders: National survey. *BMJ* 2002;324:20–23.

6. Mauksch LB, Katon WJ, Russo J, et al. The content of a low-income, uninsured primary care population: Including the patient agenda. *J Am Board Fam Pract* 2003; 16:278–289.

7. Green CR, Anderson KO, Baker TA, et al. The unequal burden of pain: Confronting racial and ethnic disparities in pain. *Pain Med* 2003;4:277–294.

8. Stewart WF, Ricci JA, Chee E, et al. Lost productive time and cost due to common pain conditions in the US workforce. *JAMA* 2003;290:2443–2454.

9. Smedley BD, Stith AY, Nelson AR. *Unequal treatment: Confronting racial and ethnic disparities in health care.* Washington, DC: National Academy Press, 2002:336–354.

10. Parrot TE. Pain management in primary-care medical practice. In: Tollison C, Satterthwaite J, Tollison J, eds. *Practical pain management.* Philadelphia: Lippincott Williams & Wilkins, 2002:729–747.

11. Litcher-Kelly L, Stone AA, Broderick JE, et al. Associations among pain intensity, sensory characteristics, affective qualities, and activity limitations in patients with chronic pain: A momentary, within-person perspective. *J Pain* 2004;5: 433–439.

12. Bertakis KD, Azari R, Callahan EJ. Patient pain in primary care: Factors that influence physician diagnosis. *Ann Fam Med* 2004;2:224–230.

13. Dersh J, Polatin PB, Gatchel RJ. Chronic pain and psychopathology: Research findings and theoretical considerations. *Psychosom Med* 2002;64:773–786.

14. Savage SR. Assessment for addiction in pain-treatment settings. *Clin J Pain* 2002;18(4 Suppl):S28–38.

15. Brunton S. Approach to assessment and diagnosis of chronic pain. *J Fam Pract* 2004;53(10 Suppl):S3–10.

16. Greco T, Eckert G, Kroenke K. The outcome of physical symptoms with treatment of depression. *J Gen Intern Med* 2004;19:813–818.

17. Barnes PM, Powell-Griner E, McFann K, et al. Complementary and alternative medicine use among adults: United States, 2002. *Adv Data* 2004;343:1–19.

18. Turk DC. Cognitive-behavioral approach to the treatment of chronic pain patients. *Reg Anesth Pain Med* 2003; 28:573–579.

19. van Tulder MW, Touray T, Furlan AD, et al. Muscle relaxants for non-specific low back pain. *Cochrane Database Syst Rev* 20032:CD004252.

20. Towheed T, Maxwell L, Anastassiades T, et al. Glucosamine therapy for treating osteoarthritis. *Cochrane Database Syst Rev* 20052:CD002946.

21. Gossec L, Dougados M. Intra-articular treatments in osteoarthritis: From the symptomatic to the structure modifying. *Ann Rheum Dis* 2004;63:478–482.

22. Arroll B, Goodyear-Smith F. Corticosteroid injections for osteoarthritis of the knee: Meta-analysis. *BMJ* 2004; 328:869.

23. Simon LS. The treatment of rheumatoid arthritis. *Best Pract Res Clin Rheumatol* 2004;18:507–538.

24. Collins SL, Moore RA, McQuay HJ, et al. Antidepressants and anticonvulsants for diabetic neuropathy and postherpetic neuralgia: A quantitative systematic review. *J Pain Symptom Manage* 2000;20:449–458.

25. Pacula RL, Chriqui JF, Reichmann DA, et al. State medical marijuana laws: Understanding the laws and their limitations. *J Public Health Policy* 2002;23(4):413–439.

26. Ibrahim MM, Porreca F, Lai J, et al. CB2 cannabinoid receptor activation produces antinociception by stimulating peripheral release of endogenous opioids. *Proc Natl Acad Sci USA* 2005;102:3093–3098.

27. Bloodworth D. Issues in opioid management. *Am J Phys Med Rehabil* 2005;84(3 Suppl):S42–55.

28. Grond S, Sablotzki A. Clinical pharmacology of tramadol. *Clin Pharmacokinet* 2004;43:879–923.

29. Fishbain DA, Cutler RB, Rosomoff HL, et al. Are opioid-dependent/tolerant patients impaired in driving-related skills? A structured evidence-based review. *J Pain Symptom Manage* 2003;25:559–577.

30. Oliver P, Keen J. Concomitant drugs of misuse and drug using behaviours associated with fatal opiate-related poisonings in Sheffield, UK, 1997–2000. *Addiction* 2003; 98:191–197.

31. Ballantyne JC, Mao J. Opioid therapy for chronic pain. *N Engl J Med* 2003;349:1943–1953.

32. Potter M, Schafer S, Gonzalez-Mendez E, et al. Opioids for chronic nonmalignant pain. Attitudes and practices of primary care physicians in the UCSF/Stanford Collaborative Research Network. University of California, San Francisco. *J Fam Pract* 2001;50:145–151.

33. Heit HA. Addiction, physical dependence, and tolerance: Precise definitions to help clinicians evaluate and treat chronic pain patients. *J Pain Palliat Care Pharmacother* 2003;17:15–29.

34. Kirsh KL, Whitcomb LA, Donaghy K, et al. Abuse and addiction issues in medically ill patients with pain: Attempts at clarification of terms and empirical study. *Clin J Pain* 2002;18(4 Suppl):S52–60.

35. Potter M. Chronic pain management: Practical tips and guidelines for primary care. *Adv Stud Med* 2004;4:31–40.

36. Heit HA, Gourlay DL. Urine drug testing in pain medicine. *J Pain Symptom Manage* 2004;27:260–267.

37. Teichman PG. A tool for safely treating chronic pain. *Fam Pract Manag* 2001;8:47–49.

38. California Pain Patient Bill of Rights. California Senate Bill No 402. Accessed March 5, 2005. Available at: http://www.paincare.org/pain_management/advocacy/ca_bill.html

Chapter 33

Principles of Caring for Alcohol and Drug Users

Alexander Y. Walley, MD, and F. Joseph Roll, MD

Objectives

- Define substance use, at-risk use, abuse, and dependence.
- Describe the burden of alcohol and substance use on individual and public health.
- Outline barriers to patient care.
- Describe screening and interviewing techniques.
- Review effective pharmacologic and nonpharmacologic treatments.

Mr. Wayland is a 45-year-old disabled ironworker. He presented to the emergency department for care after an auto accident. He was hospitalized when he began to show signs of alcohol withdrawal. While hospitalized, he learned that he had hepatitis C infection.

Alcohol and drug use burdens individuals and society through its association with acute and chronic illnesses such as overdose, trauma, liver disease, and human immunodeficiency virus (HIV) infection, and its connection to social problems such as family violence, homelessness, and poverty. Stigmatization of substance users by society in general and the health care system in particular compounds these burdens. An estimated 21 million US citizens suffer from alcohol and drug addiction. The annual economic cost of alcohol abuse alone is estimated at >$180 billion.[1] Although tobacco use is the leading cause of preventable death in the United States, the nature of addiction to alcohol and drugs reduces patients' ability to function and reduces providers' desire to provide care, making alcohol and drug dependence itself a

vulnerability in a way that smoking is not. Hence, this chapter focuses primarily on addictions other than smoking, although much of what is presented here can be used to address cigarette use as well (see Chap. 34). This chapter describes the individual and societal burdens of alcohol and drug use, and provides specific strategies to treat substance disorders and advocate for patients.

THE SPECTRUM OF SUBSTANCE ABUSE

People often begin using alcohol or drugs because they believe it will make them feel better. Indeed, limited use of alcohol and some drugs may have such health benefits as decreasing the risk of heart disease or providing pain relief. Those who are dependent on alcohol or drugs use them to avoid withdrawal. Others with underlying disorders such as chronic pain, schizophrenia, and posttraumatic stress disorder may use alcohol and drugs to cope with the symptoms of these conditions.[2] Clarifying the nature and consequences of use for each patient and then diagnosing use as at-risk, abuse, or dependence should guide clinicians' prevention and treatment efforts.

AT-RISK USE

To distinguish between safe and hazardous or harmful alcohol use, the National Institute on Alcohol Abuse and Alcoholism (NIAAA) has defined *moderate drinking* (i.e., safe) as two drinks or fewer (12 oz. of beer, 4 oz. of wine, or 1.5 oz. of liquor) per day for men under 65; and one drink or fewer per day for women and people over 65. The NIAAA defines *at-risk drinking* as >14 drinks per week or 4 drinks on any one occasion for men, and >7 drinks per week or 3 drinks on any one occasion for women. Patients in the at-risk drinking category are at greater risk for all-cause mortality and have a greater risk for developing abuse or dependence.

There are no similar "at-risk" definitions for drug use, perhaps because of the wide number and types of illicit drugs and the many ways they are used and abused. Because illicit drugs are illegal, any use is considered abuse based on the potential legal consequences.

ABUSE

The American Psychiatric Association (APA) defines abuse as recurrent use despite harmful consequences, such as inability to meet one's obligations with family, friends, or work, using in hazardous situations, and legal and interpersonal problems.

DEPENDENCE

Dependence is a synonym for addiction and can be thought of as a chronic, relapsing brain disease. The APA defines dependence as a maladaptive pattern of use with three or more of the following components occurring in the previous year: tolerance, withdrawal, using longer or more than intended, a desire or effort to stop or cut back, significant time spent using and obtaining, reduction of important activities in order to use, and ongoing use despite an understanding of physical or psychological consequences.[3] Mr. Wayland is probably alcohol dependent because he drinks despite harmful consequences (an auto accident) and he experiences withdrawal.

THE MAGNITUDE OF THE PROBLEM

Mr. Wayland started drinking alcohol at age 13. When he was working, he was fired twice for being late. After being injured at work 15 years ago, he began taking prescription pain medicines. At times, these medicines did not adequately control his pain and he started using heroin in addition to his daily drinking. Before qualifying for disability, he was homeless for a year.

For the year 2003, the National Survey on Drug Use and Health (NSDUH) estimates that of the almost 20 million people who used illicit drugs and 120 million current drinkers, about 21 million Americans meet criteria for substance abuse or dependence;[4] some argue that because of their social circumstances many more go uncounted. Surveys in primary care settings find rates of 2% to 29% for alcohol abuse or dependence,[5] 5% to 9% for current drug abuse or dependence, and 20% to 25% for lifetime illicit drug use.[6]

Concomitant alcohol and drug disorders often go unnoticed in primary care and drug treatment programs, yet "polysubstance" users have greater physical and mental health problems and higher mortality than single substance users.[7,8]

HEALTH CONSEQUENCES OF ALCOHOL AND DRUG USE

Mr. Wayland has had multiple visits to the emergency room and admissions to the hospital for trauma, alcohol withdrawal, pancreatitis, and cellulitis. Although never diagnosed with a mental illness, he overdosed on heroin after his divorce.

Substance dependence exacerbates other vulnerabilities such as race and ethnicity, poverty, mental illness, and chronic disease. Alcohol and drug users are at significantly higher risk for death and at a younger age than abstainers. These deaths result from accidental overdose, violence, and chronic diseases, and result in large numbers of years of life lost.[9,10]

MEDICAL COMPLICATIONS

Medical complications of alcohol and drug use include both acute and chronic problems. Acute problems include overdose, seizures, psychosis, endocarditis, pulmonary edema, soft tissue infections, osteomyelitis, hepatitis, pancreatitis, rhabdomyolysis, and sudden death. With chronic use, drug and alcohol addicts are at risk for chronic illnesses. Daily alcohol use of >2 drinks per day results in a twofold higher risk of hypertension, three- to fivefold higher likelihood of oral, esophageal, and liver cancer, and a ninefold higher risk of cirrhosis.[11] About half of all cirrhosis-related deaths are linked to alcohol.[9] Cocaine is associated with accelerated atherosclerosis, dilated cardiomyopathy, and chronic pulmonary toxicity (including organizing pneumonia, interstitial pulmonary fibrosis, and bullous emphysema). Cocaine users, particularly crack smokers, are at increased risk for pulmonary infections. Repeatedly injecting drugs such as heroin, cocaine, or methamphetamine is now the biggest risk factor for

HIV, and hepatitis B and C infections. About one half of new HIV infections are found in injection drug users (IDUs) and more than one third of deaths caused by AIDS occur among IDUs and their sexual partners.[12] The majority of new hepatitis C virus (HCV) infections are in IDUs.[13] Active alcohol and drug use also interferes with treatment of chronic diseases such as HIV infection.[14]

IMPACT ON THE FAMILY

Mr. Wayland's father died 5 years ago from alcoholic liver disease. His ex-wife is in recovery from alcohol dependence, and he has a brother in recovery from heroin dependence.

The consequences of substance use extend from substance users to their families and neighbors. Non–drug using individuals living with drug users are 11 times more likely to be murdered than those not living with drug users.[15] Estimates suggest that 60% to 75% of women who use substances suffer from partner violence, about three times the risk for women in general. The combination of sex, drugs, and violence brings with it increased risk for sexually transmitted infections and mental illnesses such as depression and posttraumatic stress disorder.[16]

Substance use disorders are family diseases both because of the profound burden they place on family function and because they are passed from one generation to the next through genetic and environmental means.[17,18] Children exposed to alcohol and drugs in utero risk problems such as fetal alcohol syndrome and low birth weight. In many families, alcohol abuse, domestic violence, and child abuse are linked and lead to alcohol abuse in offspring.[19]

IMPACT ON THE COMMUNITY

Although the direct medical complications of substance use are tragic for users and their families, the burdens from trauma, violence, and crime affect entire communities.[20] Drug and alcohol use are the fundamental fibers woven into the blanket of crime in the United States. In metropolitan areas across the country, 40% to 80% of people arrested test positive for drugs.[21] In 1996, more than half of criminal sentences were for drug offenses,[12] yet fewer than 11% of the prison population receives drug treatment while incarcerated.[22]

MENTAL ILLNESS

Links between substance use and mental illness abound. Substance users are more than twice as likely

to have a mental illness as non–substance users, and the mentally ill are more than twice as likely to have substance abuse or dependence. Teenage alcohol and drug use predict both chronic substance use disorders and later development of adult mental illnesses.[23] One study among drug users found that about half screen positive for depression.[24] Substance users are more likely to commit suicide.[25] For example, the increased rates of suicide among American Indian and Alaskan Native men are linked to increased rates of alcohol and drug use.[12]

DIFFICULTIES IN CARING FOR SUBSTANCE USERS

Mr. Wayland has not seen a primary care provider for 15 years. He stopped seeing his regular doctor when she refused to give him pain medicine prescriptions because he regularly ran out early.

Providers seem to derive little satisfaction from treating patients with substance use disorders,[26,27] and this is likely to result in poor care. For example, although validated tools are available to screen for alcohol abuse, providers do not often use them. Furthermore, providers frequently avoid making referral to treatment even when they identify a substance use disorder.[28] Clinicians' attitudes are not lost on substance using patients, who perceive that they receive poor access to care.[29] The alienation experienced by patients and providers can be explained by examining unrealistic expectations and mutual distrust.

Substance abusing patients do not fit health care providers' expectations: they may be too intoxicated or substance dependent to have a clear presenting complaint; they may not permit testing or a thorough examination; their symptoms may simply reflect their substance abuse; they may refuse or be unable to follow treatment recommendations. In addition, providers may fear that patients will use prescribed pain relievers recreationally or sell them. Refusing to prescribe them, on the other hand, may lead to unnecessary suffering or even increased substance use. Finally, family or personal experiences with substance abuse may unconsciously influence the response to patients.

The substance abusing patient also may have unrealistic expectations about physicians: They may expect their pain to be treated promptly and resolve quicker than is possible; they may want to be treated as if they were not intoxicated; and may want immediate treatment for their addiction. Mistrust grows as patients become disillusioned with medical care they interpret as inconsistent or intentionally poor because of their substance use.[13,29]

Common Pitfalls in the Care of Substance Users

- Underdiagnosing and undertreating substance disorders and their consequences
- Undermining the provider–patient relationship by mutual distrust
- Believing that success hinges on abstinence
- One provider trying to do all or all providers doing nothing
- Considering addiction a moral or character failing
- Perceiving relapse as failure

ALCOHOL AND DRUG DEPENDENCE ARE CHRONIC, RELAPSING BRAIN DISEASES

> After the death of his father, Mr. Wayland detoxified from heroin and alcohol and went into a halfway house. He was in recovery for 2 years until he relapsed to drinking. When asked about his drinking, he admits, "It's not fun anymore. I just drink to feel normal."

Substance abuse has been stigmatized as a moral failing; however, it is now clear that the regular use of alcohol or drugs changes brain chemistry, neuronal structure, and function, driving the cycle of tolerance, withdrawal, craving, and relapse.[18,30] With repetitive use, euphoria wanes and people use to avoid withdrawal and because they crave. Although a combination of motivation, social support, and medication often can help an addict into remission, the cycle of addiction remains hard-wired and primed for relapse. As with other chronic diseases, such as diabetes, addiction is treatable but not curable. Treatment should be considered a lifelong commitment.

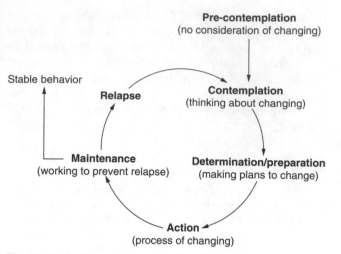

Figure 33-1. Prochaska and DiClemente's Stages of Change Model. A theoretical model of behavior change that has been the basis for developing effective interventions to promote health behavior change (see text for details). The model is often considered cyclical because most people attempting to change their health behavior relapse and have to repeat stages in order to learn how to maintain their behavior.

STAGES OF READINESS FOR BEHAVIORAL CHANGE

Although drug and alcohol dependence are chronic brain diseases, they are also behavioral disorders for which providers should seek to facilitate change. Prochaska and DiClemente's "stages of change" is a model of behavior change that has been widely adopted among providers treating drug and alcohol dependence. This model identifies six stages that patients move through when changing behavior patterns (Fig. 33-1; Box 33-1).[31,32]

Box 33-1. Stages of Change

- *Precontemplation* describes patients who deny they need to change or who feel hopeless.
- *Contemplation* describes patients who are ambivalent about change.
- *Preparation or determination* describes patients who have decided to change and are making plans.
- *Action* describes patients who are changing their behavior.
- *Maintenance or Recovery* describes patients who have changed and are stable.
- When patients in recovery start using again they are in the *Relapse* stage, which typically leads to *Contemplation* and another progression through the stages.

Representing the stages of change as a cycle (see Fig. 33-1) follows from conceptualizing addiction as a chronic, relapsing disease. By determining the stage of change, the provider can use the appropriate interviewing strategy to engage the patient.
From: Samet JH, et al. Beyond CAGE. A brief clinical approach after detection of substance abuse. *Arch Int Med* 1996;156(20):2287–2293; DiClemente CC, Velásquez MM. Motivational interviewing and the stages of change. In: W. Miller R, Rollnick S, eds. *Motivational interviewing: Preparing people for change.* New York: The Guilford Press, 2002:201–216.

Box 33-2. Conditions That Trigger Substance Use Screening

- Mental illness
- Legal, family, work or school problems
- Trauma
- Perpetrating or sustaining violence

- Physical and laboratory signs such as elevated liver enzymes, or new HIV or HCV diagnoses
- Soft tissue infections
- Sexually transmitted infections

HARM REDUCTION

Harm reduction is an approach to treatment based on the premise that, whatever its cause, drug abuse has always been part of human life and will persist. It recognizes that although substance abuse causes enormous harm, substance-using individuals are often not ready to change their behavior. As expressed by the Harm Reduction Coalition, harm reduction also "recognizes that the realities of poverty, class, racism, social isolation, past trauma, sex-based discrimination and other social inequalities affect both peoples' vulnerability to and capacity for effectively dealing with drug-related harms."[33] Proponents of harm reduction hold that clinicians should find ways to reduce the harms of drug abuse while helping patients move toward abstinence. In a practical sense, this means assessing those who are still using drugs for the greatest risks to their health and working to collaboratively minimize them. Steps as diverse as helping a patient find an Alcoholics Anonymous (AA) meeting, offering a referral for methadone treatment, linking them with a social worker for housing assistance, or arranging for a weekly Mediset containing their medications might be considered harm reduction. A successful application of harm reduction principles in the public health domain is the use of needle exchange programs for IV drug abusers; they have been shown in multiple studies to reduce the transmission of HIV infection.[34]

ADDRESSING SUBSTANCE USE IN PRIMARY CARE

About 45% of substance users believe their clinicians are unaware of their addiction; clearly, diagnosing alcohol and drug problems is an unmet challenge. Yet treating these disorders has tremendous potential for improving health. Screening for alcohol and drug use should be included in every comprehensive physical examination in every patient, and also should be triggered by specific conditions (Box 33-2).

The most commonly used screening tool for at-risk drinking, alcohol abuse, and alcohol dependence is the CAGE questionnaire. The NIAAA advises combining the CAGE questionnaire with questions about quantity and frequency to improve sensitivity and specificity (Box 33-3).[35] In 2005 the NIAA revised its screening questions, recommending that as an alternative to the CAGE questions the following single question be used: "How many times in the past year have you had 5 or more drinks (for men) or 4 or more drinks (for women) in a day?" Any answer greater than zero is considered a positive screen, worthy of further investigation. (See Resources—"Helping patients who drink too much.")

Screening tools for drug use are not as well studied as the CAGE. The CAGE-AID (CAGE Adjusted to Include Drugs) adds the phrase "or using drugs" to each of the preceding questions. A reasonable strategy is to ask

---

Box 33-3. CAGE Questionnaire + Quantity and Frequency

Step 1. Determine Whether the Patient Is an At-Risk Drinker[a]

Quantity and Frequency
On average, how many drinks do you have per week?
What is the maximum number of drinks you had in any given day in the last month?

[a]For men, at-risk drinking is 14 or more drinks per week or 4 or more drinks on any one occasion. For women, at-risk drinking is 7 or more drinks per week or 3 or more drinks on any one occasion.

Step 2. Determine At-Risk versus Abuse/Dependence
CAGE Questionnaire[b]

Have you ever felt you should **C**ut down on your drinking?
Have people **A**nnoyed you by criticizing your drinking?
Have you ever felt bad or **G**uilty about your drinking?
Have you ever taken a drink first thing in the morning (**E**ye-opener) to steady your nerves or get rid of a hangover?

[b]Two or more positive responses predict abuse or dependence in primary care settings with a sensitivity of 77% to 94% and a specificity of 79% to 97%.
From: Fiellin DA, et al. Outpatient management of patients with alcohol problems. *Ann Intern Med* 2000;133(10):815–827; National Institute on Alcohol Abuse and Alcoholism. *Helping patients with alcohol problems: A health practitioner's guide.* Bethesda, MD: National Institute on Alcohol Abuse and Alcoholism, 2004.

about any drug use in the past year. Any positive responses should lead to assessment by asking about history of withdrawal, tolerance, use despite wanting to quit, or use despite understanding the consequences. For patients who report no current or recent alcohol or drug use, it is important to ask about a history of drinking or drug use in order to support their recovery.

Prognosis and intensity of treatment are determined in part by the substance disorder. With at-risk drinkers, providers should regularly address substance use. Patients with substance abuse or dependence should be referred for substance treatment in addition to primary care–based brief intervention, as described in the following.

BRIEF INTERVENTION: ADVISE TO QUIT AND DETERMINE READINESS TO CHANGE

Brief intervention is a technique based on motivational interviewing principles and relies on a series of brief (i.e., 5- to 15-min) counseling sessions in which the provider expresses concern about the patient's substance use, acknowledges that the patient may not see it as a problem, recommends quitting, and offers to help the patient change the behavior when he or she is ready. The United States Preventive Services Task Force (USPSTF) recommends brief intervention in primary care populations for the purpose of reducing morbidity from alcohol use. Screening combined with brief intervention results in a net reduction of 3 to 9 drinks per week after 6 to 12 months of follow-up.[36,37] Among IDUs, brief intervention has been shown to decrease rates of injection, increase abstinence, and lower arrest rates.

Once it is clear that a patient has substance use disorder, the physician should express concern about the alcohol or drug use and advise the patient to stop or cut back. Provider advice to decrease use takes little time and is a useful and efficient way to assess a patient's readiness to change (see Core Competency).

PRECONTEMPLATION: ADDRESS DENIAL AND RESISTANCE

Unfortunately, physician advice to stop or cut back does not often lead to an agreement between the provider and patient about a treatment strategy. When the patient is resisting the physician's advice or denying he or she has a problem (*"I am not addicted; I can quit any time"*), further physician advice often begets more resistance and/or denial and potentially undermines the provider–patient relationship. In this precontemplative stage, a person is very unlikely to change his or her behavior. A more appropriate goal is to move him or her into a contemplative stage where the patient can acknowledge good and bad things about the behavior change the provider is advising. The underlying message to the patient should be one of support for the patient and his or her life ambitions, as well as encouragement to continue seeking care.

CONTEMPLATION: EXPLORE AMBIVALENCE

In the contemplation stage, the patient is aware that substance abuse is causing a problem but is ambivalent about quitting (*"Part of me wants to stop, but I am not sure it will be worth it"*). Monitoring the patient's health so that he or she gets individualized feedback on negative effects is important and probably more effective than simply providing general patient education in the form of pamphlets or lectures.

DETERMINATION: SUPPORT CHANGE

When the patient decides to get treatment (*"I want to stop"*), health care providers should praise the decision, assist the patient in choosing the right treatment, and make appropriate referrals. Choice of treatment depends on a number of variables: the type and severity of substance use, the treatment programs available in the area, and the patient's insurance status.

ACTION

At this stage, the patient is in some form of treatment (*"I stopped this week"*). Communication among the provider, treatment program, and patient is extremely helpful and may be facilitated by more frequent office visits. Most patients begin to notice symptoms that were masked by their substance abuse, such as pain or depression, and facilitating care for co-occurring vulnerabilities is important.

MAINTENANCE IS RELAPSE PREVENTION

Providers often see patients for medical issues when the patient is in recovery (*"I have been clean and sober for 25 days"*). Because primary care providers see patients over time, they are in a unique position to observe when a patient may be headed toward relapse, and preventing it should be a fundamental goal. Relapse prevention strategies include maintaining a therapeutic relationship and nonjudgmental attitude, communicating empathy (*"that must be hard"*), reinforcing positive behavior change (*"I know you can do this"*), identifying triggers, promoting coping strategies, and working with the patient's family. During this stage, most patients have a support network such as a social worker, counselor, AA contact, or family member who can help as they try to maintain abstinence. Providers should be familiar with local resources such as residential or daytime therapeutic communities focused on maintaining recovery.

Because addiction is a chronic, relapsing disease, relapse should be expected. The health care provider can assist by reminding the patient that relapse is a normal part of recovery, the provider will not think less of the patient if he or she relapses, he or she will be seen promptly if a relapse occurs, and he or she will not be judged.

Nonpharmacologic Options

Although a single provider may be able to move a patient along the stages of change, the patient will also require community-based substance treatment resources. AA and Narcotics Anonymous (NA) are widely available group therapy abstinence programs that are self-supporting and nondiscriminating. Halfway houses or sober houses, where people in treatment and recovery live together, are particularly valuable resources for patients who are homeless or whose use is triggered by their residential environment. Residential or therapeutic communities are programs in which patients stay for weeks to months and that provide more structure, usually restricting patients to the community grounds. The treatment effectiveness of these programs may be confounded by the fact that more motivated patients enter treatment; however, coercive measures via institutions such as drug courts, in which drug offenders are offered treatment in lieu of incarceration, also have proved successful.[22]

Pharmacologic Treatment

Despite many randomized controlled trials examining antidepressants, dopamine agonists, antiseizure medicines, and long-acting stimulant replacement, no pharmacotherapy has been found effective for cocaine or methamphetamine dependence.

Maintenance Treatment for Opiate Dependence

Methadone is a long-acting opioid agonist that reduces physical withdrawal and psychological craving in opioid-dependent patients. Methadone maintenance therapy (MMT) has been shown to reduce mortality, reduce HIV transmission, improve function and productivity, and reduce crime. A 1998 NIH Consensus Conference recommended access to MMT for all opioid-dependent patients.[38] MMT may only be distributed through federally licensed clinics; therefore, there are limited numbers of treatment slots. Buprenorphine is a newly available safe and effective, partial opioid agonist taken sublingually. It may be prescribed by certified physicians through primary care clinics. Because it is a partial agonist, it has a ceiling effect that reduces its abuse potential and the potential for respiratory depression. Both methadone and buprenorphine are effective for detoxification in addition to maintenance. Both should be prescribed in conjunction with nonpharmacologic treatments.

Therapies for Alcohol Dependence

Naltrexone, an opioid antagonist, and acamprosate, a gamma-aminobutyric acid (GABA) analog, are both effective at reducing craving and relapse in alcohol dependence. They may be used alone or in combination and should be considered adjuncts to a comprehensive treatment plan that includes counseling, group therapy, or self-help participation. Disulfiram reduces relapse in alcohol dependence by causing adverse autonomic and gastrointestinal symptoms after drinking alcohol.

Detoxification

Although detoxification (detox) is rarely enough to maintain abstinence, it is often the first step to recovery, that is, action. Detox can occur with or without medical management. Detox from heavy alcohol use is best done with medical management in a supervised setting because of the risk of seizures, autonomic instability, and delirium. Opioid withdrawal may be treated with methadone or buprenorphine tapered over days to weeks. Although no medicines are reliably effective for stimulant withdrawal symptoms, temporary inpatient respite may be helpful for initiating treatment.[39]

SUSTAINING HOPE WHILE CARING FOR ALCOHOL AND DRUG USERS

> Mr. Wayland learns about hepatitis C from his primary care provider. They discuss his alcohol and heroin use and choose these as their focus. Over the next 2 years, he relapses on heroin a few times and he enters a methadone maintenance treatment. With support, he attends AA regularly and decreases his alcohol use.

Providers who incorporate the stages of change model and harm reduction into their practices may feel greater satisfaction in caring for substance users. Providers' roles and expectations change, and as they support patients in the gradual process of quitting, providers can relish the small victories that occur.

Substance abuse, and its causes and consequences, are usually so complex that a single provider cannot address it alone. Case management teams that include drug and alcohol abuse counseling, social workers, and psychiatrists have been shown to reduce substance abuse and its harms. If a formal case management team is not available, providers can try to assemble an ad hoc team by referring patients to treatment programs and community social service agencies. Sharing tasks, insights, and rewards as well as frustrations increases the chances of successful treatment and is helpful to the medical provider.

As providers gain competency in caring for people with substance use, they will find that, as with all medical care, the most compelling reward is getting to know the patient and developing a relationship. Engaging with people as they struggle with addiction, sharing in the tragedy of continued use, and witnessing the triumph of recovery can be profoundly satisfying.

KEY CONCEPTS

- Addiction is a chronic, relapsing brain disease.
- With support, patients have the potential to change their behavior.
- Establish trust as a first step to facilitating behavior change.
- Screen for at-risk use, abuse, and dependence.
- Express concern and advise the patient to stop or cut back.

- Assess the patient's readiness to change and use the appropriate interviewing approach.
- Assemble a care plan that accounts for:
—Level of use
—Readiness for change
—Other vulnerabilities (i.e., mental illness, HIV infection)
- Appreciate any positive change.

CORE COMPETENCY

Interview Approaches Based on the Patient's Readiness for Behavior Change

Stage of Readiness	Interview Approaches
Precontemplation	• Express concern about the patient and substance use (SU). • State nonjudgmentally that SU is a problem. • Agree to disagree about the severity of the problem. • Consider a trial of abstinence to clarify the problem. • Suggest bringing a family member to an appointment. • Emphasize the importance of seeing the patient again.
Contemplation	• Elicit positive and negative aspects of SU. • Ask about positive and negative aspects of past periods of abstinence. • Summarize the patient's comments on SU and abstinence. • Clarify discrepancies between the patient's expressed values and his or her actions. • Consider a trial of abstinence.
Determination/Preparation	• Acknowledge the significance of a decision to seek treatment. • Support self-efficacy. • Affirm the patient's ability to successfully seek treatment. • Help the patient decide on appropriate, achievable action. • Caution that the road ahead is tough but very important. • Explain that relapse should not disrupt the patient–physician relationship.
Action	• Be a source of encouragement and support. • Acknowledge the discomforting aspects of withdrawal. • Reinforce the importance of remaining in recovery.
Maintenance/Recovery	• Anticipate the difficulties as a means of relapse prevention. • Recognize the patient's struggle. • Support the patient's resolve. • Reiterate that relapse should not disrupt the medical care relationship.
Relapse	• Explore what can be learned from the relapse. • Express concern and even disappointment about the relapse. • Emphasize the positive aspect of the effort to seek care. • Support the patient's self-efficacy so that recovery seems achievable.

Adapted from Samet JH, et al. Beyond CAGE. A brief clinical approach after detection of substance abuse. *Arch Int Med* 1996;156(20):2287–2293.

DISCUSSION QUESTIONS

1. When seeing a patient with alcohol and cocaine dependence, HIV infection, depression, and homelessness, how do you focus your efforts? What resources can you mobilize to help in this patient's care?

2. Five minutes into your first visit, a new patient accuses you of minimizing her pain and belittling her as an "addict." How do you begin to build trust?

3. If you were caring for Mr. Wayland as an inpatient, how could you use the described interviewing approaches during his inpatient stay? What is a

realistic goal in addressing his motivation to change his substance use?

RESOURCES

www.psych.org/psych_pract/trcatg/pg/pg_substance.cfm
American Psychiatric Association practice guideline for the treatment of patients with substance use disorders: Alcohol, cocaine, opioids

www.harmreduction.org
Harm Reduction Coalition

www.jointogether.org/resources/helping-patients-who-drink.html
Helping patients who drink to much: A clinician's guide, 2005 Edition. National Institute on Alcohol Abuse and Alcoholism. National Institutes of Health. US Department of Health and Human Services.

www.mdalcoholtraining.org
Helping Patients with Alcohol Problems: A Web-based Curriculum for Primary Care Physicians

1-800-662-HELP or http://findtreatment.samhsa.gov
National Drug and Alcohol Treatment Referral Routing Service

Available free of charge at: www.rwjf.org/publications/otherlist.jsp
Substance abuse: The nation's number one health problem. Robert Wood Johnson Foundation, 2001.

www.jointogether.org
Support for people working on substance abuse treatment

REFERENCES

1. Harwood H. *Updating estimates of the economic costs of alcohol abuse in the United States: Estimates, update methods, and data.* Rockville, MD: National Institute on Alcohol Abuse and Alcoholism, National Institutes of Health, and Department of Health and Human Services, 2000.

2. Khantzian EJ. The self-medication hypothesis of substance use disorders: A reconsideration and recent applications. *Harv Rev Psychiatry* 1997;4(5):231–244.

3. American Psychiatric Association. *Practice guideline for the treatment of patients with substance use disorders: Alcohol, cocaine, opioids.* Arlington, VA: American Psychiatric Association, 2004.

4. Substance Abuse and Mental Health Services Administration. *Overview of findings from the 2003 national survey on drug use and health.* NSDUH Series H–24. Rockville, MD: Office of Applied Studies, Substance Abuse and Mental Health Services Administration, 2004.

5. Fiellin DA, et al. Outpatient management of patients with alcohol problems. *Ann Intern Med* 2000;133(10):815–827.

6. Manwell LB, et al. Tobacco, alcohol, and drug use in a primary care sample: 90-day prevalence and associated factors. *J Addict Dis* 1998;17(1):67–81.

7. Gossop M, et al. Dual dependence: assessment of dependence upon alcohol and illicit drugs, and the relationship of alcohol dependence among drug misusers to patterns of drinking, illicit drug use and health problems. *Addiction* 2002;97(2):169–178.

8. Gossop M, et al. A prospective study of mortality among drug misusers during a 4-year period after seeking treatment. *Addiction* 2002;97(1):39–47.

9. Horgan CM, et al. *Substance abuse: The nation's number one problem key indicators: Update.* Waltham, MA: Schneider Institute for Health Policy, Heller Graduate School, Brandeis University, 2001.

10. Hser YI, et al. A 33-year follow-up of narcotics addicts. *Arch Gen Psychiatry* 2001;58(5):503–508.

11. Rehm J, et al. Alcohol-related morbidity and mortality. *Alcohol Res Health* 2003;27(1):39–51.

12. National Institute on Drug Abuse. *Drug use among racial/ethnic minorities.* Bethesda, MD: US Department of Health and Human Services, National Institutes of Health, National Institute on Drug Abuse, Division of Epidemiology, Services & Prevention Research, 2003.

13. Merrill JO, et al. Mutual mistrust in the medical care of drug users: The keys to the "narc" cabinet. *J Gen Intern Med* 2002;17(5):327–333.

14. Arnsten JH, et al. Impact of active drug use on antiretroviral therapy adherence and viral suppression in HIV-infected drug users. *J Gen Intern Med* 2002;17(5):377–381.

15. Rivara FP, et al. Alcohol and illicit drug abuse and the risk of violent death in the home. *JAMA* 1997;278(7):569–575.

16. Gilbert L, et al. The converging epidemics of mood-altering-drug use, HIV, HCV, and partner violence: A conundrum for methadone maintenance treatment. *Mt Sinai J Med* 2000;67(5–6):452–464.

17. Bierut LJ, et al. Familial transmission of substance dependence: alcohol, marijuana, cocaine, and habitual smoking: A report from the Collaborative Study on the Genetics of Alcoholism. *Arch Gen Psychiatry* 1998;55(11):982–988.

18. Cami J, Farre M. Drug addiction. *N Engl J Med* 2003;349(10):975–986.

19. Miller BA, Downs WR. Violent victimization among women with alcohol problems. *Recent Dev Alcohol* 1995;12:81–101.

20. Gentilello LM, et al. Alcohol interventions in a trauma center as a means of reducing the risk of injury recurrence. *Ann Surg* 1999;230(4):473–480; discussion 480–483.

21. White House Office of National Drug Control Policy, Clearinghouse. *Drug-related crime fact sheet.* Washington, DC: White House Office of National Drug Control Policy, 2000.

22. White House Office of National Drug Control Policy Clearinghouse, ODPI. *Drug treatment in the criminal justice system fact sheet.* Washington, DC: White House Office of National Drug Control Policy, 2001.

23. Brook DW, et al. Drug use and the risk of major depressive disorder, alcohol dependence, and substance use disorders. *Arch Gen Psychiatry* 2002;59(11):1039–1044.

24. Johnson ME, et al. Hepatitis C virus and depression in drug users. *Am J Gastroenterol* 1998;93(5):785–789.

25. Oyefeso A, et al. Suicide among drug addicts in the UK. *Br J Psychiatry* 1999;175:277–282.

26. Roche AM, Richard GP. Doctors' willingness to intervene in patients' drug and alcohol problems. *Soc Sci Med* 1991;33(9):1053–1061.

27. Saitz R, et al. Professional satisfaction experienced when caring for substance-abusing patients: Faculty and resident physician perspectives. *J Gen Intern Med* 2002;17(5): 373–376.

28. Friedmann PD, et al. Screening and intervention for alcohol problems. A national survey of primary care physicians and psychiatrists. *J Gen Intern Med* 2000;15(2): 84–91.

29. Chitwood DD, et al. Satisfaction with access to health care among injection drug users, other drug users, and nonusers. *J Behav Health Serv Res* 2002;29(2):189–197.

30. McLellan AT, et al. Drug dependence, a chronic medical illness: Implications for treatment, insurance, and outcomes evaluation. *JAMA* 2000;284(13):1689–1695.

31. Samet JH, et al. Beyond CAGE. A brief clinical approach after detection of substance abuse. *Arch Int Med* 1996; 156(20):2287–2293.

32. DiClemente CC, Velásquez MM. Motivational interviewing and the stages of change. In: W. Miller R, Rollnick S, eds. *Motivational interviewing: Preparing people for change.* New York: The Guilford Press, 2002:201–216.

33. Marlatt GA. *Harm reduction: Pragmatic strategies for managing high-risk behaviors.* New York: The Guilford Press, 1998.

34. Vlahov D, Junge B. The role of needle exchange programs in HIV prevention. *Public Health Rept* 1998;113 (Suppl 1):75–80.

35. National Institute on Alcohol Abuse and Alcoholism. *Helping patients with alcohol problems: A health practitioner's guide.* Bethesda, MD: National Institute on Alcohol Abuse and Alcoholism, 2004.

36. Beich A, et al. Screening in brief intervention trials targeting excessive drinkers in general practice: Systematic review and meta-analysis. *BMJ* 2003;327(7414):536–542.

37. U.S. Preventive Services Task Force. Screening and behavioral counseling interventions in primary care to reduce alcohol misuse: Recommendation statement. *Ann Intern Med* 2004;140(7):554–556.

38. National Consensus Development Panel on Effective Medical Treatment of Opiate Addiction. Effective medical treatment of opiate addiction. *JAMA* 1998;280(22): 1936–1943.

39. Kosten TR, O'Connor PG. Management of drug and alcohol withdrawal. *N Engl J Med* 2003;348(18):1786–1795.

Chapter 34

Tobacco Use

Clemens Hong, MD, MPH, Suzanne Harris, RN, Paul G. Brunetta, MD, and Neal Benowitz, MD

Objectives

- Review the epidemiology of patients who smoke.
- Describe the health effects of smoking.
- Describe the challenges presented to patients and providers interested in smoking cessation.
- Identify strategies to enhance smoking cessation, including patient, provider, and system-level interventions.

Clarence Cool is a 44-year-old African-American man brought to the emergency room via ambulance in respiratory distress. He has had five admissions within the past year for chronic obstructive pulmonary disease (COPD) exacerbations and has been intubated during each admission. He has been smoking since he was 8 years old and smokes up to two packs a day.

Cigarette smoking is the leading cause of preventable, premature morbidity and mortality in the United States and in many countries around the world. Smokers, on average, die 10 years earlier than non-smokers.[1] Tobacco use is a major cause of death from cancer, cardiovascular disease, and pulmonary disease. Smoking accounts for at least 6% to 8%, if not more, of total American medical costs.[2] Patterns of tobacco use are the result of the complex interactions of a multitude of factors, including socioeconomic status, culture, acculturation, poor access to medical care, targeted advertising, relative affordability of tobacco products, and varying capacities of communities to mount effective tobacco control initiatives. It is clear that helping smokers quit may be the most important acts health care providers do. This chapter reviews the epidemiology

and health effects of smoking, and the challenges it presents to patients, health care providers, and communities. It discusses some strategies for confronting these challenges.

EPIDEMIOLOGY OF TOBACCO USE

In 2003, an estimated 70.8 million Americans reported use of a tobacco product, with almost two thirds of those smoking every day.[3] Almost a million children aged 12 to 17 years old reported daily smoking.[4] The number of US first-time smokers has remained >2.5 million per year in nearly every year since 1965. In 2001, there were approximately 7000 new smokers a day, and 75% were under 18 years of age.[4] The smoking prevalence among adults in the United States is estimated at 22.1%, down from 57% among men in 1955 and 34% among women in 1965.[1] Of current smokers, 70% would like to quit if an easy method were available.

RACIAL/ETHNIC MINORITIES

Cigarette smoking varies considerably among and within different racial and ethnic populations (Fig. 34-1). Native Americans and Alaska Natives have the highest prevalence of smoking among both youths and adults,

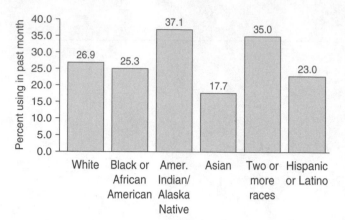

Figure 34-1. Past month cigarette use among persons aged 12 or older, by race/ethnicity. Available at: 2002 https://nsduhweb.rti.org/

although tobacco use varies widely by region, with rates of 36.1% in those 12 years old or older.[5] Asians at 12.6 % have the lowest rate of tobacco use; whites, African Americans, and Latinos all have similar smoking rates.[5,6]

GENDER

The once-wide gender gap in smoking prevalence narrowed through the 1980s to about 4%[1] and has remained stable since then. In 2004, 35.7% of men reported some tobacco use, and 27% reported smoking; 23% of women reported using tobacco products, and 22% reported smoking. Girls 12 to 17, however, are more likely to start smoking than boys of this age.[7,8]

PREGNANCY

There has been a steady decline in the prevalence of smoking during pregnancy; however, only about one third of women who stop smoking during pregnancy are still abstinent 1 year after the delivery.[8] Younger women, white or Native American women, women with <12 years of education, and women with low incomes consistently report the highest rates of smoking during pregnancy.[9] Hispanic women are more likely than non-Hispanic women to abstain from smoking use during the last 3 months of pregnancy.[9]

SOCIOECONOMIC FACTORS

College graduates are less likely than those without a high school diploma to be current smokers (14% compared with 35.3%). Smoking prevalence in unemployed adults was 42.7% in 2003 compared with 29.5% and 25.2% in full- and part-time workers, respectively.[10]

HEALTH CONSEQUENCES OF TOBACCO USE

Tobacco use causes approximately 440,000 preventable deaths each year in the United States, and more than 8.6 million people have at least one serious illness caused by smoking. If current patterns of smoking persist, 6.4 million people currently younger than 18 will die prematurely of a tobacco-related disease (Table 34-1).[10]

Table 34-1. Health Hazards of Tobacco Use (Risks Increased by Smoking)

Cancer
  Lung
  Urinary tract
  Oral cavity
  Oropharynx and hypopharynx
  Esophagus
  Larynx
  Pancreas
  Nasal cavity, sinuses, nasopharynx
  Stomach
  Liver
  Kidney
  Uterine cervix
  Myeloid leukemia
Infection
  Pneumococcal pneumonia
  Legionnaire's disease
  Meningococcal disease
  Periodontal disease
  Helicobacter pylori
  Common cold
  Influenza
  Human immunodeficiency virus infection
  Tuberculosis
Cardiovascular disease
  Sudden death
  Acute myocardial infarction
  Unstable angina
  Stroke
  Peripheral arterial occlusive disease
    (including thromboangiitis obliterans)
  Aortic aneurysm
Pulmonary disease
  Lung cancer
  Chronic bronchitis
  Emphysema
  Asthma
  Increased susceptibility to pneumonia
  Increased susceptibility to pulmonary tuberculosis and
    desquamative interstitial pneumonitis
  Increased morbidity from viral respiratory infection
Gastrointestinal disease
  Peptic ulcer
  Esophageal reflux
Reproductive disturbances
  Reduced fertility
  Premature birth
  Lower birth weight
  Spontaneous abortion

Table 34-1. Health Hazards of Tobacco Use (Risks Increased by Smoking) (*Continued*)

> Abruptio placentae
> Premature rupture of membranes
> Increased perinatal mortality
> **Oral disease (smokeless tobacco)**
> Oral cancer
> Leukoplakia
> Gingivitis
> Gingival recession
> Tooth staining
> **Other**
> Non–insulin-dependent diabetes mellitus
> Earlier menopause
> Osteoporosis
> Cataract
> Tobacco amblyopia
> Age-related macular degeneration
> Premature skin wrinkling
> Aggravation of hypothyroidism
> Altered drug metabolism or effects

Adapted from: Benowitz N, Brunetta P. Smoking hazards and cessation. In: Mason R, Broadus C, Murray J, et al, eds. *Murray and Nadel's textbook of respiratory medicine.* Philadelphia: Saunders, 2005, 2453–2465.

SECOND-HAND SMOKE

Second-hand smoke exposure is estimated to be responsible for approximately 3000 lung cancer deaths annually in nonsmokers in the United States,[11] and 40,000 cardiovascular deaths.[12] Each year, 280 children die from respiratory illness caused by second-hand smoke; and another 300 children suffer from injuries caused by smoking-caused fires.[13,14] Ingestion of cigarettes, cigarette butts, and other tobacco products found by young children around the house, in ashtrays, or in the garbage is another important source of toxic exposure.[15,16]

COMORBIDITIES LINKED TO SMOKING

Smokers are more likely to develop alcoholism (including binge drinking) or use illicit drugs than nonsmokers.[17] In addition, more than half of all children who start smoking before they are 15 years old use an illicit drug in their lifetime, compared with one fourth of those who wait until they are 17 years old.[17,18]

PSYCHIATRIC ILLNESS

Smokers are more likely to have a history of major depression and depressed smokers are more highly dependent on nicotine with resultant lower quit rates. When smokers with a history of depression do quit, they more frequently have depression as a prominent withdrawal symptom. Smoking rates in schizophrenia

have been estimated between 58% and 88%, two- to threefold the rate found in the general population.[18a] Schizophrenics also have significantly lower quit rates than the general population. Theories abound explaining the association between schizophrenia and cigarette smoking. Some posit that nicotine improves symptoms of schizophrenia and helps mitigate anti-psychotic medication side-effects. Others postulate that smokers are more likely to become schizophrenics either through common predisposing risk factors or as an etiologic risk factor itself.[18a]

DIFFICULTIES IN MANAGEMENT OF TOBACCO ABUSE

NICOTINE ADDICTION

Direct pharmacologic actions of nicotine and avoidance of withdrawal symptoms play a predominant role in tobacco addiction. Nicotine is as addictive as heroin or cocaine. It produces numerous gratifying effects, including pleasure, arousal, improved task performance, and anxiety relief. With long-term use of tobacco, physical dependence develops. When tobacco is unavailable, even for only a few hours, withdrawal symptoms occur and can be profound; for example, tobacco craving, anxiety, irritability, restlessness, difficulty concentrating, impaired task performance, hunger, weight gain, drowsiness, fatigue, malaise, anhedonia, disturbed sleep, and (in some people) frank depression. Learned associations also play a role in cigarette addiction. The need for hand and mouth stimulation or deep breathing has been described. Young smokers use cigarettes to cope with or modulate the stresses, pleasures, and complex emotions of adolescence, a strategy they often do not abandon as they mature.

A single cigarette rapidly relieves withdrawal symptoms. Nicotine moves to the brain within 10 to 15 seconds, where it acts on nicotinic cholinergic receptors and triggers the release of multiple neurotransmitters, including dopamine. Although tolerance can develop after long-term use, nicotine sensitivity returns quickly. This explains the appeal of the first morning cigarette, which quickly increases nicotine levels in the brain and brings morning arousal.

MEDIA AND TOBACCO MARKETING

Television and movies present smoking as a socially acceptable and "cool" thing to do. This places immense pressure on young people to start smoking and continue smoking. The tobacco industry spends billions of dollars—more than $41 million a day—on advertising campaigns that target teenagers, women, and minority populations.[19] Advertising and promotional campaigns target approximately 1.63 million new smokers a year to compensate for the market-loss that occurs when people quit or die.[20]

Targeting of Youth

Each day, more than 4000 children smoke their first cigarette, and half of them become regular daily smokers.[3] Smoking in the movies is the top recruiter of new adolescent smokers in the United States, estimated at 390,000 children a year; 120,000 of these children will die from tobacco-related diseases.[21] Similarly, children ages 10 to 15 who watched >5 hours of TV daily were more likely to initiate smoking than those who watched <2 hours daily.[22] Thirty-four percent of teens begin smoking as a result of tobacco company marketing efforts.[23] Restrictions on Internet advertising do not yet exist; therefore, as advertising expands here, numbers of teen smokers may increase.

Racial/Ethnic Minority Groups

Tobacco products are promoted disproportionately to racial/ethnic minority groups. The tobacco industry's pursuit of minority smokers has been relentless: advertising heavily in minority neighborhoods and publications; supporting cultural events such as rodeos and powwows for Native Americans; making contributions to minority institutions (e.g., historically African-American colleges and universities), elected officials, civic community organizations and scholarship programs; and the production of culturally targeted brands ("Rio" and "Dorado" for Latinos, and the "American Spirit" for Native Americans).[6] This close association of tobacco with significant events and rituals in many racial/ethnic communities, along with the tobacco industry's long history of providing employment opportunities and contributions to community groups and leaders, undermines tobacco prevention and control efforts in these communities.[6]

Women

The tobacco industry spends >$5 billion yearly to market to women in the United States alone.[24] Market research is done to better target the psychological and emotional needs of female smokers. Tobacco ads and promotions are designed to associate smoking with women's freedom, emancipation, sexual appeal, and empowerment.[24] Philip Morris' launching of the Virginia Slims brand in 1968, for example, significantly increased the numbers of women smokers.[25]

Disparities in Smoking Cessation Efforts

Despite the fact that smoking cessation interventions are equally efficacious for all populations and the desire for smoking cessation is higher in minority populations, even fewer minority patients are able to quit smoking. For example, more than 70% of African-American adult smokers want to quit, and African Americans are more likely than white smokers to have quit for at least 1 day during the past year. However, the prevalence of cessation (percentage of people who have smoked at least 100 cigarettes and quit) is significantly higher among whites than African Americans (50.5% versus 35.4%). Multiple factors might account for this disparity in cessation rates. Racial/ethnic minority populations commonly have less access than whites to culturally and linguistically appropriate anti-smoking educational materials, media messages, cessation services, and pharmacologic treatment.[5] Moreover, racial/ethnic minority populations have long been targets of tobacco industry marketing efforts.[5] Physicians also may be less likely to recommend smoking cessation to their poor and minority patients.[26,27]

CHALLENGES HEALTH PROVIDERS FACE IN SMOKING CESSATION EFFORTS

More than 70% of smokers report a desire to quit, and smokers cite a physician's advice to quit as an important motivator for attempting to stop smoking.[28] The majority of smokers see at least one or more health professionals each year; however, most smokers are not asked about their smoking status, urged to quit, or offered effective assistance in quitting.[28]

Many health care providers are unfamiliar with the available treatments for smoking, or their efficacy, administration, and side-effects.[28] Many physicians harbor fears that they do not have enough time and their counseling will be ineffective.[29] Training is often lacking, further adding to the hopelessness of physicians in addressing smoking cessation in their clinics. This is particularly true of providers counseling adolescents, arguably the most important group to target for prevention efforts.[30] Even when a health care provider is armed with adequate knowledge, conflicting priorities and time pressures make it extremely difficult to address tobacco use and cessation. In practices that serve vulnerable populations, these challenges—aggravated by language barriers, scarce resources, and poor access to care resulting in missed appointments—make the clinic visit increasingly more demanding.

Common Pitfalls in Smoking Cessation

- Nicotine is extremely addictive.
- Smoking continues to hold a seductive allure for many people (minority populations, the young, women) that is fostered and exploited by tobacco companies.

- Hopelessness and feelings of failure, shame, and embarrassment can undercut a person's resolve. Patients and providers alike feel that quitting is likely to fail.
- Providers are inadequately trained in smoking cessation treatments and techniques.
- Systematic screening is rarely employed
- Underserved patients have limited access to effective treatments.
- Preventive counseling is rarely reimbursed.
- Comorbid conditions of mental illness and other addictions may complicate cessation and prevention efforts.

STRATEGIES FOR MANAGING TOBACCO ABUSE

> Mr. Cool is contacted numerous times before he attends a smoking cessation class. He is prescribed nicotine patches and bonds with others in the class. He is eventually able to quit smoking. In the year after he quits smoking he has no admissions to the hospital. He becomes a cofacilitator of the cessation class.

PRIMARY PREVENTION

The vast majority of smokers initiate tobacco use prior to 18 years of age.[28] Delaying the age when children first experiment with smoking can reduce the risk that they become regular smokers and increase their chances of quitting if they become regular smokers. All adolescents should be asked about tobacco use among their peers as well as within their home environment. Risk factors for youth smoking include peer greater than parental smoking, behavioral problems, poor school performance, low self-esteem, rebelliousness or risk-taking behaviors, depression, anxiety, lack of ability to resist influences to tobacco use, and living in families of lower socioeconomic status or single-parent homes.

Counseling and behavioral interventions used in adults also are useful in adolescents. However, given their developmental stage, many teens do not respond to warnings about the long-term adverse health outcomes of tobacco use, but may respond to short-term effects such as halitosis, skin wrinkling, and erectile dysfunction. Messages pertaining to the dangers of second-hand smoke and the addiction potential of nicotine along with anti–tobacco industry messages are the most highly effective messages to use when trying to reach teen smokers.[31] Policies such as prohibiting sales to minors and particularly high cigarette taxes are also very effective components of decreasing youth smoking.

BENEFITS OF QUITTING

Health benefits to cessation begin almost immediately after the last puff of a cigarette.[1] Within weeks patients have improvement in their respiratory symptoms and exercise tolerance, although initially the excretion of excess mucus and tobacco residue may increase cough. Immune suppression in smokers resolves within 6 weeks after cessation, and smoking cessation is highly effective in prevention of infection in a short period of time.[31a] Just 1 year after quitting, the risk of coronary artery disease drops to half that of persistent smokers. Fifteen years later, the risk of coronary artery disease falls to the rate of people who have never smoked. Only 2 years after cessation, death from any cause begins to decline significantly, and the risk of stroke begins to approach the risk of never-smokers. Ten years after smoking cessation, the risk of pneumococcal disease declines to rates of nonsmokers,[31] and although risk of cancer never declines to rates of nonsmokers, it falls by 50% after a decade of abstention.[1] Smoking cessation occurring 6 to 8 weeks before elective surgery decreases overall perioperative complications.[32] Even smokers who quit after 65 years of age add 4 years to their lives when compared with people who continue to smoke.[1]

TREATING TOBACCO DEPENDENCE

Screening

Asking and recording smoking status as another vital sign has been suggested as one method of assuring that smoking does not drop off providers' radar as a problem, so those who have relapsed will be discovered and assisted. The Agency for Healthcare Research and Quality (AHRQ) guidelines recommend that clinicians begin by using the five As mnemonic to initiate a brief intervention in every patient presenting to the clinical setting (Box 34-1; Fig. 34-2).

Smoking Cessation

Intensive counseling, including cognitive and behavioral therapy, is associated with a 22% quit rate compared with a 13% quit rate with minimal counseling of less than 3 minutes. A strong dose–response relationship between length of person-to-person contact and quit rates also has been shown, and treatment delivered in four or more sessions has been shown to increase abstinence rates. Treatments delivered by multiple types of providers and in multiple types of formats are more effective than interventions by a single type of clinician in a single type of format.[28] Nevertheless, even brief interventions have been shown to have a significant benefit in helping patients quit smoking.

Box 34-1. The *Five A's* Mnemonic

Ask

- Screen patients for smoking at each and every visit. Consider making it a vital sign.

Advise

- Clearly advise patients to quit at every visit
- Personalize the message: Tie tobacco use to a current health problem, its cost, or the impact on others.
- Stress total abstinence as the goal.

Assess

- Assess each smoker's willingness to quit at every visit.
- If willing, offer behavioral and pharmacologic treatment, including intensive treatment if available.

- If unwilling, provide a motivational intervention (see five Rs).
- Provide information/resources tailored to the patient (*adolescent, pregnant smoker, racial/ethnic minority*).

Assist

- Assist patient in making a quit attempt (see STAR mnemonic).

Arrange

- Arrange follow-up tailored to the patient.

Smoker Willingness to Quit

When it is determined that a patient is ready to quit, the provider should help with a quit plan. The STAR mnemonic may be used to address all the major components to an effective quit plan (Box 34-2).

The Smoker Who Is Unwilling to Quit

The smoker may lack information about the harmful effects of tobacco because of poor health literacy or language barriers, or because no one has ever taken the time to tell him or her. Additionally, he or she may lack the required financial resources, may have concerns about quitting including fears of withdrawal symptoms, or may be demoralized because of previous relapse.

Disinterest in quitting or protest that smoking is enjoyable may mask a profound doubt in ability to overcome the habit. Reasons for continued smoking may be expressed in a number of ways, from indifference to

anger. However, challenging this assumption prematurely may be met with resistance to quitting. Promoting motivation to quit is most likely to be successful when the clinician is empathic, promotes patient autonomy, avoids arguments, and supports the patient's self-efficacy by identifying previous success in behavior change efforts (Box 34-3) (see Chap. 7).

THE SMOKER WHO HAS RECENTLY QUIT: PREVENTING RELAPSE

> Mr. Cool abstains from smoking for over 15 years. When his daughter dies, he relapses and needs to be hospitalized for a COPD exacerbation. At first he is ashamed of smoking again, but when he returns to facilitating the group, he discusses his relapse as predictable. His doctor does not ask about the smoking relapse as she assumes he no longer smokes, but when Mr. Cool brings up what happened, they decide to restart nicotine patches and bupropion.

Often in busy clinical practices it is easy to assume that once the provider has successfully helped a smoker quit, smoking no longer needs to be addressed. However, it is essential to continue to address the issue of smoking with the patient to prevent relapse. Most relapses occur within the first 3 months after quitting, although some relapses occur months or even years after the quit date.[28] Consequently, follow-up through clinic visits and telephone calls is critical during the first 3 months. Encourage patients to report any difficulties promptly, including lapses, depression, and medication side-effects while continuing efforts to quit. Congratulate the recovering smoker on success and encourage continued abstinence. Smokers respect the opinions of

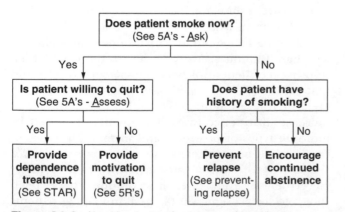

Figure 34-2. Algorithm for treating tobacco dependence.

Box 34-2. STAR Mnemonic

*S*et a quit date.

- Set a quit date, ideally within 2 weeks.
- The goal is for total abstinence.

*T*ell family, friends, and coworkers.

- Elicit support by telling family, friends, and coworkers about the quit plan. Request understanding and support.
- Solidify resolve.

*A*nticipate challenges.

- Ask open-ended questions and discuss past quit attempts to elicit the triggers for smoking.
- Problem solve ways to overcome triggers to smoking.
- Create a plan to prevent relapse and orchestrate support.
- Encourage house mates to quit with patient or not smoke in the patient's presence.
- Review nicotine withdrawal symptoms.
- Recommend abstention from alcohol during quit attempt.

- Recommend pharmacologic treatment.
- Encourage the patient to seek help before relapse.

*R*emove tobacco products.

- Before the quit date, get rid of all cigarettes and tobacco products.
- Avoid smoking in places where the smoker spends a lot of time (home/car/work).

Follow-up for quit attempt

- Follow-up 1 week after quit date.
- Follow-up 1 month after quit date.
- Phone interventions may be helpful.
- Congratulate successes.
- If relapse occurs, review circumstances and recommit to the quit process by setting a new quit date.
- Use the relapse as an opportunity to assure success.
- Review medication use and side-effects.
- Consider referral to more intensive treatment.

health care providers and these short interventions are well received.

WHEN TO INTERVENE

Although providers should not wait for special circumstances to discuss smoking cessation, there may be times when a patient is more motivated to quit, such as at the onset of new medical symptoms, a hospitalization, a myocardial infarction, impending surgery, a friend recently diagnosed with lung cancer, pregnancy, the recent birth of a child, a new child at home, or diagnosis of asthma in a child. Tailoring any event to a patient's circumstances can be used as a motivating factor. For

Box 34-3. The Five R's

*R*elevance

- Encourage the patient to reflect on why quitting is personally relevant.
- Use reflective listening and open-ended questions.

*R*isks (Cons: see Health Consequences of Smoking section)

- Ask the patient to identify the negative consequences of tobacco use.
- Highlight the risks that are most relevant to the patient.
- Discuss short-term, long-term, and environmental risks.

*R*ewards (see Pros and Cons in Core Competency)

- Ask the patient to identify the benefits of smoking.
- Highlight the benefits that are most relevant to the patient. Discuss the pros of smoking for the patient.

- Add health benefits if the patient does not articulate these.

*R*oadblocks

- Ask the patient to identify barriers and impediments to quitting.
- Problem solve with the patient by noting elements of treatment that could address barriers.

*R*epetition

- Perform a motivational intervention at every encounter.
- If past failure is a concern, notify the patient that most people make repeated quit attempts before success.
- Stress relapse as an opportunity to plumb for success.
- Schedule follow-up.

instance, smoking cessation before middle age is associated with a more than 90% reduction in tobacco-attributable cancer risk;[33] hence, the mid-life birthday of a patient is a perfect time to bring up quitting.

PHARMACOTHERAPY

In addition to counseling, all smokers making a quit attempt should receive pharmacotherapy, except in the presence of special circumstances. Additionally, long-term smoking cessation pharmacotherapy can be considered as a strategy to reduce the likelihood of relapse. It is important to remember when choosing a pharmacotherapeutic regimen that patient preferences and expectations regarding outcome are important in guiding the choice of a specific pharmacotherapy.[34] Six first-line pharmacotherapies are approved by the US Food and Drug Administration to be safe and effective for tobacco dependence treatment: bupropion SR, nicotine gum, nicotine patch, nicotine lozenge, nicotine nasal spray, and nicotine inhaler. See Table 34-2 for a summary of the dosing, recommended usage, cost, contraindications, side-effects, and other notes.

PREGNANCY

Use of pharmacotherapy is controversial during pregnancy, because none of the medications have been tested in pregnant women. A number of studies have shown that nicotine presents risks to the fetus, including neurotoxicity.[28] Treating a woman with nicotine replacement, however, may actually reduce the amount of nicotine she is absorbing if she is a heavy smoker and avoids exposing the fetus to the other toxic compounds

Table 34-2. Review of Clinical Use of Pharmacotherapies for Smoking Cessation

Pharmacotherapy	Precautions/ Contraindications	Adverse Effects	Dosage	Duration	Availability	Cost per Day
First-line						
Sustained-release Bupropion hydrochloride	History of seizure History of eating disorders	Insomnia Dry mouth	150 mg every morning for 3 days, then 150 mg twice daily (begin treatment 1–2 weeks prequit)	7–12 weeks maintenance up to 6 months	Prescription only	$3.33
Nicotine gum	Temporomandibular joint disorder	Mouth soreness Dyspepsia	1–24 cigarettes/d; 2 mg gum (up to 24 pieces/d) ≥25 cigarettes/d; 4 mg gum (up to 24 pieces/d)	Up to 12 weeks	Over the counter only (OTC)	$6.25 for 10 2–mg pieces $6.87 for 10 4–mg pieces
Nicotine inhaler		Local irritation of mouth and throat	6–16 cartridges/d	Up to 6 months	Prescription only	$10.94 for 10 cartridges
Nicotine nasal spray	Chronic nasal disorders, including rhinitis, polyps, and sinusitis	Nasal irritation Throat burning	8–40 doses/d	3–6 months	Prescription only	$5.40 for 12 doses
Nicotine patch	Skin diseases, such as atopic or eczematous dermatitis	Local skin reaction Insomnia	21 mg/24 h 14 mg/24 h 7 mg/24 h 15 mg/16 h	4 weeks then 2 weeks then 2 weeks 8 weeks	Prescription and OTC	$4.22 $4.51
Second-line						
Clonidine	Rebound hypertension	Dry mouth Drowsiness Dizziness Sedation	0.15–0.75 mg/d	3–10 weeks	Prescription only (oral formulation) Prescription only	$0.24 for 0.2 mg $3.50
Nortriptyline	Risk of arrhythmias	Sedation Dry mouth	75–100 mg/d	12 weeks	Prescription only	$0.74 for 75 mg

Adapted from: A clinical practice guideline for treating tobacco use and dependence: A US. Public Health Service Report. The Tobacco Use and Dependence Clinical Practice Guideline Panel, Staff, and Consortium Representatives. *JAMA* 2000;283:3244–3254.[45]

found in smoke. Intermittently dosed nicotine products are probably safer in pregnancy than the patch, with its continuous release of nicotine.

HARM REDUCTION

In harm reduction strategies, tobacco users alter or decrease, rather than eliminate, their use of nicotine or tobacco. Although total abstinence from cigarettes is a goal, as increased health risks have been documented even in smokers who smoke less than five cigarettes per day,[35] there is evidence that reduction in smoking is helpful. Patients who reduce smoking may eventually quit,[36] and in the meantime asthma symptoms,[37] worsening lung function and risk of lung cancer have all been shown to decrease.[33] Shifting to low-tar and -nicotine cigarettes or other forms of tobacco show no reduction in risk because smokers compensate by increasing the frequency or depth of inhalation per cigarette.[38]

SYSTEM-BASED APPROACHES TO SMOKING CESSATION

System-based approaches—referral to telephone quit lines or smoking cessation specialists or group classes to help patients quit smoking—are most useful. Creating smoking cessation consult services; implementing systematic screening and tobacco-user identification systems; and ensuring adequate training in smoking cessation for personnel and availability of appropriate resources are all important interventions. Health care facility chart audits, electronic medical records, and computerized patient databases can be used to evaluate the degree to which health care providers are identifying, documenting, and treating smokers. Feedback can be provided to providers in the form of "report cards" to remind providers about the importance of addressing tobacco use in their practices. Guaranteeing that pharmacotherapies are covered or provided for patients at minimal cost is particularly important.

Lastly, reimbursement for tobacco cessation programs is essential. Insurers and purchasers of insurance must make certain that all insurance plans include a reimbursement benefit for smoking cessation counseling and pharmacotherapy as well as a reimbursement for clinicians providing tobacco dependence treatment. In 2002, only 36 state Medicaid programs offered coverage for at least one form of tobacco-dependence treatment for all Medicaid recipients, and only 12 states covered some form of tobacco cessation counseling services to all Medicaid recipients. Given that smoking prevalence in the Medicaid population is 50% greater than in the non-Medicaid adult populations and smoking cessation has been shown to be more cost effective

than the treatment of mild or moderate hypertension or hypercholesterolemia, failure to cover these services makes no sense.[28]

TELEPHONE QUIT LINES

Toll-free telephone quit lines connect smokers with trained counselors who take an individual smoking history, prepare a customized cessation plan that includes pharmacotherapy, and provides follow-up telephone calls to assess progress. Toll-free telephone quit lines are currently available in over 42 states.[1] The American Cancer Society and the Cancer Information Service of the National Cancer Institute provide national services. The Department of Health and Human Services has a national number (1-800-QUITNOW) that forwards callers to services in their area.

Telephone counseling is effective in promoting cessation. In a large, randomized controlled trial of over 3000 patients, telephone counseling through the California state quit line (1-800-NOBUTTS) nearly doubled abstinence rates.[39] Telephone quit lines offer convenience, the ability to serve diverse and multilingual populations, and anonymity. The majority of patients also prefer using quit lines to clinic visits.[1] Internet programs to help people quit smoking are a newer variation on telephone counseling.

POLICY-BASED APPROACHES TO SMOKING CESSATION

As health care providers and patient advocates, providers have the opportunity to take part in many community-based and broader initiatives to combat the epidemic of tobacco in the United States. Many of these policy-based initiatives have been shown to be more effective in tobacco cessation than any clinic-based intervention practitioners can provide. Therefore, it is useful to review some of these policy-based initiatives.

PRIMARY PREVENTION AND POLICY-BASED APPROACHES IN CHILDREN

Primary prevention of smoking in US youth is the focus of many legislative and programmatic interventions. Effective legislative methods useful in decreasing initiation of smoking among youth include use of excise taxes to increase the cost of cigarettes, restricting tobacco advertising and promotional activities (including bans on point of purchase and print advertising as well as sponsorship of events by tobacco companies), mandating tobacco education in schools, banning representation of smoking on television and in the movies, and making tobacco access laws for minors more strict (including requirements to keep tobacco products behind the counter and bans on cigarette vending machines). Antismoking media campaigns and counter-advertising, merchant education and training, school-based tobacco use prevention programs that help model for children the identification and resistance of social influences that lead to smoking, and bans on smoking on school grounds have all been shown to be effective. Restrictions on indoor smoking, campaigns to discourage family and friends from providing cigarettes to youth, and promoting smoke-free homes also work.[40] Evidence supports the use of multiple modalities in combination in a comprehensive program against tobacco use and initiation. The prevalence of smoking among youth has declined most rapidly in states that have used the most extensive paid media campaigns in combination with other antitobacco activities in their comprehensive antitobacco campaigns.[40]

POLICY-BASED APPROACHES TO SMOKING CESSATION IN ADULTS

Policy-based interventions used to decrease smoking in adults are also important interventions. Tobacco-free work places are an example of an effective policy-based intervention in adults. In addition to protecting both workers and patrons from second-hand smoke exposure; smoke-free workplace policies are associated with decreased cigarette consumption and possibly with increased cessation rates among workers and members of the general public. These measures are supported by the general public and do not decrease business revenues in restaurants and bars.[41]

Language-appropriate, culturally competent, targeted education campaigns are being waged to combat tobacco company advertising and promotional activities in minority and low socioeconomic status populations. Continued monitoring of tobacco industry attempts to target these populations is necessary to develop a comprehensive understanding of the influences that encourage individuals in these high-risk populations to smoke and design effective counter-marketing campaigns.

CONCLUSION

Tobacco use is a scourge on the health of the United States. Helping current smokers quit and keeping people, particularly young people, from starting should be top priorities for all health professionals. Achieving these goals will require a spectrum of responses from efforts of individual providers, clinics, hospitals, and health care systems to antismoking media campaigns, legislative restrictions on promotion and sale of tobacco products, and smoking in public places.

KEY CONCEPTS

- Smoking is the leading cause of preventable death in the United States.
- The poor, the mentally ill, and minorities bear the brunt of poor health caused by cigarette smoking.
- Primary prevention in the young is best tackled through comprehensive public policies and medical counseling of children, teens, and their parents.
- All health professionals should address smoking cessation at every opportunity.
- Systems-based interventions are essential to support tobacco cessation efforts.
- Public policies are needed to combat the powerful and pervasive promotion of tobacco products by cigarette companies.

CORE COMPETENCY
Practical Smoking Cessation Tips and Exercises

GENERAL APPROACH
- *Avoid* "shoulds." Use alternatives, such as, "Consider becoming smoke free."
- Be *empathetic* and *respectful* about the difficulty of quitting.
  - *Remember:* Shame about smoking may actually inhibit cessation.
  - *Acknowledge* smoking as an addiction, not a filthy habit or deficit in the person.
  - *Fear-based motivation* may cause feelings of powerlessness and hopeless. Fear may break a person out of denial, but as a constant motivational tool is often counterproductive.
  - *Desire-based motivation* can be more powerful than avoidance.
  - Smoking cessation takes time and is a process. Do not get discouraged.

EXERCISES
Awareness
- Ask patients to pay attention to how they feel when inhaling the cigarette.
- Rate the four components of addiction to cigarettes on a scale of 1 to 5 in importance:
  - Nicotine (although remember that nicotine effects and psychological reasons for smoking may be intertwined and impossible to distinguish)
  - Hand and mouth stimulation
  - Psychological and emotional impulses for smoking
  - Review conditioned cues: smoking after meals, during break times, when angry or upset, etc.
- Use this information to focus interventions such as stress management.

Deep breathing
- Deep breathing can help manage stress and eliminate cigarettes.

 Deep breathing instruction: Purse lips and exhale as though blowing out a candle. Keep blowing until you can no longer exhale, and then allow a natural inhalation. The inhalation will be deep and go to the abdomen. Practice a minimum of three times daily with 5 to 10 deep breaths each time. Use this to postpone or eliminate cigarettes.

Delaying
- Cut drinking straws into the length of a cigarette. Put several into your cigarette pack. When you pull up a straw, deep breathe instead of smoke.

Pros and Cons
- Reviewing an individual's reasons for smoking provides the basis for exploring new responses to important needs. For example:
—Smoking helps a woman establish boundaries with men. She can use the lit cigarette to indicate "don't come closer than this."
—Smoking gives a person a reason to go outside and take a break from being with people, especially if he or she tends to be shy.
—Smoking lets you feel cool and rebellious.
—Smoking helps keep you awake, relaxed, and calm, and controls anger, hunger, and loneliness.
- *Desire-based motivation*: List the cons about smoking. Turn the cons into the pros about being smoke free. For example, feeling like a bad mother and nurse because of smoking can be turned into, "I am devoted to my children and health and can be fearless and proud and smoke free."

DISCUSSION QUESTIONS

1. Why do you think that health care professionals in your field do not tackle smoking cessation as frequently as they should? What strategies could you use in your setting to improve smoking cessation efforts?
2. Some argue that without the production and sale of tobacco our economy would suffer tremendously and that public policies to restrict tobacco use hurt the economy. Discuss.
3. Practice and role-play with your neighbor using the five As, five Rs, and STAR techniques.
4. Compare and contrast the health benefits of quitting smoking with other treatments that are often prescribed.

RESOURCES

http://www.cdc.gov/tobacco/
http://www.ahrq.gov/
Many hospitals have smoking cessation services available that enable referral of smokers as necessary. Many states have toll free quit lines (e.g., in California, 1-800-NO-BUTTS), and the national number (1-800-QUITNOW) forwards callers to services in their area.

Comprehensive information from patient aides to clinical recommendations to information on how to develop or fund comprehensive tobacco programs are available on the Centers for Disease Control and Prevention and the Agency for Health Care Research and Quality web sites.

http://www.quitnet.com
Internet-based programs such as QuitNet can provide online chat rooms and can give smokers with access to a computer a sense of community with other smokers. If patients do not have their own computer, the public library is a smokefree environment in which they can access computers.

http://www.lungusa.org/tobacco
The American Lung Association has significant information and an online program called "Seven Steps to a Smoke-Free Life" to which patients can be referred.

REFERENCES

1. Schroeder SA. What to do with a patient who smokes. *JAMA* 2005;294(4):482–487.
2. Warner KE. The economics of tobacco: Myths and realities. *Tob Control* 2000;9(1):78–89.
3. Cigarette smoking among adults: United States, 2003. *MMWR Morb Mortal Wkly Rep* 2005;54(20):509–513.
4. Centers for Disease Control and Prevention (CDC). Cigarette use among high school students—United States, 1991–2003. *MMWR Morb Mortal Wkly Rep* 2004; 53(23):499–502.
5. Centers for Disease Control and Prevention (CDC). Prevalence of cigarette use among 14 racial/ethnic populations—: United States, 1999–2001. *MMWR Morb Mortal Wkly Rep* 2004;53(3):49–52.
6. Surgeon General. Tobacco use among U.S. racial/ethnic minority groups—African Americans, American Indians and Alaska Natives, Asian Americans and Pacific Islanders, Hispanics. Executive summary. *MMWR Recomm Rep* 1998;47(RR-18):v–xv, 1–16.
7. Substance Abuse and Mental Health Services Administration. *Results from the 2003 national survey on drug use and health.* Available at: http://www.oas.samhsa.gov/nhsda/2k3tabs/PDF/2k3TabsCover.pdf
8. Centers for Disease Control and Prevention (CDC). Cigarette smoking among adults: United States, 2000. *MMWR Morb Mortal Wkly Rep* 2002;51:637–660.
9. Phares TM, Morrow B, Lansky A, et al. Surveillance for disparities in maternal health-related behaviors—selected states. Pregnancy Risk Assessment Monitoring System (PRAMS), 2000–2001. *MMWR Surveill Summ* 2004;53(4):1–13.
10. Centers for Disease Control and Prevention (CDC). Cigarette smoking among adults—United States, 2002. *MMWR Morb Mortal Wkly Rep* 2004;53(20):427–431.
11. Environmental Protection Agency. Respiratory Health Effects of Passive Smoking: Lung Cancer and Other

Disorders. Washington, DC: Office of Research and Development, US Environmental Protection Agency, 1992.

12. Glantz SA, Parmley WW. Passive smoking and heart disease. Epidemiology, physiology, and biochemistry. *Circulation* 1991;82:1–12.

13. Li JS, Peat JK, Xuan W, et al. Meta-analysis on the association between environmental tobacco smoke (ETS) exposure and the prevalence of lower respiratory tract infection in early childhood. *Pediatr Pulmonol* 1999; 27(1):5–13.

14. DiFranza JR, Lew RA. Morbidity and mortality in children associated with the use of tobacco products by other people. *Pediatrics* 1996;97(4):560–568.

15. Centers for Disease Control and Prevention (CDC). Ingestion of cigarettes and cigarette butts by children: Rhode Island, January 1994–July 1996. *MMWR Morb Mortal Wkly Rep* 1997;46(6):125–128.

16. American Academy of Pediatrics Committee on Environmental Health. Environmental tobacco smoke: A hazard to children. *Pediatrics* 1997;99(4):639–642.

17. Substance Abuse and Mental Health Services Administration. *Summary of findings from the 1998 National Household Survey on Drug Abuse.* Washington, DC: U.S. Department of Health and Human Services. March, 2000. Available at: http://www.oas.samhsa.gov/NHSDA/98MF.pdf

18. Center on Addiction and Substance Abuse (CASA), Columbia University. *Cigarettes, alcohol, marijuana: Gateways to illicit drug use.* October 1994. Available at: www.casacolumbia.org

18a. Kelly C, McCreadie R. Cigarette smoking and schizophrenia. Adv Psychiatric Treat 2000;6:327–331.

19. Federal Trade Commission. *Cigarette Report for 2003.* Washington, DC: Federal Trade Commission, 2005. Available at: http://www.ftc.gov/reports/cigarette05/050809cigrpt.pdf

20. Surgeon General. *Reducing tobacco use.* Atlanta: Centers for Disease Control and Prevention, 2000.

21. Dalton MA, Sargent JD, Beach ML, et al. Effect of viewing smoking in movies on adolescent smoking initiation: A cohort study. *Lancet* 2003;362(9380):281–285.

22. Gidwani PP, Sobol A, DeJong W, et al. Television viewing and initiation of smoking among youth. *Pediatrics* 2002;110:505–508.

23. Pierce JP, Choi WS, Gilpin EA, et al. Tobacco industry promotion of cigarettes and adolescent smoking. *JAMA* 1998;279(7):511–515.

24. Toll BA, Ling PM. The Virginia Slims identity crisis: An inside look at tobacco industry marketing to women. *Tob Control* 2005;14(3):172–180.

25. Anderson SJ, Glantz SA, Ling PM. Emotions for sale: Cigarette advertising and women's psychosocial needs. *Tob Control* 2005;14(2):127–135.

26. Houston TK, Scarinci IC, Person SD, et al. Patient smoking cessation advice by health care providers: The role of ethnicity, socioeconomic status, and health. *Am J Public Health* 2005;95:1056–61.

27. Doescher MP, Saver BG. Physicians' advice to quit smoking. The glass remains half empty. *J Fam Pract* 2000; 49(6): 543–547.

28. Fiore MC, Bailey WC, Cohen SJ, et al. *Treating tobacco use and dependence: A quick reference guide for clinicians.* Rockville, MD: US Department of Health and Human Services, October 2000. Available at: http://www.surgeongeneral.gov/tobacco/tobaqrg.htm

29. Vogt F, Hall S, Marteau TM. General practitioners' and family physicians' negative beliefs and attitudes towards discussing smoking cessation with patients: A systematic review. *Addiction* 2005;100(10):1423–1431.

30. Kaplan CP, Perez-Stable EJ, Fuentes-Afflick E, et al. Smoking cessation counseling with young patients: The practices of family physicians and pediatricians. *Arch Pediatr Adolesc Med* 2004;158(1):83–90.

31. Glantz SA, Jamieson P. Attitudes toward second-hand smoke, smoking, and quitting among young people. *Pediatrics* 2000;106(6):E82.

31a. Arcavi L, Benowitz NL. Cigarette smoking and infection. *Arch Intern Med* 2004;164(20):2206–2216.

32. Warner MA, Divertie MB, Tinker JH. Preoperative cessation of smoking and pulmonary complications in coronary artery bypass patients. *Anesthesiology* 1984;60:380–383.

33. Godtfredsen NS, Prescott E, Osler M. Effect of smoking reduction on lung cancer risk. *JAMA* 2005;294(12): 1505–1510.

34. Hughes J. Recent advances in the pharmacotherapy of smoking. *JAMA* 1999;281(1):72–76.

35. Rosengren A, Wilhelmsen L. Coronary heart disease, cancer, and mortality in male middle-aged light smokers. *J Intern Med* 1992;231(4):357–362.

36. Pisinger C, Vestbo J, Borch-Johnsen K, et al. Smoking reduction intervention in a large population-based study. The Inter99 study. *Prev Med* 2005;40(1):112–118.

37. Tonnesen P, Pisinger C, Hvidberg S, et al. Effects of smoking cessation and reduction in asthmatics. *Nicotine Tob Res* 2005;7(1):139–148.

38. *The FTC cigarette test method for determining tar, nicotine, and carbon monoxide yields of US cigarettes: Report of the NCI expert committee.* Washington, DC: National Institutes of Health Publication, 1996. Available at: http://cancercontrol.cancer.gov/tcrb/monographs/7/m7_complete.pdf

39. Zhu SH, Anderson CM, Tedeschi GJ, et al. Evidence of real-world effectiveness of a telephone quit line for smokers. *N Engl J Med* 2002;347:1087–1093.

40. Centers for Disease Control. Effect of ending an antitobacco youth campaign on adolescent susceptibility to cigarette smoking: Minnesota, 2002–2003. *MMWR Morb Mortal Wkly Rep* 2004;53(14): 301–304.

41. Centers for Disease Control. State smoking restrictions for private-sector worksites, restaurants, and bars: United States, 1998 and 2004. *MMWR Morb Mortal Wkly Rep* 2005;54(26):649–653.

42. Benowitz N, Brunetta P. Smoking hazards and cessation. In: Mason R, Broadus C, Murray J, et al, eds. *Murray and Nadel's textbook of respiratory medicine.* Philadelphia: Saunders, 2005, 2453–2456.

43. US Public Health Service. The Tobacco Use and Dependence Clinical Practice Guideline Panel, Staff, and Consortium Representatives. A clinical practice guideline for treating tobacco use and dependence. *JAMA* 2000;283(24): 3244–3254.

Chapter 35

Dental Care: The Forgotten Need

Matthew Nealon, DDS, and Francisco Ramos-Gomez, DDS, MS, MPH

Objectives

- Discuss the epidemiology of dental disease.
- Define dental caries and periodontal disease.
- Review the factors in caries development.
- Identify the link between periodontal disease and other health problems.
- Review methods of identifying and preventing early childhood caries.
- Identify strategies for assuring dental health

Juana is a 33-year-old immigrant from Mexico with diabetes. Juana complains that her molar on the lower right is loose and wants to have it pulled. This is the fourth tooth she has had extracted in the last year, and does not connect the loss of her teeth to her uncontrolled diabetes and poor oral hygiene.

Oral care is a vital part of providing comprehensive care to all patients. However, the relationship of oral health to the overall health of patients is often overlooked. Factors such as age, economic status, low education and literacy, the existence of mental or physical handicaps, and ethnicity all contribute to risk for dental caries and periodontal disease. Chronic illnesses, poor nutritional and lifestyle habits, and a lack of dental knowledge also put many patients at risk not only for the loss of teeth, but also the degradation of their overall health and quality of life. Consequently, what amounts to "a silent epidemic" of oral diseases is affecting the most vulnerable citizens: poor children, the elderly, and many members of racial and ethnic minority groups.[1]

This chapter discusses the importance of dental health to general health, identifies risk factors associated with dental caries and periodontal disease, and suggests methods of educating patients about oral health.

THE IMPORTANCE OF DENTAL CARE

People with poor dental health may have increased difficulty speaking, chewing, and swallowing. In addition to the social isolation and psychological pain that these problems can bring, general health may suffer as well. In extreme cases, nutrition may be compromised. Poor dentition also may lead to recurrent systemic infections such as pneumonia or endocarditis. Other conditions, such as worsening diabetes, cardiovascular disease, and preterm birth also may be exacerbated or increased by poor dental health.

The preservation of natural dentition is critical at all ages. In children, the prevention of early cavities is not only important for the development of the permanent teeth, but also for their quality of life and appropriate development. The loss of teeth can bring negative social stigma, especially when tooth loss occurs at a young age. In addition, chewing with partial and complete dentures is difficult for patients and in no way compares with natural dentition (Box 35-1).

Box 35-1. Major Findings of the Surgeon General's Report on Oral Health

- Oral diseases and disorders in and of themselves affect health and well-being throughout life.
- Safe and effective measures exist to prevent the most common dental diseases, dental caries and periodontal diseases.
- Lifestyle behaviors that affect general health, such as tobacco use, excessive alcohol use, and poor dietary choices, affect oral and craniofacial health as well.
- There are profound and consequential oral health disparities within the US population.
- More information is needed to improve America's oral health and eliminate health disparities.

- The mouth reflects general health and well-being.
- Oral diseases and conditions are associated with other health problems.
- Scientific research is key to further reduction in the burden of diseases and disorders that affect the face, mouth, and teeth.

From: US Department of Health and Human Services. *Oral Health in America: A Report of the Surgeon General.* Rockville, MD: US Department of Health and Human Services, National Institute of Dental and Craniofacial Research, National Institutes of Health, 2000.

DEFINITION OF ROUTINE DENTAL PRACTICE

General dentists provide three main areas of routine care: (a) prevention and treatment of periodontitis (also known as periodontal disease and commonly referred to by the public as gum disease), (b) prevention and treatment of dental caries (cavities), and (c) assessment of oral pathology.

Periodontal disease is an inflammation of the gums with corresponding destruction of bone around the teeth, secondary to bacterial infection of the gingival sulcus. Over a period of time, attachment tissue (bone and gums) is lost. Teeth loosen and can eventually fall out. Most adults have evidence of gingivitis (inflammation of the gums that is thought to be a precursor to periodontal disease) or periodontal disease.

Dental caries can be described as the dissolution of tooth structure by acidic bacterial by-products. The process requires fermentable carbohydrates, bacteria, and a susceptible host. Cariogenic (cavity-causing) bacteria adjacent to the tooth consume carbohydrates in the form of dental plaque. As a by-product of this consumption, acids are produced, which dissolve the adjacent tooth structure. Caries formation is countered in the healthy mouth by saliva. Saliva helps to clear the carbohydrate substrate, neutralize the acid by-products, and provide building blocks for the remineralization of tooth structure. When the delicate balance between caries formation (demineralization) and remineralization is continually tipped in favor of bacterial growth and acid production, cavities occur.[2] If left unchecked, dental caries also may lead to pain, the loss of teeth, and orofacial infections, occasionally with potentially life-threatening consequences.

Oral pathology deals with the nature, identification, and management of diseases affecting the oral and maxillofacial regions. It is a science that investigates the causes, processes, and effects of these diseases. The practice of oral pathology included research and diagnosis of diseases using clinical, radiographic, microscopic, biochemical, or other examinations.

EPIDEMIOLOGY: WHO IS AFFECTED?

PREVALENCE OF ORAL DISEASE

The prevalence of *dental caries* is widespread in the United States, and can be classified as a communicable disease.[3] Tooth decay is the most chronic infectious, transmissible, and preventable childhood disease, with nearly 20% incidence of caries in children ages 2 and 4. In fact, children are five times more likely to have tooth decay than asthma and it is seven times more prevalent than hay fever. By the age of 17, nearly 80% of the population has had a cavity or filling. More than two thirds of adults between the ages of 35 and 44 have lost at least one permanent tooth.[1] It is critical to prevent disease early in the primary dentition. Healthy baby teeth assist in the development of the permanent dentition, with implications for the proper placement of permanent teeth, speech, mastication of food and nourishment, self-esteem, and school readiness.

Severe *periodontal disease,* in which more than 6 mm of attachment around the teeth is lost, is present in 14% of the population aged 45 to 54 years, increasing to 23% in those aged 65 to 74 years.[1]

SOCIOECONOMIC STATUS AND THE UNINSURED

Juana has no insurance and few economic resources. She took time off from her work as a nanny to come to the dental office. She speaks only Spanish, and says she seeks medical care only when something hurts.

Despite overall improvements in oral health status in the United States, profound disparities remain in some population groups as classified by sex, income, age, and race/ethnicity. Many people do not access dental care because of the financial barriers. In fact, Juana's practice of seeking dental care on an emergency-only basis has been shaped by her experience of inaccessibility, and is representative of many who live below the poverty line in the United States.

The prevalence of oral disease is significantly higher in those living below the federal poverty line. Poor children are twice as likely to have dental caries when compared with those from an affluent background. The elderly population living in poverty is more likely to be edentulous.[1]

More than 108 million Americans lack dental insurance, 2.5 times more in number than those lacking medical insurance. Additionally, the likelihood of seeking dental care is 2.5 times greater in children with dental coverage than those without.[1] In a separate study, 76% of Latino participants with dental insurance used dental services, compared with 47% of those without coverage.[4]

Once dental care is sought by low-income patients (often only when a patient is in pain), the cheapest alternative for treatment may be the only one financially feasible. In the case of a toothache, this may be extraction, even though the tooth could be treated and maintained in the mouth by other therapeutic treatment.

RACE/ETHNICITY

Juana saw a dentist 5 weeks ago, but became frustrated in attempting to communicate with a non-Spanish-speaking provider. Since her last visit, she has had a swelling next to her lower right molar. She says the swelling comes and goes, as does the pain, but recently it has worsened. Although she knows she needs dental attention, she's discouraged because of the language/cultural barrier.

Many minority patients have great difficulty accessing dental care. In addition to financial constraints, language barriers, fear of jeopardizing immigration status, and the lack of minority providers also may be deterrent factors to seeking care. Hispanics, now officially the nation's largest minority group, are particularly at risk for dental disease and are most likely to be underserved.[5] In a study of Latino immigrants in Southern California, nearly 70% had no dental insurance, and Latino children were the least likely to have dental insurance coverage.[6]

The presence of dental disease is rampant among Hispanic youth. Of those living below the federal poverty line, Mexican-American children were significantly more likely to have untreated caries when compared with non-Hispanic whites and non-Hispanic blacks. In those aged 2 to 4 and 6 to 8, Mexican Americans have the highest number of decayed and filled surfaces in primary dentition. Many studies reveal that Latino children are at particular risk for early childhood caries (ECC) (Fig. 35-1). ECC is defined as a condition of demineralization of the enamel with different degrees of cavitation in the primary dentition.[7] The prevalence of ECC in Latino children is likely a result, at least in part, of a lack of dental education and awareness within Hispanic communities.

ECC is the most common chronic infectious disease in young children and may develop as soon as teeth erupt. In a study of young children near the California–Mexico border, 58% had ECC. Bacteria, predominantly mutans streptococci and lactobacilli, metabolize simple sugars to produce acid that demineralizes enamel, resulting in cavities.

THE ELDERLY

Elderly Americans are significantly at risk for dental disease. Living on a fixed retirement income and the termination of benefits associated with employment prevents many elders from seeking care. In addition, the elderly are more likely to have chronic disease, take medications, and be physically unable to care for their dentition.

As people age, their salivary gland function naturally decreases. A decrease in salivary gland function also may be exacerbated by medications whose side-effects dry the oral cavity or by particular disease processes. Those with a history of radiation to the oral structures also may

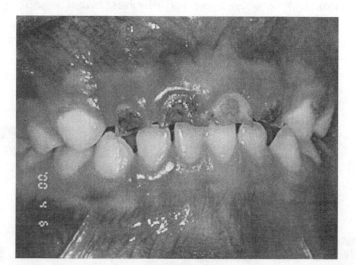

Figure 35-1. Severe early childhood caries.

have xerostomia. Without the antimicrobial and acid neutralizing effect of saliva, the demineralization–remineralization balance tips toward caries production. The likelihood of exposed root structure (the part of the tooth that is significantly softer and more prone to caries) resulting from periodontal disease increases the propensity for dental caries in the elderly. Lack of adequate home care because of physical impairments (e.g., a patient with arthritis who is unable to hold a toothbrush) may add to the propensity for caries and periodontal disease.

THE CHRONICALLY ILL AND THOSE WITH PHYSICAL OR MENTAL BARRIERS

> A review of Juana's medical history reveals a family history of diabetes and early tooth loss. Her mother was a diabetic and died at the age of 48.

Some chronic illnesses add another barrier for the maintenance of healthy tissues. It has been suggested that periodontal disease *may* be linked to cardiovascular disease[8] and preterm low birth weight.[9] A link between diseases that affect the immune system, such as human immunodeficiency virus/acquired immunodeficiency disease (HIV/AIDs) and diabetes and periodontal disease has been well established.[10,11] Observational studies have linked glycemic control in diabetics to the prevalence of periodontal disease. As diabetic control worsens, the likelihood, progression, and severity of periodontal disease increases. Current theory suggests a bidirectional relationship between diabetes and periodontal disease; control of periodontal disease helps control diabetes and vice versa.[11] More investigation is needed to shed light on the relationship between these two diseases, but it is sufficiently clear that health care providers caring for diabetics must include dental care in their comprehensive care plans. Some have referred to the dental extractions commonly seen in diabetics as another kind of "amputation" that providers should seek to prevent.

Quadriplegic patients and patients with physically impairing conditions such as Parkinson's disease, multiple sclerosis, and stroke are likely to have more difficulty with brushing and flossing. The mentally impaired, such as those with Down's syndrome and autism, may rely solely on their caretakers for oral care. In some cases, access to care is difficult because many dental offices are unequipped to manage patients with these physical and mental conditions. In some cases, these patients must be admitted to a hospital and placed under general anesthesia to administer care.

Common Pitfalls in Treating Dental Disease

- Most patients seek help only for acute dental problems.
- Many health care providers other than dentists do not incorporate dental health into their care.
- Access to dental care is limited for many.
- Many patients and providers have limited knowledge as to how to prevent dental illness.

ASSURING DENTAL HEALTH

Perhaps the most difficult challenge to assuring dental health is motivating patients to both value and seek dental care in a preventive and nonsurgical mode. Clinicians should emphasize a proactive approach, encouraging patients to have routine checkups, maintenance, and preventive services. Routine fluoride varnish applications have been found to significantly reduce the incidence of tooth decay,[2] and should be used rather than waiting until surgical repair is necessary (Box 35-2).

Box 35-2. Keys to a Successful Program of Prevention

- Stress the importance of oral hygiene and the importance of establishing a dental home, a regular place where oral care is received, especially among children.
- Educate parents and health care providers that oral health is a key to overall health.

- Provide nutrition counseling to prevent caries in children and adults.
- Use fluoride and sealants as caries-preventive measures.
- Reach out to underserved groups and incorporate dental screenings into medical examinations.

ORAL HYGIENE AND REGULAR VISITS TO THE DENTIST

| Juana has had few interactions with dentistry in her lifetime and has never been taught the importance of home care and diet. Neither her friends nor her extended family value dentistry, and tooth extraction is a common means of treating tooth pain. Her two sons have never seen a dentist.

Without adequate brushing and flossing, the incidence of dental caries and gingivitis/periodontitis increases dramatically. The presence of plaque or biofilm produced by bacterial fermentation of carbohydrates is a critical component of the dental caries and periodontal disease process. Microorganisms associated with periodontal disease also propagate and invade the sulcus and tissues surrounding the teeth. The resulting immune response to this invasion causes the breakdown of the dental attachment and bone. If left undisturbed, this breakdown continues and ultimately leads to the loss of teeth.

Health care providers should examine children's teeth for defects and cavities at every well-child visit (see Core Competency). Any child with significant risk factors for caries, such as poor oral hygiene, inadequate home dental care, premature birth, a mother with many cavities, a high sugar intake, enamel defects, special health care needs, low socioeconomic status, and/or spot lesions should be referred to a dentist by 12 months of age for preventive services. Promoting appropriate use of topical and systemic fluoride and providing early oral hygiene instruction can help reduce caries in young patients, as can regularly counseling parents on anticipatory guidance.

At-risk adults, especially those with conditions that may affect oral health, should have oral examinations as well. Newly diagnosed diabetics should be referred to a dentist for examination and counseling. At this visit the dentist will review the increased risk of periodontal disease with the patient and emphasize the importance of home care and an increased frequency of office visits. The elderly and the physically and mentally disabled should visit the dentist on an annual basis because they are at greater risk for caries. Tobacco users should be screened for oral cancers and encouraged to quit. In particular, tobacco use is a risk factor for oral cavity and pharyngeal cancers, periodontal diseases, candidiasis, and dental caries, among other diseases. Importantly, tobacco-related oral lesions are prevalent in adolescents who currently use smokeless tobacco. Patients undergoing radiation or chemotherapy therapy for cancer, especially head and neck cancers, should be referred immediately for an oral evaluation. These therapies may damage salivary glands and increase the likelihood of ulcers, fungal infections, and caries in the mouth.

Incorporation of home care and regular visits to the dentist is vital for the maintenance of a healthy mouth. Those patients with little or no home care because of lack of dental knowledge, a physical or mental handicap, or habitual poor oral hygiene, are the most at risk for oral disease. Tooth brushing removes plaque (or biofilm) from the teeth and gums, limiting the fermentable carbohydrates used by bacteria to proliferate and produce acid. The use of an American Dental Association–approved toothpaste containing fluoride adds an antibacterial action, as well as a remineralization source for cavitated teeth. Flossing removes plaque between the teeth, where most adult cavities occur. As a general guideline, dentists recommend that their patients floss once a day and brush at least twice daily, after breakfast and dinner.

Regular visits to a dentist allow providers to check for disease present in or around the oral structures. Many dentists begin their evaluation by performing an extraoral screening: an examination of the extraoral tissues of the head and neck, and palpation of these tissues to confirm health. Radiographs, if deemed necessary, are taken of the patients' teeth and/or jaws. An intraoral examination follows to assess the patient's home care and presence or absence of disease. Treatment appointments are then scheduled.

It should be the goal of health care providers to encourage patients to establish a dental home (an office or clinic in which the patient establishes a relationship with the dental providers through repeated visits) by age 1. Regular care instills patient–provider trust and increases the chance of returning for regular care. Incorporation of tooth brushing and a sealants program into public schools and day care programs can benefit children of all communities.

EDUCATING PATIENTS AND HEALTH CARE PROVIDERS

The importance of early detection of oral disease cannot be overstated. In addition, the incorporation of a visual examination of the oral structures by any health care provider can help patients tremendously. The presence of white spot lesions, broken teeth, oral pain, swelling, and bad breath can all indicate the presence of dental disease and mandate a referral to a dentist. Physicians should not be afraid to educate at-risk patients on the importance of oral care and, when possible, provide a list of dental resources for the patient.

NUTRITIONAL COUNSELING

> As the dentist discusses the factors leading to caries, Juana begins to understand her sons' risk because of their diet.

Nutritional counseling is an important aspect of preventive dental care. Both diet and frequency of consumption of foods affect one's likelihood of developing cavities. As fermentable carbohydrates are ingested, the pH of the mouth drops because of acid production. Saliva then acts as a buffer and neutralizes the acid. Each drop of the mouth pH and subsequent neutralization can be described as a cariogenic episode. Foods high in sugar (e.g., sodas, cookies) produce a strong carious episode, and should be eaten sparingly. However, the amount of sugar intake is not as important as the frequency of intake. Multiple cariogenic episodes spaced closely together are more likely to cause tooth decay. When counseling patients regarding diet, limiting the frequency of snacking should be emphasized. Minimizing the length of exposure to sugars also should be given special importance, especially with children. Slowly drinking sodas and eating sticky candies are considered to be long exposures. Particularly harmful are those situations where parents put their infants to bed with juices or milk. The sugars present in milk and juices sit on their teeth overnight and provide ample food for cariogenic bacteria. Baby bottle tooth decay can quickly decimate a child's dentition and require extensive dental treatment. Nutritional counseling is a powerful facet of preventive dentistry that any health care worker can provide (Table 35-1).

THE USE OF FLUORIDES AND SEALANTS

Fluoride is a powerful tool to fight cavities. Water fluoridation in particular is very effective at reducing caries incidence.[12] A 1-ppm fluoride concentration in water sources is recommended as therapeutic without causing fluorosis and mottled teeth.[1] A public health plan to fluoridate community water supply began in 1945 in Michigan and New York. Nevertheless, more than 108 million people today have no access to fluoridated water.

Health care providers should evaluate their communities' water sources for fluoride content and supplement with oral tablets to children, accordingly. The presence of fluoride during tooth development (from birth to approximately age 16) creates teeth with stronger enamel and a higher caries resistance. Application of fluoride gels and varnishes (FV) at schools and medical facilities can greatly reduce caries rate among children.

FV efficacy in this age group provides additional rationale for an early dental visit, especially for children in high caries risk groups, because applying FV at this first visit and counseling based on anticipatory guidance will help reduce future dental disease in young children (http://www.ucsf.edu/cando/).

The application of sealants to children's permanent first molars also has been highly successful as a means of preventing biting surface decay.[13] Teeth deemed susceptible to decay on the occlusal (biting) surface, usually first molars in children and adolescents, are cleaned with a pumice, etched with phosphoric acid, and painted with a resin that flows into the fissures of the tooth. The covered fissures now prevent food collection in this area and make cleaning these teeth easier.

THE IMPORTANCE OF OUTREACH TO UNDERSERVED AREAS

Reaching the underserved population is important. A shortage of dental care workers in rural areas is evident. Many have no physical access to dental care, and no opportunity for dental education. Preschools are a great forum to educate teachers as well as children on the importance of diet and oral hygiene. Preschool and grade school visits also allow for dental screenings and the distribution of toothbrushes and toothpaste to children. Because low-income and poorly educated persons are more at risk for dental disease, these populations should be focused upon (Box 35-3).

Box 35-3. 2003 US Surgeon General's National Call to Action to Promote Oral Health

Action 1: Change Perceptions of Oral Health (Establishing a dental home, preventive care rather than reactive care, link between oral health and overall health)

Action 2: Overcome Barriers by Replicating Effective Programs and Proven Efforts (water fluoridation, sealant programs, no sleeping with the bottle)

Action 3: Build the Science Base and Accelerate Science Transfer

Action 4: Increase Oral Health Workforce Diversity, Capacity, and Flexibility

Action 5: Increase Collaborations (educate not only children and parents, but also pediatricians, nurses, health care providers, and day care providers)

Table 35-1. Anticipatory Guidance

	Prenatal	Birth to 1 Year	2 to 3 Years	3 to 5 Years
Take home message for caregivers	• Baby teeth are important! • Parents'/caregivers' oral health affects baby's oral health. • Parents/caregivers should obtain regular dental check-up and get treatment if necessary. • Schedule child's first dental appointment by age one. • Use of fluorides, including tooth brushing with fluoride toothpaste, is the most effective way to prevent tooth decay	• Baby teeth are important! • Parents'/caregivers' oral health affects baby's oral health. • Parents/caregivers should obtain regular dental check-up and get treatment if necessary. • Parents/caregivers should avoid sharing with their child things that have been in their mouths. • Schedule child's first dental appointment by age one. • Prevention is less costly than treatment. • Use of fluorides, including tooth brushing with fluoride toothpaste, is the most effective way to prevent tooth decay.	• Baby teeth are important! • Parents'/caregivers' oral health affects baby's oral health. • Parents/caregivers should obtain regular dental check-up and get treatment if necessary. • Parents/caregivers should avoid sharing with their child things that have been in their mouths. • Schedule child's first dental appointment by age one. • Prevention is less costly than treatment. • Use of fluorides, including tooth brushing with fluoride toothpaste, is the most effective way to prevent tooth decay.	• Baby teeth are important! • Parents'/caregivers' oral health affects child's overall health. • Parents/caregivers should obtain regular dental check-up and get treatment if necessary. • Parents/caregivers should avoid sharing with their child things that have been in their mouths. • Prevention is less costly including tooth treatment. • Use of fluorides, including tooth brushing with fluoride toothpaste, is the most effective way to prevent tooth decay.
Oral health and hygiene	• Encourage parents/caregivers to obtain dental check-up and, if necessary, treatment before birth of baby to reduce cavity-causing bacteria that can be passed to the baby. • Encourage parents/caregivers to brush teeth with fluoride toothpaste.	• Encourage parents/caregivers to maintain good oral health and get treatment, if necessary, to reduce spread of bacteria that can cause tooth decay. • Encourage parents/caregivers to avoid sharing with their child things that have been in their mouths. • Encourage parents/caregivers to become familiar with the normal appearance of child's gums. • Emphasize using a washcloth or toothbrush to clean teeth and gums with eruption of the first tooth. • Encourage parents/caregivers to check front and back teeth for white, brown, or black spots (signs of cavities).	• Encourage parents/caregivers to maintain good oral health and get treatment, if necessary, to reduce spread of bacteria that can cause tooth decay. • Encourage parents/caregivers to avoid sharing with their child things that have been in their mouths. • Review parent's/caregiver's role in brushing toddler's teeth. • Discuss brush and toothpaste selection. • Problem solve on oral hygiene issues. • Schedule child's first dental visit by age one.	• Encourage parents/caregivers to maintain good oral health and get treatment, if necessary, to reduce spread of bacteria that can cause tooth decay. • Encourage parents/caregivers to avoid sharing with their child things that have been in their mouths. • Discuss parents/caregivers continued responsibility to help children under age eight to brush their teeth. • Encourage parents/caregivers to consider dental sealants for primary and first permanent molars. • Emphasize importance of baby teeth for chewing, speaking, jaw development and self-esteem.
Oral development	• Describe primary tooth eruption patterns (first tooth usually erupts between 6 and 10 months old). • Emphasize importance of baby teeth for chewing, speaking, jaw development and self-esteem.	• Discuss primary tooth eruption patterns. • Emphasize importance of baby teeth for chewing, speaking, jaw development and self-esteem. • Discuss teething and ways to soothe sore gums, such as chewing on teething rings and washcloths.	• Emphasize importance of baby teeth for chewing, speaking, jaw development and self-esteem. • Discuss teething and ways to soothe sore gums, such as teething rings, washcloths.	• Emphasize importance of baby teeth for chewing, speaking, jaw development and self-esteem.

(Continued)

369

Table 35-1. Anticipatory Guidance (*Continued*)

	Prenatal	Birth to 1 Year	2 to 3 Years	3 to 5 Years
Fluoride adequacy	• Evaluate fluoride status in residential water supply • Review topical and systemic sources of fluoride • Encourage mother to drink fluoridated tap water.	• Evaluate fluoride status of residential water supply. • Review topical and systemic sources of fluoride. • Encourage drinking fluoridated tap water. • Consider topical needs (e.g., toothpaste, fluoride varnish).	• Re-evaluate fluoride status of residential water supply. • Review topical and systemic sources of fluoride. • Encourage drinking fluoridated tap water. • Review need for topical fluorides.	• Re-evaluate fluoride status in residential water supply. • Review sources of fluoride. • Review need for topical or other fluorides.
Oral habits	• Encourage mother to stop smoking	• Encourage breastfeeding. • Advise mother that removing child from breast after feeding and wiping baby's gums/teeth with damp washcloth reduces the risk of ECC. • Review pacifier safety.	• Remind mother that removing child from breast after feeding and wiping baby's gums/teeth with damp washcloth reduces the risk of ECC. • Begin weaning of non-nutritive sucking habits at 2 years old.	• Discuss consequences of digit sucking and prolonged non-nutritive sucking (e.g., pacifier) and begin professional intervention if necessary.
Diet and nutrition	• Emphasize eating a healthy diet and limiting number of exposures to sugar snacks and drinks. • Emphasize that it is the frequency of exposures, not the amount of sugar, which affects susceptibility to caries. • Encourage breastfeeding. • Remind parents/caregivers never to put baby to bed with a bottle with anything other than water in it or to allow feeding "at will."	• Remind parents/caregivers never to put baby to bed with a bottle with anything other than water in it or allow feeding "at will." • Emphasize that it is the frequency of exposures, not the amount of sugar, which affects susceptibility to caries. • Encourage weaning from bottle to cup by 1 year of age. • Encourage diluting juices with water.	• Remind parents/caregivers never to put baby to bed with a bottle or allow feeding "at will." • Discuss healthy diet and oral health. • Emphasize that it is the frequency of exposures, not the amount of sugar, which affects susceptibility to caries. • Review snack choices and encourage healthy snacks.	• Review and encourage healthy diet. • Remind parents/caregivers about limiting the frequency of exposures to sugar. • Review snacking choices. • Emphasize that child should be completely weaned from bottle and drinking exclusively from a cup.
Injury prevention	• Encourage childproofing of home including electrical cord safety and poison control. • Emphasize use of properly secured car seat. • Encourage caregivers to keep emergency numbers handy	• Review child proofing of home including electrical cord safety and poison control. • Emphasize use of properly secured car seat. • Encourage caregivers to keep emergency numbers handy.	• Review childproofing of home including electrical cord safety and poison control. • Emphasize use of car seat. • Emphasize use of helmet when child is riding tricycle/bicycle or in seat of adult bike. • Remind caregivers to keep emergency numbers handy.	• Emphasize use of properly secured car seat. • Have emergency numbers handy. • Encourage safety in play activities including helmets on bikes and mouth guards in sports. • Remind caregivers to keep emergency numbers handy.

From: Dr. Ramos-Gomez.

370

CONCLUSION

Health care workers act as a valuable bridge between scientific research and the public need. Periodontal disease has been linked to diabetes and cardiovascular diseases. Caries remains a transmissible infectious disease. An understanding of current measures to treat dental disease and the preventive roles that providers can take will allow more effective care of patients.

KEY CONCEPTS

- Instruct patients that caries is a transmissible disease.
- Incorporate oral screenings into overall physical examinations.
- Emphasize that nutrition is critical to caries prevention.
- Encourage patients to minimize frequency of sugar intake.
- Encourage patients to establish a dental home, especially if:
  - They have diabetes.
  - They are in an at-risk group.
- Assess caries in children by looking for white spot lesions or brown spots.
- Discuss fluoridation and its importance in caries prevention with your patients.
- Prescribe fluoride tablets for children in communities whose water is unfluoridated.
- Consider fluoride varnishes for children in school.
- Explain the importance of preventive dental care.

CORE COMPETENCY

An Oral Examination for the Non-Dentist

Extraoral Examination:

- Examine the face and neck for symmetry, skin lesions, swelling, and overall appearance.
- Cancer screening: Palpate the lymph nodes along the sternocleidomastoid muscles and under the chin for edema or indurated masses.
- Temporomandibular Examination: Place your pointer and middle fingers just in front of the patient's ears and have them open. Popping and clicking are a variation of normal. Ask the patient:
  - Have you ever had any pain in this region?
  - Have you ever had your jaw lock open or shut?
  - Do you wake up with their jaw muscles tight?
  - Do you get headaches?
  - Does you partner ever tell you that you grind your teeth?
  - Is there any deviation of the mandible upon opening?
  - Is there any limitation on opening?

  A "yes" answer to any of these questions indicates referral to a dentist.

Intraoral Examination:

- Examine the soft tissues of the mouth, tongue, and throat for cancer.
  - Look inside along the cheeks for anything unusual: white, red, or mixed lesions, swelling.
  - Examine under the tongue. Palpate the floor of the mouth digitally with one hand, using the other extraorally under the chin. Feel for indurated masses.
  - Examine the lateral borders of the tongue, the roof of the mouth (palate), and back of the throat for abnormalities.
- Examine the condition of the dentition.
  - Children: Look for black spots on the biting surfaces of the teeth (Fig. 35-2). These may be cavities. Ask the parent if the child is eating well or if they have any pain in his or her mouth.
  - Adults: Look for cavitations in the teeth (black staining of grooves in the teeth is not abnormal in adults.) Does the patient have unusually bad breath? Feel the teeth: Are they loose? Look at the gums. They should look pink and flat. Red, swollen, and inflamed gums indicate gingivitis or periodontal disease (Fig. 35-3).

  If in doubt, call your local dentist!

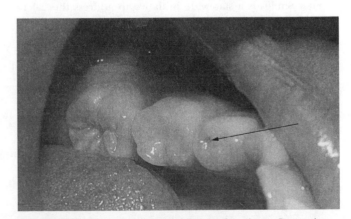

Figure 35-2. Early caries (cavity) lesion of a primary first molar (arrow).

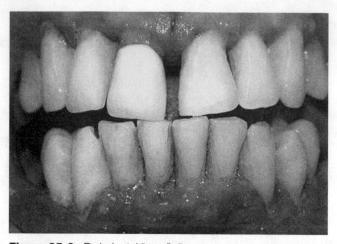

Figure 35-3. Periodontal "gum" disease.

DISCUSSION QUESTIONS

1. Why is the treatment of dental disease important, considering the goal of treating the whole patient?
2. In what ways can rural health care providers impact oral health in their communities?
3. If Juana walked into your office, what recommendations would you give her regarding her oral care? What concerns would you have with her children, understanding Juana's own medical and social history?

RESOURCES

http://www.ada.org
The American Dental Association

http://www.adha.org/oralhealth/
American Dental Hygienists' Association

http://www.ucsf.edu/cando/
The Center to Address Disparities in Children's Oral Health

http://www.first5oralhealth.org/
First Smiles is a statewide initiative to address the "silent epidemic" of Early Childhood Caries affecting children ages 0 to 5.

http://www.nidcr.nih.gov/
National Institute of Dental and Craniofacial Research

http://www.nidcr.nih.gov/HealthInformation/DiseasesAndConditions/OralSystemicHealthConnection/OralSystemic.htm

The oral-systemic health connection. National Institute of Dental and Craniofacial Research, National Institutes of Health. Accessed June 1, 2006.

REFERENCES

1. US Department of Health and Human Services. *Oral Health in America: A Report of the Surgeon General.* Rockville, MD: US Department of Health and Human Services, National Institute of Dental and Craniofacial Research, National Institutes of Health, 2000.
2. Mellberg J, et al. *Fluoride in preventive dentistry: Theory and clinical applications.* Hanover Park, IL: Quintessence Publishing Co., 1999.
3. Keyes PH. Infectious nature of experimental dental caries—findings and implications. *Arch Oral Biol* 1960;1: 304–320.
4. Marcus M, et al. *Policy implications of access to dental care for immigrant communities.* California Policy Research Center, University of California and California Program on Access to Care. Los Angeles, 2002. Available at: http://www.ucop.edu/cprc/dentalaccess.pdf
5. Cohn D. Hispanics are the nation's largest minority. *Washington Post,* June 18, 2003.
6. *The Oral Health of California's Children: Halting a Neglected Epidemic.* The Dental Foundation, 2000.
7. Shiboski CH, et al. The association of early childhood caries and race/ethnicity among California preschool children. *J Public Health Dent* 2003;63(1):38–46.
8. Scannapieco TA, et al. Associations between periodontal disease and risk for atherosclerosis, cardiovascular disease, and stroke. A systematic review. *Ann Periodontol* 2003; 8(1):38–53.
9. Scannapieco TA, et al. Periodontal disease as a risk factor for adverse pregnancy outcomes. A systematic review. *Ann Periodontol* 2003;8(1):70–78.
10. Taylor G, et al. Diabetes, periodontal diseases, dental caries, and tooth loss: A review of the literature. *Compendium* 2004;25(3):179–190.
11. Vastardis SA, Yukna RA, Fidel PL Jr, et al. Periodontal disease in HIV-positive individuals: Association of periodontal indices with stages of HIV disease. *J Periodont* 2003;74(9): 1336–1341.
12. Dean HT. Epidemiological studies in the United States. In: Moulton FR, ed. *Dental caries and fluorine.* Washington, DC: American Association for the Advancement of Science, 1946:5–31.
13. Ahuvuo-Saloranta A, et al. Pit and fissure sealants for preventing decay in the permanent teeth of children and adolescents. *Evid Based Dent* 2004;5(4):93–94.

Chapter 36

Chronic Disease

Margaret B. Wheeler, MS, MD, Teresa J. Villela, MD,
and Thomas S. Bodenheimer, MD

Objectives

- Define chronic disease.
- Describe the morbidity and mortality of chronic disease.
- Review quality and costs of chronic disease care.
- Outline challenges to patient care, including patient, provider, and system factors.
- Suggest interventions to improve care.

> Mrs. Gonzalez is a 65-year-old housekeeper. She learns that she has high blood pressure and high blood sugar. Like many with chronic illness, she is not prepared for how radically the diagnoses of hypertension and diabetes will affect her life.

Achronic disease is any illness that has a prolonged course and neither resolves spontaneously nor is curable. Chronic illnesses may be mild or severe; may have constant or remitting courses; and their long-term consequences can be unpredictable. They range in severity from mild problems (e.g., seasonal allergies) to life-changing illnesses (e.g., cancer). Implied is that chronic illnesses cause ongoing discomfort and need for medical care. Chronic illness can bring significant disability and early death and affect every aspect of life—how one eats, works, and loves. This chapter discusses the care of adults with chronic illnesses and interventions designed to improve that care.

EPIDEMIOLOGY: WHO IS AFFECTED?

> Mrs. Gonzalez is representative of many with chronic illness: She is elderly, has more than one chronic illness, is from an ethnic minority group, and is poor.

Chronic disease is common in people of all ages. About 100 million people in the United States, or almost half the population, have at least one chronic illness. Ninety percent of people over 65 have one chronic illness and about 6.5% of children are disabled by chronic conditions.[1,2] Indeed, having more than one chronic condition is common: Almost 20% of Americans have more than one chronic disease.[1] Hence, it is not surprising that three fourths of US health care dollars go to caring for those with chronic illness.[4]

Chronic conditions are the most significant causes of morbidity and mortality in the United States (Fig. 36-1). More than one in ten Americans is significantly disabled by a chronic illness. Four diseases alone—asthma, depression, diabetes, and congestive heart failure—afflict half of all those with chronic illness.[3,4] Chronic diseases cause 70% of all deaths in the United States.[4]

RACE/ETHNICITY AND SOCIOECONOMIC STATUS

The risks of developing chronic diseases and their complications are highest in people from ethnic minority populations and the poor. These translate into higher mortality and morbidity rates as well.[5]

For people in low-income groups suffering from chronic disease, the old adage rings true: People are

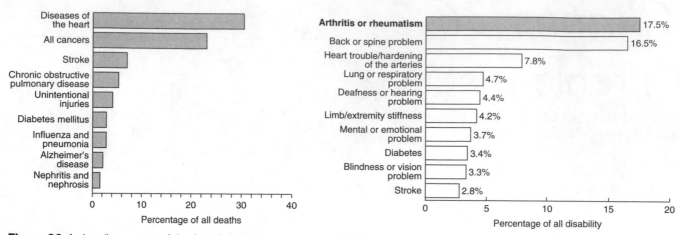

Figure 36-1. Leading causes of death and disability among American adults.
(From: Centers for Disease Control and Prevention (CDC). Prevalence of disabilities and
associated health conditions among adults—United States, 1999. *MMWR Mobid Mortal
Wkly Rep* 2001;50:120–125.)[56]
(From: Mokdad A, JS Marks, et al. Actual causes of death in the United States, 2000. *JAMA*
2004;291(10):1238–1245.)[57]

poor because they are sick and sick because they are poor. Chronic illness may make it more difficult to remain employed, leading to lower socioeconomic status; in turn, lack of insurance and poverty make it more difficult for patients to obtain appropriate care.

The Uninsured

Not having health insurance is one of the most obvious barriers to care, and can be devastating for someone with a chronic condition. Younger patients, the poor, and minority patients are the most likely to lack insurance. The uninsured tend to have their diseases diagnosed at more advanced stages, receive less preventive care and, once diagnosed, receive less therapeutic care. Predictably, the uninsured chronically ill are more likely to have poorly controlled illnesses.[6,7]

Quality of Care

Despite the large expenditures on care, even patients with adequate access do not always receive fully appropriate care. How poorly the US system manages the care of the chronically ill is well documented and sobering. Most patients with hypertension, coronary artery disease, diabetes, hyperlipidemia, congestive heart failure, atrial fibrillation, asthma, and depression are inadequately treated.[8] To cite a few examples in a long litany: Only 27% of patients have their hypertension controlled;[9] only 14% of patients with coronary artery disease have low-density lipoprotein (LDL) cholesterol controlled;[10] fewer than 35% of eligible patients with atrial fibrillation are anticoagulated;[11] and clini-

cians counsel only half of patients who smoke to quit.[12] In one national evaluation of physician performance for 30 medical conditions, patients were shown to receive only 55% of the recommended care.[13] Minority and poor patients seem to get the worst care.[14,15] For example, even within Medicare plans African Americans are less likely than whites to receive breast cancer screening, eye examinations if they have diabetes, beta-blockers after myocardial infarction, and follow-up after hospitalization for mental illness.[16]

CHALLENGES

LIFE WITH CHRONIC DISEASE

Mrs. Gonzalez finds it difficult to keep medical appointments and to refill her medicines. She does not eat regularly at work, so often does not take her medications at all.

Having a long-term illness can demand profound life changes. Managing symptoms, changing diet, taking medications, and interacting with the medical care system are but a few of the tasks entailed. Controlling the inevitable emotional reactions to the disease—anger, fear, and isolation—is also no easy feat.[17] Furthermore, juggling life's tasks is more difficult because people often feel unwell and their ability even to do basic activities may be affected.[18]

Indeed, many patients with chronic diseases become socially isolated. Most feel that someone would help them in an emergency, but only about half feel that they would be able to count on family and friends to assist with daily chores and housekeeping.[18] Learning how to garner support from friends, family, and community without exhausting them is one crucial task to living successfully with a chronic illness. This support may be as important for health as it is for happiness. Patients with supportive families report better health,[18] and have better diabetic control[19] and lower mortality rates than their disease severity might predict.[20]

Habitual Behavior

Not only are chronic diseases difficult for patients because they are ongoing, unpredictable, and pervasive, but because they may be extensions of the ways people have lived their lives. Indeed, the chronic diseases most likely to kill people—heart disease, stroke, chronic obstructive pulmonary disease (COPD), and diabetes—often are associated with smoking, obesity, and lack of exercise. For most conditions, the risky behavior is not immediately related to symptoms and is deeply ingrained and difficult to change, even for knowledgeable and motivated people. Complicating matters further, this association with behavior may lead many patients to be blamed for their illnesses by everyone from their doctors and family members to themselves.

Getting Health Care

> Mrs. Gonzalez is often put on hold for prohibitively long periods of time when she tries to make follow-up appointments or call for refills.

Navigating the medical system is another challenge for the chronically ill. Having a regular doctor can make this easier, and patients with a regular source of care get more preventive care and more chronic disease care.[21] Getting medications, necessary support services and coordinating medical care are common difficulties for those with chronic illness.[18]

Patients' Knowledge

Many with chronic disease are ill informed about their illness and do not feel equipped to deal with their condition. One survey of chronically ill patients found that they did not feel confident of their ability to make decisions about even the most basic questions, such as how to take medications or when to see a doctor. It is sobering to read how little patients understand of their disease: 42% of diabetics report not understanding diabetes management; 30% of asthmatics do not know what to do in the case of a severe attack; and those with coronary disease often do not understand the importance of taking an aspirin or lowering their blood pressure.[18]

Patients' Beliefs and Expectations

Expectations and beliefs of both patients and providers complicate all medical interactions. Diseases that are incurable or that can lead to death and disability are especially likely to be imbued with meaning by patients, doctors, and society.

Attitudes toward disease can encourage or dissuade individuals from seeking diagnosis and treatment of disease. Not all patients share the biomedical model of illness, and different beliefs may be active within one ethnic, racial, or even family group. For example, a study of African-American women with hypertension found two distinct beliefs about hypertension: One group of women referred to their condition as "high tension" and attributed it to transient stresses and related "tensions"; the other viewed their condition as one of "high blood pressure" and regarded it as a more persistent condition. As a result, the former group took their antihypertensive medications less consistently than the latter group.[22] Fatalism toward disease, belief in more traditional remedies, and suspicion of multiple medications (often justified!) are other frequently encountered obstacles to treatment.

Explanatory models of disease and treatment are particularly important in chronic disease care. Cure is a common expectation among patients with chronic diseases. A recent study of patients with hypertension, for example, found that close to 40% expected to be cured, did not expect to take their medications for life, or took their medications only when experiencing symptoms.[23] When treatments are long term, patients' attitudes are also understandably different than those related to short-term treatments. For example, patients may believe that taking medications long term might make them worse or make them "drug dependent" or more like "guinea pigs."[24]

Other Barriers

Other barriers, such as low literacy levels, poverty, difficulty speaking and understanding English, and distrust of the medical system also can contribute to patients receiving substandard care and are addressed in other chapters. The costs of care even for those who are insured are often prohibitive. Moreover, because many patients have more than one chronic illness, the number and complexity of problems, not to speak of medications, may overwhelm both patient and provider. Psychiatric illnesses or substance use, common comorbid conditions that often go unrecognized or unaddressed, also can undermine care.

The Role of Community

It can take a village to care adequately for those with chronic illness. Communities have varying attitudes toward health, and allocation of resources and where a person lives can influence diagnosis and treatment. Governmental support of screening, treatment, and prevention efforts can be crucial. Churches, community centers, and schools may become places where people can get information, form support groups, or be screened for diseases. Even the neighborhood a patient comes from is important: neighborhoods with no grocery stores in which one can buy fresh fruit or few safe places to exercise pose difficulties for even the most motivated patients.

CARING FOR THE CHRONICALLY ILL

Caring for acute medical problems and curing disease are the dominant paradigms of modern medicine. Health care providers, whose training is largely in the acute care paradigm and setting, do not adequately emphasize addressing long-term illness and promoting prevention. The US health care system, structured to care for acute disease, often thwarts rather than supports clinicians caring for the chronically ill.[25]

Providers' Knowledge and Skills

Both recent graduates and practicing doctors often feel incompetent to care for patients with complex chronic illness. Graduating residents often report feeling unprepared to care for patients with many of the most common chronic illnesses and lack the skills essential to caring for the chronically ill, such as collaborating with other providers, participating in quality assurance, or managing populations of patients.[26,27]

Communication skills are another area in which physicians have been found wanting. Not only do physicians interrupt their patients seconds into their initial statements,[28] but they fail to assess patients' concerns,[29] educate patients,[30,31] or assess their understanding of instructions.[32] Not surprisingly, miscommunication between doctor and patient is the most common reason that patients do not take their medications as prescribed.[33] Minority patients are even less likely than white patients to receive information about prognosis and treatment.[34] Given the poor communication between doctors and patients, it is not surprising that fewer than 50% of patients follow physician instructions about their chronic illnesses.[35]

Providers' Beliefs and Expectations

In general, doctors actually prefer to care for healthy patients.[36] Asked to define "difficult" patients, doctors describe characteristics that may be especially prevalent in chronically ill patients: repeated visits, unexplained symptoms, coexisting social problems, aims that differ from the doctor's, and distress or lack of satisfaction.[37] This is understandable. The role of doctor as heroic protagonist in the fight against disease is predicated on cure. When cure is elusive, doctors and patients are dissatisfied. Making an acute intervention to save a life is more immediately rewarding than accompanying a patient struggling with lifelong behavioral changes.

Providers' Cultural Awareness and Sensitivity

Health care providers receive little training in how to care for patients from different cultures and backgrounds. The care of poor patients, those who do not speak English well, and minority patients may suffer as a consequence. For example, physicians have been shown to recommend different treatments based on the race and gender of their patients.[38] Many physicians think poor and minority patients, the very patients most likely to be suffering from chronic conditions, are more likely to engage in risky behaviors and are less intelligent.[39] Providers' beliefs about patients can also influence how they interpret patients' symptoms.[39] Health care providers commonly interpret these patients' inability to adhere to treatments as lack of cooperation, for example.[29] To quote one participant in a study on primary care providers' attitudes toward caring for the poor: "You just don't get the positive feedback and reward for trying to make these people well . . . they're hard to work with . . . hard to help. And you get tired."[40]

Another common perception physicians have of poor patients is that they are less likely to change their behavior based on their physician's recommendations.[40] Although poorer patients may have more difficulty adhering to complex treatment regimens,[41] low-income patients are more likely than wealthy patients to report attempting to change their behavior based on their physician's advice.[42] If doctors feel that poor and minority patients are less likely to follow their advice, they may not dispense it in the first place. Studies show that doctors are less likely to discuss things like diet and exercise,[42] prenatal advice,[43] smoking cessation,[44] or mammography[45] with their minority and low-income patients. Thus, fatalism toward a patient's disease may be held not only by the patient, but also by the physician.

Providers Navigating the Medical System

Navigating the medical system may be as difficult for providers as it is for patients. Health care providers often are unaware of the intricacies of Medicare and Medicaid rules, health plan regulations, pharmacy formularies, and the like. Good medical recording and information systems are crucial. When multiple health care providers are involved, the risk of having conflicting or redundant plans is great. Linking patients with other services and community resources is often beyond the ken of many physicians. (To understand how important this can be, consider the difference between an elder struggling with daily tasks, and one who has been linked with a senior center where she can have a meal, do laundry, visit a nurse, and participate in social events.)

THE HEALTH CARE SYSTEM

> At a follow-up visit a year later, Mrs. Gonzalez discusses her grandson's health and reports that her back hurts. Her doctor addresses the back pain. Somehow, she forgets to review Mrs. Gonzalez's blood pressure or give her a flu vaccine.

Despite the myriad challenges to patients and health care providers in chronic illness care, most patients have a high regard for their doctors and most doctors are dedicated professionals. Health care systems provide the framework in which health care providers and patients interact. At their best, systems can organize care to support physicians and patients to overcome the inevitable oversights and miscommunications. At their worst they can compound them.

Most health care systems in the United States have been organized to support acute rather than chronic illness care. Managing chronic illness within a model and system created to respond to acute illness is fraught with difficulty. It is common for more urgent problems and concerns to be all-consuming, leaving chronic issues unaddressed. Preventive measures, such as the influenza vaccine, are easily forgotten. Often there seems to be no time to discuss the chronic problems at all, like Mrs. Gonzalez's blood pressure, let alone teach patients how to care for their illnesses themselves.

This phenomenon, referred to as "the tyranny of the urgent,"[25] arises from the way health care is delivered and shapes provider–patient encounters. The timing and expectations of visits often do not allow for comprehensive exchanges. This is equally true in the hospital as it is in the clinic. Patients hospitalized with exacerbations of chronic illnesses are often helped with the acute event and then discharged with little to prevent the next hospitalization. It is no wonder that patients are often inadequately treated and hospital readmission rates are high for many chronic illnesses.[11,46–48]

Coordination of Care

Health care providers and patients also may be challenged by the complexity imposed by a multiplicity of medical problems. If practitioners, subspecialists, and allied health providers are not communicating and integrating their care, patients may receive conflicting advice and treatments. In addition, without tracking the care delivered to groups of patients with similar diagnoses, there will be little opportunity to create systems to overcome the understandable negligence of harried providers.

In summary, the US health care system produces patients who are uninformed about their illness and not empowered to care for themselves. Health care professionals receive little training in caring for the chronically ill and work in systems that are inadequately organized to support either patient or provider. Is it any wonder that the quality of chronic care is poor?[49]

Common Pitfalls

- Applying acute illness model to chronic care
- Forgetting preventive measures and lifestyle changes
- Not addressing patient goals, beliefs, and expectations
- Allowing multiple problems to overwhelm comprehensive care
- Allowing poor coordination among providers to complicate care
- Not detecting substance use and mental illness
- Not addressing community resources and barriers

IMPROVING THE CARE OF THE CHRONICALLY ILL

> Mrs. Gonzalez's clinic begins a chronic care improvement program. When she reveals that she often runs out of medications, the clinic arranges to have her medicines sent to her home once a month.

NEW MODELS OF CARE

New models of care are being developed to address the inadequacy of care in the chronically ill. These models recognize the long-term nature of chronic disease and assure that urgent medical needs will not overwhelm the need for ongoing care of chronic problems. The new models are patient-centered, specifically enlisting the patients themselves in formulating plans and managing disease.

Acknowledging the impact of chronic illnesses on people's lives is at the heart of many innovations in chronic illness care. Patients with chronic diseases, from sickle cell disease to diabetes, have a greater sense of well-being, report less severe symptoms, and require fewer clinic visits and hospitalizations if they feel able to cope with their illness themselves.[50,51] Moreover, patients who are actively involved in their own care have better clinical outcomes. In one study of diabetics, patients who were taught to discuss medical decisions with physicians dropped their hemoglobin A1c levels and had significantly lower average HbA1c levels than patients who were not taught these skills.[52]

Active patients work as partners with providers to define problems, set goals, and fashion management solutions. Together they establish priorities and the steps required to fulfill them. A hierarchy of goals allows success in small steps to bring confidence that larger issues can be tackled; and both provider and patient are liberated from defining ultimate success as the only commendable achievement. Although a blood pressure of less than 130/80 mmHg might be the long-term goal, learning how to get refills or recognize pills may be an important first step in achieving control.

Creating strong partnerships requires that providers work collaboratively with patients, abandoning the dictatorial style common in acute care, and addressing the full panoply of challenges facing the chronically ill, from how to manage symptoms and use medicines to the emotional upheavals of being sick. Nevertheless, the collaboration must avoid being too "patient-centered:" by ceding complete control to patients, practitioners could actually abrogate their responsibility to provide care.

THE CHRONIC CARE MODEL

One successful multidimensional approach to caring for patients with chronic illness within primary care is "the chronic care model."[53] This model includes system changes designed to provide both patient and provider with support for disease management. Examples include programs linking patients with community resources; accessible guidelines to inform providers' clinical decisions, and clinical information systems that foster integrated care and track actual disease management.

Registries are one fundamental component of these new systems. Registries are lists of patients with a particular condition. Clinical information about these patients is used to create tracking systems to evaluate an organization or provider's panel and create reminder systems. Registries help a health care system transcend the traditional focus on an individual patient, focusing rather on a population of patients. For example, through a registry a community clinic could track how many of their diabetics are receiving annual eye examinations and could design systems for ensuring that patients receive proper referral. The registry also might identify those patients at high risk or failing conventional care. These patients then could be targeted for intensive interventions such as referral to case management programs.

Case management programs are an example of another important innovation: forming teams of providers, including nonphysicians, to care for patients. Physicians have neither the time nor the skills to manage all aspects of chronic care. Teams with many allied health providers working in concert can form a rich network of support for patients and providers. Planned visits and group visits, during which only chronic problems are addressed, or influenza vaccines given, for example, are modes of health care delivery that have been shown to improve chronic care and often depend on nurses, nutritionists, pharmacists, or health educators.[54]

The care of patients hospitalized with chronic illnesses can also be improved using similar interventions. Preprinted orders increase the likelihood that recommended treatments will not be overlooked. Practice guidelines can direct high-quality care. Use of teams of providers, case management, discharge planning, and patient education are all techniques that may prevent patients with chronic illness from returning to the hospital.

A majority of studies reviewing outcomes, utilization of health services, and costs of care show that programs using chronic care techniques tend to reduce emergency room visits, hospital admissions, and costs. Programs that focus on patients with the most severe disease are often the most effective.[52] Half of all patients hospitalized with congestive heart failure, for example, are readmitted in 90 days. A program in which nurses followed up with patients post-hospitalization not only reduced subsequent admissions by 56%, but also costs, when compared with randomized controls.[55]

CONCLUSION

Learning about and addressing the particular needs of those with chronic illnesses is important for patients, providers, and health care systems and can help improve the quality of medical care. Involving patients directly in managing their health; redesigning systems to facilitate effective care; integrating care of multiple problems; using multidisciplinary teams; and designing interventions to manage populations of patients are promising strategies.

Despite the many challenges, caring for the chronically ill can be deeply rewarding. The time frame of the treatment is long, and rich relationships often develop. Preventing the severely debilitating consequences of chronic illness, prolonging life and health, or accompanying a patient through disability and death fulfill the loftiest goals of medicine, and can bring sustaining satisfaction to health care providers.

KEY CONCEPTS WHEN CARING FOR THOSE WITH CHRONIC ILLNESS

- Create provider–patient partnerships.
  - —Ask about and validate health beliefs.
  - —Engage patient to generate an action plan.
  - —Teach self-management skills.
  - —Reward positive behavior changes, no matter how small.
  - —Garner familial support.
- Discuss chronicity of the disease explicitly.
- Remember lifestyle changes and risk reduction.
- Screen for depression and substance use.
- Integrate treatments of coexisting illnesses.
- Assess community for resources and barriers.
- Avoid the "tyranny of the urgent" through systemwide changes.
- Create systems to deliver preventive care.
- Create systems to support self-management.
- Remember the time frame:
  - —Establish and nourish your relationship with patients.
  - —Have a hierarchy of priorities.
- Approach ultimate goals with appropriate intermediate steps.
- Always assess for adherence.

DISCUSSION QUESTIONS

1. Discuss the differences between acute and chronic medical illness and what forms of care are most appropriate for each.
2. Describe a difficulty in navigating the medical system that you have experienced or witnessed. What system changes could be made to rectify the problem?
3. Mrs. Gonzalez is your patient. After following her for 3 years, you note that her blood pressure, hemoglobin A1c, and LDL are all still very high. Describe what approaches you might take to address these problems.

RESOURCES

www.qualityhealthcare.org/IHI/
www.improvingchroniccare.org/resources/resources.htm
www.guideline.gov

REFERENCES

1. Bodenheimer T, Wagner E, Grumbach K. Improving primary care for patients with chronic illness: The chronic care model, parts 1 and 2. *JAMA* 2002;288(14): 1775–1779; (15):1909–1915.

CORE COMPETENCY
Chronic Disease

Setting realistic goals and outlining the steps patients can take to achieve them is an important aspect of promoting patient self-management. Making action plans with patients supports their self-management skills.

Problem Solving

Agree on a problem. Remember problems might include how to get a follow-up appointment, how to enlist familial support as well as how to eat or take medicines.

Define an Attainable Goal

- What are the steps that might be taken to reach the goal?
- Brainstorm possible steps. The patient should take the lead, and there should be several options.

Make an Action Plan

- Ask the patient to choose something *he* thinks he should do.
- Choose something reasonable and accomplishable.
- Make the intervention *behavior-specific.*

NOT *"I will lose weight this week"*
BUT *"I will drink mineral water instead of sodas this week."*

- Make specific plans: *What* will be done? *When? How often? How much?* "I will walk one half hour after dinner every evening."
- Assess the patient's sense of the importance of the action plan: if unimportant, change the plan.
- Assess the patient's confidence that he or she can carry it out. Change the plan if the patient lacks confidence. (Using a 1 to 10 scale can be helpful to assess importance and confidence. Ratings of 7/10 or more are more likely to be successful.)
- Brainstorm reminders: signs on the refrigerator, pill bottles at the bedside, etc.
- Have a written record of the plan for both the patient and provider.
- Consider each action plan a model for the next plan. Build on success and create success from failures.
- Be an ally. Praise success, use difficulties as opportunities for further understanding.
- Assess the results.
- Have action plans for every goal.
- See http://www.action-plans.org/ for more tips and forms you can download.

2. Newacheck P, Halfon N. Prevalence and impact of disabling chronic conditions in childhood. *Am J Public Health* 1998;88(4):610–617.

3. Anderson G, Knickman JR. Changing the chronic care system to meet people's needs. Health Affairs 2001;20(6):146–160.

4. Centers for Disease Control and Prevention. *The burden of chronic disease and their risk factors.* Washington, DC: 2004. Available at: www.cdc.gov/nccdphp/burdenbook2004/pdf/burden_book2004.pdf (Accessed 5/12/06).

5. Smedley B, Stith A, Nelson A. *Unequal treatment: Confronting racial and ethnic disparities in health care.* Washington, DC: National Academic Press; Institute of Medicine, 2002.

6. Hadley J. *Sicker and poorer: The consequences of being uninsured.* Washington, DC: The Urban Institute and Kaiser Commission on Medicaid and the Uninsured, 2002 (updated Feb. 2003). Available at: http://www.kff.org/uninsured/loader.cfm?url=/commonspot/security/getfile.cfm&PageID=13971

7. Ayanian JZ, Weissman JS, Schneider EC, et al. Unmet health needs of uninsured adults in the United States. *JAMA* 2000;284(16):2061–2069.

8. Richardson W, Berwick D, Bisgard JC, et al. *Crossing the quality chasm: A new health system for the 21st century.* Washington, DC: National Academy Press, 2001.

9. Joint National Committee on Prevention, Detection, Evaluation, and Treatment of High Blood Pressure. Sixth report. *Arch Int Med* 1997;157:2413–2446.

10. McBride P, Schrott HG, Plane MB, et al. Primary care practice adherence to national cholesterol education program guidelines for patients with coronary heart disease. *Arch Intern Med* 1998;158:1238–1234.

11. Samsa GP, Matchar DB, Goldstein LB, et al. Quality of anticoagulation management among patients with atrial fibrillation. *Arch Int Med* 2000;160:967–973.

12. Perez-Stable E, Affleck-Fuentes E. Role of clinicians in cigarette smoking prevention. *West J Med* 1998;169:23–29.

13. McGlyn E, Asch S, Adams J. The quality of health care delivered to adults in the United States. *N Engl J Med* 2003;348:2635–2645.

14. AHRQ, National Health Care Quality Report, 2003. Available at:__http://www.ahrq.gov/qual/nhqr03/nhqrsum0>3.htm

15. Fiscella K, Franks P, Gold M. Inequality in quality: Addressing socioeconomic, racial and ethnic disparities in health care. *JAMA* 2000;283:2579–2584.

16. Schneider E, Zaslavsky A, Epstein A. Racial disparities in the quality of care for enrollees in Medicare managed care. *JAMA* 2002;287(10):1288–1294.

17. Lorig K, Holman H, Sobel D, et al. *Living a healthy life with chronic conditions.* Palo Alto, CA: Bull Publishing Co, 2000.

18. FACCT, RWJ Foundation. *A portrait of the chronically ill in America, 2001: A report from the Robert Wood Johnson Foundation National Strategic Indicator Surveys.* www.facct.org://facct/facct/site/facct/facct/home

19. Fisher L, Chesla CA, Mullan JT, et al. Contributors to depression in Latino and European-American patients with type 2 diabetes. *Diabetes Care* 2001;24(10):1751–1757.

20. Coyne JC, Rohrbaugh MJ, Shoham V, et al. Prognostic importance of marital quality for survival of congestive heart failure. *Am J Cardiol* 2001;88(5):526–529.

21. Schneider EC, Zaslavsky AM, Landon BE, et al. National quality monitoring of Medicare health plans: The relationship between enrollees' reports and the quality of clinical care. *Med Care* 2001;39(12):1313–1325.

22. Heurtin-Roberts S, Reisin E. The relation of culturally influenced lay models of hypertension to compliance with treatment. *Am J Hypertens* 1992;5(11):787–792.

23. Ogedegbe G, Mancuso C, Allegrante J. Expectations of blood pressure management in hypertensive African-American patients: A qualitative study. *J Natl Med Assoc* 2004;96(4):442–449.

24. Carder P, Vuckovic N, Green CA. Negotiating medications: Patient perceptions of long-term medication use. *J Clin Pharmacol Ther* 2003;28(5):409–417.

25. Wagner E, Austin B, von Korff M. Organizing care for patients with chronic illness. *Milbank Q* 1996;74:511–544.

26. Greiner AC, Knebel E, eds. *Institute of Medicine Committee on the Health Professions. Education Summit on Health Professions Education: A bridge to quality.* Washington, DC: National Academies Press, 2003.

27. Blumenthal D, Gokhale M, Campbell EG, et al. Preparedness for clinical practice: Reports of graduating residents at academic health centers. *JAMA* 2001;289(9):1027–1034.

28. Beckman H, Frankel R. The effect of physician behavior on the collection of data. *Ann Int Med* 1984;101:692–696.

29. Marvel MK, Epstein RM, Flowers K, et al. Soliciting the patient's agenda. Have we improved? *JAMA* 1999;281:283–287.

30. Clement S. Diabetes self-management education. *Diabetes Care* 1995;18:1204–1214.

31. Roter D, Hall JA. Studies of doctor–patient interaction. *Annu Rev Public Health* 1989;10:163–180.

32. Schillinger D, Piette J, Grumbach K. Closing the loop. Physician communication with diabetic patients who have low health literacy. *Arch Intern Med* 2003;139:907–915.

33. Hulka B, Kupper LL, Cassel JC, et al. Doctor–patient communication, and outcomes among diabetic patients. *J Commun Health* 1975;1(1):15–27.

34. Stewart A, Napoles-Springer A, Perez-Stable E. Interpersonal processes of care in diverse populations. *Milbank Q* 1999;77:305–339.

35. Lutfey K, Wishner W. Beyond compliance is adherence. *Diabetes Care* 1999;22:635–639.

36. Hall JA, Epstein AM, DeCiantis ML, et al. Physicians' liking for their patients: More evidence for the role of affect in medical care. *Health Psychol* 1993;12(2):140–146.

37. Sharpe M, Mayou R, Seagrott V, et al. Why do doctors find some patients difficult to help? *Q J Med* 1994;87(3):187–193.

38. Schulman KA, Berlin JA, Harless W, et al. The effect of race and sex on physicians' recommendations for cardiac catheterization. *N Engl J Med* 1999;340(8):618–626.

39. Van Ryn M, Burke J. The effect of patient race and socioeconomic status on physicians' perception of patients. *Soc Sci Med* 2000;50(6):813–828.

40. Komoromy M, Lurie N, Bindman AB. California physicians' willingness to care for the poor. *West J Med* 1995; 162(2):127–132.

41. Singh N. Determinants of compliance with antiretroviral therapy in patients with human immunodeficiency virus: Prospective assessment with implications for enhancing compliance. *AIDS Care* 1996;8:261.

42. Taira D, Safran D, Seto T. The relationship between patient income and physician discussion of health risk behaviors. *JAMA* 1997;278:1412.

43. Kogan MD, Kotelchuck M, Alexander GR, et al. Racial disparities in reported prenatal care advice from health care providers. *Am J Public Health* 1994;84:82–88.

44. Doescher M, Saver B. Physician's advice to quit smoking. The glass remains half empty. *J Fam Pract* 2000;49: 543–547.

45. O'Malley M, Earp J, Harris R. The association of race/ethnicity, socioeconomic status and physician recommendation for mammography: Who gets the message about breast cancer screening? *Am J Public Health* 2001;91:49–54.

46. Ni H, Nauman DJ, Hershberger RE. Managed care and outcomes of hospitalization among elderly patients with congestive heart failure. *Arch Int Med* 1998;158: 231–236.

47. Clark N, Gong MB. Management of chronic disease by practitioners and patients: Are we teaching the wrong things? *BMJ* 2000;320:572–575.

48. AHRQ. *Diabetes disparities in ethnic and racial minorities.* 2004. Available at: http://www.ahrq.gov/research/diabdisp.htm

49. Wagner E. Chronic disease management: What will it take to improve care for chronic illness? *Effect Clin Pract* 1998;1:2–4.

50. Edwards R, Telfair J, Cecil H, et al. Self-efficacy as a predictor of adult adjustment to sickle cell disease: One-year outcomes. *Psychosom Med* 2001;63(5):850–858.

51. Anderson L, Zimmerman M. Patient and physician perceptions of their relationship and patient satisfaction: A study of chronic disease management. *Patient Educ Couns* 1993;20(1):27–36.

52. Greenfield S, Kaplan SH, Ware JE Jr, et al. Patients' participation in medical care: Effects on blood sugar control and quality of life in diabetes. *J Gen Intern Med* 1988;2:448–457.

53. Bodenheimer T, Lorig K, Holman H, et al. Patient self-management of chronic disease in primary care. *JAMA* 2002;288(19):2469–2475.

54. Bodenheimer T. Interventions to improve chronic illness care: Evaluating their effectiveness. *Disease Manag* 2003;6(2):63–69.

55. Rich MW, Beckham V, Wittenberg C, et al. A multidisciplinary intervention to prevent readmission of elderly patients with congestive heart failure. *N Engl J Med* 1995;333:190–195.

56. Centers for Disease Control and Prevention (CDC). Prevalence of disabilities and associated health conditions among adults—United States, 1999. *MMWR Morb Mortal Wkly Rep* 2001;50:120–125.

57. Mokdad AH, Marks JS, Stroup DF, et al. Actual causes of death in the United States, 2000. *JAMA* 2004;291(10): 1238–1245.

Chapter 37

Disability and Patients with Disabilities

Margot Kushel, MD, and Lisa I. Iezzoni, MD, MSc

Objectives

- Define the concept of disability.
- Review the epidemiology of disabilities among community-dwelling persons.
- Describe key social, legal, and health policy issues relating to disability.
- Describe issues raised by disabilities related to vision, hearing, and lower extremity mobility difficulties and strategies to improve these.

Ever since humans began coalescing into social networks, people realized that some among them might need special assistance—those who could not hunt, gather, or subsist for themselves because of sensory, physical, or other impairments. However, along with that realization came the need to distinguish "deserving from undeserving" persons. After all, lazy people could fake disabilities to avoid work. In the 19th century physicians assumed the role as arbiter of eligibility for disability-related social programs.

Disabilities are diverse in their causes, nature, timing, pace, and personal and social implications. Some are congenital, others acquired. Some arrive suddenly with injury or accident; others progress slowly over time. Some gradually limit but do not threaten life; others hasten death. Some are visible to outsiders; others remain hidden. Some engender stigmatization and blame; others prompt pity and paternalism. Some are seen primarily as "diseases" (e.g., end-stage cancer, emphysema, schizophrenia), even when profoundly disabling. Anyone can become disabled, and in the fullness of time, most people do.

Given this diversity, speaking of "persons with disabilities" as a single subpopulation is almost meaningless.

Even within categories of impairments—such as lower extremity mobility difficulties—the causes, manifestations, and clinical implications are wide ranging. This chapter does not discuss specific medical conditions that cause disabilities. Instead, it offers an overview of the key social and health policy issues and selected major practice concerns raised by disability, focusing on persons with disabilities related to seeing, hearing, and walking. For convenience, this chapter uses the term "disability" when referring to sensory or physical impairments. Nonetheless, it makes no presumption that individuals with these conditions are, in fact, disabled, however they choose to define the word.

DEFINING DISABILITY

Judy, in her late twenties, was born to deaf parents who themselves had deaf parents. Judy is third-generation deaf. Judy's family speaks American Sign Language (ASL), which also was the language used at her Deaf school. She later learned English and now works in the hearing world, relying on lip reading and ASL interpreters. Judy does not view herself as disabled, but instead as belonging to the Deaf linguistic minority culture.

Identifying individuals as disabled is complex, with multilayered personal, administrative, legal, and societal ramifications. Over the last century, various definitions of disability have appeared for diverse purposes, with little consensus across definitions. A "medical model" treats disability "as a problem of the person, directly caused by disease, trauma or other health condition, which requires medical care. Management of the disability is aimed at cure or the individual's adjustment and behavior change."[1,2] In the last 40 years, a "social model" has viewed disability "mainly as a socially created problem, and basically as a matter of the full integration of individuals into society. Disability is not an attribute of an individual, but rather a complex collection of conditions, many of which are created by the social environment."[2] Judy, for example, sees communication problems she confronts in her workplace not as her personal deficit, but as failures of the majority hearing world to accommodate communication with a linguistic minority.

In 2001, the World Health Organization approved the *International Classification of Functioning, Disability and Health* (ICF), which attempts to integrate medical and social models of disability.[2,3] The ICF identifies three interrelated concepts: "Impairments are problems in body function or structure such as a significant deviation or loss. Activity is the execution of a task or action by an individual. [and] Participation is involvement in a life situation." The ICF defines disability as an "umbrella term for impairments, activity limitations or participation restrictions," conceiving "a person's functioning and disability . . . as a dynamic interaction between health conditions (diseases, disorders, injuries, traumas, etc.) and contextual factors," including environmental and personal attributes.[2] As discussed in the following, the Americans with Disabilities Act (ADA, P.L. 101-336) adopted an even more expansive definition of disability.

> Whenever she goes to the doctor, Judy says, the first question is always about why she is deaf: "I was just born that way." She wants the first question to address her chief complaint.

Today's broad definition of disability carries important lessons for clinicians, primarily because of potential effects on patient–clinician communication and incorporating the disability appropriately into treatment plans. Clinicians should approach clinical encounters with patients with disabilities just as they do with other patients, starting with the chief complaint and then, as necessary, learning more about any impairments when asking history questions. It is useful for the clinician to learn the patient's view of the impairment. In some instances, impairments may be irrelevant to the reason patients seek care. For example, Judy's identification as a linguistic minority rather than as someone with a disability should be known and respected, regardless of how social programs or legal mandates would categorize her.

In addition, the social definition highlights the relationships between patients and their daily environments. Interventions that affect the interplay between them (e.g., various assistive technologies) or even the environment itself (e.g., grab bars in bathrooms) may prove extremely efficacious in restoring persons to safe and independent functioning; thus, the physician's role in "treating" disability includes adjustments not only to the impairment, but in recommended adjustments to the environment and the interplay between them.

EPIDEMIOLOGY

Varying definitions impede efforts to determine the population prevalence of disability. Patterns of disability (e.g., by age, sex) vary depending on perspective. Nearly 20% of community-dwelling, civilian, US residents age 5 years and older report at least some disabling condition, with rates rising sharply (to 41.9%) among persons age 65 and older. Disability frequently tracks with personal attributes that characterize vulnerable populations, including minority race and ethnicity, low educational attainment, high level of unemployment, and poverty.

Conditions relating to aging are the most common causes of sensory and physical disabilities. Cataracts and glaucoma, along with presbyopia, are the main causes of vision loss;[4] presbycusis is the most common reason for hearing loss;[5] and arthritis is the single most disabling condition among adult Americans.[5] Overall, because of very high rates of hearing problems among white men, white persons are more likely than African-American, Hispanic, and other race individuals to report any sensory or mobility disability. However, African Americans report higher rates of mobility disabilities than do whites; relative rates for Hispanics vary depending on the nature of the physical impairment.

OVERVIEW OF SOCIAL, LEGAL, AND HEALTH POLICY ISSUES

> Jimmy, a man in his mid-40s, has painful arthritis in his hips and knees, which sometimes causes him to fall. He worked moving boxes in a warehouse, but the physical demands of his job seemed too much for him and his employer fired him. Out of a job, Jimmy is unable to sustain his level of living and seeks public assistance. He asks his physician to write a disability letter in support of his Social Security Disability Insurance (SSDI) application.

SOCIAL SECURITY PROGRAMS

In the late 1950s, Social Security began two programs authorizing cash benefits for persons, such as Jimmy, who cannot work because of disability: SSDI (under Title II of the Social Security Act); and Supplemental Security Income (SSI, under Title XVI). SSDI gives benefits to persons who are "insured" by virtue of having worked and contributed to the Social Security trust fund through withholdings on their earnings (SSDI also covers certain disabled dependents of insured persons). The 1972 Social Security Act amendments granted eligibility for Medicare to individuals who have received SSDI cash benefits for 2 years. Title XVI provides SSI payments to persons, including children, who are disabled, blind, or elderly and have passed a means test documenting limited income and resources. Persons qualifying for SSI immediately receive Medicaid coverage. Poor persons receiving SSDI also can obtain SSI benefits after passing the means test; some states supplement the federal income benefit with additional cash payments.

SSDI and SSI use identical definitions to determine whether working-age adults are "disabled": Under a yes/no standard, persons either can or cannot engage in "substantial gainful activity" because of medically proven sensory, physical, or mental impairments.[6] As codified by 1968 regulations, the disability evaluation starts with the "Listings of Impairments" (the so-called "List"), which itemizes impairments, grouped by body system, that should be sufficiently severe to preclude substantial gainful employment among adults.[7] The List stipulates specific tests (e.g., radiographs) and physical examination findings (e.g., joint range of motion) required to validate each condition. Musculoskeletal conditions are the leading cause of disability eligibility.[7]

PHYSICIAN ROLE IN ELIGIBILITY ASSESSMENT

Typically, officials determining eligibility seek information from applicants' own physicians, presuming that they have the greatest clinical knowledge of their patients' conditions. Thus, when Jimmy sought benefits from Social Security he was referred to his physician for an evaluation and completion of the appropriate paperwork. This sometimes causes tensions between patients and physicians, especially when physicians think that patients can still work and the patient disagrees. After all, physicians must document all forms honestly, based on their professional judgments. In such instances, physicians should thoroughly explore the reasons why persons wish to stop working. For example, in Jimmy's case his physician might believe that he is not significantly impaired and could work at another job requiring less physical labor.

How disagreements between patients and physicians are handled often depends on the nature of the inter-

personal and professional relationships. When there is disagreement, one strategy is to show the patient the final evaluation, asking if he or she would like the physician to submit it. Often, if the patient is unhappy, he or she may simply seek the advice of another physician. Finally, it is important to note that in the final analysis it is not the clinician who grants disability, it is the agency or courts (see Core Competency).

Gaps in Coverage

When Jimmy asked his doctor to complete the disability evaluation form, she readily agreed with his decision, and he was awarded SSDI. Jimmy will get Medicare 24 months after he first receives SSDI cash benefits, which happens 5 months following his disability determination. During that 29-month wait, he plans to use COBRA provisions to retain health insurance, but Jimmy is very worried about paying the premiums.

SSI recipients immediately get Medicaid coverage. However, SSDI beneficiaries have a 29-month waiting period before they receive Medicare. Consequently, during this waiting period these beneficiaries often have a difficult time. They can no longer work, few carry insurance from their employers, and SSDI cash benefits are often insufficient to cover living costs and premiums of private coverage. In 2002, this population included an estimated 1.26 million individuals; approximately one third lacked health insurance entirely, whereas roughly 40% enrolled in Medicaid.[8] Relatively little is known about the health and health care of SSDI beneficiaries during the waiting period. During the waiting period, many persons put off doctor visits, forego necessary medications, and get little rehabilitation therapy.[9] Among those newly entitled to SSDI in 1995, 11.8% died during the waiting period, whereas 2.1% recovered.[10]

Even once persons with disabilities receive Medicare, they face additional challenges. A 2004 survey of Medicare beneficiaries found that 48% of persons under age 65 reported significant difficulties paying for prescription drugs, compared with 17% of older beneficiaries.[10] Another study found that 34% of persons with disabilities blamed inability to pay prescription medication for their failure to follow prescribed regimens.[11] It is unclear how this will be impacted by Medicare Part D.

AMERICANS WITH DISABILITIES ACT

Given his financial straits, Jimmy sometimes wonders whether he should have tried to continue working, suing his company under the Americans with Disabilities Act for a job that would have been less physically demanding.

According to its opening statement, the aim of the Americans with Disabilities Act is "to provide a clear and comprehensive national mandate for the elimination of discrimination against individuals with disabilities." Title I charges the Equal Employment Opportunity Commission, established initially with the Civil Rights Act of 1964, with ensuring that employers do not discriminate because of disability against otherwise qualified individuals "in regard to job application procedures, the hiring, advancement, or discharge of employees, employee compensation, job training, and other terms, conditions, and privileges of employment" (Sec. 102(a)). Discrimination includes "not making reasonable accommodations to the known physical or mental limitations" (Sec. 102(b)(5)(A)). Title II prohibits discrimination or denial of services provided by public entities, while Title III prohibits discrimination involving public accommodations and services operated by private entities, including the "professional office of a health care provider, hospital, or other service establishment" (Sec. 301(7)(F)).

The ADA defines disability as: "(A) a physical or mental impairment that substantially limits one or more of the major life activities of such individual; (B) a record of such an impairment; or (C) being regarded as having such an impairment" (Sec. 3(2)). In operationalizing this definition, the ADA differs fundamentally from other civil rights laws. For instance, to sue for racial or gender discrimination, plaintiffs do not need to prove that they belong to a particular race or gender group. However, to litigate under the ADA, individuals must prove, sometimes to a skeptical judiciary, that they are disabled before they can broach questions about discrimination.

Through various cases (*Sutton et al.* v. *United Air Lines, Inc.* and *Murphy* v. *United Parcel Service, Inc.*, 1999; *Toyota Motor Manufacturing Inc.* v. *Williams*, 2002), the US Supreme Court has further constrained the ADA's reach, largely by delimiting the "major life activities" clause. Therefore, it is unclear that, even with his physician's assertions about his debilitating lower extremity arthritis, Jimmy would pass muster as "disabled" under Title I of the ADA. After all, he still functions around home, doing light chores and preparing meals. However, as noted later in this chapter, Titles II and III of the ADA carry important implications for public and private health care providers, respectively.

Common Pitfalls: Having a disability can have a profound effect on the health care one receives. Providers often:

- Fail to seek the patient's perspective on his or her impairments.
- Assume that the disability is the reason the patient is seeking care.
- Are unfamiliar with the assistive devices that may help their patient.
- Are not adequately trained to assess the disability.
- Do not work in settings that accommodate people with disabilities.
- Medical insurance coverage often lags behind attainment of SSI and is often inadequate.
- Poor and disadvantaged people are more likely to be disabled.
- Applying for disability benefits can be difficult for patient and provider.

LOWER EXTREMITY MOBILITY DIFFICULTIES

Tom's wife is both irritated and worried. Tom, a shop clerk in his mid-forties, refuses to acknowledge the foot drop that is making him fall ever more frequently. He will not even tell the clinic doctor about it.

Walking not only physically moves persons at will from point A to point B, but also it carries tremendous cultural significance. The US ethos assumes citizens are free to move at will, act independently, be self-reliant, and take control; not be a burden to others. Bipedal, upright movement permeates US aphorisms, connoting independence, autonomy, perseverance, strength, achievement: "standing on your own two feet," "walking tall," "standing up for yourself," "taking things in stride," and "climbing the ladder of success." If their walking progressively fails, people can become embarrassed, ashamed, terrified of losing control, and afraid of being called lazy. Especially when older, people can feel that worsening walking is inevitable, something to be borne without complaint and hidden from view, something physicians can do little to help.[12] Some, such as Tom, believe they can beat the problem by sheer willpower. In addition, Tom fears, not without reason, that he will lose his job if his boss notices his increasing debility.

THE ACT OF WALKING

Walking involves multiple interactive components, including gait, balance, strength, and endurance. Gait is the physical action of walking—a repeating cycle of movements encompassing one step with each foot. The gait cycle involves the stance phase (about 60% of the gait cycle) and the swing phase (the other 40%). The stance phase splits further into the double-leg stance (both feet contacting the ground) and the single-leg stance. One way to increase stability is to increase the time spent in double-leg stance. As people age, stride length shortens, thus resulting in larger proportions of walking time spent with two-leg support.

During the gait cycle, a person's center of mass (COM, located midway between the hips) moves rhythmically up-and-down and side-to-side, while transferring weight from one leg to the other. People naturally adjust their limb and trunk muscles, counterbalancing arm swings and walking speeds to minimize COM movements and maintain their balance (the ability to control upright posture). Abnormalities that distort smooth, wavelike COM movement, such as the hemiplegic gait of strokes or efforts to avoid weight-bearing on painful hips or knees, increase the energy required to walk. Walking slowly actually demands more energy for muscles and other structures to provide additional balance. If persons with impairments walk slowly, they therefore consume more energy than do others while walking the same distance.

TAKING A WALKING HISTORY AND EVALUATING MOBILITY

Asking about physical activity should be part of a complete primary care evaluation. Physicians have long used patients' abilities to walk distances or perform other physical activities as explicit clinical indicators of cardiorespiratory endurance. Carefully questioning patients with, for example, congestive heart failure or chronic obstructive pulmonary disease about how far they can walk before becoming short of breath provides important information about the severity of those diseases. Sometimes clinicians walk patients around the office while monitoring their oxygenation via an oximeter. However, this does not constitute a formal gait analysis.

Major primary care textbooks say little about evaluating gait, and primary care physicians often fail to recognize fully patients' functional deficits. Some primary care physicians observe patients as they walk into examining rooms or climb onto examining tables; however, these efforts are neither rigorous nor consistent. Only a few ask their patients to walk down the corridor and formally evaluate their gait. Evaluation tools do exist to assess walking, requiring nothing more sophisticated than a hallway, chair, and stopwatch. One that has been validated for elderly populations is the "Get Up and Go Test."[13] At a minimum, assessments provide a critical baseline evaluation (Box 37-1).

Getting patients such as Tom to describe their difficulty walking can take careful questioning, cautiously circling the issue. Clinicians could begin with a series of questions: Do you ever have trouble walking across the street before the light changes? Tell me about the last time you walked around your neighborhood. What do you hold onto when you walk around your house? How many times a day do you walk up and down stairs? Do you ever find yourself unexpectedly on the floor? How much do you worry about falling? Family members, such as Tom's wife, can volunteer important insight, albeit sometimes at the cost of interpersonal harmony. Obviously, additional questions should target specific diagnostic possibilities (e.g., asking about pain, muscle weakness). As in Tom's case, if patients report falls, questions should address potential precipitants and elicit information that could assist in designing strategies to prevent falls.

Tip: Standard cross-walks are timed to normal adult gait speed. If your patient regularly has difficulty crossing the cross walks prior to the "Don't Walk" signal, he or she may have a gait disorder.

REFERRALS TO REHABILITATION SPECIALISTS

His physician plans to work up Tom's drop foot, but in the meantime he refers Tom to a physical therapist for evaluation, potential strengthening and balance exercises, and to learn how to prevent falls or at least minimize injury when falls do occur.

Box 37-1. The "Get Up and Go" Test

Instruct patient to:	Taking more than 30 seconds to complete this task suggests higher rates of dependence and risk of falls; less than 20 seconds suggests independence for transfers and mobility.
• Rise from sitting position • Walk 10 feet • Turn around • Return to seated position in chair	Podsiadlo D, Richardson S. The timed "Up & Go": A test of basic functional mobility for frail elderly persons. *J Am Geriatr Soc* 1991;39(2):142–148.[14]

Primary care clinicians are not typically trained to perform detailed functional evaluations or recommend specific exercises or other clinical interventions or assess persons for assistive technologies, such as mobility aids.[14]

When patients have important and active medical issues affecting their function, physical medicine and rehabilitation (PM&R) physicians (also known as physiatrists) can help. They assess functional needs and provide nonsurgical interventions, frequently working alongside physical and occupational therapists. By fully understanding complex medical factors as well as the nature of impairments, PM&R specialists aim to construct care plans that maximize health and independent functioning. Table 37-1 shows guidelines of appropriate referral to physical or occupational therapists.

AMBULATION AIDS AND WHEELED MOBILITY AIDS

Tom's physician recommends a cane to assist with balance and help prevent falls.

Mobility aids fall into two broad classes, depending on whether they assist or replace ambulation. These aids can restore functional independence to persons unable to walk safely without them. The proper choice depends on the cause of the mobility difficulty, the setting in which the person will use the aid, and the person's physical condition (e.g., endurance, upper and lower body strength, hand strength and dexterity, balance, truncal stability), cognition, judgment, vision, and hearing. Some people may benefit from having more than one type of aid for use in different circumstances. Ambulation aids include canes, crutches, and

Table 37-1. Guidelines for Appropriate Referrals to Rehabilitation Specialists

Referrals to physical therapists are appropriate when patients:
  Are adapting to new disability
  Have significant balance or gait disturbance
  Have significant range of motion or strength impairments
  Need assessment for a mobility aid
  Need training in use of ambulatory aid
  Have seating or positioning problems with a wheelchair
Referrals to occupational therapists are indicated when patients:
  Are adapting to new disability
  Need assistance with basic or instrumental activities of daily living
  Display limited judgment about safety
  Need splint or orthotic fabrication
  Need adaptive equipment for work
  Require assessment of home environment for possible modification to improve safety and usability

walkers, whereas wheeled mobility aids include manual and power wheelchairs and scooters. To use ambulation aids, persons must have adequate shoulder, arm, and hand functioning.

Historically, mobility aids had distinctly institutional appearances, underscoring images of debility. Now, diverse manufacturers compete to provide mobility aids meeting all consumer demands and needs, including children's crutches in fluorescent colors, canes decorated with elaborate carvings or paintings, rolling walkers with seats and baskets useful at the mall, lightweight manual wheelchairs in rainbow hues, and specialized wheelchairs for sports from racing to basketball. Language is also shifting. The phrases "wheelchair bound" and "confined to a wheelchair" imply passivity and are simply wrong (i.e., no one spends every minute in a wheelchair). Today's preferred phrase—"wheelchair user"—is simple and accurate, reflecting action.

Canes

Canes can aid balance and offload weight. Although multiple styles of canes exist (standard, offset, and multilegged), little research has explored the optimal cane for different situations, and often the choice comes down to personal preference and availability. All canes offer an additional point of contact with the ground and thus widen persons' base of support. Offset canes bear weight better than standard canes, but multilegged canes may be best for that purpose. Regardless of the style, canes must be the proper height and used correctly to maximize their utility. For increasing balance, patients should place the cane in their dominant hand; the extra sensory input from the hand-cane-ground contacts helps improve balance. For offloading weight, persons hold the cane in the hand opposite the weak or painful leg (e.g., persons with right knee problems should use the left hand). When taking a step, persons should advance their cane along with their problem leg, allowing some weight to shift from that leg to their arm and the cane.

Crutches

Unlike canes, crutches can bear a person's full weight, assuming the individual has sufficient upper body strength. Crutches also increase the lateral base of support and thus improve stability. The two classes of crutches are axillary and forearm models. Because they require considerable upper body strength, axillary crutches are most appropriate for temporary complete weight bearing following an injury. Forearm crutches, also called Canadian crutches, require triceps strength but allow the hands to be free when not walking. Persons with partial paralysis or lower extremity amputations can use forearm crutches to offload weight.

Walkers

Numerous models of walkers now exist: standard four-point walkers without wheels; walkers with wheels in front but not in the back; and walkers with three or four wheels, brakes on their handlebars, seats, and baskets. Depending on their style, walkers greatly increase stability and balance. Wheeled walkers minimize the energy demands of their use, but require greater attention and care from users. As with canes and crutches, walkers must be set to an appropriate height for the individual user, and optimally physical therapists would train persons in proper use of their walker.

> Tom's leg weakness worsens, preventing him from walking long distances. His wife has an old, institutional wheelchair hidden away, left behind from her mother's final illness. Would that help Tom?

Most assume that when people are seated they are safe and comfortable. Nothing is further from the truth. Standard chrome wheelchairs, with plastic sling backs and seats used to ferry people around hospitals and airports, generally are uncomfortable to occupy for lengthy periods. "Seating" is now a science. Engineers and materials specialists design wheelchairs and wheelchair cushions specifically to maximize safety, comfort, and functionality, with adequate back supports, padding for vulnerable sites (e.g., ischial tuberosities) to minimize risks of pressure ulcers, and maximal maneuverability and stability. For people with money or generous insurance coverage, countless options exist. However, inexpensive and suboptimal models are all some people can afford. Many, such as Tom, end up using equipment left behind by others and likely inadequate to their needs.

Numerous types of wheeled mobility aids are now available. Different models generally fall into one of four categories: manual wheelchairs, in which the user is either pushed from behind or provides all the propulsive power, made from standard or ultra-lightweight materials; new power assist wheelchairs, which are basically manual models with a switch that temporarily turns on power, boosting the propulsion of the wheels as the user pushes; four-wheel power (battery-powered) wheelchairs, with a wide range of different controls (e.g., a joystick on the armrest, controls operated by the user's mouth or breaths) and features (e.g., tilt devices); and three- or four-wheeled scooters, in which users sit in a captain's chair, affixed to a platform and positioned behind the controls. Although manual wheelchairs seem optimal for maximizing the physical fitness of persons who can use them, long-term self-propulsion can cause rotator cuff injuries, carpal tunnel syndrome, and shoulder pain. Careful evaluation by specialists, preferably in a seating clinic, is essential to ensure choice of equipment that maximizes independent function and minimizes physical risks.

> Tom does not have the upper body strength to self-propel a wheelchair for any distance and seeks coverage for a power wheelchair from Medicare.

Medicare and other insurers typically will not pay for items or services unless they are deemed "medically necessary." Insurers often reduce the arguments to a simple question: Is the item or service medically necessary to treat a disease, disorder, or injury or is it primarily desired for convenience? This question poses a vexing problem for mobility aids, which by definition are not "treating" a condition but are explicitly recognizing that a permanent deficit might exist. Medicare adds to their evaluation the "in-home" rule: Items are covered only if persons must use them in their home. In Tom's case, he "furniture surfs" at home and uses the wheelchair only outdoors to travel longer distances; therefore, Medicare would view a power chair as a "convenience item" and deny Tom's request.

> Tom initially refused to use a cane, worried about how people would see him. Later Tom said, "I won't be seen dead in a wheelchair." Now Tom finds the wheelchair improves his independence.

A lingering sense of social stigma and other complex emotions often make people reluctant to use mobility aids. Primary care physicians may wish to work closely with rehabilitation specialists to find the optimal options for individual patients. When patients like Tom hesitate to use equipment that could potentially improve their safety, physicians should avoid "all-or-nothing" recommendations. Many patients successfully and appropriately use mobility aids intermittently. For example, Tom successfully "furniture surfs" at home but would benefit from using his cane outdoors or when in large crowds. Physicians should take care to avoid "all-or-nothing" declarations, making it clear that patients may use equipment in different ways at different times. In addition, physicians should help reframe issues for patients, emphasizing the ways in which aids will increase mobility for patients, rather than serving as an indicator of debility.

Tip: When providing documentation for insurance, letters must be specific and contain all relevant information, including:

1. Diagnoses that lead to impairment
2. Documentation of physical limitations, including impact on daily functioning
3. Specific description of equipment and how used: what activities were limited; when and where will equipment be used
4. Clear rationale justifying benefits

Note that Medicare pays only for equipment that is needed within the patient's house. Also note that for power equipment, Medicare demands that the patient receive prescription from (depending on cause of the impairment) a rheumatologist, orthopedist, neurologist, or physiatrist, unless going to one would place an undo burden on the patient.

BLINDNESS AND LOW VISION

Lorna, in her late forties, has many medical problems, especially diabetes, which has limited her vision.

About 1.3 million Americans, roughly 5 in 1000 persons, are legally blind (central visual acuity of (20/200 in the better eye with correction or a field of vision of (20 degrees), although about 80% of them have some useful vision.[15] Blindness does not mean total loss of vision; many blind people can still see shadows, light, colors, or images, albeit sometimes within extremely narrowed visual fields. Many others have low vision not fully corrected by eyeglasses. Vision problems can compromise mobility and activities of daily living, heighten risks of falls, and contribute to depressed mood. However, new technologies and consumer products, such as computer screen readers, books on tape, and "talking" appliances, have dramatically expanded options and quality of life for many persons with impaired vision. When vision cannot be restored by glasses, medications, or surgery, focusing on making the most of the remaining vision to maintain independence is crucial.

Lorna comes to the clinic for a routine visit, using a white cane to assist independent ambulation.

Office staff and clinicians should be trained about communicating appropriately with persons who are blind or have low vision. Introducing oneself and asking what kind of assistance persons might want are the first steps. At the front desk, persons may need assistance completing routine paperwork. Finding a private place to give this assistance is essential to protect patients' privacy. Offering to assist persons in getting around facilities is also appropriate, but let the person make the first move. Persons who are blind typically use several strategies to navigate spaces: lightly holding the arm, just above the elbow, of a sighted guide; or proceeding independently with a white cane or guide dog and following a sighted guide who walks a few steps ahead. The ADA requires public and private facilities to allow service animals, such as guide dogs, on the premises even if pets are excluded. Facilities should have Braille and raised print signage marking doors and passageways so that persons can get around independently, should they choose.

Blindness or low vision may not be the person's chief complaint. Physicians should therefore not automatically assume that vision should be the first topic discussed. For patients such as Lorna, who has diabetes, physicians obviously should routinely question them about their vision and refer them to appropriate specialists. Limited evidence supports the value of routine questioning about visual functioning during primary care visits for all patients. However, depending on the clinical context, questions about sight may identify important problems. Useful questions include asking persons whether (with their glasses) they have trouble driving at night, seeing someone across the street, reading a newspaper, seeing details on the television screen, or going up stairs.

Lorna lives alone. She would like a glucose monitor that would allow her to test her blood sugars at home. However, she reports trouble distinguishing her many different pill bottles.

Lorna's independence should not come as a surprise. Persons who become blind or develop low vision can continue living productive and independent lives. Rehabilitation programs specifically targeting vision loss can train persons in independent ambulation (e.g., using a white cane), in Braille (a system using raised dots to represent letters, numbers, punctuation, and certain words), and various assistive technologies to assist reading, writing, and other activities. As persons begin losing vision, large print materials (i.e., 14-point font or larger) can allow them to read printed materials, such as prescription labels on pill bottles or medication instructions. With more impaired vision, other devices may help. Health insurance usually will not pay for assistive devices for enhancing vision, although some Medicaid programs might pay for prescription eyeglasses. However, Medicare and other insurers now typically pay for selected health-related items such as home glucose monitors that "talk" (i.e., convey information orally).

Web sites such as those sponsored by the American Foundation for the Blind (www.afb.org) and National Federation of the Blind (www.nfb.org) offer extensive listings of various products and services to assist persons with visual disabilities. Some large health plans offer telephone information hotlines that provide recorded messages containing general information about health problems or conditions. Web sites designed to be accessible to all users, such as those of agencies within the US Department of Health and Human Services, offer growing volumes of accessible health information.

Unfortunately, clinicians rarely provide information in accessible formats, such as prescription drug or postdischarge instructions, test results, or appointment slips. At home, patients can sometimes use technologies to access this information, for example, by magnifying print manyfold using video magnifiers or closed circuit television systems. However, depending on individual preferences, giving patients information in large print, Braille, audiotape, or digital formats (e.g., sending appointment reminders, test results, and other information through secure Internet portals) could readily improve the accessibility of information. If high-tech formats are unavailable, clinicians should discuss with patients who are blind or have low vision alternative ways of conveying critical information even by such low-tech means as telephone calls (e.g., to make sure patients understand medication instructions, provide visit reminders).

Other adaptive devices are critically helpful, albeit sometimes expensive. Synthetic speech systems (a synthesizer that does the speaking and a screen reader that tells the synthesizer what to say) allow persons with visual disabilities to "hear" texts that appear on computer screens. Text-to-speech software contains all the phonemes and grammatic rules of the designated language, producing fairly natural pronunciations. Keyboard commands instruct these systems to perform various functions, such as reading specific portions of texts, identifying the cursor location, and finding strings of text.

Optical character recognition technologies scan printed texts then speak the words using synthetic speech or save it on a computer. Technology does not yet exist that conveys graphic or pictorial information into accessible formats for persons with impaired vision. Nonetheless, current optical character recognition programs contain logic to identify and correct errors, such as major grammatic or spelling mistakes, before speaking the texts. For persons with low vision who can see enlarged images, screen magnification programs offer access without speech, although users can focus only on one part of the screen at a time.

Tips for helping patients who are blind or have low vision manage their medications:

1. Record all pertinent information about their medications in a form useful for them: Braille, large print, audiocassette.
2. Ask pharmacist to dispense medications of similar shape in different sized bottles to help differentiate and keep this consistent.
3. Wrap rubber bands or other tactile clues around the bottle corresponding to the number of times a day they are to take that medication. Remove one band with each dose. At end of day, replace all bands for the next day.

DEAF AND HARD OF HEARING

Jerry, an auto mechanic in his early fifties and father of four, is growing increasingly hard of hearing. His children are frustrated that he will not admit and "deal with" his hearing loss.

Roughly, 9% of Americans have hearing loss, 10% of them with profound deficits. Age-related hearing loss (presbycusis) is the most common cause. At birth, 1 in 1000 children have severe to profound hearing loss, with four to five children having hearing deficits that impair verbal communication. Persons who are deafened prelingually (before the onset of speech, usually at age 3 years) typically have different communication patterns and preferences than postlingually deafened individuals, such as Jerry. In the former group, those who attend Deaf schools and interact with others through sign language often develop a strong cultural identity. In contrast, persons such as Jerry can feel that "going deaf" is embarrassing or an inevitable sign of aging and refuse to admit progressive impairments. Often, they feel isolated and alone.

Tip on language: Persons who are "deaf" or "hard of hearing" generally prefer these terms to other labels. Many view such phrases as "hearing impaired" are well intentioned but inappropriate, because they imply that hearing loss requires cure. Phrases such as "deaf and dumb" or "deaf and mute" are offensive. When spelled with a capital D, Deaf represents a cultural or linguistic view of deafness; an understanding of deafness not as an impairment but rather as a cultural identity.

ASSISTIVE DEVICES

Jerry's children convince him to get a hearing aid, although his health insurance does not cover it. However, he rarely wears the hearing aid because he feels it does not work.

Depending on the nature of the hearing impairment, some persons may find individual mechanical interventions useful.

Hearing Aids

Hearing aids aim to amplify sounds, with different settings to target sounds within particular wavelengths, depending on the person's needs and physical setting (e.g., quiet rooms for private conversations, settings with significant background noise). Hearing aids range widely in their prices, quality, and capabilities. Health insurance rarely covers these devices (Medicare explicitly does not cover them), so persons' financial resources largely determine the type of device they can obtain. Persons seeking hearing aids should undergo careful assessments by audiologists skilled specifically in these devices, and they must recognize that months of trial and error may ensue before they figure out how to make the hearing aid work well for them. Not surprisingly, because of these complexities, many people use their devices only intermittently and some abandon them altogether.

Assistive Listening Devices

Assistive listening devices (ALDs) aim to improve the "signal to noise ratio," thus allowing listeners to hear better. The process is technically equivalent to putting listeners' ears closer to the sound source. ALDs come in different types depending on their mechanisms for enhancing sound. These technologies are widely used in public settings, such as theaters and concert halls. Personal amplified ALDs represent the most basic technology, consisting of a pocket-sized, lightweight amplifier with a microphone, either attached to the unit or connected by a wire. During conversations, users place the microphone near the speaker's mouth and hear the amplified sounds via earphones or headphones. Having one or more ALD units available in a clinic could assist people with hearing loss and may be acceptable even to patients who generally hesitate to admit difficulty hearing.

Cochlear Implants

Persons with sensorineural hearing losses, regardless of when they occur, can find that cochlear implants restore much of their hearing. Hair cells of the cochlea, positioned in the inner ears, normally transmit sounds to the brain. With a cochlear implant, sounds picked up by an external microphone are transmitted to electrodes that stimulate remaining nerve cells in the cochlea, which are then recognized by the brain as sounds. Experiences with cochlear implants are highly variable and the technology is very controversial, especially among Deaf parents who wish their deaf children to be raised entirely in the Deaf culture they themselves inhabit.

TELECOMMUNICATIONS TECHNOLOGIES

Many devices are available to assist persons with hearing impairments, such as those displayed in Web sites sponsored by the Gallaudet University Technology Access Program (tap.gallaudet.edu) and Self Help for Hard of Hearing People (www.shhh.org). Examples of useful devices include vibrator beepers or watches, flashing lights to indicate ringing telephones or emergency alarms, amplified headsets for telephones, baby monitors that vibrate the parent's bed, closed captioning decoders on television sets, and telecommunications equipment and services.

Teletypewriter

The teletypewriter (TTY), also called a telecommunications device for the Deaf, is a keyboard with an alphanumeric display that, when linked through a telephone outlet or appropriately configured computer, can communicate directly with another TTY. TTY users then type their messages back and forth, often using shorthand phrases. ADA regulations require installation of TTYs in specified settings within health care facilities. TTYs come in portable, lightweight models that some persons carry with them and simply plug into available telephone outlets. In some Deaf communities, however, handheld text messaging devices are gradually replacing TTYs, although the price of this equipment and monthly fees pose a barrier to their use.

Telephone Relay Services

Anyone with a telephone or TTY can use telephone relay services (TRS), which by law are available free at all times under Title IV of the ADA. Dialing 7-1-1 nationwide connects directly to the local TRS, which uses operators called "communications assistants" (CAs), to facilitate telephone calls for people who have difficulty hearing or speaking. A TTY user types a message that the CA then reads aloud to a hearing person who answers the telephone. The hearing person speaks a return message to the CA, who types this response to the TTY user. Some regions now offer video relay services, in which a Deaf caller signs to the CA with the use of video equipment (e.g., computer cameras with broadband connections); the CA voices what is signed to the called hearing person; and then signs back the spoken response to the Deaf caller.

COMMUNICATION APPROACHES

Persons like Jerry, who lose their hearing later in life, typically have speaking skills comparable to persons who are not hard of hearing. However, the communication skills of prelingually or early deafened individuals depend very much on their early education. Methods for teaching deaf children have generated considerable controversy for well over a century, with some educators advocating completely "oral" approaches (i.e., forcing children to learn speech and lip reading, precluding use of visual or sign languages). Today, although deaf children frequently start with sign language training, they go on to "total communication" or "bilingual-bicultural" training, learning both sign languages (which do not have written forms) and spoken and written languages, such as English.

American Sign Language

ASL, used by approximately 500,000 Americans, is a unique language grammatically and linguistically distinct from English; it is not simply English translated into hand signals. Instead, ASL uses hand signals, facial expressions, and body movements to convey concepts as effectively as spoken languages. When persons who started life using ASL later learn a spoken and written language, typically English, their English knowledge is frequently comparable to that of others for whom English is their second language. In other words, they may have limited vocabulary, perhaps making note writing with their clinicians an ineffective strategy for communication. Importantly, sign languages vary from country to country. British Sign Language, for instance, differs fundamentally from ASL.

Lip (Speech) Reading

Many deaf and hard of hearing individuals rely, at least in part, on lip or speech reading. Someone such as Jerry, who lived his life speaking English, typically finds lip reading easier than someone whose first language is ASL. Lip reading is inevitably imperfect. Only about 30% of English words are clearly readable on the lips, because many English words form at the back of the throat. Therefore, people who rely on lip reading may not necessarily know when they misunderstand or misinterpret spoken words.

Primary care providers receive little training about the diversity of experiences faced by persons who are deaf or hard of hearing and strategies to overcome communication barriers. The limited training generally focuses on pathology of hearing loss. Therefore, clinicians can carry erroneous assumptions about methods for communicating effectively with persons with hearing disabilities. For instance, they may believe that note writing and lip reading provide effective communication, but in many instances, they do not.

Tip: Important questions when taking a hearing history include:

- Age at onset (prelingually versus postlingually)
- Preferred language, communication modality (e.g., sign language, lip reading, English using assistive device)
- Cultural identification
- Educational history, including level of understanding of spoken and written English

COMMUNICATION ACCOMMODATIONS

> Judy's doctor did not have an ASL interpreter during her first Pap test, so she did not understand the procedure. She felt so traumatized that she refuses to have another Pap test.

The ADA requires accommodations to ensure effective communication unless doing so would cause significant difficulty or expense. The law stipulates that patients' preferences for communication accommodations should receive primary consideration. However, the physicians have the final authority to determine what constitutes effective communication. At the most basic level, accommodations involve facing the person while speaking, keeping the mouth visible; speaking naturally but clearly, without shouting or rushing; ensuring adequate lighting, especially of the face; and eliminating background noise. When clinicians must wear surgical masks, choosing clear or transparent fog-free masks could assist lip readers. However, many people need additional communication accommodations, such as a sign language interpreter.

The ADA does not require health insurers to cover sign language interpreter costs, and it prohibits providers from charging patients for this expense. Sometimes, sign language interpreter fees can exceed health insurance reimbursement for the visit, posing a financial disincentive for clinicians to hire interpreters. Nevertheless, legal experts caution physicians against using ineffective communication strategies. Courts have held physicians legally liable for failing to accommodate communication needs, especially when medical injury ensues.

NEED FOR ACCESSIBLE EQUIPMENT

> Angela had a high thoracic spinal cord injury in her teens. Now in her late twenties, she is married and thinking of having a child.

Since her injury, Angela has not been weighed, and she has not had a complete physical examination, including a Pap smear, by her primary care physician. Her physician's office has neither a wheelchair accessible scale nor an examining table that lowers automatically to wheelchair height for easy transfer. No one feels comfortable lifting Angela out of her wheelchair onto the fixed-height examining table, designed for the convenience of a standing clinician. Once she becomes pregnant, following her weight and conducting comprehensive physical examinations will become even more important. Regulations relating to the ADA Titles II and III stipulate certain requirements for accessibility to public and private structures, but they say nothing about equipment or furnishings. The law requires that persons with disabilities receive equal services as those without disabilities, but does not specify exactly how to achieve that goal.

Access problems in health care settings are readily apparent. For instance, when Judy, who is deaf, goes in for radiologic procedures, she will not hear spoken instructions from the radiologist or technician, who is often positioned behind opaque radiation shields. Lorna, who is blind, will not be able to see the instructional video on breast self-examinations on view in the mammography center waiting room. Tom, with his foot drop and propensity to fall, may find lengthy hospital corridors hazardous without railings along the walls. Angela even has trouble getting into her physician's office, because the heavy plate glass door has no automatic opener.

KEY CONCEPTS

- Never make assumptions about the abilities, preferences, or expectations of persons with disabilities: Ask how you may assist them, and as much as possible, comply with their wishes.
- Disability marks an interaction between a person's functional abilities and the environmental demands placed on them.
- Disability can be lessened by modifications in the environment.
- Many assistive devices and adaptive technologies exist to eliminate the gap between functional ability and environmental demands.
- Physical therapists, occupational therapists, and physiatrists are important resources for both physicians and patients. Clinicians should make appropriate referrals.
- Health care providers should seek to alter their practice environment to make it accessible to persons with disabilities by eliminating physical and communication barriers.

CORE COMPETENCY
The Disability Process

Understand the steps:

- A patient initiates a claim by filing with the Social Security Office.
- The state-based Disability Determination Service (DDS) gathers evidence to support claims of disability. They will request records of previous clinic visits and hospitalizations. They can request medical evaluation either from the treating physician or from a physician consultant who contracts with the SSA.

- A board consisting of medical and nonmedical personnel at the DDS reviews the full application, including the medical documentation. Approximately 30% receive SSDI at this stage. If not approved, the applicant can appeal within 60 days. Approximately 15% of denied claims are reversed at this stage. If still denied, applicants can appeal to an administrative law judge; new information can be included and the applicant can have a lawyer. Approximately one half of denials are reversed at this stage.

Concepts:

- Physicians are not expected to decide whether or not the patient is disabled; rather they are to provide information regarding the impairment.
- Physicians can familiarize themselves with the "Disability Evaluation Under Social Security," also known as the "Blue Book," which lists the medical criteria that the SSA uses to determine impairment and disability for common causes (available online at www.ssa.gov).
- Referral to lawyers or advocates can help patients.

Writing the letter: The letter should detail the following:

- Duration of impairment
- How the impairment affects ability to work and function
  —Be detailed and give specific examples
  —Include functional, sensory, emotional, and cognitive examples:
  > *Mrs. B cannot be expected to lift more than 10 pounds or walk further than 15 feet.*
  > *During his last manic episode, Mr. B drove the delivery truck to Mexico and did not return it.*

  —Include documenting evidence: diagnostic tests, radiographs, laboratory, or functional testing
  —Expected duration of impairment
  —Likelihood of recovery

DISCUSSION QUESTIONS

1. What is a disability?
2. Name three examples of assistive devices for persons with lower extremity mobility impairments, hearing loss, or low vision.
3. What steps can clinicians take to make their offices more accessible to persons with sensorimotor disabilities?
4. What is ASL? How does one use an ASL interpreter?
5. What are key components for insurance documentation of a mobility aid?

RESOURCES

http://www.afb.org
American Foundation for the Blind

http://tap.gallaudet.edu
Gallaudet University Technology Access Program

http://www.shhh.org
Self Help for Hard of Hearing People

http://www.nfb.org
National Federation of the Blind

7-1-1 nationwide connects directly to the local TRS, which uses operators called "communications assistants" (CAs), to facilitate telephone calls for people who have difficulty hearing or speaking.

REFERENCES

1. Pope A, Tarlov A. *Disability in America: Toward a national agenda for prevention.* Washington, DC: National Academy Press, 1991.
2. *Towards a common language for functioning, disability and health.* ICF. Geneva, Switzerland: World Health Organization, 2002.
3. Ustun TB, Chatterji S, et al. WHO's ICF and functional status information in health records. *Health Care Financ Rev* 2003;24(3):77–88.
4. Goldzweig CL, et al. Preventing and managing visual disability in primary care: clinical applications. *JAMA* 2004; 291(12):1497–502.
5. Bogardus ST Jr, et al. Screening and management of adult hearing loss in primary care: Clinical applications. *JAMA* 2003;289(15):1986–1990.
6. *Disability evaluation under Social Security.* Washington, DC: Social Security Administration, 2003.
7. Wunderlich GS, et al. *The dynamics of disability: Measuring and monitoring disability for Social Security programs.* Washington, DC: National Academies Press. National Research Council Committee to Review the Social Security Administration's Disability Decision Process Research, 2002.
8. Dale S, Verdier J. *Elimination of Medicare's waiting period for seriously disabled adults: Impact on coverage and care.* New York: Commonwealth Fund, 2003.
9. Williams B, et al. *Waiting for Medicare: Experiences of uninsured people with disabilities in the two-year waiting period for Medicare.* New York: The Commonwealth Fund, 2004.
10. Riley GF. The cost of eliminating the 24-month Medicare waiting period for Social Security disabled-worker beneficiaries. *Med Care* 2004;42(4):387–394.
11. Kennedy J, Erb C. Prescription noncompliance due to cost among adults with disabilities in the United States. *Am J Public Health* 2002;92(7):1120–1124.
12. Iezzoni LI. *When walking fails: Mobility problems of adults with chronic conditions.* Berkeley, CA: University of California Press, 2003.
13. Podsiadlo D, Richardson S. The timed "Up & Go": A test of basic functional mobility for frail elderly persons. *J Am Geriatr Soc* 1991;39(2):142–148.
14. *Guidelines for the use of assistive technology: Evaluation, referral, prescription,* 2nd ed. Chicago: American Medical Association, Department of Geriatric Health, 1996.
15. Kirchner C. Prevalence estimates for visual impairment: Cutting through the data jungle. *J Vis Impair Blind* 1999;93(4):253–259.

Chapter 38

HIV/AIDS: Impact on Vulnerable Populations

Meg D. Newman, MD, and Margaret B. Wheeler, MS, MD

Objectives

- Define human immunodeficiency virus (HIV) infection and acquired immunodeficiency syndrome (AIDS) and the vulnerabilities associated with this disease.

- Describe how stigma affects prevention and treatment efforts.

- Describe groups at highest risk for morbidity and mortality of HIV/AIDS.

- Describe challenges to patient care including patient, provider, system, and disease factors.

- Identify interventions to improve HIV prevention efforts.

- Identify interventions to improve care for vulnerable patients with HIV or AIDS.

Don Sterr is a 34-year-old man with bipolar disease and AIDS. When off his bipolar medications he develops mania and becomes hypersexual. He uses amphetamines, adheres poorly to HIV medications, and engages in high-risk sex. As a consequence, Don has developed pan-resistance to his HIV medications and a falling CD4 count. When he was 16, his parents discovered he was gay and forced him to leave their house.

Despite major advances in human immunodeficiency virus (HIV) medicine, living with HIV infection or acquired immunodeficiency syndrome (AIDS) remains a major challenge. In the United States, HIV/AIDS is disproportionately found in minorities, especially African Americans and Latinos, men who have sex with other men (MSM), injection drug users, those with mental illness, and the poor. Untreated HIV infection is fatal. HIV treatments, when available, may be life sustaining, but are not devoid of complications. A powerful stigma is attached to the illness that burdens those who are infected and stymies prevention and treatment efforts. This chapter reviews the challenges of living with HIV/AIDS and focuses on strategies for improving care for those with the disease.

DEFINING HIV AND AIDS

Isaiah Grant is a 24-year-old man unaware of his HIV infection until he is diagnosed with Pneumocystis carinii pneumonia (PCP). He became infected after having unprotected sex with a man.

HIV is transmitted through the exchange of bodily fluids: during unprotected vaginal or anal sex; by direct

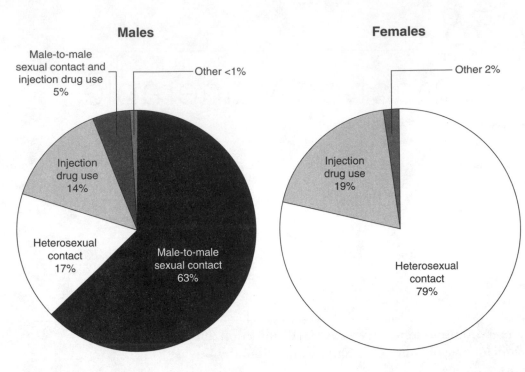

Figure 38-1. Exposure categories of adults and adolescents who received a diagnosis of HIV/AIDS in 2003. HIV/AIDS includes persons with a diagnosis of HIV infection (not AIDS), a diagnosis of HIV infection and a later diagnosis of AIDS, or concurrent diagnoses of HIV infection and AIDS (Data are from 33 areas with long-term, confidential name–based HIV reporting; males, n = 23,153; females, n = 8733). (From: Centers for Disease Control and Prevention. *HIV/AIDS fact sheet. A glance at the HIV/AIDS epidemic, June 2005.* Available at: http://www.cdc.gov/hiv/PUBS/Fact/At-A-Glance.htm#ref1)[16]

inoculation of the virus (e.g., through contaminated needles, blood products, or transplanted organs); or through mother to child transmission (MTCT) during pregnancy, birth, or breastfeeding. It is defined by having a positive antibody test to HIV (Fig. 38-1).

Individuals with HIV infection may be asymptomatic and hence unaware of their infection for many years, although a person infected with HIV can transmit the infection from the time he or she becomes infected. Medications that effectively suppress viral load diminish but do not eliminate infectivity. In the absence of antiretroviral medication, rates of progression to clinical illness are quite variable: few individuals progress within 2 years; however, approximately 50% develop clinical symptoms within 10 years of infection. Eventually, the loss of immune function caused by the HIV virus leads to overwhelming infections and death. One is defined as having AIDS when severe immunologic compromise is evident, which generally occurs when the CD4 count is below 200/mL and is characterized by the appearance of opportunistic infection (e.g., PCP, tuberculosis, parasitic or fungal infections), HIV wasting syndrome or malignancy (e.g., lymphoma, cervical cancer, Kaposi's sarcoma).

EPIDEMIOLOGY OF HIV AND AIDS

In 2003, an estimated 1,185,000 persons in the United States were living with HIV/AIDS, and about one fourth of these were undiagnosed and unaware of their HIV infection. Changes in behavior have radically altered the incidence of the disease throughout the United States, with new infections occurring in fewer than 40,000 persons a year.[1]

Fortunately, advances in treatment of the disease have slowed the progression to AIDS and decreased mortality rates.[2] However, closer looks at the epidemiologic trends show that not all groups have shared equally in the advances of the last 20 years. MSM, minorities, the poor, and intravenous drug users (IVDU) account for most HIV/AIDS diagnoses and deaths.

RISK FACTORS AND BARRIERS TO PREVENTION AND TREATMENT

Even two and a half decades into the epidemic, having HIV/AIDS is associated with great stigma, perhaps considered most shameful in the communities in which it is most prevalent. HIV/AIDS is viewed as an illness that individuals bear direct control over.[3] The very factors that put people at risk for contracting HIV also constitute barriers to prevention and optimal care. Neither society nor the health care system has been successful at combating the poverty, low education, recklessness of youth, substance use, or discrimination that underlie the risks of contracting and living with HIV/AIDS.

STIGMA AND HIV

"People who got AIDS through sex or drug use have gotten what they deserve" describes the sentiment of about 20% of those surveyed by the Centers for Disease Control and Prevention (CDC). Its association with drugs and sex, its contagious nature, severity, and the disfigurement that occurs with wasting or Kaposi's sarcoma all contribute to its stigma.[4] Those at highest risk for HIV—MSM, IVDU, and prostitutes—are treated as pariahs by society.[4] Efforts to engage these groups and mitigate their risk are opposed by some who fear this condones or encourages their risky behavior. As a consequence, effective prevention measures such as needle exchanges or over-the-counter purchase of syringes are illegal in some places, and messages about condoms and their distribution have been diluted.

Heterosexuals with HIV/AIDS fear they will be thought gay, bisexual, transgendered, or an IVDU because of their infection. In particular, women who were infected through a single partner, often their husbands, may have great internalized stigma that results from concern that others will perceive them as a commercial sex worker or promiscuous even if that is far from the truth. Lack of social support, especially from family and uninfected friends, often correlates both with greater suffering and faster progression of HIV/AIDS and an increased sense of stigma.

Support from the health care system for "people living with HIV and AIDS" (PWHA) may not always be forthcoming. Indeed, over one fourth of HIV-infected patients believe their health care providers have discriminated against them, 8% report having had services denied,[5] and others felt their sexual preference influenced the likelihood of being placed on medications by their physician.[6] Nationally, almost one fourth of physicians caring for HIV patients have negative attitudes toward IVDUs, and those with these attitudes are less likely to start IVDU patients on antiretrovirals.[7] Finally, health care providers who care for PWHA may themselves face social and professional exclusion.

POVERTY

Poverty is a unifying characteristic found in those at highest risk for HIV/AIDS. More than 40% of AIDS diagnoses made in 1999 were made in residents from the poorest counties in the United States, although these contained only 25% of the US population.[8] Substance use, sexually transmitted diseases, incarceration, violence, and poor access to preventive education and services are both risk factors for HIV transmission and often related to poverty. Young people who have dropped out of school are at higher risk for early and unsafe sexual activity.[9] Once infected, people put needs such as food, shelter, and immediate safety above seeking medical care for their infection;[10] and not surprisingly HIV-positive people who are poor or less educated die sooner than their wealthier, more educated counterparts.[11,19] Disparities in treatment of those who are infected also have been widely documented. Blacks, Latinos, women, the uninsured, and those with public insurance are less likely to receive optimal treatment

(antiretroviral medications or preventive care) and are hospitalized more often.[13,14]

MEN WHO HAVE SEX WITH MEN

In 2003, men accounted for 72% of all HIV/AIDS patients among adults and adolescents. Over two thirds of these were exposed to the virus through sex with another man. Other important categories of exposure among men are heterosexual contact (17%) and intravenous drug use (14%). The risk of transmission of HIV in MSM has been related to having multiple sexual partners, using alcohol and drugs, and being uncircumcised. Although MSM are still the most affected group, in the early 1980s the incidence of seroconversion in MSM was up to 20/100 per year and now, despite some concerning increases, that rate is down to between 2 and 5/100 per year.[8,15] Behavior change caused this radical reduction in transmission.

About 50% of the MSM diagnosed with HIV/AIDS in 2003 were white, about 33% African American, and a little over 10% Hispanic.[2] Almost half of African-American MSM are infected and over 65% of them are unaware of their infection,[16] a fact with grave implications for continued transmission of the disease.

Transgendered persons also have high rates of HIV. Although not segregated in CDC statistics, a study of transgendered persons (male to female) in San Francisco suggests that 35% of the community is infected with HIV. In most communities, transgendered persons are a marginalized group; consequently, HIV-infected transgendered people are at risk for isolation and victimization.[17]

RACE/ETHNICITY

People from ethnic and racial minority populations are diagnosed with HIV/AIDS more frequently, and once diagnosed have worse outcomes. For example, African Americans accounted for 50% of all HIV/AIDS cases diagnosed in 2003 (Fig. 38-2). African Americans are diagnosed with AIDS at 10 times the rate of whites and three times the rate of Hispanics. The death rate for African Americans in 1999 was 11 times that of whites.[8] Native Americans represent only 1% of AIDS cases; however, they are diagnosed with AIDS at a rate that is less than African Americans but higher than whites. Native Americans die from AIDS at about the same rate as African Americans.[2]

WOMEN AND CHILDREN

Early in the epidemic, few women were infected, but by 2001 HIV/AIDS had become one of the top killers of young African-American and Hispanic women).[18]

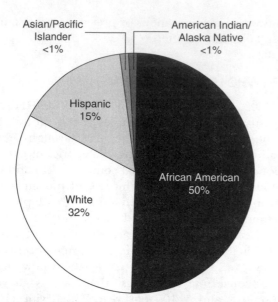

Figure 38-2. Race/ethnicity of persons (including children) who received a diagnosis of HIV/AIDS in 2003. Data are from 33 areas with long-term, confidential name–based HIV reporting. Includes persons of unknown race or multiple races (*n* = 32, 048). (From: Centers for Disease Control and Prevention. *HIV/AIDS fact sheet. A glance at the HIV/AIDS epidemic, June 2005*. Available at: http://www.cdc.gov/hiv/PUBS/Facts/At-A-Glance.htm#ref1)[16]

Women now comprise about 20% of those diagnosed with HIV/AIDS. African-American and Hispanic women make up only about 25% of the women in the United States; however, 83% of women infected with the HIV virus are from these two groups.[2]

Women are overwhelmingly infected through heterosexual contact (see Fig. 38-1). Many women may not be aware of their partner's possible risk for HIV.[19] This may be especially true for minority women. Studies show that among MSM, African-American and Latino men are more likely to identify themselves as heterosexual and report having sex with women.[20] Therefore, women frequently have limited knowledge about their partner's risk factors for HIV/AIDS and often have the misperception that they are at low risk of contracting AIDS. Unknowingly they may contract and spread the disease to other partners and children. Women also may not feel empowered to insist on safe sex practices. Fear of emotional or physical abuse or the withdrawal of financial support, as well as substance use, prevents some women from consistently using condoms. Women who want to get pregnant do not insist on condom use and may discover that they are infected only when they seek care for their pregnancy. Minority women also face a number of structural factors that place them at high risk for infection: High rates of incarceration among minority men, residential segregation and lack of medical services, and condemnation of homosexuality all contribute to women's vulnerability.

Moreover, as women are infected, so are children: Close to 70% of the babies diagnosed with HIV/AIDS in 2003 were African American.[2] Importantly, from 2000 through 2003, the estimated number of HIV cases decreased slightly among children less than 13 years of age. In addition, the estimated number of AIDS cases and deaths decreased among children.[2]

SEXUALLY TRANSMITTED DISEASES

People with sexually transmitted diseases (STDs) other than HIV are also at higher risk to get HIV. This is partly because the unsafe sex that has exposed them to the STD also exposes them to HIV, and STDs can cause physical changes such as genital lesions that increase the transmission of HIV. Transmission of HIV can be increased as much as five times by the presence of some other STDs.[21] Hence, those at high-risk for STDs—MSM, adolescents, substance users, and minorities—also are at high risk for HIV.

SUBSTANCE USE

Injection drug use accounts for about one third of the cases of HIV in the United States,[2] but the effect of substance use on the spread of HIV is not limited to sharing needles. Both the sexual partners and the children of IV drug users are at high risk for the disease. Other types of drug abuse also increase risk of HIV because substance users in general are more likely to engage in high-risk behaviors, such as unprotected sex, especially when they are "high."[22] Exchanging sex for drugs or using drugs to enhance the sexual experience also contribute to risk.[23] Indeed use of crystal methamphetamine, poppers, and even Viagra have been associated with unprotected serodiscordant sex in MSM.[24] Drug users also often have multiple sexual partners.[22] Drug use also may increase the risk for sexual violence and coercion among drug-using couples[25] and hence transmission.

For those who are already infected, drug use also can affect the adherence that is so crucial to treatment success. Drug use itself adds medical risks beyond the disruption of HIV treatment (see Chap. 33). Injection drug use exposes patients to multiple infections that can be life threatening given HIV's immunosuppression. Tuberculosis is particularly deadly when combined with HIV. Evidence is accumulating that substance use with cocaine may contribute to atherosclerotic cardiovascular disease.[26] Worsening mental health issues are well documented during marked substance use. Indeed, in patients living with HIV, marked substance use may inform the provider about underlying mental illness, personality disorders, or inability to adequately cope with life circumstances.

TRAUMA, MENTAL ILLNESS, AND INCARCERATION

Besides those characteristics (IVDU, sexual practices) that place people at risk for transmission, other characteristics (history of trauma, mental illness, incarceration) increase the likelihood of HIV infection. Trauma of all varieties, including sexual abuse, increases the risk of poor self-care, inability to insist on condoms, or lack of access to care. Indeed, history of trauma and victimization is common in HIV/AIDs patients; consequently, routine screening is recommended. Among individuals living with mental illness, the prevalence of HIV infection is dramatically increased when compared to the general population. Estimates vary, but HIV is thought to be more than five times higher in those living with mental illness.[27,28] Given the consequences of mental illness—poverty with concomitant homelessness or marginal housing, sexual abuse, trauma, social isolation, and substance use—it is easy to envisage how HIV infection is more likely to occur. The presence of mental illness also portends difficulty with treatment of this complex disease. Indeed, depression is remarkably common in patients with HIV and is underdiagnosed, although treatment of depression may improve ability to adhere to medications.[29]

BARRIERS TO TESTING

Without knowing their diagnosis, people cannot access life-saving treatment or prevent transmission. Data show that people reduce their risk behaviors if they know they are positive.[30,31] Nevertheless, multiple barriers to diagnosis exist, including lack of awareness of the risk, substance use, fear, and denial. With limited access to health care, it is harder for the poor, the homeless, or those living in rural areas to be tested. Moreover, in any small, close-knit community, people may be hesitant to be screened because they fear encountering a friend, relative, or town gossip when seeking testing. For Native-American patients, this may be of particular concern.[32] Interestingly, most PWHA from rural areas seek care in cities.[33]

Common Pitfalls in the Care of Patients with HIV/AIDS

- Comorbid conditions that accompany HIV disease— mental illness and substance use are not adequately addressed.
- Other problems, such as poverty, victimization, and homelessness interfere with prevention, diagnosis, and treatment.
- HIV's stigma undermines prevention, treatment, and care.
- Providers miss opportunities to screen patients for HIV.

- Providers often neglect to give patients important information on how to prevent transmission.
- Providers are inadequately trained to provide the complex care HIV/AIDS patients require.
- Many health care systems are not organized to support optimal care for HIV patients.
- HIV prevention efforts are politically charged.

PREVENTION AND CARE FOR VULNERABLE PATIENTS

PREVENTION AND SCREENING

Counseling and testing for HIV infection is a basic step to prevention and treatment. Prevention messages that are tailored specifically to an individual's behavior have been shown to be effective. Novel outreach models also may be required, such as mobile outreach to homeless youth or offering counseling to a wide range of patients, including monogamous women and others living in communities where the prevalence of infection, and therefore risk of transmitting or contracting HIV infection, is extraordinarily high. Rapid HIV screening that allows for immediate disclosure of the results may be particularly useful for people who may have difficulty in returning for testing results or for inpatients.

HARM REDUCTION

Practitioners hope to develop an effective vaccine for the eradication of HIV; this is an active area of investigation. In the absence of definitive measures, preventing or lessening the negative impacts of the disease and its associated comorbidities (while pursuing the ultimate goal of prevention and elimination) has become the focus of many interventions. This approach, termed harm reduction, minimizes the vulnerability of unhealthy behaviors that may not be easily or rapidly treated and are socially unacceptable. Harm reduction strategies raise tricky questions. For example, do advances in HIV treatment that prolong life diminish the fear of the disease and increase willingness to engage in risky behavior? Although investigation of these issues for individual strategies is crucial, many such interventions (indeed HIV treatment itself) have proved very powerful.

Public health strategies employing this philosophy have had dramatic results. Multiple approaches have been employed in HIV care: needle exchange, rectal and vaginal microbicides, antiretroviral treatment to lessen infectivity, needle disinfection, and techniques for successful negotiation of condom use. Cities that created early responses to the spread of HIV through IVDU with outreach workers to at-risk communities and assured legal access to sterile needles and drug treatments, including methadone and buprenorphine, have been able to curtail spread of the disease. Conversely, cities that applied more punitive approaches have seen HIV prevalence skyrocket from 5% to more than 40% of IVDU in less than 1 year.[34]

ACCESS TO HIV/AIDS CARE

Once patients are diagnosed with HIV/AIDS and embark on treatment, they are confronted with a host of challenges, including accessing and negotiating medical care and confronting the terminal nature of their illness if left untreated. There is no doubt that barriers to quality care still exist in both inner city and rural areas, but HIV/AIDS is unique in the range of insurance coverage provided for clinical care, medications, and some ancillary services. Through federal and state Medicaid programs and initiatives, such as the AIDS Drug Assistance Program (ADAP), patients with HIV/AIDS can receive timely clinical care and medications in most states. Some states may have waiting lists for the ADAP program leading individuals to move to another state to obtain coverage. The Ryan White care funding covers ancillary services such as case management, urgent entrance into care programs, and dental services for people living with HIV and AIDS.

Although access is more open, variability of the quality of care has been well documented. Practitioners who see a paucity of patients are often ill equipped to manage the complexity of antiretroviral, pharmacokinetic, and metabolic conundrums that are common in HIV medicine. Multiple studies have documented that having a well-trained HIV practitioner improves both the quality of care and survival among patients living with HIV/AIDS.[35,36]

CARE FOR VULNERABLE HIV PATIENTS: CHALLENGES AND APPROACHES

Despite a myriad challenges, providing outstanding care for vulnerable HIV patients is occurring in most inner cities.[28] The cornerstone of successful medical care for vulnerable HIV patients is the formation of a system of care that addresses the multiple medical and social issues of PWHA.

Multidisciplinary Teams

Multidisciplinary teams (MDT) of care providers with a primary goal of addressing underlying comorbidities such as psychiatric illness and substance use; integrating primary care with urgent and subspecialty care; and linking patients to community resources and entitlement services are important components of successful systems. Case management using MDT

has been demonstrated to improve care of particularly high-risk patients.[37]

Multidisciplinary teams that maintain consistency with patients and develop appropriate care are mutually beneficial for patients and staff. Patients are assisted with the full panoply of issues, and providers are less likely to become overwhelmed by complicated patients. Integration of specialty and social services, such as mental health and substance use treatment and social work services (preferably offered on-site), is maximized through the team approach.

Urgent Care Clinic

Having a daily urgent care clinic as part of the HIV clinic can make a profound difference in helping engage and maintain patients in HIV care. It allows patients to avoid emergency departments (EDs) in which the waiting times are so long that patients may forgo a critical visit. ED staff also may be unfamiliar with the unique, uncommon, and dangerous complications of HIV therapy. Coming to an HIV urgent care clinic allows the multidisciplinary team to build relationships with patients and patients to avail themselves of clinic resources. Often these spontaneous visits are another opportunity to offer drug treatment referrals, reinforce adherence, review medication side-effects, address other needs, schedule primary care appointments, and complete housing or medical benefits forms. Most importantly, this type of service emphasizes that the clinic as an accessible resource.

Treatment Challenges

Adherence to complicated HIV treatment regimens is required to suppress viral load and avoid resistance. Providers fearing patients will not be able to adhere to the complex medication regimens may hesitate to offer them to patients.[38] Moreover, a wide array of complications may occur in patients who are HIV infected, some of which are directly linked to the medications used to treat HIV/AIDS and or HIV itself. The morbidity from the HIV-related metabolic syndrome, mitochondrial toxicity, avascular necrosis, and Fanconi's syndrome are examples. Finally, the long-term efficacy for antiretroviral medications (ARV) has not been ascertained.

Mechanisms of improving adherence are an active area of research. Simplification of regimens is one important step. More and more combination pills are now available and highly potent regimens can be taken by swallowing 2–4 pills one time a day. Ironically, despite the fact that treatment options in the United States have saved countless lives, US pharmaceutical companies have resisted the development of combination pills (produced abroad often by disregarding patents) that dramatically simplify regimens. Using structured interview techniques can help providers more accurately assess adherence.[39] Outreach treatment services, treatment linked to methadone dosing and use of interactive technologies to cue patients, are some examples of other techniques in use.[40] Finally, even despite chaotic and stressed lives, many patients are capable of taking medications appropriately. Homeless patients have been shown to be able to adhere as strictly to highly active antiretroviral therapy (HAART) as more stable clinical populations.[41]

Provider Challenges

Caring for patients with HIV/AIDS is demanding, putting those who care for patients with HIV at risk of burnout. Integrating what traditionally have been considered "nonmedical" problems and keeping abreast of treatment advances are formidable tasks even for the most diligent providers. Reviewing the guidelines and having structured protocols for starting medications and assessing adherence may assist in decreasing the disparities in treatment that have been documented. Easy access to up-to-date information through web sites and consultation can help manage the barrage of new information (see Resources). Multidisciplinary teams and well-integrated systems can support providers' efforts to provide comprehensive care.

Many HIV/AIDS providers consider advocacy an essential dimension of their practice (see Chap. 41). This is not easy work: As noted, those at highest risk may be ostracized in their own communities. Further, many high-risk groups have reason to distrust the medical establishment and many efforts such as needle exchange, condom distribution, or frank sexual discussions have faced political opposition.

Community Challenges

Addressing prevention and care in disparate communities can be complex. Each community requires its own approach. Prevention efforts that are most successful are fueled by input and direction from affected community members and leaders; that is, people who can convey a sincere interest in an affected or at-risk group. Many ethnic and racial minorities look for prevention efforts to be led by people who are like them and not the ethnic and racial majority.

Some generalizations about prevention and care efforts can be made about each risk group, although refinements are necessary for each specific community. Common to all groups is the need for respect, confidentiality, and safety. Those who are infected and those seeking screening need to know that their illness will not be a judged and that they will be well cared for. In tight-knit communities, a patient may be afraid to be seen in an HIV clinic; therefore, discretion is another hallmark of appropriate outreach and care. Safety from legal prosecution is a concern for undocumented immigrants, substance users, and prostitutes. Drug users may engage in care despite continued illicit drug use and often need to know that accessing care is not dependent on cessation of all IVDU or substance use. Simultaneously, many drug users in HIV care want to address their drug addiction. Making drug treatment available and linked to HIV care is an enticing reason for some drug users to engage in care.

MSM as a group have been vilified over the unsafe sexual practices of some members. As a result, years of struggle for "gay liberation" have been threatened. Like other affected groups, engaging MSMs in care is done most successfully by ensuring that their culture will be respected.

One approach to care has been to establish clinics that focus on a single community: Hispanics, African Americans, women, adolescents, or MSM. Like all risk groups, ethnic and racial minorities may want to know that their language or customs will be recognized and respected in care. Having providers from the targeted community or of the same ethnic/racial background as the patient has been shown to decrease the time to initiating antiretroviral treatment.[42] Women need to know that they will be sensitively cared for as well, despite the fact that most HIV patients are men. HIV-infected women may be intimidated by being in a clinic full of mostly male patients. Establishing clinic times when a critical mass of women can be seen and accommodating children lowers the barrier for engaging and remaining in care.

Tragically, sometimes whole families are infected. Even when they are not, a diagnosis in one member of the family has profound repercussions for all. Clinics focusing on the care of families integrate medical and social needs of all family members.[43] Adolescents too have special needs, consequently, specific media campaigns or outreach to homeless shelters targeted to high-risk teens (such as runaways) are effective venues for risk-reduction education in teens.

CONCLUSION

Preventing the transmission of HIV and caring for people living with HIV/AIDS is a formidable task. Eliminating the social injustices that put patients at risk and complicate treatment is ambitious and cannot be accomplished by health care workers alone. Eradicating transmission of the HIV virus through development of an HIV vaccine will be one of the greatest human achievements. In the interim, however, the combination of the medical knowledge and commitment to nonjudgmental, patient-centered care that is evolving in caring for and preventing HIV in high-risk groups can be seen as a model of care to which everyone can aspire.

KEY CONCEPTS

Create multidisciplinary teams (MDT) to care for patients.

- Successful teams include social workers, mental health professionals, case managers, primary care providers, nurses, and clinic staff.

Make mental health and substance use issues a priority.

- Case management is the foundation for helping patients access and succeed at mental health care.
- Attempt to develop on-site psychiatric services.
- If unavailable, develop MDT that interact on a regular basis with chosen mental health services.

Establish urgent care drop-in clinics for patients.

- Use to develop longitudinal primary care relationships.

Become an advocate for access to health care.

- This maximizes resources and minimizes the powerlessness the provider may feel.

Learn about people who define themselves differently than you define yourself.

- People living with HIV/AIDS are everyone and everywhere

CORE COMPETENCY

HIV Prevention Counseling

Effective HIV prevention counseling combines elements important to behavior change generally: education, assessment of the particular patient's risks and needs, and negotiating an action plan. Increasing the patient's sense of self-efficacy and empowerment are important goals. Delicate discussions of sexual conduct and drug use require trust.

Steps in prevention counseling:

- Establish rapport.
  —Convey positive regard, respect, and empathy. Review parameters of conversation. Explain rationale for delving into private concerns and ask permission to do so. Confirm confidentiality.
- Explore the patient's risk behavior, beliefs, and concerns.

- Identify areas in which the patient's concerns and actions or beliefs and safety are at odds. Assess concern.
  —Tell me what you know about HIV.
  —Tell me what types of things have you done that would put you at risk for HIV.
  —Do you practice safe sex? What does safe sex mean to you?
  —How has/will testing/diagnosis change what you do?
  —Identify and explain when beliefs and behavior put the patient at high risk. *"You can get infected if you have unprotected sex with an HIV+ person, even if he or she is on medications."*
  —*"When are you worried that you might become infected?"*
  —Explore any areas of ambivalence or discordance. *"You say you are very worried about getting HIV, but often have unprotected sex or share needles. Help me understand this."*
- Explore a specific, recent incidence of risky behavior.
  —Assess who, how, what, where, and when of recent incident. Discuss barriers, contributors/triggers of behavior; communication about HIV with others. *" Tell me about the last time you had unprotected sex. . . ." "Did anything increase the chance of doing something risky?"*
  —Assess how common an occurrence this incident was.
- Review past prevention/risk reduction techniques used.
  —*"Have there been times when you have been able to practice safer sex? How was it different from other times?"*
  —Assess barriers. *"How does alcohol affect what you do?"*
  —Assess sense of ability/self-efficacy to prevent transmission. *"Do you feel you could ask your partner to use a condom?" " What could you do to decrease your risk?" "Tell me about situations in which it is harder to be safe."*
  —*"Have you discussed HIV status with your partners? How did it go?"*
  —Explore areas of ambivalence or discordance.
- Synthesize, recap information, and educate the patient about misconceptions.
  —*"It seems that . . .* (use patient information, including pattern, frequency, contributors) *are putting you at risk. X and Y make you more likely to take greater risks. You are/are not concerned about transmitting or contracting HIV. Do you agree? Have I left anything out?"*
  —Explore areas of ambivalence, discordance, or concern.
- Develop concrete steps to decrease risk and negotiate a risk reduction action plan (see Core Competency in Chap. 36).
  —*"What steps do you think you could take to reduce your risk of getting/transmitting (for positives) HIV?* Break down into concrete steps, identify barriers to implementation, and problem solve together.
  —Identify supports and resources.
  —Agree and document plan

Adapted from: *RESPECT-2 counseling guidelines.* Available at: http://www.cdc.gov/hiv/projects/respect-2/counseling.htm[44]

DISCUSSION QUESTIONS

1. Describe a patient with poorly controlled mental illness and how this illness made it difficult for this patient to manage his or her HIV/AIDS.
2. What are some strategies that can be useful in managing patients who are triply diagnosed with HIV/AIDS, depression, and addiction to cocaine?
3. Most HIV-infected women in the world had HIV transmitted through heterosexual contact. Describe how you might help a woman whose only sexual partner was her husband come to accept her HIV infection.

RESOURCES

http://www.aegis.com/
AEGiS: AIDS Information Global Information System provides wide-ranging information on HIV/AIDS.

http://www.aids-ed.org/
AIDS Education and Training Center contains tips for care of HIV/AIDS patients, including comorbid conditions.

http://www.aidsinfo.nih.gov/
AIDSinfo is a service of the U.S. Department of Health and Human Services. They provide information on treatment, prevention and research.

http://www.AIDS.org
AIDS.org is a site for both PWHA and practitioners who want to learn more about HIV.

http:www.gmhc.org/
Gay Men's Health Crisis, founded in 1981, offers a wide array of educational services.

www.hivinsite.org
HIVinsite provides information on all aspects of HIV/AIDS treatment and research.

www.iasusa.org
International AIDS Society-USA offers CME training opportunities for providers that they can utilize online or attend.

http://thewellproject.org/
The Well Project maintains an online site for PWHA and practitioners who want information specifically about women and HIV care and research.

http://aidsmeds.com
http://www.projectinform.org/
These two online sites that provide PWHA and practitioners easy programs about HIV medications:

REFERENCES

1. Glynn M. *Estimated HIV prevalence in the United States at the end of 2003*. National HIV Prevention Conference, 2005. Atlanta, GA.
2. Centers for Disease Control and Prevention. *HIV/AIDS surveillance report, 2003*. Atlanta: US Department of Health and Human Services, Centers for Disease Control and Prevention, 2004. Available at: http://www.cdc.gov/hiv/stats/hasrlink.htm
3. Crawford AM. Stigma associated with AIDS: A meta-analysis. *J Appl Soc Psychol* 1996;26:398–416.
4. Herek G, Capitanio J. AIDS stigma and sexual prejudice. *Amer Behav Sci* 1999;42:1126–1143.
5. Schuster MA, Collins R, Cunningham WE, et al. Perceived discrimination in clinical care in a nationally representative sample of HIV-infected adults receiving health care. *J Gen Intern Med* 2005;20(9):807–813.
6. Melendez RM, Exner TA, Ehrhardt AA, et al. Health and health care among male-to-female transgender persons who are HIV positive. *Am J Public Health* 2006;96:1034–1037.
7. Ding L, Landon BE, Wilson IB, et al. Predictors and consequences of negative physician attitudes toward HIV-infected injection drug users. *Arch Intern Med* 2005;165(6):618–623.
8. Karon JM, Fleming PL, Steketee RW, et al. HIV in the United States at the turn of the century: An epidemic in transition. *Am J Public Health* 2001;91(7):1060–1068.
9. Office of the Surgeon General, 2001.
10. Cunningham WE, Andersen RM, Katz MH, et al. The impact of competing subsistence needs and barriers on access to medical care for persons with human immunodeficiency virus receiving care in the United States. *Med Care* 1999;37(12):1270–1281.
11. Cunningham WE, et al. The effect of socioeconomic status on the survival of persons receiving care for HIV infection in the United States. *J Health Care Poor Underserved* 2005;16(4):655–676.
12. McFarland W, Chen S, Hsu L, et al. Low socioeconomic status is associated with a higher rate of death in the era of highly active antiretroviral therapy, San Francisco. *J AIDS* 2003;33(1):96–103.
13. Fleishman JA, Gebo KA, Reilly ED, et al. Hospital and outpatient health services utilization among HIV-infected adults in care 2000–2002. *Med Care* 2005;43(9 Suppl III):40–52.
14. Moore RD, Stanton D, Gopalan R, et al. Racial differences in the use of drug therapy for HIV disease in an urban community. *N Engl J Med* 1994;330(11):763–768.
15. Koblin B, Chesney M, Coates T. Effects of a behavioural intervention to reduce acquisition of HIV infection among men who have sex with men: The EXPLORE randomised controlled study. *Lancet* 2004;364(9428):41–50.
16. Centers for Disease Control and Prevention. *HIV/AIDS fact sheet. A glance at the HIV/AIDS epidemic, June 2005*. Available at: http://www.cdc.gov/hiv/PUBS/Facts/At-A-Glance.htm#ref1
17. Clements-Nolle K, Marx R, Guzman R, et al. HIV prevalence, risk behaviors, health care use, and mental health status of transgender persons: Implications for public health intervention. *Am J Public Health* 2001;91(6):915–921.
18. Anderson RN. Deaths: Leading causes for 2001. *Natl Vital Stat Rep* 2003;52(9):32–33, 53–54.

19. Hader SL, Smith DK, Moore JS, et al. HIV infection in women in the United States: Status at the millennium. *JAMA* 2001;285(9):1186–1192.

20. Centers for Disease Control and Prevention. HIV/AIDS among racial/ethnic minority men who have sex with men: United States, 1989–1998. *MMWR Morbid Mortal Wkly Rep* 2000;49:4–11.

21. Fleming D. From epidemiological synergy to public health policy and practice: The contribution of other sexually transmitted diseases to sexual transmission of HIV infection. *STIs* 1999;75:3–17.

22. Booth RE, et al. Sex related HIV risk behaviors: Differential risks among injection drug users, crack smokers, and injection drug users who smoke crack. *Drug Alcohol Depend* 2000;58(3):219–226.

23. Fernando D, Schilling RF, Fontdevila J, et al. Predictors of sharing drugs among injection drug users in the South Bronx: Implications for HIV transmission. *J Psychoactive Drugs* 2003;35(2):227–236.

24. Colfax GN, Mansergh G, Guzman R, et al. Drug use and sexual risk behavior among gay and bisexual men who attend circuit parties: A venue-based comparison. *J AIDS* 2001;28(4):373–379.

25. El-Bassel N, Gilbert L, Rajah V. The relationship between drug abuse and sexual performance among women on methadone. Heightening the risk of sexual intimate violence and HIV. *Addict Behav* 2003;28(8):1385–1403.

26. Lai S, Lima JA, Lai H, et al. Human immunodeficiency virus 1 infection, cocaine and coronary calcification. *Arch Intern Med* 2005;165:690–695.

27. Weiser SD, Wolfe WR, Bangsberg DR. The HIV epidemic among individuals with mental illness in the United States. *Curr Infect Dis Rep* 2004;6(5):404–410.

28. Treisman GJ, Angelino AF, Hutton HE. Psychiatric issues in the management of patients with HIV infection. *JAMA* 2001;286(22):2857–2864.

29. Asch SM, Kilbourne AM, Gifford AL, et al. Underdiagnosis of depression in HIV: Who are we missing? *J Gen Intern Med* 2003;18(6):450–460.

30. Fernyak SE, Page-Shafer K, Kellogg TA, et al. Risk behaviors and HIV incidence among repeat testers at publicly funded HIV testing sites in San Francisco. *J AIDS* 2002;31(1):63–70.

31. Colfax GN, Buchbinder SP, Cornelisse PG, et al. Sexual risk behaviors and implications for secondary HIV transmission during and after HIV seroconversion. *AIDS* 2002;16(11):1529–1535.

32. Bertolli J, McNaghten AD, Campsmith M, et al. Surveillance systems monitoring HIV/AIDS and HIV risk behaviors among American Indians and Alaska Natives. *AIDS Educ Prev* 2004;16(3):218–237.

33. Schur CL, Berk ML, Dunbar JR, et al. Where to seek care: An examination of people in rural areas with HIV/AIDS. *J Rural Health* 2002;18(2):337–347.

34. Ball AL, Crofts N. HIV risk reduction in injection drug users, 2001. In: Lampety P, Gayle H, eds. *HIV/AIDS prevention and care in resource constrained settings: A handbook for the design and management of programs.* Family Health International, Arlington VA. (Available online at: http://www.fhi.org/en/HIVAIDS/pub/guide/HIVAIDSPreventionCare.htm.)

35. Kitahata MM, Van Rompaey SE, Dillingham PW, et al. Primary care delivery is associated with greater physician experience and improved survival among persons with AIDS. *J Gen Intern Med* 2003;18(2):95–103.

36. Valenti WM. The HIV specialist improves quality of care and outcomes. *AIDS Read* 2002;12(5):202–205.

37. Katz MH, Cunningham WE, Fleishman JA, et al. Effect of case management on unmet needs and utilization of medical care and medications among HIV-infected persons. *Ann Intern Med* 2001;135(8 Pt 1):557–565.

38. Wong MD, Cunningham WE, Shapiro MF, et al. Disparities in HIV treatment and physician attitudes about delaying protease inhibitors for nonadherent patients. *J Gen Intern Med* 2004;19(4):366–374.

39. Bangsberg DR, Hecht FM, Clague H, et al. Provider assessment of adherence to HIV antiretroviral therapy. *J AIDS* 2001;26(5):435–442.

40. Bamberger JD, Unick J, Klein P, et al. Helping the urban poor stay with antiretroviral HIV drug therapy. *Am J Public Health* 2000;90(5):699–701.

41. Moss AR, Hahn JA, Perry S, et al. Adherence to highly active antiretroviral therapy in the homeless population in San Francisco: A prospective study. *Clin Infect Dis* 2004;39(8):1190–1198.

42. King WD, Wong MD, Shapiro MF, et al. Does racial concordance between HIV-positive patients and their physicians affect the time to receipt of protease inhibitors? *J Gen Intern Med* 2004;19(11):1146–1153.

43. Rotheram-Borus MJ, Flannery D, Rice E, et al. Families living with HIV. *AIDS Care* 2005;17(8):978–987.

44. *RESPECT-2 counseling guidelines.* Available at: http://www.cdc.gov/hiv/projects/respect-2/counseling.htm

Chapter 39

Care of Ill Socially Complicated Patients in the Hospital

Jeffrey M. Critchfield, MD, and Mark V. Williams, MD

Objectives

- Review the trend toward transitioning hospitalized patients to home care.
- Outline challenges to providing care to inpatients with complicated social circumstances.
- Identify interventions to improve care, both at provider and systems levels.
- Describe the importance of establishing and maintaining trust during hospitalization.
- Review the concepts of patient capacity and competency, and methods of assessing these.

Mr. Garcia is a 66-year-old man who emigrated from El Salvador. He completed approximately 6 years of school. He learned to speak and read some English while working in restaurants. The manager of his residential hotel found him passed out on the floor of his room. The paramedics transport Mr. Garcia to the hospital to evaluate his altered mental status and labored breathing.

Severe illness necessitating admission to the hospital is a time of great emotional and physical vulnerability for all patients. It is even more traumatic when the medical illness is complicated by social circumstances such as poverty, isolation, minority status, legal difficulties, mental disability, or substance abuse. Moreover, there is evidence that the most vulnerable patients, that is, patients living at 200% below the poverty level, have a higher rate of hospitalization and also receive a lower standard of care while hospitalized.[1,2]

This chapter highlights issues and challenges in the care of vulnerable patient populations unique to the hospital, including medical evaluation in the emergency department, ongoing care throughout the hospital course, and discharge planning from the hospital. After providing a framework to understand the issues, this chapter offers examples of interventions designed to address the challenges raised.

EPIDEMIOLOGY OF HOSPITAL-BASED CARE

In 2003, of the $1.6 trillion spent on health care in the United States, 30% went for the treatment of hospitalized patients.[3] Over the past two decades the number of hospitalizations has decreased from 39 million to 32.1 million.[1] However, the patients admitted to the hospital are sicker, with nearly one third of all hospitalized patients having two or more comorbidities.[1,4] Despite enriching for increasingly complicated patients, from

1985 to 2001 the average length of stay fell by 20%, from 6.6 to 4.9 days.[2,4]

Technological advances, such as minimally invasive surgical approaches, explain some of this marked reduction in length of stay. Another important change involves the transfer of acute care from the hospital to the outpatient setting. Development of in-home health services coupled with increased use of skilled nursing facilities contributes to the discharge of patients much sooner than before. Indeed, in 1997, nearly 20% of all discharges involved one of these strategies.[1]

Poor patients have a hospitalization rate nearly twice that of the non-poor.[2] Among the uninsured, regardless of age, three of the top 10 most common reasons to be admitted involve substance abuse or mental health conditions.[1] Ironically, these higher rates of admission represent delivery of the most expensive care to those who have been deprived of more cost-effective preventive measures.

Among the vulnerable, unstable housing, limited access to outpatient health providers, insufficient financial resources, social isolation, or a fundamental distrust of institutional intrusion into one's personal life, make the transition from acute hospitalization to outpatient care exceedingly challenging. These factors contribute to the longer length of stay of poor patients compared with the non-poor (5.1 days versus 3.7 days, respectively).[2]

CHALLENGES AND BARRIERS TO QUALITY CARE FOR THE ACUTELY ILL, VULNERABLE PATIENT

In the emergency department the triage nurse notes Mr. Garcia's heart rate is 118 with an oxygen saturation of 91%. He is mumbling in what she guesses is Spanish. The odor of alcohol emanates from him. She finds no record that Mr. Garcia has ever visited the hospital or clinics before. He has no insurance. Despite insisting that he be allowed to return to his hotel, Mr. Garcia eventually agrees to be admitted to the hospital.

THE VULNERABLE PATIENT IN THE EMERGENCY DEPARTMENT

The emergency department (ED) is the sole option for care for many patients with limited financial and social resources. These patients typically present for care only when they suffer from symptoms preventing them from continuing their usual activities. Moreover, lack of trust in physicians is also associated with reluctance to seek care and is more common in minority patients without continuity relationships than whites or those followed by primary care physicians.

Rapid collection and effective exchange of information between provider and patient is a central concern in the delivery of quality care in the ED. Discordant language abilities between patient and provider represent a tangible barrier to communication (see Chap. 26), yet trained interpreters are rarely used. Multiple studies demonstrate that non–English speaking patients report less satisfaction with ED care, have a more limited understanding of their treatment and evaluation, are submitted to increased laboratory and imaging tests, and are admitted to the hospital at a higher frequency than English-speaking patients with the same chief complaint.[5–7]

Shame or fear of a diagnosis that involves substance misuse or psychiatric illness that clouds mental capabilities can profoundly limit effective interactions among providers and patients. Provider bias also can contribute to treatment differences between white and non-white patients presenting to an ED with the same condition. For instance, studies have found that Hispanic patients with long bone fractures received less analgesia than white patients,[8] and poor patients are often thought to be substance users when they are not.[9]

Because Mr. Garcia has not had access to primary care, no documentation of prior health status is available to the ED provider. The provider–patient interaction then takes on even greater importance. Nevertheless, there are extensive data that providers, despite evidence that screening can improve outcomes, often do not screen for crucial information such as histories of alcohol use or domestic violence.[9] When available, information from family members, friends, or other members of the patient's social support network can provide invaluable data but often are not pursued.

In the ED, the most pressing question is, "Does this patient need to be admitted?" or "Is this patient sick enough to require hospitalization?" The answer to this question requires a global assessment of the patient's circumstances. One must also ask, "Is this patient capable of caring for himself and his illness if I discharge him?" For individuals living in poverty, particularly those lacking housing, the absence of resources to care for themselves requires lowering the threshold for admission. Hence having "means" in the context of discharge (from the ED or hospital) refers to resources to support timely recovery, including shelter, someone to help with care, and safe administration of discharge medicines, access to regular meals, use of a phone, ability to seek help should the treatment fail, and transportation to allow participation in follow-up programs.

THE VULNERABLE PATIENT DURING THE HOSPITAL COURSE

> Once admitted to the hospital, Mr. Garcia wanted to be released from the hospital. Interpreting his agitation as a sign of early alcohol withdrawal the team gave Mr. Garcia sedatives. When he pulled out his IV and began to leave, the team requested that the psychiatry consult declare him lacking in decision-making capacity. After talking with Mr. Garcia the consultants determined that he wanted to return home to care for his 12-year-old nephew who was living alone.

Building and maintaining trust throughout the course of the admission is one of the central challenges to caring for hospitalized patients.[10] When hospitalized, even empowered individuals can experience feelings of loss of control, abandonment, and confusion heightening a sense of vulnerability around their care.

As with the ED, a medical ward is fertile terrain to cultivate misunderstandings based on assumptions, biases, and alternative belief systems between patients and the health care team. Ethnic minorities, after experiencing disproportionately unjust treatment by social institutions such as public schools, law enforcement services, housing and work opportunities, may be wary of social institutions such as large public hospitals. Those using illegal substances, undocumented immigrants, or victims of domestic violence may fear legal consequences of seeking care or being forthcoming about their medical histories. These fears can influence decisions and behaviors of hospitalized patients. Mentally ill patients, for example, have recorded that their concerns will not be taken seriously if they do not exaggerate their symptoms.[11] What appears to the provider to be an irrational refusal of an offered diagnostic intervention or treatment may seem very rational to the patient who harbors unspoken concerns, for example, fear that the cost of care will be too expensive and lead to financial ruin.

Trust, comfort, and reassurance are enhanced by effective communication and active participation in the decision-making process.[10,12] At the time of admission, the patient possesses the majority of critical information that needs to be passed on to the provider, but during the hospital course, providers accumulate tremendous quantities of information that in turn need to be passed effectively back to the patient. This crucial communication (more about this in the following) is often neglected.

The structure of the hospital day is organized for the convenience of medical professionals. Many patients, regardless of their social standing, complain of the disruptions of hospital life—being awakened, long waits for assistance, and loss of privacy. For the patient plagued by addiction or mental illness, the disruptions of routine or the pangs of withdrawal can lead to difficult interactions with the health care team. Such tensions erode a sense of trust and can contribute to a patient's reluctance to participate with the providers' treatment plan.

As seen with Mr. Garcia, a crisis can ensue when the patient disagrees with the plan presented by the treatment team. Providers assume that refusal of their treatment indicates the patient lacks decision-making capacity.[13,14] When unsuccessful at convincing a patient to cooperate, a provider may look to his or her psychiatric consultant to deem the patient incompetent so as to assume decision-making responsibilities to pursue the provider's own plan. When available, psychiatric consult and liaison teams are a tremendous resource; however, nonpsychiatric practitioners are empowered by law and practice standards to perform this evaluation themselves (see Core Competency). Studies investigating reasons for psychiatric consultation on a medical service indicate providers frequently have misconceptions about what constitutes lack of capacity.[15,16] Providers incorrectly assume that the presence of a psychiatric disease such as schizophrenia or dementia indicates the patient lacks capacity. Providers often fail to ensure that the patient has been given sufficient time or information to make a decision, or they give greater weight to the final decision with little attention to the process by which it was reached. Perhaps most importantly, the treating team may not bring thoughtful inquiry to understanding why the patient may not be aligned with the team's plan. The psychiatric consult discerned a very understandable reason for Mr. Garcia's seemingly inappropriate behavior.

TYRANNY OF THE URGENT

The inpatient setting is perhaps at greatest risk for what has been called the "tyranny of the urgent," wherein the most pressing concerns subvert the clinician's ability to implement a proactive strategy for promotion of health. Pursuit of diagnosis and treatment of acute problems overwhelm consideration of the psychosocial conditions that may contribute to the patient's illness and recovery. Providers must intentionally engage patients, particularly those less able to advocate for themselves, in their own care. Regrettably, the tyranny of the urgent, ubiquitous in the high-volume, high-acuity setting of the hospital, undermines a thoughtful, interactive approach to care.

With time management at a premium, the inpatient provider spends the most energy on those who are either very sick or most able to demand their attention, or may limit patient responses and dictate treatment. Vulnerable patients are at greatest risk for being alienated and left out of the discussion, reinforcing the experience that the health care system is not designed for their needs and thus is not to be trusted.

CHALLENGES AND BARRIERS TO QUALITY CARE FOLLOWING HOSPITALIZATION

> After several days of rest and antibiotics, Mr. Garcia is certain he is ready to go home, although he is slightly short of breath while walking. He does not want home health services because he fears they will tell the apartment manager that his nephew is surreptitiously living with him. He feels comfortable taking some antibiotics and following up with a primary care provider.

DISCHARGE PLANNING FOR THE SOCIALLY COMPLICATED PATIENT

The transition from the hospital, where care is fully supported, to home can be precarious for all patients. However, effective communication at time of discharge is an obviously crucial but commonly neglected step. Physicians tend to overestimate how well their patients understand discharge instructions.[17] In one study, fewer than half of the patients were able to list their diagnoses, or their medications, purposes, or side-effects at time of discharge.[18] For patients with language skills discordant with their providers, effective exchange of communication is even less likely and use of interpreter services to explain the medications, treatment plans, and follow-up appointments is not common (see Chap. 26). Other barriers to effective communication (e.g., limitations in health literacy or health care beliefs) are also important considerations when formulating discharge plans. Importantly, lack of hospital discharge education is associated with unanticipated readmission.[19]

IN-HOME HEALTH SERVICES

At discharge the patient with limited means is sent back to his or her marginal circumstances with only a small fraction of the thought and resources that went into hospital evaluation and management. Multiple studies show that patients who are poor, from ethnic minority groups, or have meager social support or confounding mental illness have inferior posthospital outcomes compared with their counterparts with more resources.[20–22] The push toward significantly shorter length of stays further exacerbates this tension. Individuals of higher socioeconomic status (SES) have the security of insurance-supported home services, sick leave from work, safe housing, higher education with commensurate ability to be a self-advocate, and family members who can take off from work to help; however, poor patients often leave the hospital with little more than distant follow-up appointments.

Some cities finance in-home health services for low SES patients. These services are not a panacea: Homelessness or ambivalence over the intrusion of social services are barriers to this form of added support. Nevertheless, home follow-up has been shown to be an effective intervention improving function, quality of life, and reducing hospitalizations and uncovering problems (see Chap. 11).[23,24]

Consequently, at discharge, as at admission, the practitioner must ask, "Is this patient capable of caring for himself and his illness if I discharge him?" Discharge plans not only need to be properly communicated, but they should also integrate knowledge of what resources are available to patients (see preceding discussion for the ED). For low SES patients, particularly those lacking housing, raising the threshold for discharge may be appropriate. For example, the homeless patient with pneumonia, might require additional hospital days to recover pulmonary capacity sufficient to walk multiple blocks from his campsite to a soup kitchen. This is no doubt one of the reasons that homeless patients tend to be hospitalized for longer times than their housed counterparts.[25]

Common Pitfalls:

At the time of admission

- Neglecting appropriate communication with the patient, including the use of interpreters
- Discharging patients from the ED without considering the psychosocial challenges that impede their ability to care for themselves

During the hospital course

- Underestimating how confusing and frightening the hospital environment can be to patients
- Underestimating the degree to which patients experience the hospital as another untrustworthy social institution
- When addressing the patient who disagrees with the treatment plan, assuming he or she lacks capacity, rather than exploring his or her unspoken concerns
- Allowing the acuity of other patients to distract one's full attention from the development of a successful discharge plan for the stabilized patient ready to leave the hospital

- Neglecting appropriate communication with the patient, including the use of interpreters

At time of discharge from the hospital

- Failing to consider the importance of stable housing and social support in improving the patient's health
- Failing to assess the patient's ability to adhere to the discharge plan, including access, understanding, and functional capacity to take medications or change dressings
- Incompletely appreciating the patient's deficient understanding about how to take his or her medications
- Neglecting appropriate communication with the patient, including the use of interpreters

IMPROVING THE CARE OF THE SOCIALLY COMPLICATED INPATIENT

Any factor that hinders patients' ability to advocate for themselves, whether physical, emotional, or social, heightens their vulnerability when they interact with the health care system. At the core of any potential solution is an awareness of the challenges faced by patients, and willingness and competence to address them. Medical schools and residency programs recently have designed curricula to provide trainees with greater exposure to attitudes, knowledge, and skills and community immersion experiences in the hopes of improving care of vulnerable patient populations.[26,27] When validated, in some cases learners who have participated in these types of experiences have improved perceptions of these patients and are more likely to work with them in the future.[10,28]

PATIENT-CENTERED APPROACH TO CARE OF THE SOCIALLY COMPLICATED INPATIENT

The Institute of Medicine, in their report, *Crossing the Quality Chasm,* proposes using the patient-centered approach as one solution to close the gap between ideal care and actual care.[29] Patient-centered, holistic care requires that the provider bring thoughtful, or "mindful" inquiry to the interaction.[30–32] Validated and designed in the outpatient setting, the patient-centered approach can be applied to the care of hospitalized patients as well.

Figure 39-1 illustrates a schema incorporating concerns of cultural competency to care, particularly integrating a bearing of cultural humility.[33] For less empowered patients, a commitment must be made to create an environment in which the concerns of the vulnerable patient can be voiced and appreciated. Using this approach to address Mr. Garcia's demands for immediate discharge despite his persistent shortness of breath would have revealed Mr. Garcia's concern for his nephew. Instead, the hospital team assumed he was agitated from early alcohol withdrawal and intervened with sedatives.

The patient-centered approach enjoys great support among training institutions because studies suggest it yields outcome benefits, including medication adherence and reduced use of diagnostic tests. Patient-centered inquiry requires engaging the patient in his or her own care. The research around a patient-centered approach indicates patients respond positively when their views are sought and incorporated into plans.[34] Over the course of one hospitalization, the patient who experiences recurring interactions with providers that reinforce a dynamic of thoughtful, informed engagement not only will "get better," but also might begin to

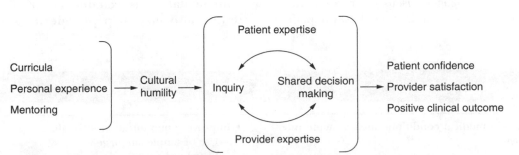

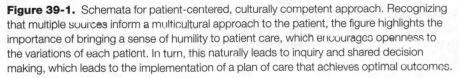

Figure 39-1. Schemata for patient-centered, culturally competent approach. Recognizing that multiple sources inform a multicultural approach to the patient, the figure highlights the importance of bringing a sense of humility to patient care, which encourages openness to the variations of each patient. In turn, this naturally leads to inquiry and shared decision making, which leads to the implementation of a plan of care that achieves optimal outcomes.

develop trust for the provider and the system he or she represents. Inherent in the approach of shared decision making is the powerful message that the provider has enough regard for the patient to invest in discussion.

Using this approach appears to have benefits for both patients and providers: Data suggest that heightened awareness of the patient's expectations and concerns can increase provider satisfaction.[31] Biases held by providers also may contribute to the observed disparities in health care for patients of varied ethnic backgrounds. Sadly, data indicate that providers are less likely to involve minority and poor patients in care decisions.[35] Teaching and practicing patient-centered models of shared decision making may help decrease disparities in health care.

Indeed, true patient-centeredness includes recognizing that not all patients may be comfortable with the approach and thus open to any possible benefits.[36] Thus, application of the patient-centered approach involves taking the time to assess the patient's wishes and expertise in his or her own care. The nature and degree of patients' involvement with shared decision making varies. The wishes and ability of the hospitalized patient to participate in shared decision making may change from day to day with the progress of the illness. As enthusiasm for teaching the patient-centered approach grows, two significant questions need to be addressed. First, are the outcome benefits robust in varying patient populations and treatment settings? Second, can patient-centered skills be taught successfully?

APPLYING THE PATIENT-CENTERED SCHEMA: APPROACH TO THE UNCOOPERATIVE PATIENT

The patient who refuses to comply with the team's treatment plan creates a particularly vexing situation for the inpatient practitioner. This situation is an ideal time to implement the schema represented in Figure 39-1. Often the act of this engaged discussion reveals underlying concerns, which once addressed allow the patient to feel comfortable moving forward with the proposed plan of care.

Refusal (and indeed, acceptance!) of medical treatments need careful assessment if clinicians question the patient's decision-making capacity. Informing patients about treatment decisions and optimizing their ability to respond are crucial. Legal standards for competence (see the following for distinction from capacity) include the ability to communicate a choice, understand relevant information, appreciate the current situation and its consequences, and manipulate information rationally.[37] Legally, competence can only be determined by the court; consequently, the clinician's role is to gather enough information to decide whether it is necessary to proceed with an adjudication of incompetence. Practically, practitioners do this by determining decision-making capacity.

DETERMINING DECISION-MAKING CAPACITY

Decision-making capacity can be a dynamic state. Treating the patient to improve his or her ability to understand and function is crucial.[16,38] Box 39-1 outlines a useful approach to improve a patient's decision-making capacity.

Once the clinician feels assured that the patient's ability to comprehend and interact has been maximized, mindful inquiry into assessing capacity requires that the provider determine the patient's: (a) awareness of his or her medical situation; (b) appreciation for the relative benefits and risks inherent in the treatment plan; (c) understanding of the consequences of forgoing treatment; (d) understanding of alternatives; and (e) rational thought process as he or she articulates the decision and its consequences. If the clinician questions the patient's ability to do any of these steps, he or she should review methods of increasing capacity. Performance on tests such as the mini-mental status examination or neuropsychiatric testing also may help provide insight. Sometimes

---

Box 39-1. Interventions to Improve Decision-making Capacity

- Treat reversible medical conditions such as acute infections and hypoxia.
- Treat pain.
- Review medications as causes for sedation or confusion.
- Maximize emotional and psychiatric functioning.
  —Treat underlying mental illness or psychosis.
  —Involve or remove family as appropriate.
- Make sure the patient can hear or read.

- Improve communication through:
  —Use of simple language
  —Visual or hearing aids
  —Trained interpreters, including sign language interpreters
  —Low literacy materials
  —Recurring discussions
  —Patience

Box 39-2. Documentation of Patient's Decision-making Capacity

- Patient's ability to communicate a consistent choice
- Patient's understanding of relevant diagnostic and treatment information
- Patient's appreciation of situation and its consequences
- Patient's rational use of the information

  For example:

  —The patient understands his or her present condition to be . . .
  —The patient understands the treatment offered is . . .
  —The patient feels the following will happen with acceptance of treatment . . .

—The patient feels the following will happen without treatment . . .
—The patient understands the alternatives and their consequences.

Note any others who are present during this discussion, materials used, and the stability of the decision over time.

Adapted from: Appelbaum PS, Grisso T. Assessing patients' capacities to consent to treatment. *N Engl J Med* 1988;319:1635–1638;[37] Miller SS, Marin DB. Assessing capacity. *Emerg Med Clin North Am* 2000;18:233–242;[41] Annas GJ, Densberger JE. Competence to refuse medical treatment: Autonomy versus paternalism. *Univ Toledo Law Rev* 1984;15:561–592.[42]

---

neuropsychiatric testing can help suggest methods of communication (e.g., visual, pictorial) that might improve understanding.

Several points are important to appreciate when assessing decision-making capacity. First, decision-making capacity is referable only to the decision being considered. It is not a global judgment on the ability of the patient to speak on his or her own behalf. Patients with mental illness, substance abuse, and mild forms of dementia still retain the right to decision-making autonomy, and studies indicate that they retain the ability to execute this right.[16,38] Finally, as caretakers of sick inpatients, it is also the job of clinicians to try to help prevent patients from becoming more confused during hospital stays. Protocols for preventing delirium in the elderly, particularly in high-risk postoperative situations, have been shown to be effective.[39] Simply implementing standard orders to raise the head of the bed to 30 degrees in all patients who have a risk of aspiration (many of whom also are at high risk for developing delirium while in the hospital because of stroke, alcohol withdrawal, overdose, or brain injury to name a few) may prevent aspiration pneumonia, confusion, and intubation.[40] Protocols for treatment of alcohol withdrawal and opiate dosing, as well as specialized pain management, palliative care, and pharmacy consult teams are other methods of providing patient-centered care and preventing complications.

The evaluation of capacity can yield two outcomes for the patient refusing treatment. If after implementing the preceding strategies the provider is convinced that the patient has capacity but continues to refuse treatment, then the provider is obligated to respect the patient's autonomy and not pursue the proposed intervention.

It is wise for the provider to document this discussion in the chart and also communicate this to the patient's other providers (Box 39-2).

How stringently one applies these steps and documents them depends on their medical importance, with refusals that pose significant risk to the patient requiring the most rigorous application. Assent to treatments with minimal risk and great benefits; for example, treatment of urinary tract infection with antibiotics, or refusal of a risky treatment of little proven benefit require that the patient only have a general sense of the situation. Of course, in life-threatening situations, if the patient is unable to consent because of trauma or illness that undermines his or her ability to make a reasoned judgment, then treating the patient to stabilize him or her is justified. Patients need to have a greater comprehension of the risks and benefits when the treatment is more uncertain, is one of several therapeutic options, or is not necessary to sustain life.[41]

MEDICAL PROBATE

If the patient is deemed to lack decision-making capacity and refuses a treatment that clinicians feel is beneficial but not emergently required, then seeking court adjudication of incompetence is appropriate if there are no advance directives or other surrogate decision makers who can consent on the patient's behalf.

In California, providers may apply for a short-term determination of incompetence for medical decisions, termed *medical probate*. These privileges, if granted by the court, give the team the authority to serve as a surrogate decision maker for the patient around issues relevant to the care they proposed for the patient. If the patient demonstrates capacity for other medical decisions, then the medical probate does not override his or her autonomy in that realm. Medical probate does not allow providers to use psychoactive medicines to treat an underlying psychiatric illness against the patient's will, for example. Nor does medical probate allow providers to make decisions around housing or placement in rehabilitation facilities against the patient's will. These decisions require court authority provided through the *conservatorship* process.

CAPACITY VERSUS COMPETENCE

Although often used synonymously with decision making, "capacity" and "competence" are distinctly different entities. *Capacity* is the ability of a person to understand and make judgments based upon that understanding. *Competence,* on the other hand, is a legal concept that requires that a person have "sufficient ability or skill" and the legal authority to exercise it.[43] A patient who is deemed incompetent to manage his or her financial affairs, for example, may nevertheless have sufficient decision-making capacity to consent to medical treatment.

Using the concept of competence as a patient's practical ability to carry out the steps required to fulfill a goal can be useful to providing more effective patient care. Decision making, cognition, psychiatric stability and functional abilities all contribute to competence in this sense. Competence at its fullest also can be associated with community resources and the ability to access them.[44]

Competence is particularly important for medical providers to consider at the time of discharge, when care becomes dependent on the patient and his or her family or support system. Providers can help ensure a patient's competence to care for himself or herself by assessing not only the understanding but the actual functional ability to carry out discharge plans. Physical and occupational therapists have important roles to play in assessing competence and offering treatments and interventions to improve it. For example, the Kohlman Evaluation of Living Skills (KELS test) is performed by occupational therapists. It determines functional ability in living skills, from the ability to manage money and medicines or to take the bus or use the telephone. Other tools, such as the development of checklists to aid in the assessment of important realms like housing, entitlements, and psychiatric treatment, also have been developed by some systems.[45] Linking patients with resources that allow them to care for

themselves is important to success. Case management programs (see the following) can be seen as one way of remediating deficiencies in competence.

IMPROVING SYSTEMS OF CARE FOR VULNERABLE POPULATIONS

Systems changes designed to address needs of vulnerable populations must be implemented. Policy discussions relevant to health care financing, provision of health care coverage, and issues such as housing are also important considerations. This section focuses on systems changes at the level of hospitals and their affiliated training institutions. Systems have responded with changes in several areas loosely organized as patient education and direct services, targeted case management programs, and optimized use of the information infrastructure.

Patient Education and Direct Services

Because some specific needs of certain vulnerable populations can be anticipated, hospitals and their associated clinics can develop resources targeted for these populations. Hospitals serving patients whose language is discordant with their provider can hire interpreters or create opportunities for multilingual providers and staff to undergo professional medical interpreter training. Supplying written materials translated into the appropriate language with cultural relevance can greatly facilitate communication around commonly encountered hospital scenarios.

Institutional Cultural Competence

Recognizing that certain vulnerable patient populations are frequently encountered in the acute setting, hospitals have responded by forming specific teams or initiatives to meet the needs of these groups. Palliative care suites or consult teams provide expertise in end-of-life care for patients and families with benefits ranging from improved quality of life to patient and family and decreased length of stay (LOS). Expertise consolidated in this way creates an atmosphere of support for both the patient and the provider. Treatment guidelines for specific diseases, such as alcohol withdrawal, represent a variation on this theme.

Case Management

The case management strategy is an even more comprehensive and typically longitudinal approach to address the concern of inadequate self-advocacy among the vulnerable populations it represents (see Chapter 15). Although each program has a different focus, requiring different interventions, common to each is the systematic delivery of resources, including professionals, who can support the patient and offer advocacy on their behalf when they are unable. Case management programs targeting the high user of inpatient services can reduce admissions to the hospital, while also connecting these patients to continuity of care with primary providers.[46]

Improving the Health Care Delivery Infrastructure

In addition to these more direct patient contact approaches, hospitals can better serve vulnerable patients by altering fundamental aspects of their health care delivery infrastructure. Efficient information exchange among providers is valuable for all patients, but particularly critical for those patients at greatest risk for falling through the cracks.

Many institutions use electronic messages to notify primary providers that their patient was admitted to the hospital. For the vulnerable patient fortunate enough to have a longitudinal relationship with a provider, involvement with a primary care provider contributes vital medical and social information and the voice of a longstanding advocate. Electronic information systems can be configured to include mandatory alerts that cue the admitting provider to contact surrogate decision makers or import members of the patient's support system. Details of advanced directives or end-of-life care wishes can be similarly noted, and thus become accessible to acute providers meeting the patient for the first time.

The electronic record also can improve the transition from the inpatient to outpatient setting. Electronic access to details of hospital-based evaluations, including discharge summaries noting any changes in medication regimen, greatly enhances the continuation of any treatment plan.[47]

Discharge planning is a key component to the successful completion of an acute hospitalization.[7,17–19] Working with social services, rehabilitation, and primary care physicians, the team can craft an appropriate discharge plan.

CONCLUSION

Admission to the hospital frames a time of significance, if not crisis, for most patients and their loved ones. Many inpatient providers, or hospitalists, choose to practice in this setting because of the rewards of caring for the most ill and unstable patients. These rewards take the form of intellectual challenges, collegial interactions, and the opportunity to have a significant impact in a patient's life in a short amount of time. The fast pace of hospital care can insidiously erode the core of medical care, i.e., engaging with your patient. The challenge and potential great opportunity for hospitalists is to see this moment of acute distress as an entry into the longer-term issues of patient care. The hospitalization can then become an opening for educating a patient about improved health behavior, inclusion in a chronic disease management program, or further engagement of the patient in his or her own medical care. If successful in this challenge, the hospital provider can reap both the satisfaction of helping getting a patient back on the road to recovery and helping set a direction that keeps him or her moving along that road.

KEY CONCEPTS

- Develop the discipline to consider how the patient's social circumstances may challenge his or her ability to optimally manage his or her health.
  - —Determine stability and safety of housing.
  - —Use professional interpreters as available.
  - —Consider the possibility that substance abuse is affecting the patient's decision-making capacity.
  - —Consider the possibility that mental illness is affecting the patient's decision-making capacity.
  - —Consider the possibility that the socially marginalized patient is concerned that social institutions, such as hospitals, are unreliable.
  - —In the emergency department, consider the patient's ability to care for himself or herself when making a decision to admit or discharge.
- Consider outside social pressures that may be contributing to the anxiety or agitation of your hospitalized patient.
- Always consider the possibility of drug withdrawal in the hospitalized patient.
- Make every effort to contact continuity providers to elicit more information while laying the foundation for a successful discharge plan.
- Support the development and use of electronic record initiatives to extend the distribution of important patient care data to all providers.
- Support the development of case management teams, with strong social service and nursing support to address the multiple needs of the vulnerable patient

CORE COMPETENCY

Process to determine decision making capacity

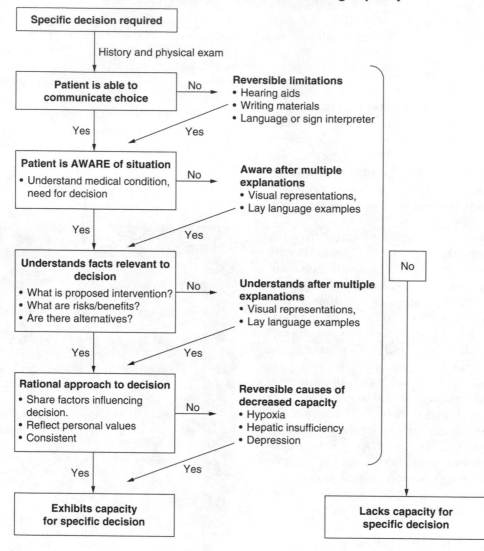

DISCUSSION QUESTIONS

1. Consider from your own experience how an acute illness and the recovery from that illness affected the life and family of a loved one or friend. How might financial limitations have affected the outcome?
2. You are admitting a very ill patient from the emergency department who does not speak English and your hospital does not have a suitable interpreter to facilitate the interaction. What strategies might you pursue to get further information?
3. Consider any patient admitted to the hospital. What vulnerabilities might he or she experience? How are these vulnerabilities common to many patients, compounded among patients who do not speak English well; among patient plagued by mental illness?
4. What factors must be considered at the time of discharge for patients who are homeless; who have limited English ability?

RESOURCES

http://www.ahrq.gov/data/hcup/#h1
   Link to clearinghouse of utilization of health resource including hospitalized populations

http://www.ahrq.gov/research/cbprrole.htm
   Link describing strategies for community linkage and outreach

http://www.diversityrx.org/HTML/models.htm
Resource for multicultural, multilingual practices and strategies of care

REFERENCES

1. Elixhauser A, Bierman A. *Hospitalization in the United States, 1997.* HCUP Fact Book No. 1. AHRQ Publication No. 00-0031, 2000.
2. Centers for Disease Control and Prevention. *Health, United States, 2003 with chartbook on trends in the health of Americans.* Atlanta, GA: D.O.H.A.H. Resources, 2003.
3. Smith C, Cowan C, Sensenig A, et al. Health spending growth slows in 2003. *Health Aff (Millwood)* 2005;24: 185–194.
4. Popovic JR, Hall MJ. *1999 National hospital discharge survey. Advance data from vital and health statistics.* Report No. 319. Hyattsville, MD: National Center for Health Statistics, 2001.
5. Hampers LC, McNulty JE. Professional interpreters and bilingual physicians in a pediatric emergency department: Effect on resource utilization. *Arch Pediatr Adolesc Med* 2002;156:1108–1113.
6. Carrasquillo O, Orav EJ, Brennan TA, et al. Impact of language barriers on patient satisfaction in an emergency department. *J Gen Intern Med* 1999;14:82–87.
7. Baker DW, Parker RM, Williams MV, et al. Use and effectiveness of interpreters in an emergency department. *JAMA* 1996;275:783–88.
8. Todd KH, Samaroo N, Hoffman JR. Ethnicity as a risk factor for inadequate emergency department analgesia. *JAMA* 1993;269:1537–1539.
9. Gentilello LM, Villaveces A, Ries RR, et al. Detection of acute alcohol intoxication and chronic alcohol dependence by trauma center staff. *J Trauma* 1999;47: 1131–1135;discussion 1135–1139.
10. Thom DH. Physician behaviors that predict patient trust. *J Fam Pract* 2001;50:323–328.
11. Lester H, Tritter JQ. Listen to my madness: Understanding the experiences of people with serious mental illness. *Sociol Health Illn* 2005;27:649–669.
12. Stewart AL, Napoles-Springer A, Perez-Stable EJ. Interpersonal processes of care in diverse populations. *Millbank Q* 1999;77:305–339, 274.
13. Umapathy C, Ramchandani D, Lamdan RM, et al. Competency evaluations on the consultation-liaison service. Some overt and covert aspects. *Psychosomatics* 1999;40: 28–33.
14. Stotland NL. Refusal of medical treatment: Psychiatric emergency? *Am J Psychiatry* 1997;154:106–108.
15. Ganzini L, Volicer L, Nelson W, et al. Pitfalls in assessment of decision-making capacity. *Psychosomatics* 2003; 44:237–243.
16. Wong JG, Clare CH, Holland AJ, et al. The capacity of people with a "mental disability" to make a health care decision. *Psychol Med* 2000;30:295–306.
17. Calkins DR, Davis RB, Reiley P, et al. Patient–physician communication at hospital discharge and patients' understanding of the postdischarge treatment plan. *Arch Intern Med* 1997;157:1026–1030.
18. Makaryus AN, Friedman EA. Patients' understanding of their treatment plans and diagnosis at discharge. *Mayo Clin Proc* 2005;80(8):991–994.
19. Marcantonio ER, McKean S, Goldfinger M, et al. Factors associated with unplanned hospital readmission among patients 65 years of age and older in a Medicare managed care plan. *Am J Med* 1999;107:13–17.
20. Ottenbacher KJ, Smith PM, Illig SB, et al. Characteristics of persons rehospitalized after stroke rehabilitation. *Arch Phys Med Rehabil* 2001;82:1367–1374.
21. Philbin EF, Dec GW, Jenkins PL, et al. Socioeconomic status as an independent risk factor for hospital readmission for heart failure. *Am J Cardiol* 2001;87:1367–1371.
22. Rao SV, Kaul P, Newby LK, et al. Poverty, process of care, and outcome in acute coronary syndromes. *J Am Coll Cardiol* 2003;41:1948–1954.
23. Stuck AE, Egger M, Hammer A, et al. Home visits to prevent nursing home admission and functional decline in elderly people: Systematic review and meta-regression analysis. *JAMA* 2002;287:1022–1028.
24. Naylor MD, Brooten D, Campbell R, et al. Comprehensive discharge planning and home follow-up of hospitalized elders: A randomized clinical trial. *JAMA* 1999;281: 613–620.
25. Salit SA, Kuhn EM, Hartz AJ, et al. Hospitalization costs associated with homelessness in New York City. *N Engl J Med* 1998;338:1734–1740.
26. Betancourt JR. Cross-cultural medical education: conceptual approaches and frameworks for evaluation. *Acad Med* 2003;78:560–569.
27. Tervalon M. Components of culture in health for medical students' education. *Acad Med* 2003;78:570–576.
28. O'Toole, TP, Kathuria N, Mishra M, et al. Teaching professionalism within a community context: Perspectives from a national demonstration project. *Acad Med* 2005;80: 339–343.
29. Institute of Medicine. *Crossing the quality chasm: A new health system for the 21st century.* Washington, DC: National Academy Press, 2001.
30. Boyle D, Dwinnell B, Platt F. Invite, listen, and summarize: A patient-centered communication technique. *Acad Med* 2005;80:29–32.
31. Kern DE, Branch WT Jr, Jackson JL, et al. Teaching the psychosocial aspects of care in the clinical setting: Practical recommendations. *Acad Med* 2005;80:8–20.
32. Haidet P, Paterniti DA. "Building" a history rather than "taking" one: A perspective on information sharing during the medical interview. *Arch Intern Med* 2003;163: 1134–1140.
33. Tervalon M, Murray-Garcia J. Cultural humility versus cultural competence: A critical distinction in defining physician training outcomes in multicultural education. *J Health Care Poor Underserved* 1998;9:117–125.
34. Williams S, Weinman J, Dale J. Doctor–patient communication and patient satisfaction: A review. *Fam Pract* 1998;15:480–492.
35. Johnson RL, Roter D, Powe NR, et al. Patient race/ethnicity and quality of patient-physician communication

during medical visits. *Am J Public Health* 2004;94:2084–2090.

36. Swenson SL, Buell S, Zettler P, et al. Patient-centered communication: Do patients really prefer it? *J Gen Intern Med* 2004;19:1069–1079.

37. Appelbaum PS, Grisso T. Assessing patients' capacities to consent to treatment. *N Engl J Med* 1988;319:1635–1638.

38. Ness DE. Discussing treatment options and risks with medical patients who have psychiatric problems. *Arch Intern Med* 2002;162(18):2037–2044.

39. Milisen K, Lemiengre J, Braes T, et al. Multicomponent intervention strategies for managing delirium in hospitalized older people: A systematic review. *J Adv Nurs* 2005;52:79–90.

40. Cook DJ, Meade MO, Hand LE, et al. Toward understanding evidence uptake: Semirecumbency for pneumonia prevention. *Crit Care Med* 2002;30:1472–1477.

41. Miller SS, Marin DB. Assessing capacity. *Emerg Med Clin North Am* 2000;18:233–242.

42. Annas GJ, Densberger JE. Competence to refuse medical treatment: Autonomy versus paternalism. *Toledo Law Rev* 1984;15:561–592.

43. *Merriam-Webster online dictionary,* 2005.

44. Pepper-Smith R, Harvey WR, Silberfeld M. Competency and practical judgment. *Theor Med* 1996;17:135–150.

45. Gantt AB, Cohen NL, Sainz A. Impediments to the discharge planning effort for psychiatric inpatients. *Soc Work Health Care* 1999;29:1–14.

46. San Francisco Trauma Recovery Center. *Report to the state legislature.* California Victim Compensation and Government Claims Board and University of California, SFSFGHDoP. May, 2004.

47. Bates DW, Gawande AA. Improving safety with information technology. *N Engl J Med* 2003;348(25):2526–2534.

Chapter 40

Caring for Oneself While Caring for Others

Lee Lipsenthal, MD

Objectives

- Describe challenges that lead to practitioner burnout when caring for vulnerable patients.
- Describe how people's personalities put them at risk for burnout and health problems.
- Outline specific personal strategies for avoiding burnout.
- Review how connection with others enhances one's work and home life.

Sherry is a 43-year-old physician employee of a community clinic and the mother of two children, aged 10 and 12. She prides herself on being very good at both. However, she finds it tougher each day to go to work. Her "fuse" is growing shorter and shorter, and she has more generalized fatigue and frequent headaches.

The practice and delivery of medical services to the underserved and vulnerable populations of US society is difficult at best. Despite burgeoning demands and high community expectations, health systems are increasingly unable to meet the demands of the community, and in many cases are becoming financially disabled. Within this system, health care workers try to deliver the best possible health care with severely limited resources. Very often, practitioners' own lives and health suffer while they attempt to fulfill this mission. Consequently, health professionals—physicians, nurses, social workers, dentists, emergency service staff members, mental health workers, physical therapists, occupational therapists, and speech pathologists—are at particular risk of burnout. Burnout represents a deterioration of values, dignity, spirit, and will.[1] There is growing concern that the high risk for burnout

among health care professionals threatens the sustainability of the health care enterprise.

This chapter reviews some of the challenges that lead health care practitioners to feel overwhelmed by caring for vulnerable patients. It concentrates largely on ways that practitioners can find balance in their lives by cultivating their own physical, emotional, mental, and spiritual well-being while confronting the intellectual and emotional forces that inspire yet undermine their professional lives.

CHALLENGES TO HEALTH CARE WORKERS' WELL-BEING

Bernard, an internist, works in an inner-city, university-based, outpatient clinic. He often feels harried and worries that he is not really helping his patients. His patients often have multiple problems, and he is expected to deal with each patient in a 15-minute office visit.

WHAT ARE YOU ACCOMPLISHING?

Physicians and nurses caring for the underserved are frequently overloaded with the demands of caring for

---

Box 40-1. Risk Factors for Health Care Worker Burnout

- Dislocation between what people are doing compared with what they are expected to do
- Consistent work overload
- A perceived lack of control over the extent to which the load exceeds their capacity
- Unrewarding work

- Community breakdown
- The belief that one is being treated unfairly
- Being confronted with conflicting values

Adapted from: Spickard A Jr, Gabbe SG, Christensen JF. Mid-career burnout in generalist and specialist physicians. *JAMA* 2002;288: 1447–1450.[1]

---

these sick patients while facing increasing constraints of fewer organizational resources. In trying to help those with limited resources they often wonder, "What good are we actually doing?" Their labors begin to seem like those of Sisyphus (i.e., condemned to an eternity of rolling a boulder uphill then watching it roll back down again). In addition, physicians are increasingly being forced to adopt a business mentality that conflicts with their idealistic concept of providing the best possible professional care for their patients.[2] Despite these structural impediments, they often view the inability to meet the many demands of their patients and health system as a personal failure. The difficulty of their patients' lives is great, and there is much they cannot change. Yet, they often feel they need to fix all their problems, which is an impossible task, even if they had the time, training, and resources to do so. Surviving these constant challenges with a sense of grace and humor and with one's core values intact is challenging (Box 40-1).

WORK DEMANDS AND FINANCIAL REWARDS

Jennifer, a family physician in a public health clinic, makes roughly half of what her husband Larry (a cardiologist) makes on a daily basis. She does 90% of her own paperwork, often draws her own labs, and is on the phone making arrangements for patients many hours a day. She feels that she is taking care of "real people with real problems," whereas he is treating "rich people with angina." She is frustrated that her work efforts are far greater than his and she gets less money for them.

Choosing to care for the underserved, like every decision about work, income, and personal satisfaction, can be viewed in terms of tradeoffs (Table 40-1). Everyone needs to decide for himself or herself what balance of work, income, time, and professional satisfaction works best. Physicians in public service often earn less than those in private practice. Multiple factors cause this

---

Table 40-1. Occupational Stressors in the Medical Profession

Common Occupational Stressors in Physicians	Stressors Unique to the Medical Profession
Excessively high patient-to-caregiver ratio	Pressures of time; long years of preparation
Lack of time outs for a temporary breather	Inherent uncertainty involved in patient care
Excessive continuous direct contact with patients	Chronic fatigue
No system for caregivers to "cover" for each other	Dealing with life-and-death or difficult issues
Limited access to a social–professional support system	Difficult, demanding, or chronically ill patients
Limited time and place to share personal feelings with colleagues	Maintaining clinical competence
Inadequate training for working with people	Government regulation
Tendency in the work setting to blame people rather than the situation when care or service deteriorates	Third-party intrusions
Repetitive single tasks	Increase in malpractice litigation
Problems without solutions	Pressure to practice defensive medicine
Time pressures and demands	Diminished public image of physicians
Indispensable syndrome	Breakdown of doctor–patient relationship
	Inadequate support personnel
	Fear of violent patients
	Decreased compensation
	Managing business aspects of practice

Adapted from: Regional Education Team of the TMA Committee of Physician Health and Rehabilitation. *Physician stress and burnout.* Austin, TX: Texas Medical Association, 2005. Accessed at: http://www.texmed.org/Template.aspx?id=1828

disparity: lower income generated per patient; less control over the type of patients seen (often treating all patients regardless of health plan coverage); and dependence on state, federal, and private funding to meet overhead costs. Private practices have the ability to accept or reject patient populations based on insurance coverage and do this in order to stay afloat.[3]

As Jennifer noted, one positive side of caring for the underserved is taking care of real people with real problems whose needs might not otherwise be met. However, this is bound to raise profound emotional issues for health care workers. Witnessing the suffering of others may occasion responses that can affect professional and personal satisfaction and even patient care. A sense of failure at being unable to provide a cure or fear and grief may lead to a sense of helplessness and desire to escape these feelings, as well as the patients. Frustration, isolation, loss of satisfaction with medicine, and even poor judgment are possible results.[4]

Working with others who share a similar commitment or mission can create an energizing work environment that helps mitigate discontent with hardships. The challenges and rewards of working with people from diverse backgrounds also may prove to be profoundly intellectually and emotionally satisfying.

PERSONALITY FACTORS

> Esteban, a 42-year-old general internist, is a driven, compulsive doctor dedicated to his work. He attended medical school on a National Health Service Corps scholarship. Following residency, he joined the staff of a rural health center. After he finished his 2-year commitment, and because of his dedication to the health center and its patients, he was asked to remain on as medical director. He spends many evenings and weekends in the office or at the hospital. He feels he cannot, in good conscience, take time off for the long vacations that his wife and children want. He faults the demands of his work, the fact that it is difficult to attract new physicians to the practice, and the needs of his patients. As the years pass, his family backs away from him, and it seems they share all their fun times without him.

Emotional stress or distress is one of the primary causes of life imbalance. Conversely, emotional well-being is one of the strongest antidotes. Much of one's emotional imbalance is rooted in personality structure. Certain personality traits may increase the risk of burnout by influencing an individual's response to the stressors of medical training or the workplace. Both environments put a premium on intense work, expertly and competitively executed. Thus, the seeds of burnout may be sown in medical school and residency training, in which fatigue and emotional exhaustion often are the norm. By the time they are ready to enter practice, physicians are often exhausted, isolated from family and friends, in debt, nontrusting, egocentric (the expression of insecurity), and emotionally dissociated (numb). This is a recipe for burnout in residency and practice (Box 40-2).[5-7]

Compulsiveness

The psychological makeup of health care professionals, particularly a physician-to-be, compounds the problem. Physicians are intelligent, caring, inquisitive, and people oriented. This is a natural fit with their intended careers. Physicians are commonly type A, compulsive, perfectionist, and competitive. Although these are not considered, by most, to be positive attributes, it would seem to be very difficult to survive the current structure of medical school and postgraduate training without these qualities. Fear of failure exacerbates type A and competitive behaviors. Fear of error elevates perfectionism to obsessive levels; although physicians deal with serious issues, obsession is neither healthy nor productive.

Resistance to Change

Individuals attracted to a career in medicine also tend to be safety seeking or change averse. This made sense 20 years ago, when medicine was a stable career path. However, medicine has changed dramatically over the last few decades and will continue to do so. This change can be a significant source of anxiety. Awareness of change does not necessarily reflect adaptability or flexibility. Inflexibility and resistance to

---

Box 40-2. Personality Factors That Increase Risk for Burnout

- Compulsiveness
  - Doubt
  - Excessive, unrealistic guilt
  - Exaggerated sense of responsibility
- Perfectionism
- Resistance to change
- Need for control

- Difficulty asking for help
- Suppression of feelings
- Difficulty taking vacations and enjoying leisure time

Adapted from: Regional Education Team of the TMA Committee of Physician Health and Rehabilitation. *Physician stress and burnout.* Austin, TX: Texas Medical Association, 2005. Accessed at: http://www.texmed.org/Template.aspx?id=1828[2]

change can lead to frustration and anxiety about the future. Physicians also tend toward social isolation. Many are shy or quiet and a bit "nerdy" as well. Isolation can make change more difficult to accept.

> Cindy, a 47-year-old pediatrician, is highly dedicated to taking care of her patients. Her charts are immaculate, her notes are precise and well written, and her diagnostic testing is always rigorous. She loves complex cases and will spend evenings poring over her textbooks at home. She always works later than the other physicians, she is always running behind and she never seems able to catch up. She wakes up at night worried about patients and is concerned that she might have missed something in her evaluation of them. She is fatigued and frustrated. Her husband is very frustrated as well but does not say anything because medicine is so important to Cindy.

Perfectionism

Like Cindy, many physicians and other health care professionals strive for perfection, an all-pervasive attitude that whatever you attempt in life must be done letter perfectly with no deviation, mistakes, slip-ups, or inconsistencies. As physicians move forward in their careers, they often try to find approval—from mentors, colleagues, and even patients—by seeking perfection. Perfectionists tell themselves that their determination to be perfect will win success, acceptance, love, and fulfillment. However, because none will ever achieve perfection, many remain unsatisfied with their performance and themselves.

In a positive form, perfectionism can provide the driving energy that leads to great achievement. Clearly, meticulous attention to detail often is necessary for scientific investigation. Also, setting high standards is not in itself a bad thing. However, this striving to be the best, reach the ideal, and never make a mistake may doom one to failure, cripple the imagination, kill the spirit, and so handicap performance that an individual may never achieve at the level expected.[8] This outcome seems especially likely when one is working in a profession where there is constant change, complicated and needy patients, and a system that only sometimes works. Consequently, it is better both for one's professional growth and emotional well-being to focus on improvement rather than the unattainable state of perfection.

Because clinicians often deal with life and death issues, mistakes are seen as inexcusable. Yet they are often put into situations that make mistakes more common. In studies of interns on an every-third-night call schedule versus those who sleep every night, the on-call group made 35.9% more serious errors than the sleep group.[9] This paradox can create significant stress, particularly because there are few forums in which to discuss mistakes. Indeed, many physicians do not discuss their mistakes, either with colleagues or spouses, for fear of being judged. Often, this reflects insecurity about their abilities. Perfectionism thus can erode collegial communication. If physicians have to be right all the time, then they become afraid to hear others' opinions of their work.[10] Although physicians who have made mistakes find the greatest relief in talking to others, the sense of vulnerability is often so great that they actually stop talking to others.[11,12]

The Need to Be Needed

In their book, *The HeartMath Solution,* Doc Childre and Howard Martin describe a state of emotional being very common in physicians: the state of "overcare," or caring run amok.[13] Caring for someone and being cared for is energizing. Overcaring, however, is energy depleting. This need to be needed makes physicians believe they are the only ones who can "do it right," and therefore often prevents them from delegating patient care to others. Some physicians are desperate for patients and their families to tell them how great they are. However, this gratification is often not forthcoming and is only intermittent. Physicians then overextend themselves in order to be appreciated. Consequently, many physicians are so busy caring for others that they no longer take care of themselves. To overcome this, physicians must learn to love themselves.

Physical Well-Being

> It is no use walking anywhere to preach unless their walking is preaching. (St. Francis of Assisi)

Statistics on physician health have only recently begun being evaluated. They smoke less, exercise more, and eat healthier than their patients, yet their overall mortality is not much better than any other professional group. In earlier studies their per capita rates of heart disease and stroke were higher than any other working group.[14,15] One reason may be their high rates of stress and depression, which increase risk of cardiovascular mortality.[16] Although these data on physician mortality are a bit frightening, more recent data suggest that their overall mortality is improving. Physicians now live roughly 5 years longer than other professionals.[17]

Despite being in better health than many, poor health behaviors are substantial, even early in physician training; however, they worsen over time. One study evaluated a cross-section of 512 medical students. The outcome measures were self-reported health behaviors and ratings of the importance of prevention. A linear decreasing trend was noted with first-year students, who rated the importance of prevention the highest, and fourth-year students, who rated it the lowest. Additionally, this study attempted to correlate health behaviors with perceptions. The results show significant relationships between student-reported behaviors and corresponding perceptions. The authors went on to state that "the attrition of interest in prevention during undergraduate medical training is cause for concern; future clinical practice will be strongly motivated by their perceptions." Medical students are learning how not to be healthy and therefore become the worst possible teachers for their future patients.[18]

EMOTIONAL WELL-BEING

Burnout is a health care professional's occupational disease that must be recognized early and treated.[19] Burnout occurs during training or after. It can be transient, lasting for days or months, or it can be a long-term state. Most of us do not recognize it when it comes. The proportion of doctors showing above threshold levels of stress is remarkably constant at around 28%, whether the studies are cross sectional or longitudinal, compared with around 18% in the general working population.[20] Women physicians are more likely than male physicians to report signs or symptoms of burnout.[1] Female physicians tend to have more responsibility for the management of domestic responsibilities and, if they have children, must balance the role of mother with career demands.[1]

For people accustomed to functioning at high levels of energy, this often can be experienced as depression. The rates of depression and suicide among physicians are higher than those of the general population.[15] In a 2004 meta-analysis of physician suicide studies, it was found that the aggregate suicide rate ratio for male physicians compared to the general population was 1.41, whereas for female physicians the ratio was 2.27.[21]

In medical school, rates of depression average 25%, and are highest at the end of the second year.[22] Depressed medical students do not tend to seek help for the following reasons: lack of time (48%), lack of confidentiality (37%), stigma associated with using mental health services (30%), cost (28%), fear of documentation on academic record (24%), and fear of unwanted intervention (26%).[23] These reasons are also likely to be true for the depressed resident or practicing physician. Physicians do not want to be found out, vulnerable (less than perfect), or labeled.

Common Pitfalls Leading to Physician Burnout

Blaming and judging others
Putting the health of others before one's own
Worrying excessively about one's patients
Believing that "perfect" exists

- MYTH: Believing that you are the only one who can get it right
- MYTH: Physicians should be all knowing
- MYTH: Uncertainty is a sign of weakness
- MYTH: Technical excellence will provide satisfaction
- MYTH: To reveal emotions is a sign of weakness
- MYTH: Physicians do not have needs

Not sleeping
Not spending time with family and friends to recharge
Trying to please everyone (home, work, play)
Avoiding stress management

FINDING BALANCE: A PERSONAL APPROACH

Esteban not only missed out on family fun, he rarely exercised and always ate on the run. At age 47 he suffered a myocardial infarction and required a bypass operation. During his recuperation, Esteban spent more time with his family. He began cooking, exercising, and going to church with them. When he returned to work, he made changes in his schedule to allow him to continue many of these activities. He began to feel that he had gotten his life back.

It is difficult for physicians to maintain a sense of sanity and control when their lives feel truly out of balance. The extreme pressure to perform, life and death responsibility of medicine, pressure to keep up with the literature, and fear of litigation often lead practitioners to forget to take care of themselves or their families. How can health care providers gain a reasonable sense of life balance and therefore be better teachers to their patients? First, physicians must accept the fact that there will be a certain level of stress in their life and work to manage it in a way that avoids or minimizes the negative consequences of the stress. Second, they must realize that life balance is a process, not a goal. One day you may feel as if you have "got it," and then something unexpected occurs, throwing you into imbalance once more. The process of balance includes paying attention to the four key areas of one's personal life and development: physical, emotional, mental, and spiritual. If they are well, they can approach their work with grace, humor, and intact values.

"MEDICAL" APPROACH TO RECOGNITION OF EMOTIONAL PROBLEMS AND BURNOUT

In studies of medical students early in their career, those with proactive coping mechanism do far better than those with avoidant coping mechanisms.[24] Avoidant mechanisms include introversion, social isolation, and alcohol and drug use. Proactive mechanisms can include, but are not limited to, exercise, meditation, yoga, social interaction, and recreational activities—in essence, self-care.

Women physicians who work fewer hours and have support from colleagues and family in balancing work and home life also do better.[25] A 1990 study of physicians in practice found that those involved in personal growth processes did well at achieving a more balanced life.[26] The authors described five general requirements for personal growth: (a) self-awareness, (b) sharing of feelings and responsibilities, (c) self-care, (d) developing a personal philosophy, and (e) nontraditional coping skills of reframing and limit setting.[26]

Meier and colleagues suggest a "medical" approach that includes steps to recognize emotional problems and respond to them.[4] "Diagnosis" of the problem is aided by: (a) Recognizing risk factors for emotionally difficult patient situations; (b) recognizing the signs of unexamined emotional responses to patients, such as avoidance or excessive engagement; and (c) recognizing the symptoms of unexamined emotions (e.g., anger, contempt, sense of blame, failure, sense of victimization). "Treatment" follows several steps including naming the feelings, normalizing them, considering their effect on patient care and discussing these issues with trusted colleagues (see Core Competency).

KEYS TO LIFE BALANCE

Avoid Complaining, Moaning, and Whining

Think of these as warning symptoms. Try to evaluate what you might change to make things more tolerable for yourself, reach out to colleagues, and reassess your goals and motivations. Recognize that to some extent all practitioners must be "pessimists of the intellect and optimists of the will."[27]

Accept That Life Is Change

Change in medicine and in life is normal, inevitable, and often for the best. Be an agent of change rather than its victim. "Never doubt that a small group of thoughtful, committed citizens can change the world; indeed it is the only thing that ever has."[28]

Be Willing to Give Up Some Control

Practitioners live and work within a large, interdependent system, and need to be realistic about what they can change. "The arch of history is long, but it bends toward justice."[29]

Learn to Reflect

Learn to reflect upon the profundity and complexity of your work. Discuss it with others, colleagues, and family. Health care providers are exposed to the richest moments in people's lives in large and small ways.

Forgive Yourself the Errors You Have Made

In medicine, practitioners make multiple decisions throughout their days and nights. Who does not make multiple mistakes in the course of a year? It is reasonable to review these errors in order to learn from them, create systems that will eradicate them, and maintain honest relationships with patients (making lawsuits less likely). They need also to create a culture of medicine that allows practitioners to make the process of reviewing mistakes the norm rather than the exception.

Learn to Manage Stress

There are multiple ways to manage stress; yoga, meditation, prayer, hobbies, and exercise are just a few.

KEY CONCEPTS

- Be realistic about what you can and can not control.
- Learn to accept and appreciate your own limitations.
- Have the willingness and courage to evaluate yourself and make changes when needed.
- Remember to love those people in your life who give you meaning and purpose.
- Find reasons to love even the difficult people in your life.
- Learn to love yourself. You may be one of the difficult ones.
- Remember that the other person might be right (and it is okay to be wrong).
- Learn to understand, love, and embrace the parts of your personality with which you struggle.
- Care for yourself first so you can take care of your family and serve your patients.
- Listen with your heart.
- Take care of the body you have been given.
- Know that you will make mistakes and learn from them.
- Be open to new ways of thinking.
- Explore and learn.
- See the big picture through love and spirituality.
- Perform service.
- Know that today is a good day to die; that you have lived fully, lovingly, and without remorse.

CORE COMPETENCY

Diagnosis and Treatment of the Health Care Provider Who Is Experiencing Emotional Conflict

Identify Risk Factors for Emotions That May Cause Burnout or Impact Patient Care	Identify Signs and Symptoms of Emotional Conflict	Treatment
PHYSICIAN FACTORS	SIGNS (BEHAVIORS)	PROCESS OF REFLECTION/SELF-MONITORING
Provider identification with patient or family	Avoiding patient and family	Name and search for potential source of emotion
Provider sense of failure	Not communicating with colleagues	Identify behaviors resulting from emotion
Time pressure and demands; lack of time outs for a temporary breather	Overlooking details of patient care	RESPOND CONSTRUCTIVELY
Conflicting obligations	Excessive involvement with patient or family	Make connections and find support. Loners do not do well in difficult work environments. Use a therapist, friend, or support group for this. Create a sense of shared mission at work. Discuss with valued colleagues, friends, intimates, or professional counselors.
Fear of illness, disability, or death	Tension/stress when seeing patient or family	
Difficulty tolerating ambiguity	Providing different level of care for one patient rather than another	
Provider illness such as depression	Dismissive or belittling remarks about patient or colleagues	
Provider with recent illness, death in family	SYMPTOMS (EMOTIONS)	Avoid seeing crises as insurmountable problems.
Inadequate training for working with people	Anger at the patient or family	Accept that change is a part of living.
Limited access to a social–professional support system	Feeling you are the only one who can adequately care for the patient	Adopt practices that help deal with an ever-changing and difficult work environment. This can include meditation, yoga, support groups, or individual counseling.
Limited time and place to share personal feelings with colleagues	Feeling imposed upon by patient or family	
SITUATIONAL OR PATIENT FACTORS	Contempt or disdain for patient or family	Take decisive actions.
Close relationship with patient or family	Intrusive thoughts about patient or family	Look for opportunities for self-discovery
Long hospitalization or frequent rehospitalizations	Sense of failure or self-blame, guilt	Nurture a positive view of yourself.
Difficult communication with family or patient	Feeling you are the patient's savior	Keep things in perspective. Evaluate your own emotional responses to your work. Are you helping or hurting yourself and your colleagues and family? Consider doing this with a counselor or in a support group.
Disagreements with family or colleagues about goals of care	Frequently feeling victimized by the demands of the practice of medicine	
Excessively high patient-to-caregiver ratio or continuous direct contact with patients	Increased use of tobacco, alcohol, prescription medications, and/or illicit substances "to help cope with stress"	Maintain a hopeful outlook.
No system for caregivers to "cover" for each other		Take care of yourself.
Familial stressors, which can arise from relationship problems with parents, spouses, and children.		Evaluate your income and time spent with work. It would be very helpful to speak with physicians in other environments and settings. Compare the time and effort you spend at work with your life needs. If it is working for you, stay there, but be proactive.
		Take time to evaluate your role as a physician in your environment. Is the work you are doing of value? If yes, continue. If not, consider your alternatives.

Adapted from: Regional Education Team of the TMA Committee of Physician Health and Rehabilitation. *Physician stress and burnout. Austin,* TX: Texas Medical Association, 2005. Accessed at: http://www.texmed.org/Template.aspx?id=1828[2]; Meier DE, Back AL, Morrison RS. The inner life of physicians and care of the seriously ill. JAMA 2001;286:3007–3014.[4]

Learn to Love Yourself

This may be the biggest emotional task of all. Self-love is not easy for most health care providers, not because they are bad people, but because they hold themselves to higher standards than they do others. If they learn to lower their standards a bit, they can allow themselves to be imperfect and can love themselves, flaws and all. Then they can truly love and care for others.

Attend to Your Mental Well-Being

Their learning and mental growth are critical to their survival. It is useful to allow themselves to enjoy learning again by setting aside one uninterrupted hour per week to read the literature. Allow yourself the time to learn about subjects outside of medicine, such as art, history, or music, which allows for an enhanced sense of personal growth and development.

Learn to Say, "I Don't Know"

Physicians are taught, through adverse conditioning in residency, never to utter these words, but obviously you can not know everything. If a physician does not know the answer to a patient's question, she can tell the patient she will find it out. This can mean searching the Internet or other resource, or consulting a colleague. The physician provides excellent patient service, and learns something new in the process.

Enhance Your Spiritual Well-Being

For many, spirituality provides energy. In Erica Frank's study of women physicians, she found that those women who had a religious or spiritual life were happier in their work life than those who did not.[30] Spirituality and religion are not always connected. In a simple way, spirituality is a sense of connection with something greater than oneself. This can be family, community, mission, or a supreme being. The common thread is that it is not "all about you."

Connect with Others

Cultivate your intimate relationships and make time for them. Deep connection with others will lead to a greater sense of humanity and a richer sense of a "larger" meaning. Connection is especially critical in a difficult workplace. Spending time with your staff and colleagues at work is a key to sanity when working hard under stressful circumstances. Recognizing the contributions of others in the health care team will enhance everybody's morale. Socialize with those you like. Bring humor into the workplace. Bring treats for your friends. Thank your staff for their hard work and acknowledge your colleagues for a job well done.

Remember to Love

Everyone needs to love and be loved. One who gives more love will receive more love. With a loving home environment, the little annoying things at work will not balloon into larger problems. "We are not held back by the love we didn't receive in the past, but by the love we're not extending in the present."[31]

DISCUSSION QUESTIONS

1. Discuss the key personality traits of people who choose a career in medicine.
2. Describe how the physician's need to be needed makes burnout more likely.
3. Identify occupational "anticipated" stressors when entering the medical profession and those "unanticipated" stressors unique to the medical profession.
4. List the key components to life balance.

RESOURCES

www.cma.ca/index.cfm/ci_id/25541/la_id/1.ht
The Canadian Medical Association Centre for Physician Well-Being (1-877-262-4968)

www.commonweal.org
The Healer's Art: The Institute for the Study of Health and Illness at Commonweal. (415-868-2642). The Healer's Art Program pioneered by Rachael Naomi Remen is an elective course in relationship-centered care for first- and second year medical students. The program's educational objectives include reinforcing the human dimensions of the student physician, preventing burnout, and strengthening a sense of personal mission and meaning in professional work.

www.Healthclassics.com
Lipsenthal K. *Finding balance in a medical life program.* 805-898-0089. The Finding Balance Project, a study at University of Minnesota, is being tested in residents in family practice and surgery. This project teaches stress management, psychosynthesis (self-analysis), yoga, meditation, emotional shifting, and emotional intelligence as well as strategies to enhance communication and manage medical error.

www.umassmed.edu/cfm/
The Finding Balance in a Medical Life Program has been successfully delivered in a large independent practice association (IPA) model and has reduced practicing physician stress, decreased burnout, and enhanced communication.[32]

Mindfulness-based meditation. Center for Mindfulness in Medicine, Health Care, and Society (508-856-2656).

Ferrucci P. What we may be: *Techniques for psychological and spiritual growth through psychosynthesis.* New York: Jeremy P. Tarcher, 1982.

Peterkin AD. *Staying human during residency training.* Toronto: University of Toronto Press, 2004.

Sotile WM, Sotile MO. *The resilient physician: Effective emotional management for doctors & their medical organizations.* Chicago: American Medical Association, 2001.

REFERENCES

1. Spickard A Jr, Gabbe SG, Christensen JF. Mid-career burnout in generalist and specialist physicians. *JAMA* 2002;288:1447–1450.
2. Regional Education Team of the TMA Committee of Physician Health and Rehabilitation. *Physician stress and burnout.* Austin, TX: Texas Medical Association, 2005. Accessed at: http://www.texmed.org/Template.aspx?id=1828
3. Grumbach K, Dower C, Mutha S, et al. *California physicians 2002: Practice and perceptions.* San Francisco: California Workforce Initiative at the UCSF Center for the Health Professions. December 2002. Available at: http://www.futurehealth.ucsf.edu/pdf_files/Phass2ES.pdf
4. Meier DE, Back AL, Morrison RS. The inner life of physicians and care of the seriously ill. *JAMA* 2001;286: 3007–3014.
5. Frank E, McMurray JE, Linzer M, et al. Career satisfaction of US women physicians: Results from the Women Physicians' Health Study. *Arch Intern Med* 1999;159: 1417–1426.
6. Shugerman R, Linzer M, Nelson K, et al. Pediatric generalists and subspecialists: Determinants of career satisfaction. *Pediatrics* 2001;108:E40.
7. Thomas NK. Resident burnout. *JAMA* 2004;292: 2880–2889.
8. Roedell WC. Vulnerabilities of highly gifted children. *Roeper Rev* 1984;6:127–130.
9. Landrigan CP, Rothschild JM, Cronin JW, et al. Effect of reducing interns' work hours on serious medical errors in intensive care units. *N Engl J Med* 2004;351:1838–1848.
10. Akre V, Falkum E, Hoftvedt BO, et al. The communication atmosphere between physician colleagues: Competitive perfectionism or supportive dialogue? A Norwegian study. *Soc Sci Med* 1997;44:519–526.
11. Christensen JF, Levinson W, Dunn PM. The heart of darkness: The impact of perceived mistakes on physicians. *J Gen Intern Med* 1992;7:424–431.
12. Newman MC. The emotional impact of mistakes on family physicians. *Arch Fam Med* 1996;5:71–75.
13. Childre DL, Martin H, Beech D. *The HeartMath solution: The Institute of HeartMath's revolutionary program for engaging the power of the heart's intelligence.* New York: HarperCollins, 1999.
14. Arnetz BB. White collar stress: What studies of physicians can teach us. *Psychother Psychosom* 1991;55:197–200.
15. Heim E. Job stressors and coping in health professions. *Psychother Psychosom* 1991;55:90–99.
16. Rozanski A, Blumenthal JA, Kaplan J. Impact of psychological factors on the pathogenesis of cardiovascular disease and implications for therapy. *Circulation* 1999; 99:2192–2217.
17. Frank E, Biola H, Burnett CA. Mortality rates and causes among U.S. physicians. *Am J Prev Med* 2000;19:155–159.
18. Delnevo CD, Abatemarco DJ, Gotsch AR. Health behaviors and health promotion/disease prevention perceptions of medical students. *Am J Prev Med* 1996;12:38–43.
19. Felton JS. Burnout as a clinical entity—its importance in health care workers. *Occup Med (Lond)* 1998;48:237–250.
20. Firth-Cozens J. *Stress in health professionals: Psychological and organizational causes and interventions.* London: Wiley, 1999.
21. Schernhammer ES, Colditz GA. Suicide rates among physicians: A quantitative and gender assessment (meta-analysis). *Am J Psychiatry* 2004;161:2295–2302.
22. Clark DC, Zeldow PB. Vicissitudes of depressed mood during four years of medical school. *JAMA* 1988; 260:2521–2528.
23. Givens JL, Tjia J. Depressed medical students' use of mental health services and barriers to use. *Acad Med* 2002;77:918–921.
24. Stewart SM, Betson C, Lam TH, et al. Predicting stress in first year medical students: A longitudinal study. *Med Educ* 1997;31:163–168.
25. McMurray JE, Linzer M, Konrad TR, et al. The work lives of women physicians results from the physician work life study. The SGIM Career Satisfaction Study Group. *J Gen Intern Med* 2000;15:372–380.
26. Quill TE, Williamson PR. Healthy approaches to physician stress. *Arch Intern Med* 1990;150:1857–1861.
27. Gramsci, Antonio. *Selections from the Prison Notebooks,* New York: International Publishers, 1971.
28. Margaret Mead.
29. Martin Luther King, Jr.
30. Frank E, Brogan DJ, Mokdad AH, et al. Health-related behaviors of women physicians vs other women in the United States. *Arch Intern Med* 1998;158:342–348.
31. Marianne Williamson.
32. Barron V, Lipsenthal L. Engendering and marketing physician wellness: Creating a healthier delivery system. *Group Practice Journal* 2004;53:13–16

Chapter 41

Advocacy

Thomas P. O'Toole, MD

Objectives

- Discuss a historical perspective on health care advocacy.
- Describe current challenges to effective physician advocacy.
- Identify core elements and a typology of health care advocacy.

Mrs. Brown, who has always had well-controlled hypertension and diabetes, presents with elevated blood pressure and hyperglycemia. Her insurance carrier changed their formulary and she has had difficulty paying for her medications out-of-pocket. She reluctantly reports that following the recommended diet is difficult because "that food doesn't come cheap." The rent on her apartment has increased. She has nearly depleted her savings.

Advocacy in medicine involves taking action, as an individual or organization, on behalf of the patient or the profession to assure the delivery of quality care and to promote professional standards of practice. Advocacy is a venerated medical tradition as old as the Hippocratic Oath. Health care advocacy derives its legitimacy and power from the unique relationship providers have with their patients.

The recent attention focused on advocacy by medical providers is an effort to restore prestige to a profession tarnished by scandal and misuse of trust. In addition, health care advocacy serve as a "call to arms" to address the growing disenfranchisement of vulnerable populations in an increasingly proprietary and market-driven health care environment.

This chapter reviews the roles and contexts of advocacy to demonstrate the breadth of engagement required if providers are to pursue medicine's highest ideals. This is followed by a description of core competencies necessary to sustain commitment, effectiveness,

and idealism. The chapter closes with specific recommendations for developing more effective medical advocacy efforts. Although the focus is placed on physician advocacy, the general principles described in this chapter apply to all health care workers.

WHAT IS ADVOCACY?

Mrs. Brown's case exemplifies the common balancing act of many patients in their struggle to stay healthy. It also illustrates the need for advocacy that extends beyond the strictly clinical. Clinician advocacy starts with providing holistic care that is mindful of the patient's full spectrum of needs. However, it extends beyond the provision of good clinical care to include work that also addresses interpersonal, structural, and systemic inequities and abuses. Key skills for successful health care advocacy include mediating, coordinating, clarifying, resolving conflict, and assisting the patient to acquire, interpret, and use health care information.

Robert Coles, in his book, *A Call to Service*, writes eloquently about altruistic service that transcends social status, stature, and professional rankings to provide basic human needs, promote dignity and respect, seek justice, or provide a good or service not otherwise available.[1] An important element of this definition of advocacy is that its purpose is not driven by narrow self-interest. Lack of self-interest is a critical measure of advocacy, particularly when issues benefiting medical providers (e.g., better reimbursement, fewer practice restrictions) are often framed, appropriately or not, in terms of patient care, safety, and outcomes. Defining who truly benefits can help distinguish between true advocacy on behalf of a patient and exploitation of the patient for self-serving ends (Box 41-1).

Advocacy can be further complicated when clinicians share complicity for the problem. Health care providers are in an awkward position when they, or their institutions, are at least partially to blame for the very situations they oppose. Clinics and physicians alert to problems like Mrs. Brown's might have been able to help her before she went without medications. In another example, Saha and Bindman, commenting on access to care for uninsured patients, argue that to the extent that office policies toward uninsured patients create an illusion of adequate access, clinicians are partly responsible for continued complacency toward the problem.[2]

Health care in the United States is projected to be a $3.4 trillion dollar industry by the year 2017, representing the largest employer and economic sector in many regions. The myriad financial incentives and disincentives in health care often pit the clinician's personal welfare against the welfare of his or her patient, exaggerate clinician's financial expectations, impair judgment, erode professionalism, and ultimately harm patients.[3]

Finally, it is important to understand the role of clinician advocacy in advancing an open and civil society. Karl Popper in his seminal book, *The Open Society and Its Enemies,* argues that an open society is defined in terms of how it promotes equal opportunity for all of its citizens and protects the weakest from the untoward consequences of a market economy.[4] The realization of an open society is contingent on equal opportunity for all people based on strong and unequivocal roles for four societal institutions and professions: education, law and jurisprudence, a free press, and medicine. The inherent challenge in US medicine is how to accomplish the ideals of the open society when medicine itself is structured as a market economy driven by demand and supply-side economies, innovations, and increasingly segregated care.

DISSECTING CLINICIAN ADVOCACY: TYPES OF ADVOCACY

Although it is critically important not to place the proverbial bar for defining true advocacy so high that it dissuades some from becoming involved, it is useful to employ some metrics for defining and describing what providers do. One approach is to ask four basic questions about the advocacy effort: For whom are you advocating? To whom are you advocating? What are you advocating? How are you doing it? (See Fig. 41-1.)

FOR WHOM ARE YOU ADVOCATING? THE ROLE OF THE CLINICAL ENCOUNTER AND THE PROVIDER–PATIENT RELATIONSHIP

In considering the question, "For whom are you advocating?" three themes emerge: (a) advocacy must be clearly and unequivocally on behalf of patients; (b) the provider–patient relationship is critical to informing, legitimizing, and holding the advocacy process accountable; and (c) this relationship provides a unique opportunity to connect a clinical encounter with social determinants of health and justice.

The challenge to the health provider is twofold: first, to develop a trusting relationship with his or her patient so that open and broad-ranging discussions about nonmedical issues can occur. This requires cultural competency and sensitivity that conveys a safe environment for patients to discuss issues of concern without fear of blame or disregard. This is part of the process of patient empowerment and shared decision making that has been shown to make a difference in clinical outcomes (see Chapters 8 and 9).[6,7]

The next challenge is to make the connection between the clinical presentation and the patient's

Box 41-1. Definitions of Advocacy

- Speaking out on issues of concern. This can mean something as formal as sitting down and talking to your legislator; as intensive as engaging in efforts to change laws or policies; or as simple as telling your neighbor about the impact of a law. (www.npaction.org/article/articleview/381/1/124/)
- An act of pleading or arguing in favor of something, such as a cause, idea, or policy; active support. (cadca.org/CoalitionResources/PP-Documents/Glossary.asp)
- A campaign that an individual or organization undertakes to promote any measure that would broadly benefit society. (www.canadacouncil.ca/help/ lj1272287916973437 50.htm)
- Persuasive communication and targeted actions in support of a cause or issue that seek to change policies, positions, and programs. (www.rho.org/html/ glossary.html)
- The act of speaking or of disseminating information intended to influence individual behavior or opinion, corporate conduct or public policy and law. (www.voluntary- sector.ca/eng/about_us/glossary.cfm)

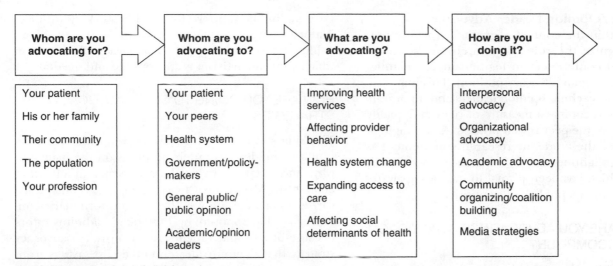

Figure 41-1. Typology of clinician advocacy.

social context. This is critical to validating the risks a patient takes in sharing issues that may be sensitive or embarrassing and in which the connection to one's health and health care is not always obvious. This also allows providers to group observations beyond a single individual and speak to the needs of families, communities, and populations (see Chapter 16).

TO WHOM ARE YOU ADVOCATING? THE SPECTRUM OF STAKEHOLDER-DEFINED ADVOCACY

Advocacy limited to circular discussions among the like-minded may be self-validating but typically changes little. The question then becomes, To whom should practitioners direct their efforts? Knowing your advocacy audience is important for matching the strategy and message to the stakeholder, and identifying the partnerships and coalitions that will be most effective in moving an agenda forward. The common advocacy audiences reviewed here are not meant to be exclusive, exhaustive, or hierarchal.

Patient-Focused Advocacy

In Mrs. Brown's case, educating her about her disease and steps she can take to better manage it is good patient care. Informing her of her rights and recourse against her landlord or insurance company or about how to effectively navigate the health care system are important elements of patient-centered advocacy. Unfortunately, both types of discussions do not occur as often as they should in current practice settings,[8–10] but may be as important as the more glamorous efforts often extolled by the media.

Peer-Focused Advocacy

Influencing one's colleagues represents the next tier in the spectrum of stakeholder targets. Preestablished

collegial working relationships play an important role in conveying ideas and inspiring action. Convincing one's partners to accept Medicaid patients or refrain from accepting pharmaceutical company gifts are two examples.

Health System–Focused Advocacy

Trying to influence a health system, insurance carrier, hospital, or provider group represents a more formal process compared with peer-based advocacy. The advocating clinician still has an established insider identity and legitimacy that facilitates access and confers a sense of "advocacy from within" that can often make change easier to accept. An example of advocacy at this level is to improve the clinic's response to problems like Mrs. Brown's, including insisting that the insurance companies and pharmacies notify providers of formulary changes.

Mrs. Brown's doctor and nurse notice that many of the older women at the clinic are stressed by caring for the grandchildren of absent parents. They decide to start a grandmother's support group. Mrs. Brown's doctor and nurse help the grandmother's group approach local and state agencies about changing eligibility requirements for child-support benefits such as food stamps to include them as caretakers of the children.

Advocacy Geared Toward the General Public and Public Opinion

Essential for effecting change is the need to change opinion and perception, raise awareness that a problem exists, or convince others that the proposed solution is the right one. Here, once again, being part of a larger coalition or movement and employing communication strategies that go beyond one's professional scope and capacity is often vital.

Academic/Opinion Leader Advocacy

Finally, within the context of medicine, it is important to recognize the role of research and scientific meetings and conferences in legitimizing, validating, and disseminating an advocacy position. This is an efficient means of reaching opinion leaders and innovators in the field, and confers a measure of rigor and quality that comes from the peer review process. An example of this is the role the academic research community has played in highlighting and defining race-based health disparities, which has been pivotal to increasing awareness and making it a public policy priority.[11,12]

FOR WHAT ARE YOU ADVOCATING? WHAT DO YOU WANT TO ACCOMPLISH?

Careful consideration of this aspect of advocacy is important for three reasons. First, you need to ensure the appropriateness of what you want to achieve. Advocacy for advocacy's sake or a hollow victory without meaningful impact on those for whom one is advocating is fruitless at best. At worst, it is exploitative and deceitful. Second, advocacy is typically not a short-term endeavor marked by watershed events and outcomes, as popularized by the media. Rather, change typically comes slowly and incrementally. Staying engaged and avoiding burnout requires establishing intermediate goals that let one know he or she is on the right track. Third, knowing what one is advocating for helps to identify the best approach. For example, a particular advocacy goal might first require coalition building and

fostering public support, followed by working with legislators and policy makers to address the problem. Table 41-1 provides a list of advocacy objectives in which clinician activism is appropriate and needed.

HOW ARE YOU GOING TO DO IT? ADVOCACY STRATEGIES

Thinking strategically involves knowing who the relevant stakeholders are, their positions on the issue and why, and what is involved or at stake in effecting change. In Mrs. Brown's case, getting her insurance carrier to change the way they amend formularies initially may be opposed by that plan's administrators because of cost and timeliness concerns. An advocacy strategy that demonstrates potential cost savings from improved health outcomes could address this. Most advocacy efforts employ several levels in promoting an issue or cause. For example, changing physician behavior may include peer-based interpersonal advocacy, use of academic profiling (an intervention combining office-based educational outreach and peer comparison data feedback generated from chart audit and health plans) and opinion leaders, and work at the health system or policy-maker level. Some strategic options include the following.

Interpersonal Advocacy

Communications with patients, peers, administrators, and key decision makers usually is crucial to effect a change. Although lending a clinician's voice

Table 41-1. Advocacy Objectives of Clinician Activism

Objective	Recognized Needs of Vulnerable and Disenfranchised Patients
Improving health services	Lack of access to routine or population-targeted primary and preventive health promotion and disease prevention interventions Default reliance on emergency departments Overriding urgency of acute care issues on presentation Lack of resources Insensitiveness and lack of awareness of the social, cultural, and language-based discordances that exist in the clinical encounter
Affecting physician behavior	Studies show that clinician behavior (types of patients seen, what they are charged, and ways of interacting and communicating) is a determinant of health outcomes and access and an appropriate focus for change.
Health system change	Wide spectrum of system change goals ranging from how a health system accommodates those most vulnerable and disenfranchised, to the way in which services are charged and billed to patients
Expanding access to care	There are a myriad of barriers to patients receiving adequate care including: cultural, ethnic, racial, language, and literacy biases, and geographic hurdles, and means to pay for that care.
Affecting social determinants of health	This underscores the importance of advocacy efforts that are empowering and not merely enabling to our patients, particularly when considering patients who lack the opportunities provided by good jobs, decent housing, affordable childcare, and good schools.

From: O'Toole TP, Arbelaez JJ, Dixon BW. Full disclosure of financial costs and options to patients: The role of race, age, health insurance, and usual source of care. *J Health Care Poor Underserved* 15(2004):52–62[14]; Cooper LA. Health disparities. Towards a better understanding of primary care patient-physician relationships. *J Gen Intern Med* 2004;19(9):985–986[15]; Thorpe KE, Seiber EE, Florence CS. The impact of HMOs on hospital-based uncompensated care. *J Health Polit Policy Law* 2001;26(3):543–555[16]; O'Toole TP, Simms PM, Dixon BW. Primary care office policies regarding care of uninsured patients. *J Gen Intern Med* 2001;16(10):693–696.[17]

and perspective to an advocacy effort often can be crucial, it is not always so. Sometimes patients and their families can articulate an issue best.

Organizational Advocacy

Working through established channels and within professional societies and organizations is often less divisive than more public advocacy approaches. Trying to effect change from within an organization often can be more effective and less threatening than approaching it as an outsider. However, sometimes this also comes with its own set of risks that need to be factored into the advocacy strategy.

Academic Advocacy

The best example of this is in the role researchers have played in studying, validating, and further defining an issue, giving it scientific merit and heightened legitimacy. Many journals and professional associations make special accommodations to include advocacy-related scholarship. Navigating the time span often needed to achieve positive outcomes in this arena can be a challenge.

Community Organizing and Coalition-Building

Patient- and population-centered advocacy is sustained and legitimized by patient and community engagement and leadership. Several excellent texts elaborate on community organizing efforts.[13]

Media Strategies

Print, television, radio, Internet, and other media outlets are often key to information dissemination and have been successfully used as well as inadvertently misused or misdirected in many advocacy campaigns. Knowing your message and staying on message are critical to effectively using these venues. Here again, coalition-building can be key to having an effective communications strategy.

CORE ELEMENTS TO SUCCESSFUL PHYSICIAN ADVOCACY

Successful advocacy requires a deliberate, decisive, and focused approach with full knowledge of the risks involved and understanding that there may not be a second chance if the first attempt comes up short. More importantly, it requires the ability to stay effective and credible not only on this issue but on future issues as well. It also requires a level of preparedness and competency that should not be taken for granted.

Suppose in this case that the clinician advocating on behalf of Mrs. Brown determines that the focus for his advocacy should be the management company that has imposed unfair housing practices upon fixed-income seniors. He decides to hold a press conference with Mrs. Brown that centers on her poorly managed blood pressure and why she can not pay her medical bills (which to most outside observers appear to be too high in the first place) and launches a pointed barrage of accusations at the management firm. A skeptical press attending the event finds it ironic that he is lambasting the management firm while doing nothing to change his own billing practices and openly wonder why other groups working in this area are not present. Those attending the conference may dismiss his efforts as economically self-serving and exploitative of Mrs. Brown's plight (Box 41-2).

This worst case scenario highlights several "do's" and "don'ts" essential to the clinician advocacy effort.

1. *Know your issue.* You should always corroborate your findings or assertions, and do some fact-finding before you begin communicating. The clinician must ensure that his or her efforts are put to good use rather than exploited. Conversely, one must not assume or assert expertise beyond one's knowledge base or sphere of legitimacy.
2. *Know who is involved.* Who are the current stakeholders? Where do they stand on this issue? Whose decision

---

Box 41-2. Do's and Don'ts of Clinician Advocacy

Do's	Don'ts
Know your issue.	Don't become bigger than your issue. A little humility can go a long way.
Know who is involved.	Don't isolate or let your cause consume you.
Develop your skills.	Don't assume that your medical training is adequate.
Partner, organize, and build coalitions.	Don't be a "lone ranger" in your advocacy.
Be strategic; set benchmarks and realistic goals.	Don't forget what it is you want to do, and why you are doing it.

will determine the outcome? Who is currently work-ing on this issue and what are they doing? Can you join them in this effort? Being aware of and sensitive to these questions can help avoid the kinds of prob-lems described in the preceding case. It also helps ensure that one's efforts complement ongoing work, facilitate coalition-building, and enhance a strategic effort.

3. *Develop your skills.* Nothing about a medical educa-tion or degree makes physicians uniquely qualified as advocates. In fact, the opposite may be true. This underscores the importance of having a mentor, partnering with individuals, joining a coalition, or affiliating with an agency or organization with the complementary skill sets needed for the advocacy effort.

   Topping the list of skills needed for effective advo-cacy is effective communication (see Chapter 6). For clinicians, this means not talking down to or patron-izing those outside the health care field and avoid-ing the use of medical jargon. Additional skills include writing in a clear, succinct, accurate, and per-suasive way, whether it is advocacy research for peer-reviewed publications, op-eds for a local paper, press releases, information packets, or issue briefs for legis-lators. Knowing how policy is made, regulations are drafted, and laws are enacted is also vital if trying to effect change at this level. This requires reading, attending meetings and conferences, and talking to people outside of one's professional circles.

4. *Partner, organize, and build coalitions.* The maxim "there is strength in numbers" could not be truer in this instance. The effectiveness of an advocacy effort is often driven by the number of people and the diversity of their perspectives. Coalition building and collaborating with other groups and organizations also reduces the likelihood of being dismissed as purely self-serving in one's intent. Involving directly affected or victimized patients in the partnering process empowers them. This does not always come naturally to physicians, who are used to leading or working independently. The process of partnering with or joining a coalition requires willingness to sometimes follow or cooperate.

5. *Be strategic.* Finally, and perhaps most importantly, it is essential to be strategic in approaching an advo-cacy agenda. Is this something that your patient wants you to do? All too often the person originally presenting with the need is long forgotten as the advocacy effort takes on a life of its own. If there is a struggle to achieve clarity with the four core ques-tions asked in the preceding, you need to step back and reconsider what you are trying to do. This should also be informed by those with a vantage point on what is realistic and what are the levers and pace for change.

SUSTAINING ONE'S EFFORT: BEING AN ADVOCATE OVER THE LONG HAUL

Avoiding burnout and frustration is as important as fueling one's passions and idealism. It is easy to become consumed by an advocacy cause and agenda to the point where it jeopardizes one's personal and profes-sional life and identity. There are four things advocates need to do in order to sustain them and prevent burnout. First, *don't become isolated.* This can be a natural by-product of the effort. It is important to stay actively engaged personally and professionally to maintain legit-imacy in the field, help maintain perspective, and sus-tain one's idealism and commitment through the difficult and bleak times. Second, *pace yourself.* Making time in a busy schedule to tend to your personal and professional needs, relax, unwind, and take a break from the action is vital to sustaining one's enthusiasm and energy over what may be a long and drawn-out process. Third, *don't let yourself become bigger than the issue.* Clinician advocacy often can be celebrated by the media and public to an extent that it overshadows the actual advocacy effort. Not only can this alienate one from his or her advocacy partners or coalition, but also it can fos-ter an unrealistic sense of self and purpose. A little humility can go a long way. Finally, *set short-term and achievable benchmarks and goals.* This includes being able to celebrate the successes of others who have picked up on your work and moved an issue forward with or with-out your assistance. Being able to justify the time and energy dedicated to a cause can help validate the effort.

WHAT NEEDS TO HAPPEN TO MAKE IT HAPPEN

There are several issues and impediments to increased advocacy efforts. First and foremost, advocacy on behalf of patients needs to be viewed and accepted as an essential, defining aspect of professionalism. However, it also takes time, requires a personal commitment, and often demands personal and professional sacrifices. In fact, there are different degrees of advocacy that clini-cians can and should become engaged in, each with different levels of required preparation, skill develop-ment, and mentoring.

Following on this theme, advocacy skills need to be taught, mentored, and nurtured, including how to do it, the ethical underpinnings of advocacy, the required lead-ership skills, and the appropriate avenues. Health profes-sional education and residency training are ideal venues for introducing and fostering this ethic. Exposure to advocacy at this stage also creates an expectation of what is possible at a very formative point in a career. This requires curricular reform, supporting faculty as mentors and role models, engaging communities-of-need in a more empowered context, and partnering with other professions and disciplines.

There are several examples of models that have been developed that merit closer inspection. The University of Pittsburgh School of Medicine has developed an innovative curriculum that involves patients and community advocates as co-mentors within a population-based curriculum. Case Western Reserve University, University of California-San Francisco, and Georgetown University have developed advocacy tracks and opportunities for their students, and the Pediatrics Residency Review Commission (RRC) includes advocacy as a core competency required during training. The Physician Advocacy Fellowship (formerly the Soros Advocacy Fellowship for Physicians) provides an opportunity for physicians to develop advocacy skills and receive targeted mentoring from experts across disciplines and professions (http://www.imapny.org/advocacy).

Finally, physicians need to both protect and institutionalize the process and commitment to advocacy within the profession. Clinicians assume risks when they take up the advocacy mantle, particularly when support of their cause includes being critical of their peers, employer, hospital, or academic institution. There are too many instances of physicians and other clinicians being fired, denied tenure, or otherwise suppressed because of a position or stance they took. This has a chilling effect not only on continuing one's advocacy efforts but also on others becoming involved. One option may be to create safe havens for advocacy through independent watchdog organizations and entities that have a protected mandate and capacity for patient- and community-centered advocacy. Examples include organizations such as Public Citizen, Physicians for Human Rights, and Physicians for Social Responsibility, and some private foundations such as the Kaiser Family Foundation, Commonwealth Foundation, or the Open Society Institute. Another option is to extend whistle-blower protections to clinicians similar to those developed in other fields.

CONCLUSION

In summary, advocacy is at the core of medical professionalism. It is uniquely defined by its selfless nature and grounding in the clinician–patient relationship. Advocacy covers a spectrum of actions and activities depending on the issue or need, the stakeholders involved, and the action being sought. Thinking strategically about the advocacy process, partnering and collaborating wherever possible, and honing one's own skills and competencies are all critical elements. As physicians look to what they need to do individually, they also need to look at how they support, institutionalize, and strengthen the environment for clinician advocacy, particularly within increasingly restrictive employment structures. Finally, as physicians enter into the 21st century and confront the new challenges facing patients and communities, it is important to remember this early-20th-century quote from Frances Weld Peabody, "One of the essential qualities of the clinician is interest in humanity, for the secret of care of the patient is in caring for the patient."

KEY CONCEPTS

- Clinician advocacy is legitimized and informed by the provider–patient relationship and a basic tenet of clinician professionalism.
- Successful advocacy requires a deliberate, decisive, and focused strategic effort and several specific skills.
- Know your issue, including what you don't know or are not qualified to speak on.
- Know who is involved, and whom you are your trying to convince or persuade. Always appreciate the other side of an issue or position.
- Know who else is working on this issue, who else has a stake in the outcome, and whom you can join forces with and organize.
- Develop your skills, get a mentor, and work with people outside your field.

CORE COMPETENCY
Becoming an Advocate

We can all be advocates.

- Recognize the many ways you can be an advocate.
- Choose ways that are a good fit for your talents.
- Assess who truly benefits from your advocacy.
- Choose your audience: patients, peers, systems, public opinion, research community, and Congress?
- Assess your allies and opposition.
- Define your goals.

Be sure to:

- Know your issue.
- Know who is involved.
- Develop your skills—media presentations, peer-education, and community building.
- Partner, organize, and build a coalition.
- Be strategic—choose your battles.

Staying an advocate:

- Don't isolate, work with others.
- Pace yourself.
- Don't let yourself become bigger than the issue.
- Set short-term and achievable intermediate goals and benchmarks.
- Have fun!

DISCUSSION QUESTIONS

1. How is physician advocacy a basic tenet of physician professionalism? Where is this being realized? Where is it most challenged?
2. In what ways are physicians well-prepared to engage in advocacy? In what ways are they poorly prepared?
3. How does society currently regard physicians who are engaged in advocacy? Should this change?
4. What are some emerging structures and dynamics to how and where physicians practice that have potential impact on their role as advocates?
5. When is advocacy not appropriate, useful, or beneficent?

RESOURCES

http://www.advocacy.org
  The Advocacy Institute

http://www.familiesusa.org
  FamiliesUSA

http://www.imapny.org
  Institute on Medicine as a Profession

http://www.sorosny.org/medicine
  Open Society Institute

http://www.phrusa.org
  Physicians for Human Rights

http://www.psr.org
  Physicians for Social Responsibility

http://www.citizen.org
  Public Citizen

REFERENCES

1. Coles R. *The call of service: A witness to idealism.* New York: Houghton Mifflin, 1993.
2. Saha S, Bindman AB. The mirage of available health care for the uninsured. *J Gen Intern Med* 2001;16(10): 714–716.
3. Kassirer JP. *On the Take: How medicine's complicity with big business can endanger your health.* New York: Oxford University Press, 2005.
4. Popper KP. *The open society and its enemies: The spell of Plato.* Princeton, NJ: Princeton University Press, 1971.
5. Rothman DJ. Medical professionalism: Focusing on the real issues. *N Engl J Med* 2000;342(17):1283–1286.
6. Johnson RL, Roter D, Powe NR, et al. Patient race/ethnicity and quality of patient-physician communication during medical visits. *Am J Public Health* 2004;94(12): 2084–2090.
7. Frosch PL, Kaplan RM. Shared decision making in clinical medicine: Past research and future directions. *Am J Prev Med* 1999;17(4):285–294.
8. Alexander GC, Casalino LP, Meltzer DO. Patient-physician communications about out of pocket costs. *JAMA* 2003;290:953–958.
9. CDC. *Fewer doctors urge weight loss.* Associated Press/CNN. Tuesday, April 20, 2004. Available at: http://www.cnn.com/2004/HEALTH/diet.fitness/04/20/obesity.doctors.ap/index.html
10. Olfson M, Tobin JN, Cassells A, et al. Improving the detection of drug abuse, alcohol abuse, and depression in community health centers. *J Health Care Poor Underserved* 2003;14:386–402.
11. Smedley BD, Stith AY, Nelson AR, et al. *Unequal treatment: Confronting racial and ethnic disparities in health care.* Washington, DC: The National Academies Press, 2002.
12. Schulman KA, Berlin JA, Harless W, et al. The effect of race and sex on physicians' recommendations for cardiac catheterization. *N Engl J Med* 1999;340(8):618–626.
13. Rinku S, Klein K. *Stir it up: Lessons in community organizing and advocacy.* San Francisco: Jossey-Bass, 2003.
14. O'Toole TP, Arbelaez JJ, Dixon BW. Full disclosure of financial costs and options to patients: The role of race, age, health insurance, and usual source of care. *J Health Care Poor Underserved* 2004;15:52–62.
15. Cooper LA. Health disparities. Towards a better understanding of primary care patient-physician relationships. *J Gen Intern Med* 2004;19(9):985–986.
16. Thorpe KE, Seiber EE, Florence CS. The impact of HMOs on hospital-based uncompensated care. *J Health Polit Policy Law* 2001;26(3):543–555.
17. O'Toole TP, Simms PM, Dixon BW. Primary care office policies regarding care of uninsured patients. *J Gen Intern Med* 2001;16(10):693–696.

INDEX

Note: Page numbers followed by *b* indicate boxed material, by *f* indicate figures, and by *t* indicate tables.